CANCER GENETICS
A CLINICAL APPROACH

CANCER GENETICS
A CLINICAL APPROACH

EDITORS

XAVIER LLOR, MD, PHD
Professor of Medicine
Yale University
New Haven, Connecticut

ERIN WYSING HOFSTATTER, MD
Associate Professor Adjunct
Yale University
New Haven, Connecticut

New York   Chicago   San Francisco   Athens   London   Madrid   Mexico City
Milan   New Delhi   Singapore   Sydney   Toronto

Cancer Genetics: A Clinical Approach

1 2 3 4 5 6 7 8 9   DSS   26 25 24 23 22 21

ISBN 978-1-260-44027-0
MHID 1-260-44027-3

This book was set in Minion Pro by MPS Limited.
The editors were Jason Malley and Christina M. Thomas.
The production supervisor was Rick Ruzycka.
Project management was provided by Rishabh Gupta, MPS Limited.
The cover designer was W2 Design.

Library of Congress Cataloging-in-Publication Data

Names: Llor, Xavier, editor. | Hofstatter, Erin Wysing, editor.
Title: Cancer genetics : a clinical approach / [edited by] Xavier Llor,
    Erin Wysing Hofstatter.
Other titles: Cancer genetics (Llor)
Description: New York : McGraw Hill, [2021] | Includes bibliographical
    references and index. | Summary: "A guide and comprehensive reference
    for the care of patients with hereditary cancer syndromes. This book is
    intended to provide the essential tools needed to understand clinical
    cancer genetics"—Provided by publisher.
Identifiers: LCCN 2021011591 | ISBN 9781260440270 (hardcover)
Subjects: MESH: Neoplasms—genetics | Risk Assessment
Classification: LCC RC268.4 | NLM QZ 210 | DDC 616.99/4042—dc23
LC record available at https://lccn.loc.gov/2021011591

McGraw Hill books are available at special quantity discounts to use as premiums and sales promotions, or for use in corporate training programs. To contact a representative, please, visit the Contact Us pages at www.mhprofessional.com.

Contents

Contributors...vii

Preface ix

1 Clinical Cancer Genetics 1

2 Risk Assessment in the Primary Care Office: Identification of
   Patients for Referral 31

3 Principles of Cancer Risk Assessment and Genetic Counseling 41

4 Laboratory Methods in Cancer Genetics Testing 59

5 Breast Cancer...71

6 Gastrointestinal Polyposis Syndromes..117

7 Hereditary Nonpolyposis Colorectal Cancers 141

8 Risk Assessment and Clinical Management – Uterine Cancer 167

9 Risk Assessment and Clinical Management – Ovarian Cancer 183

10 Pancreatic Cancer Genetics 209

11 Risk Assessment and Clinical Management – Genito-Urinary Tract Cancer........247

12 Genetic Predisposition to Gastric Cancer 269

13 Endocrine Cancers...289

14 Risk Assessment and Clinical Management – Skin Cancer 319

15 Risk Assessment and Clinical Management – Pediatric and
   Other Cancers 343

16 Ethical, Legal, and Psychosocial Issues in Cancer Genetic
   Assessment and Genetic Testing...379

17 Talking to Children and Family About Hereditary Cancer Risk and
   Genetic Test Results..415

18 Future Challenges and Opportunities in Clinical Cancer Genomics 431

Index...445

Contributors

C. Rick Boland, MD
Professor of Medicine
University of California San Diego
San Diego, California

Karina Brierley, MS, CGC
Genetic Counselor
Yale University
New Haven, Connecticut

Tobias Carling, MD, PhD
Surgeon-in-Chief
Carling Adrenal Center
Tampa, Florida

Marcia Cruz-Correa, MD, PhD
Professor of Medicine
University of Puerto Rico
San Juan, Puerto Rico

James Farrell, MBChB
Professor of Medicine
Yale University
New Haven, Connecticut

Amanda Ganzak, MS, CGC
Genetic Counselor
Yale New Haven Health
New Haven, Connecticut

Heather Hampel, MS, LGC
Professor of Medicine
Ohio State University
Columbus, Ohio

Gary M. Kupfer, MD
Professor of Oncology and Pediatrics
Georgetown University
Washington, DC

Dave J. Leffell, MD
Professor of Dermatology and Surgery
Yale University
New Haven, Connecticut

Michael F. Murray, MD, FACMG, FACP
Professor of Genetics and Pathology
Yale University
New Haven, Connecticut

Stephanie Prozora
Assistant Professor of Clinical Pediatrics
Yale University
New Haven, Connecticut

Elena Ratner, MD
Associate Professor of Obstetrics,
Gynecology and Reproductive Sciences
Yale University
New Haven, Connecticut

Preston C. Sprenkle, MD
Associate Professor
Yale University
New Haven, Connecticut

Elena Stoffel, MD, MPH
Clinical Associate Professor
University of Michigan
Ann Harbor, Michigan

Jennifer Scalia Wilbur, PhD
Clinical Program Manager
Cancer Genetics and Prevention Program
Brown University
Providence, Rhode Island

Rosa Xicola, PhD
Assistant Professor
Yale University
New Haven, Connecticut

Preface

It is hard to imagine any other field in contemporary medicine with more astonishing and rapid progress than cancer genetics. In fact, if we take a moment to recall how we used to approach patients with these conditions just a few years ago, we realize how dramatically the new landscape we are currently facing has shifted.

This book is intended to provide the essential tools needed to understand clinical cancer genetics. The emphasis on clinical practice is designed to assist practitioners in the daily challenges of caring for patients with inherited cancer predisposition. Accordingly, the content is organized in a way that assists in every step of the continuum of care, including tools to help guide the formulation of a differential diagnosis, understand available genetic testing options, enable logical and informed interpretation of results, and educate individuals and their families about strategies to prevent cancer development. Approaches on how to effectively and thoughtfully counsel patients—from pre-test counseling and relaying test results to assisting in navigating the legal implications of hereditary conditions and coping with the psychological challenges emanating from them—are also addressed.

Given the wide spectrum of different professionals involved in the care of individuals and families with inherited cancers, the aim of this book is to serve as a practical and comprehensive resource for the entire team of providers, including physicians, genetic counselors, nurses, psychologists, physician assistants, geneticists, and others. In particular, this book should be useful not only for specialized cancer genetics clinics, but also for healthcare professionals in any field who are seeking basic knowledge and tools to improve their skills in the identification of patients with possible hereditary cancer syndromes and recognize which patients should be referred to a high-risk/clinical genetics specialty program. Finally, and perhaps most importantly, we hope that this book serves as a guide and comprehensive reference for the care of patients with hereditary cancer syndromes not only at the time of diagnosis but also throughout their entire lifespan.

CHAPTER 1

Clinical Cancer Genetics

C. Richard Boland and Paivi Peltomaki

▦ CANCER IS A GENETIC DISEASE

Cancer has been recognized as a specific pathological entity since the nineteenth century, and there have been multiple proposed mechanistic explanations for this disease process. Theodor Boveri determined that cancer was a cellular process caused by a scrambling of the chromosomes, and in 1902, he proposed that physical insults such as radiation, chemical agents, or even microbial pathogens might be responsible for this. Over the past 120 years, most of Boveri's proposed triggers have been linked to cancer. Although abnormalities in chromosomes are frequently found in cancers, the degree of aneuploidy is quite diverse among tumors, and a few cancers are nearly diploid (but may be highly mutated). However, every cancer has genetic aberrations of some sort, and all investigators involved in cancer research agree that cancer is fundamentally a genetic disease. Most cancers are not a result of inherited germline mutations (or epimutations), but all cancers are driven by aberrant gene expression. The variety of ways through which cancers develop and the heterogeneity of genetic alterations in tumors have served to fascinate and perplex those who study the disease.

It is important to distinguish germline alterations (those inherited from the parents and identical in all cells of an organism) from somatic mutations (those mutations found in cancer cells but not in the germline). Germline mutations and somatic mutations are both important in cancer but for different reasons. Germline mutations are sometimes involved in creating increased risk for cancer, through a variety of mechanisms. Some cancer-associated germline mutations are in genes that normally regulate cellular proliferation; when inactivated, the progeny grow without one layer of control. Other germline mutations may occur in systems that monitor or repair deoxyribonucleic acid (DNA) damage and, when inactivated, permit an accelerated accumulation of mutations. Somatic mutations occur in a wide variety of genes and alter the biology of the affected cells, as discussed later. The combination of somatic mutations determines the nature of cancer cell growth and the ability to metastasize and determines the responses to therapies. Virtually all of the cancer-associated germline mutations can be found as somatic mutations in cancers; however, the reverse is not the case.

▓ GENETIC TERMINOLOGY

Dominant, Recessive, Dominant Negatives, and Haploinsufficiency

In traditional genetics, hereditary diseases are usually classified as autosomal dominant (only one mutant allele is sufficient), autosomal recessive (two mutant alleles are required), and sex-linked (truly recessive, but the allele is on the X chromosome, so it appears dominant in men). Based upon the study of hereditary and sporadic retinoblastomas, in 1971 Knudson proposed that the involvement of genes in cancer required "two hits" for the tumor to develop, i.e., that both alleles of the culprit gene needed to be affected. This novel concept accommodated the observation that familial cancer syndromes (like familial retinoblastoma or familial adenomatous polyposis [FAP]) can be inherited in an autosomal dominant fashion but are recessive at the tissue level, requiring a second inactivating somatic mutation for a neoplastic behavior to begin.[1] Consequently, the inheritance of a single inactive allele of *RB* or *APC* would create a dominantly inherited family pedigree with half of the offspring receiving the disease allele, but the disease is still recessive at the tissue level, requiring inactivation of the wild-type allele inherited from the unaffected parent. It was difficult to explain the mechanism behind familial inheritance of elevated cancer risk without this insight.

The Knudsonian explanation for inheriting cancer-predisposing genes becomes more complicated in certain instances. For example, some mutations are more destructive of the protein product of the gene than others. Total deletions of genes in the germline are not uncommon, and those have an unambiguous effect on abrogating gene expression. Some missense mutations may have an intermediate impact on gene expression and create a less severe phenotype based upon a reduction in the expressed dose of the gene product. Most premature termination codon mutations destroy gene expression through nonsense-mediated ribonucleic acid (RNA) decay, but the location of the termination is critical in determining whether the messenger RNA (mRNA) (and consequently, the truncated protein product) is stably expressed or subject to destruction. These mechanisms contribute—in part—to the variable phenotypes of genetic diseases when comparing families with different specific mutations in the same gene.

The concept of heterogeneous mutations in a single gene is exemplified by the locations of *APC* mutations in FAP and consequent clinical heterogeneity. Germline mutations in *APC* causing FAP are usually premature termination codons, splice site disruptors, or complete deletions of the gene.[2,3] Missense mutations in *APC* have not been shown to cause the adenomatous polyposis phenotype. *APC* is a long gene (2843 codons, 15 coding exons), and premature termination mutations between codons 1250 and 1464 are associated with more profuse polyposis (with as many as 5000 adenomas) compared with termination codons upstream of 1250 or downstream of 1464.[4] This may be due to a *dominant negative* effect. The APC protein normally functions as a homodimer. In the example of mutations associated with profuse polyposis, the truncated protein product of the mutant gene may form a heterodimer with the wild-type protein, and this complex may interfere with the normal function of the APC protein, which is to bind β-catenin, facilitate specific phosphorylation, and downregulate the signal for proliferation. If this is the case, then specific mutant protein products may be more disruptive of cellular proliferation than literally being absent (or haploinsufficient, i.e., having just one wild-type copy of the gene in each cell), leading to a more severe phenotype. This also suggests that an alteration in growth dynamics may begin prior to losing the wild-type allele of *APC* due to a lower concentration of APC protein or the dominant-negative effect, which is important, since the "second hit" is traditionally thought to be the initiating event of neoplasia in most colorectal adenomas.

Evidence in animal models of Peutz-Jeghers syndrome (caused by germline mutations in *STK11/LKB1*—two names for one gene) and juvenile polyposis syndrome (germline mutations in *SMAD4* or *BMPR1A*—two different genes in the same signaling pathway) suggests the role of *haploinsufficiency* in the development of the benign polyps that occur in childhood, whereas the classic two-hit Knudsonian dynamics may be involved later in life in the development of cancer. In both instances, polyp formation is driven by the reduced degree of gene expression and may occur through the effects of haploinsufficiency on stromal rather than epithelial tissues.

Inactivating mutations in the *STK11* gene lead to upregulation of inflammatory cytokines and promotion of *overgrowth of normal gut epithelium and stromal cells* through the *JAK-STAT* pathway. A single germline mutation in this gene in mice creates a situation of haploinsufficiency in all normal cells, which leads to immune cell proliferation in the stroma without the need for a second hit in the somatic tissue. Specifically, in animal models, conditional knockouts in the hematopoietic compartment or in the T-cell compartment is sufficient to drive the growth of gastrointestinal polyps.[5] Haploinsufficiency is when the simultaneous presence of one wild-type and one mutant allele at a functionally relevant locus leads to reduced expression of the gene product, with a detectable phenotype (which may be minor and different from the consequences of biallelic loss). Interestingly, the very high risk for cancer in Peutz-Jeghers syndrome may not occur through the same mechanism.

The evidence for the importance of haploinsufficiency is also observable in the animal model of juvenile polyposis syndrome, but with a twist. The presence of a genetically engineered inactivating germline mutation in *Smad4* in mice is associated with upregulation of the Th17-inflammatory pathway in stromal cells and a *Smad4* dose-related development of gastrointestinal juvenile polyps.[6] Moreover, selective deletion of *Smad4* in T cells leads to the development of tumors in the gastrointestinal tract, whereas epithelial-specific deletion does not.[7] It remains to be demonstrated how widespread the impact of gene dosage works in the polyposis syndromes, but haploinsufficiency appears to permit abnormalities of cell growth in certain settings. This is a somewhat complex example of haploinsufficiency, as the mechanism involves a change in behavior in the stromal cells, which then affects the growth of epithelial cells and has been termed a *landscaper effect* (see later).[8]

Terms Used to Describe Clinical Heterogeneity in Genetic Diseases

A number of unique terms are used to describe the heterogeneity of clinical expression in inherited syndromes (Table 1.1).

Penetrance refers to the likelihood that individuals will express a given phenotype when they inherit the germline mutation. In some cases, the clinical outcomes are binary, such as the presence or absence of a cancer in a *BRCA1/2* or Lynch syndrome patient. In these diseases, the penetrance for cancer is incomplete, usually ranging between 20% and 80% of those carrying the critical germline mutations, depending upon the gene involved. In Lynch syndrome, penetrance associated with germline mutations in *MSH2* and *MLH1* is quite high, over 50%, but with the *PMS2* gene, the lifetime penetrance for cancer may be <20%.[9]

TABLE 1.1: Genetic Terminology
Allele – a specific copy or sequence of a gene
Allelic heterogeneity – differences in phenotype caused by different kinds of mutations in a single gene
Allelic loss – the deletion of one of two alleles at a genetic locus; may be referred to as loss of heterozygosity (LOH)
Caretaker gene – a gene involved in maintaining the integrity of DNA
Dominant – one copy of an allele is sufficient for a phenotype to occur
Dominant negative effect – a mutant allele has a negative or suppressive effect on the wild-type allele
Driver mutations – mutations that provide a selective growth advantage in causing neoplastic behavior
Epigenetic effects – alterations in gene expression not caused by a change in the DNA sequence
Gatekeeper gene – a gene whose mutation permits the initiation of a neoplastic phenotype
Genetic heterogeneity – multiple different genes can produce the same phenotype
Genetic pleiotropy – heterogeneous phenotypes throughout the body caused by a mutation in one gene
Germline mutation – a mutation originating in the germline and present in all cells
Haploinsufficiency – loss of one copy of a gene in the germline produces a phenotype
Landscaper effect – a phenotype in which one group of cells (such as epithelial cells) are affected by an adjacent group of cells (such as stromal cells)
Locus heterogeneity – one clinical disorder caused by multiple different genes (often involved in the same physiological process)
Missense mutation – a single nucleotide substitution in the DNA sequence that changes the coding amino acid
Multistep carcinogenesis – the concept that the accumulation of multiple mutations is required for a cancer to develop; this may or may not require a specific sequence of events
Mutational signature – a pattern of mutations that indicates the involvement of a specific class of mutagens or the loss of a specific DNA repair or maintenance system
Nonsense mutation – a mutation that creates a premature termination or stop-gain codon
Oncogene – dominantly acting driver mutations occurring in normal cellular genes
Passenger mutations – mutations found in tumors that are not drivers
Penetrance – the likelihood that an individual carrying a germline mutation will develop the phenotype
Recessive – both copies of an allele are required for a phenotype to occur
Single nucleotide polymorphisms (SNPs) – variations of single nucleotides commonly found throughout the normal genome
Somatic mutation – a mutation that occurs after the initial zygote forms and present in only the progeny of the mutant cell, typically (but not always) a tumor
Tumor suppressor gene – a gene whose function is to suppress the development of cancer
Two-hit effect – when two alterations at one locus are required for neoplasia to occur
Variable expressivity – variable phenotypes observed between individuals with a germline mutation in a single gene

In the case of FAP—which is a disease primarily based upon the risk of adenomatous polyps—the chance of developing adenomatous polyps is nearly 100% for most of the germ-line mutations. In FAP, the ultimate penetrance for cancer would probably be nearly 100%, but this complication can be avoided if the polyposis is discovered at an early stage and the colorectum is removed. This is because germline mutations in *APC* are an adenoma-initiating event, not a cancer-causing event per se. However, there are unique mutations in the *APC* gene that are associated with a sharp reduction in penetrance called attenuated FAP,[10] due to the presence of an internal ribosomal entry site at codon 184 in *APC* that permits the ribosome to reinitiate transcription downstream of some terminating mutations in the gene. So mutations upstream of that codon may be attenuated by the ability of transcription to skip the mutation and mitigate penetrance.[11]

Variable expressivity refers to the variety of clinical expression in different individuals caused by mutations in the same gene. This is a common occurrence in many of the familial cancer genes. For example, individuals with *BRCA1/2* mutations may get breast cancer, ovarian cancer, pancreatic cancer, or no cancer. Patients with the same *APC* mutation in unrelated families may have variable phenotypes through poorly understood mechanisms, presumably interactions with other genes.[12] Similarly, patients with Lynch syndrome are at risk for cancer of the colon, endometrium, small intestine, urinary tract, stomach, and other organs. Some patients develop multiple different tumors and others get none. Variable expressivity is commonly used to describe differences in the clinical extent of expression of some metabolic disorders where there may be more or less accumulation of certain metabolites. However, as mentioned earlier, not all mutations disable the gene product to the same degree, and some of the variability mentioned in the discussion of haploinsufficiency may result in variable expressivity, particularly when the disease gives rise to benign neoplasms early in the disease process and cancers later.

Genetic pleiotropy occurs when a single mutation produces heterogeneous effects in different parts of the body. Peutz-Jeghers syndrome is an example of this where patients with a mutation in *STK11* develop a cutaneous phenotype (freckling), gastrointestinal polyps in childhood, and in adult life, a severe tendency to develop a broad range of cancers (in the breast, luminal gut, pancreas, gonads, etc.).

Genetic heterogeneity is when there are two or more genes responsible for risk of the same types of tumor. For example, *BRCA1/2* and *STK11* are quite distinct genes functionally, but germline mutations in either of them increases the risk for breast cancer in women.

Allelic heterogeneity refers to variability (or similarity) in phenotype caused by mutations in different parts of an individual gene. For example, the *APC* gene encodes for a long protein with multiple functional domains. As mentioned earlier, the principal function of the protein is to regulate the intracellular concentrations of β-catenin in gastrointestinal (and other) epithelial cells by serving as a scaffold for its phosphorylation. However, the APC protein functions as a homodimer, with the amino termini dimerized. The scaffold and phosphorylation functions are in the middle portion of the gene, and the carboxy terminus of the APC protein interacts with microtubules.[13] Premature termination mutations in the mid-portion of the gene (codons 1250 to 1464) are associated with a more severe phenotype, which has been attributed to a dominant negative effect of the truncated protein dimerizing and interfering with the protein product of the wild-type allele.

Locus heterogeneity refers to a single clinical disorder caused by mutations in different genes. This typically involves multiple genes that participate in a single cellular process. For example, inactivation of any of four genes in the DNA mismatch repair (MMR) system can cause Lynch syndrome. The story is a more complex mix of locus heterogeneity and *variable* penetrance, as germline mutations in the two "major" DNA MMR genes, *MSH2* and *MLH1*, cause a more highly penetrant phenotype, whereas mutations in the "minor" MMR genes, *MSH6* and *PMS2*, cause a more attenuated phenotype because of the ability of the cell to use the proteins MSH3 and PMS1/MLH3 in place of the missing MSH6 and PMS2 proteins, respectively, to provide at least partial MMR function.[14] Similarly, biallelic inactivating mutations in any of several members of the nucleotide excision repair (NER) system can all cause xeroderma pigmentosum (see later).[15]

Epigenetics refers to heritable changes in gene expression that do not alter the DNA sequence of the gene. This usually involves covalent binding of methyl, alkyl, or other groups to DNA, which alters the conformation of chromatin and alters (increasing or decreasing) gene expression. Epigenetic changes are normal physiological events that cells use to permanently silence the expression of a gene that is not necessary for optimal cell function. In cancer, one can see inappropriate hypermethylation-induced silencing of genes through methylation of the C-G (usually called CpG sites, where the "p" refers to the phosphodiester bond between the adjacent C and G) in the promoters of many genes.[16] Some tumors have an excessive amount of apparently dysregulated promoter hypermethylation, which appears to be an important part of tumorigenesis in those tumors.[17] However, there are also instances of inappropriate hypomethylation of genes in tumors, which was a very early observation in cancer.[18]

THE HUMAN GENOME

The Human Genome Project provided an initial understanding of the organization and sequence of our DNA and provided insights into the regulation and dysregulation of gene expression. The human genome consists of about 3.23×10^9 linear, paired nucleotides (adenines, cytosines, guanines, and thymines) organized into 22 paired chromosomes, plus the sex chromosomes X and Y.[19-21] DNA sequences are about 99.9% identical among humans, which still leaves a considerable amount of heterogeneity between individuals. Much of this heterogeneity is due to single nucleotide polymorphisms (SNPs or "snips"), some of which account for the biological differences among individuals and others of which are probably completely silent. Distinguishing innocuous variations from pathological mutations is a challenging exercise.

The heterogeneity of the human genome has added to the complexity of how gene expression can be altered in cancer. Human genomes contain at least 38 million SNPs, 1.4 million short insertion-deletion variants ("in-dels"), and at least 14,000 larger insertion-deletion variants. Furthermore, much of the non-protein-coding DNA may be expressed at the RNA level, and some of this is biologically relevant.[22]

There is considerable geographical and population-based variation in DNA sequences.[23] Moreover, protein-coding genes are interrupted by introns that are spliced out during processing of mRNA, increasing the range of possibilities for protein expression from an individual gene. Determining which of these changes is essential for carcinogenesis ("driver mutations") and which are simple passenger alterations continues to be a challenge.

Moreover, cancer genomes are far from uniform within the tumor mass as the mutations accumulate and cancer evolves in the host organism.

CANCER GENOMICS

Complete sequencing of cancer genomes has been performed for many tumor types, which demonstrates a wide range of variation among tumors of different organs, as well as among tumors of the same organ from different individuals.[24,25] Some altered sequences are found in the ~1.22% of the genome that codes for proteins, but there are also alterations in the noncoding portions of the genome. Sequence variants that occur at splice sites are frequently disruptive, and epigenetic changes (i.e., cytosine methylation at CpG sequences) in the promoters can lead to abnormal gene silencing in cancer. It is also becoming clear that alterations in the noncoding DNA can be an important source of dysregulation of gene expression.

When compared to the normal human genome, cancer genomes demonstrate a diverse range of altered anatomies. For example, in the case of colorectal cancer (CRC), in a sample of 276 tumors, the number of mutations varied over a 500-fold range. This is largely driven by the fact that a subset of 16% of these CRCs were hypermutated due to the germline or acquired inactivation of one of the DNA repair systems, rendering those tumors with a very large number of passenger mutations, often in specific target sequences such as microsatellites (when DNA MMR is defective), most of which (but not all) are noncoding. When the somatic mutations were compared between the hypermutated and non-hypermutated tumors, the apparent drivers were almost completely different between the two groups, explaining why these tumors have differing behaviors.[26]

The advent of more sophisticated DNA sequencing techniques has permitted "deep sequencing," or repetitive sequencing of the DNA from tumor tissues, which permits the detection of variant sequences that are not present in all the cells of a tumor. The interpretation of the sequencing data is complicated by the fact that not all of the cellular constituents of a tumor mass are cancer cells. Some are mesenchymal cells from the stroma, blood vessels, infiltrating immune cells, etc. Moreover, tumor cells are constantly replicating and accumulate new mutations as the tumor evolves. Genetic analysis of tumors has become important, as it provides information that can increasingly be used to direct targeted therapies.

Cancer Drivers and Passengers

Given the large number of sequences and other variations in tumors, it is obvious that not all are equally important in the pathogenesis of the tumor. This has given rise to the concept of "driver mutations," which add to the fitness of a cell and are functionally essential for neoplastic behavior, and "passenger mutations," which are created by the rapid replication of tumor cells or a failure in one of several DNA repair systems. Passenger mutations do not increase the fitness of the cell and are not responsible for the pathological behavior of the tumor. In a study utilizing exome sequencing and informatics analyses of >9400 tumor samples, >3400 different missense mutations in 299 putative driver genes were identified.[27] Uniform driver mutations were not present in all tumors from any organ and were frequently shared across tumor types. Driver mutations confer fitness, mediate cellular selection, and are consequently highly enriched in the tumor; drivers are also likely to be recurring mutations in an analysis of multiple different tumors. Separating the drivers from the passengers is of critical importance in designing effective therapeutics, which will target the most important drivers. Deep sequencing and the identification of enriched and recurrent mutations can be especially valuable in understanding the mutations in a hypermutated or ultramutated tumor.[28]

One reason for a very large number of passenger mutations can be an overwhelming exposure to a mutagenic insult, such as occurs in tissues exposed to ultraviolet radiation (skin) or tobacco smoke (respiratory tract) or that is in close proximity to a concentrated microbial environment (the gut). However, a more common cause of a large number of passenger mutations is the inactivation of one of the DNA repair systems, such as the DNA MMR system, the base excision repair (BER) system, NER, and double-strand break (DSB) repair systems, including homologous recombination (HR) repair and nonhomologous end joining (NHEJ) repair. Failure of each of these creates a recognizable "mutational signature" in the tumor DNA, as discussed later.

Genes Involved in Cancer: Oncogenes, Tumor Suppressor Genes, Caretakers, and Landscapers

Genes functionally involved in carcinogenesis do not all work the same way mechanistically, and cancer-driving genes can be put into general classes depending upon the biological process involved.

The first class of cancer-causing genes discovered were *oncogenes*, proposed by Boveri in 1914 but properly characterized and interpreted by Michael Bishop and Harold Varmus in the 1970s. Oncogenes are normal cellular genes (proto-oncogenes) involved in driving cell growth or proliferation and may be permanently activated in cancer by mutation or amplification.[29] Some oncogenes were initially identified in transforming viruses, which had hijacked a mutated copy of a normal cellular gene (proto-oncogene) and produced cancer by gaining entry into a cell. These genes were discovered by extracting DNA from cancers and transfecting fragments into NIH3T3 fibroblasts, where the *in vitro* growth patterns were altered upon introduction of oncogenic DNA. The DNA responsible for the altered growth was identified, found to contain the mutant or amplified DNA, and interpreted to be oncogenes.

Oncogenes are all dominantly acting tumor drivers and include genes such as *RAS, RAF, SRC,* and *MYC,* just to name a few (of more than 100). Oncogenes are usually activated by missense mutations in a specific portion of the gene or in a portion of the gene that is interactive with a signal transduction process in the expressed protein.[30] In some important instances, oncogenes become functionally important by amplification of the gene (i.e., multiple copies of the gene are present in the tumor). In brain tumors, oncogene amplification is a major genetic mechanism driving tumor formation and progression. Extrachromosomal DNA (such as "double minutes") is not restricted to division with the chromosomal DNA, which permits independent amplification and selection of those cells with multiple copies of the driver mutation.[31]

A second class of genes mechanistically involved in cancer are the *tumor suppressor genes* (TSGs). TSGs are normally involved in restraining cellular growth, and when inactivated, their absence is permissive of neoplastic growth. Both copies of TSGs must be inactivated to release the usual restraints on growth, so these can be thought of as recessively acting genes.

One of the key conceptual components of TSGs is the accommodation of a familial predisposition to cancer, since inheriting one mutant copy of a TSG could be associated with a normal phenotype but an increased likelihood of developing cancer when the second, wild-type allele undergoes an inactivating somatic mutation—the "second hit" proposed by Knudson in 1971.[1] Some TSGs act by regulating a cell cycle checkpoint that prevents inappropriate growth and, in many instances, responds to DNA damage and prevents the replication of mutated DNA sequences. Unlike oncogenes, which are usually activated by point mutations at specific sites in the gene, TSGs can be inactivated in a broad variety of ways, including deletion of the gene, missense and nonsense mutations throughout the genetic sequence, splice site alterations, and epigenetic gene silencing. Oncogenes and TSGs are drivers of cancer, as they are mechanistically involved in mediating neoplastic growth. However, another important class of genes is involved with cancer that may not directly mediate cell growth or division, but can be drivers of cancer in an indirect way. *Caretaker genes* are involved in DNA repair processes and serve as stabilizers of the genome.[32] Caretaker genes include those involved in DNA MMR, BER, NER, HR, NHEJ, etc., as listed earlier, but also include genes involved in repair of DNA strand breaks such as *BRCA1* or *BRCA2* (double-strand breaks), *BLM* (helicase), and *ATM* (recognition of DNA strand breaks).[32] These DNA repair and maintenance systems limit the number of mutations that accumulate with each cycle of replication in some instances and in response to mutagens in others. In addition, the DNA MMR system arrests the cell cycle at the G2/S checkpoint in the face of an unrepairable mutational load.[33]

The loss of a caretaker gene may lead to a pattern of mutational burden that might be recognized as the "signature" of that pathological process. The best example of this is the generation of a very large number of mutations at microsatellite sequences that occurs after the loss of the DNA MMR system.[34-36] This mutational signature (called microsatellite instability [MSI]) is readily recognized using a simple polymerase chain reaction (PCR)–based assay,[37] and more importantly, this hypermutable phenotype provides an indication for specific immune checkpoint therapy.[38]

Finally, it has been proposed that some genetic alterations may occur in the stroma surrounding the tumor cells and function as a *landscaper*, as appears to be the case with *SMAD4* in juvenile polyposis syndrome[39] and possibly also Peutz-Jeghers syndrome.[5] In this instance, the key driver of tumor growth may not even be in the genome of the tumor cells, but rather through the influence of an abnormal stromal cell on the collaborative growth of the epithelial cells.[8,39]

How Many Mutations Does It Take for a Cancer to Develop?

Based upon the relationship between the annual incidence of some common solid cancers versus age, it was estimated over 40 years ago that a relatively small number of cumulative mutations were responsible for cancer.[40] The exponential relationship between age and the incidence of those cancers was best explained by the gradual accumulation of somatic mutations over time and the requirement for a specific number of specific types of mutations to occur. Data over the past 30 years have largely substantiated that hypothesis and demonstrated that the carcinogenesis may require some of these alterations to occur in a specific order.

Although tumors usually harbor a large number of DNA sequence variants, not to mention chromosomal deletions, duplications, and rearrangements, as well as abnormalities of methylation, it is speculated that between two and eight driver mutations, occurring in the proper sequence, are sufficient to cause cancer.[30] It appears that there may be as many different constellations of mutations as there are tumors. Moreover, mutagenesis is an ongoing process in most cancers, so the tumors continue to evolve throughout their histories. This leads to intratumoral heterogeneity, heterogeneity between different metastatic lesions in an individual, and the wide range of heterogeneity between tumors from different patients.[30]

Classes of Driver Mutations in Cancer

Driver mutations in cancer can be classified into 12 signaling pathways, each of which has multiple genes involved.[30] First, six of the pathways are involved in the regulation of cell survival. This group includes *transforming growth factor-β, MAP kinase, STAT, PI3K, RAS,* and pathways regulating the cell cycle and apoptosis. The second group of five pathways is involved with cell fate and includes members of the *NOTCH, hedgehog, APC,* chromatin modifiers, and transcriptional regulation pathways. Finally, a group of genes is involved in genomic maintenance (including all of the DNA repair pathways). Multiple genes participate in each of these pathways, and conceivably a mutation in any of the genes in the pathway could give rise to the same oncogenic mechanism. This is the best explanation for the variable mutational patterns between tumors in the same location with generally similar behaviors.

Sequence of Mutation Accumulation in Cancer (Multistep Carcinogenesis)

Cancers are driven by the sequential accumulation of mutations that inactivate DNA maintenance systems, inactivate TSGs, and activate driving proto-oncogenes. An important consideration is whether there is a required or preferred sequence for this to occur. CRC was the first cancer to have a careful cataloging of the sequence of genetic events involved in carcinogenesis.[41] This was possible because CRCs are common and evolve gradually from benign adenomatous polyps, which can be found and easily removed from humans during colonoscopy, and both benign and malignant tumors in all stages of development were available for study. This was harder to achieve in other common cancers such as the breast or prostate and nearly impossible for tumors of the brain.

In 1987, the gene for FAP, the familial disease characterized by a large number of early-onset adenomatous polyps, was mapped to chromosome 5q21-22,[42] and although the gene had not been cloned and the gene product would not be known for another four years, it was suspected that sporadic adenomatous polyps were initiated through an alteration at that locus. At the same time, it was also noted that "allelic loss" (deletion of one allele of a gene) or loss of heterozygosity (LOH) at this same locus was seen in CRCs.[43] Restriction fragment length polymorphism (RFLP) analysis was used on DNA extracted from these lesions to assay for allelic loss. Also in 1987, it had been shown that activating mutations in the *RAS* oncogene family (*KRAS, HRAS,* and *NRAS*) were commonly found in CRCs as well as adenomatous polyps, but not the normal colonic mucosa adjacent to these neoplastic lesions.[44,45] Finally, in 1989, it was noted that both point mutations and allelic losses of the *p53* gene on chromosome 17p were present in at least some CRCs.[46]

The laboratory of Bert Vogelstein, which was involved in these efforts, looked for alterations at the 5q locus, the *RAS* genes (*KRAS, HRAS,* and *NRAS*), and p53 in normal mucosa, adenomatous polyps of varying sizes and degrees of dysplasia, and CRC.[41] None of these alterations were present in normal colonic tissues. LOH was found at the 5q locus in some proportion of early adenomatous tissues, but were not more frequent in advanced adenomas or carcinoma. Therefore, losses on 5q were determined to be an *early* alteration in colorectal carcinogenesis. The *APC* gene was cloned in 1991 at the 5q locus and eventually shown to be the *gatekeeper* gene for colorectal adenomas.[47,48] *KRAS* mutations were uncommon in early adenomas but substantially more common in larger and more advanced adenomas and were not more frequently seen in CRCs than in the advanced adenomas. Therefore, *KRAS* mutations were placed as an intermediate step in the progressive process of colorectal carcinogenesis, occurring after the losses on 5q and associated with the growth in size and dysplastic appearance of the adenoma, but did not appear to be sufficient for CRC. Moreover, 88% of *RAS* mutations were in codons 12, 13, or 61 of *KRAS,* which encodes the domain of the KRAS protein that interacts with guanine nucleotide exchange. In this study, allelic losses on chromosome 18q were found (which had been an area of interest in CRC at the same time[49]), which were found to be uncommon in the early neoplastic lesions and more common in the larger, more advanced lesions. Finally, allelic deletion at 17p was rare in the adenomas but commonly seen in advanced adenomas and in 75% of CRCs. Chromosomal arm 17p is small, and only a few genes were known to be located there, one being *p53,* which had been known to be involved somehow in carcinogenesis. It was quickly recognized that many tumors had only one copy of *p53,* and it was mutated, which confirmed the biallelic inactivation of *p53* in CRC.[46]

These studies were performed using Southern blots and other techniques requiring relatively large amounts of DNA that made fine-tuning the relationship between the genetic lesions and the pathological changes in colorectal neoplasms challenging. Later work using PCR-based techniques and microdissection of a large number of specimens that simultaneously contained normal tissue, adenoma, high-grade dysplasia, and cancer confirmed that losses of the 5q locus occurred exactly at the normal-to-adenoma transition and that loss of *p53* occurred exactly at the adenoma-to-carcinoma transition.[50] Thus, multistep carcinogenesis was conceived as the stepwise accumulation of genetic alterations that explained the presence of the full pathological range of neoplastic lesions in the colon, beginning with the early adenomas (driven by loss of *APC*), followed by the appearance of *KRAS* mutations and losses on 18q as the premalignant lesions grew and became progressively more dysplastic, followed by biallelic loss of the *p53* gene as the adenoma-to-carcinoma event.

The process seemed logical, but as additional data accumulated, it became clear that there are multiple ways to achieve each "step" in the multistep pathway. For example, in about 10% to 15% of colorectal neoplasms, alternative genetic events other than biallelic loss of *APC* can initiate an adenoma. Similarly, not all colorectal neoplasms necessarily undergo activating mutations in *KRAS* or inactivation of *SMAD4* (central to signaling through the transforming growth factor-β pathway) as the benign polyp grows and becomes more dysplastic. Also, there are multiple alternatives to *p53* loss at the adenoma-to-carcinoma transition, such as mutations in *PI3K* (see Figure 1.1).[30]

How Important Is the Order of Genetic Alterations?

At least two groups have reported that when *KRAS* mutations occur in the absence of losses of *APC* (or other disruption of the WNT signaling pathway), the result is a nonprogressive hyperplastic polyp[51] or hyperplastic aberrant crypt focus.[52] However, this has been a controversial topic in part because of the changing pathological classification of hyperplastic and "serrated" lesions over time.[53]

Pathways

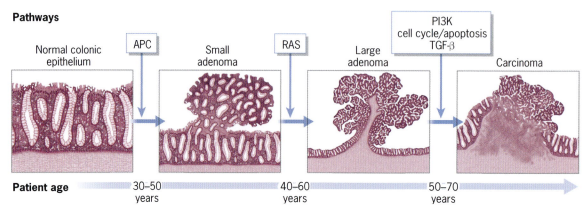

FIGURE 1.1: Multistep carcinogenesis. This is an updated version of the original multistep carcinogenesis paradigm originally proposed by the laboratory of Vogelstein in 1990. The first step on the pathway involves loss of control of WNT signaling, depicted here as loss of the *APC* gene product. This is the usual mechanism for initiation of colorectal neoplastic lesions, but other members of this pathway may achieve the same biological outcome. The subsequent steps include mutational activation of *RAS*, and ultimately the adenoma-to-carcinoma transition, which can be mediated by loss of *p53*, as initially proposed, or inactivation of the control of the transforming growth factor-β through PI3K, as shown here. The essential point is that signaling pathways involve multiple members, but progression occurs through alterations in key checkpoints in growth control.

The issue of sequence context has been clarified by more complete analyses of the genes involved in multistep carcinogenesis. Germline mutations in the *APC* gene virtually guarantee the early appearance of multiple adenomatous polyps. The fact that patients with FAP ultimately develop CRC is related to the very large number of polyps and the early age of their appearance. The gene of interest on 18q (not lost in the early lesions) has been found to be *SMAD4*, and curiously, germline mutations in that gene cause familial juvenile polyposis (as mentioned earlier, acting through the stromal and lymphatic tissues to produce benign polyps). However, CRC may occur in ~38% of those patients.[54] Germline mutations in the *p53* gene cause Li-Fraumeni syndrome, and although there is some increased risk for CRC in this disease, that is not the primary cancer risk in that setting. All of this suggests that the order of appearance of the mutations is indeed critical to the clinical outcome.

A similar stepwise sequence of genetic alterations has not been reported for many other cancers, but there are few other organs in which the full pathological range of premalignant lesions has been available for detailed analysis. Pancreatic cancer is associated with somatic mutations in *KRAS*, *SMAD4*, and *p53*, which overlap with what has been reported in CRC. Of course, there are multiple other mutated genes in pancreatic cancers. In some patients with pancreatic cancer, there is a series of pathologically recognizable lesions leading from premalignant intraductal papillary mucinous neoplasms (IPMNs) to pancreatic cancer. By analyzing tissues in which the various precursor lesions could be microdissected and analyzed by multiple techniques, it has been found that the order of accumulations is different from what occurs in CRC. *KRAS* and *GNAS* (a component of the G-protein complex) mutations appear to be early events in the multistep process, the accumulation of mutations may vary between each pancreas studied and within an individual pancreas with multiple IPMN lesions, and at least three different pathways for the evolution of IPMNs may occur[55] (see Figure 1.2). This again underscores the heterogeneity and complexity of tumor formation.

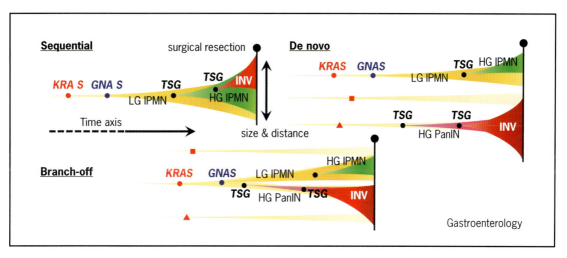

FIGURE 1.2: Multistep carcinogenesis in the pancreas. In contrast to the linear and frequently followed pathway for multistep carcinogenesis in CRC, the sequence of events in the evolution of pancreatic malignancies is different even though many of the same genes are involved. To illustrate the complexity, there are multiple routes through the development of pancreatic adenocarcinoma from intraductal papillary mucinous neoplasms (IPMNs) with differences in the genes involved and the order of accumulation of the mutations. LG = low grade; HG = high grade; TSG = tumor suppressor gene; INV = invasive cancer. Pathways may occur through a specific common sequence; and within a single pancreas; one can see new (de novo) mutations and branches off the primary pathway over time.

Somatic Mutational Signatures in Cancer

Tumors of different organs tend to have different numbers of somatic mutations, as illustrated in Figure 1.3, although there is a wide range between individual tumors from each organ.[30] A few features are particularly prominent. Generally, pediatric tumors have the smallest number of mutations, typically ranging from 4 to 14. This reflects the absence of a lifetime of collecting potential driver mutations and suggests the malignant behavior is mediated by a relatively small number of critical drivers. At the other end of the scale CRCs, lung cancers, and melanomas have a median of 66 to 163 mutations, reflecting in part long-standing exposure to a mutagenic milieu. Moreover, when one looks specifically at CRCs with defective DNA MMR (dMMR) and microsatellite instability (MSI), the median number of mutations jumps to 500 to 1000, reflecting the loss of DNA MMR activity and the accelerated accumulation of mutations—most of which are not drivers, but passengers.

This MSI phenotype is recognizable as a "mutational signature" and is overrepresented with in-del mutations at simple repetitive sequences (microsatellites).[14] At this time, finding MSI in a tumor is a diagnostic tool that can be used to screen for possible Lynch syndrome, and more importantly, this hypermutable phenotype is a potential candidate for immune checkpoint therapy when there is advanced disease.[56]

Disabling other DNA repair systems gives rise to different mutational signatures. For example, families were being investigated that had multiple adenomatous polyps in the colon but no germline mutations in the *APC* gene; moreover, the phenotype inheritance appeared to be recessive rather than dominant.[57,58] Somatic mutations in *APC* were sought in the adenomas, and these were highly prevalent, but in heterogeneous locations throughout the *APC*

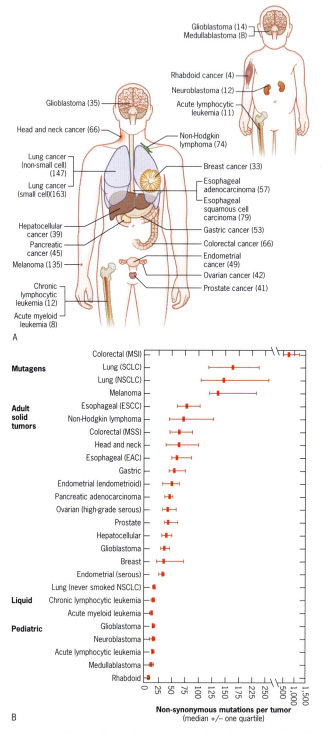

FIGURE 1.3: Tumor locations and somatic mutations. Number of somatic mutations in selected human cancers. A. The median number of non-synonymous somatic mutations per tumor in groups of childhood and adult cancers, with microsatellite unstable CRCs at the high end and all the pediatric tumors at the low end. B. The median number of non-synonymous mutations, with 25%–75% quartile bars. MSI = microsatellite instability; SCLC = small cell lung cancers; NSCLC = non-SCLCs; ESCC = esophageal squamous cell carcinomas; MSS = microsatellite stable; EAC = esophageal adenocarcinoma. (Reproduced with permission from Vogelstein B, Papadopoulos N, Velculescu VE, et al: Cancer genome landscapes, Science 2013 Mar 29;339(6127):1546–1558).

gene in individual polyps. The investigators noted that the somatic mutational profile had an excess of somatic mutations consisting of G:C>T:A in the *APC* gene, which is a predicted consequence of oxidative damage when guanine residues develop an adduct that mispairs with adenine, leading to this mutational signature. This is ordinarily repaired by the BER system, which raised the hypothesis that inactivation of the BER system might be the underlying mechanism for this disease entity.

Three gene members of the BER family, *MutYH, MTH1,* and *OGG1,* were sequenced in the germlines of affected individuals. Six affected individuals (from a group of 152 subjects) had biallelic mutations in the *MutYH* gene, leading to the discovery of *MutYH*-associated polyposis.[59] These patients had a smaller number of adenomas with later onset than classic FAP, there was recessive inheritance, and the polyps had the characteristic mutational signature.

Over time, two mutations in *MutYH* were found to be the most common germline mutations in Western European populations: Y179C and G396D. Many more mutations have been found in European populations, and there are prominent founder effects, with different mutations being present in non-Europeans. What is clinically of importance is that each of these germline variants produces a different degree of loss of function in the BER complex. Consequently, homozygotes for the Y179C mutation (the more disabled allele) have earlier ages of presentation for polyposis and increased risk of CRC compared with G396D homozygotes or the compound heterozygotes.[60] As more data are gathered, there will be an increased ability to predict neoplastic risk depending upon the relative dose-loss of BER activity in these patients.

DNA Repair and Genomic Instability

The average rate of *de novo* (new) *germline* mutations in humans is 1.2×10^{-8} mutations per base pair (bp), as determined by identifying single nucleotide variants (SNVs) present in offspring but absent in parents from family trios.[61] Sequencing single cells from cultured fibroblasts to detect *de novo* SNVs absent in bulk DNA arrived at a median *somatic* mutation rate of 2.8×10^{-7} mutations per bp—more than an order of magnitude higher than the germline mutation frequency.[61] In addition to SNVs, several types of lesions arising from endogenous or exogenous sources can affect cellular DNA and are repaired by different mechanisms. Also, germline mutations in the DNA repair systems essentially all result in familial cancer syndromes, as illustrated in Table 1.2.

Single-strand breaks (SSBs) involve one strand of the DNA double helix and are repaired by BER, NER, and MMR. BER mitigates the mutagenic properties of alkylation, oxidation, and deamination modifications in a process utilizing DNA glycosylases to recognize specific mismatches (e.g., 8-oxo-G:A mispairs) and catalyze base excision.[68] NER acts on bulky lesions that distort the DNA double helix such as cyclobutane pyrimidine dimers induced by ultraviolet (UV) radiation.[69] NER consists of two pathways: global genome repair (GG-NER) that recognizes and removes lesions throughout the genome and transcription-coupled repair (TC-NER) with preference for the transcribed and template strands.

Postreplicative MMR corrects DNA mismatches and insertion/deletion loops arising in DNA replication.[70] MMR only sees replication errors that are generated by the replicative polymerases *Polδ* and *Polε* (error rates 10^{-4} to 10^{-5} per nucleotide) and escape the proofreading activity of these polymerases. Polδ and Polε have a 3′ to 5′ exonuclease activity that proofreads the nascent strand, which is estimated to increase the replication fidelity by 100-fold.[71]

TABLE 1.2: DNA Repair and Hereditary Cancer

Gene and Function	Syndrome	Inheritance	Hereditary Tumors
MutYH (BER)	MutYH-associated polyposis	Recessive	Colorectal adenomas (oligopolyposis)[59]
MSH3 (DNA MMR)	Oligopolyposis of the colon	Recessive	Colorectal adenomas and other tumors[62]
MLH3 (DNA MMR)	Oligopolyposis of the colon	Recessive	Colorectal adenomas and other tumors[63]
Polymerase delta 1 (POLD1)	Polymerase proofreading-associated polyposis (PPAP)	Dominant	Oligopolyposis syndrome, CRC, duodenal adenomas[64]
Polymerase epsilon (POLE)	Polymerase proofreading-associated polyposis (PPAP)	Dominant	Oligopolyposis syndrome, CRC, duodenal adenomas[64]
ATM (repair of DNA DSBs)	Ataxia telangiectasia	Recessive	Breast, pancreas, leukemia, lymphoma, brain
BLM (DNA helicase)	Bloom syndrome	Recessive	Leukemia, lymphoma, skin
BRCA1/2 (HRR)	Hereditary breast and ovarian cancer	Dominant	Breast, ovarian, pancreas
FANCA/C/D2/E/F/G (HRR and interstrand crosslink repair)	Fanconi anemia	Recessive	Leukemia
NBN (broken DNA strand repair)	Nijmegen breakage syndrome	Recessive	Breast, ovarian, prostate
RECQL4 (DNA helicase)	Rothman-Thomson syndrome	Recessive	Bone, skin
WRN (DNA helicase)	Werner syndrome	Recessive	Bone, brain
MSH2 (and EPCAM), MLH1, MSH6, or PMS2 (DNA MMR)	Lynch syndrome	Dominant	Colon, uterus, ovary, renal, other[65]
Biallelic MSH2 (and EPCAM), MLH1, MSH6, or PMS2 (DNA MMR)	Constitutional DNA mismatch repair deficiency (CMMRD)	Recessive	Childhood leukemia, lymphoma, colorectal polyps, CRC, brain, other[66]
NTHL1 (DNA glycosylase)	Attenuated FAP	Recessive	Attenuated colonic adenomatous polyposis syndrome; other cancers[67]
XPA/C, ERCCA-5, DDB2 (NER)	Xeroderma pigmentosum (XP)	Recessive	Multiple skin tumors
PALB2 (HHR, BRCA pathway)	-	Dominant	Breast, ovarian
CHEK2 (signals DNA damage to p53 checkpoint)	-	Dominant	Breast, CRC
RAD51-C/D (DNA DSB repair)	-	Dominant	Ovarian
LIG4, XLF, PRKDC, or Artemis (NHEJ)	Severe combined immunodeficiency	Recessive	Lymphoid malignancies

BER = base excision repair; DNA MMR = DNA mismatch repair; DSBs = double strand breaks; HRR = homologous recombination repair; NER = nucleotide excision repair; NHEJ = non-homologous end joining.

The combined activity of polymerase proofreading and postreplicative MMR results in high replication fidelity: one incorrect base for every 10^9 to 10^{10} nucleotides replicated.[72]

Double-strand breaks (DSBs) may arise during DNA replication or as a result of exogenous damage, such as ionizing radiation.[73] Two main pathways act on DSBs. Homologous recombination repair (HRR) uses the undamaged chromosome as a template for transferring sequence information to the broken chromosome. This results in a precise, error-free restoration of the DNA sequence.[74] NHEJ does not depend on sequence homology when ligating the two ends of a DSB and is therefore error-prone.[75]

Functional DNA repair is crucial for maintaining genome stability. Genetic or epigenetic inactivation of DNA repair genes impairs the cell's ability to restore damaged DNA, leading to genomic instability or cell death. Hereditary disorders of DNA repair have provided important insights into DNA repair mechanisms and consequences of their defective function.[76] The rare autosomal recessive syndrome xeroderma pigmentosum was identified biochemically as the first DNA repair disorder in 1969.[77] In patients with xeroderma pigmentosum, NER is defective involving GG-NER, TC-NER, or both, depending on the mutant gene.[78] Faulty NER results in increased risk of skin cancer following UV exposure, and mutational signatures of tumors exhibit transcribed strand bias.[25]

Lynch syndrome–associated MMR genes have been known since the early to mid-1990s.[65] Somatic MMR defects, mostly hypermethylation of *MLH1*, occur with variable frequencies in most cancer types. MMR deficiency constitutes an important molecular classifier of CRCs and endometrial cancers, with some 15%[79] and 30%[80] of the respective cancers being MMR-defective (MSI-high, or just MSI for simplicity). MMR-deficient/MSI cancers are the most prevalent subgroup of hypermutable cancers, defined as over 12 mutations per 10^6 bases.[26] The base substitution signature 6 (C>T at NpCpG) from Alexandrov et al.,[25] combined with very frequent in-dels at simple repeat sequences, characterizes MMR-deficient tumors. Mutations in the proofreading domains of the replicative polymerase genes *POLE* and *POLD1* result in an "ultramutation" phenotype and represent another subgroup of hypermutable cancers. This characteristic signature 10 is present in 0.5% of various cancers.[25,28]

The susceptibility genes *BRCA1* and *BRCA2* associated with breast and ovarian cancer were identified in the 1990s and subsequently found to be key players in HR.[81] Their defects reduce genome integrity, resulting in distinct base substitution/in-del and rearrangement signatures.[81] Furthermore, *BRCA1/2* defects cause sensitivity to DNA-damaging agents, influencing therapeutic options (see the discussion on PARP inhibitors later).

A few recessively inherited polyposis predisposition syndromes linked to DNA repair genes are known, including those due to biallelic germline mutations in the DNA glycosylase genes *MutYH* (monoallelic germline mutations are relatively common in the population) and *NTHL1* (which is rare). Reflecting specific BER defects, tumors from biallelic *MutYH* mutation carriers display G:C>T:A transversions,[82] whereas C to T transitions at non-CpG sites (signature 30) are characteristic of tumors from biallelic *NTHL1* mutation carriers.[83]

The repair systems listed in Table 1.2 are not all-inclusive and other repair mechanisms exist. The O^6-methylguanine DNA methyltransferase (*MGMT*) enzyme removes potentially mutagenic alkyl groups from the O^6 position of guanine and provides an example of direct repair (reversion of DNA damage). The activity of *MGMT* is regulated by promoter methylation, and the methylation status of the *MGMT* promoter has been found to be an important prognostic/predictive factor when treating gliomas and metastatic CRC with alkylating drugs.[84] The poly ADP-ribose polymerase (PARP) enzymes function as posttranslational modifiers by adding poly ADP-ribose molecules to target proteins.[85] PARPs repair SSBs through the BER pathway. PARP inhibitors such as olaparib, which is used to treat *BRCA1/2*-defective ovarian cancer, prevent the repair of SSBs, leading to DSBs. While normal cells can tolerate DNA damage caused by PARP inhibition, cancer cells with defective HR (*BRCA1/2* mutations) cannot, resulting in the death of cancer cells. The concept of targeting complementary molecular defects to potentiate the killing effect of an anticancer drug is known as synthetic lethality. As more data accumulate, it is likely that somatic mutations in genes such as *BRCA1/2, EGFR,* and others, occurring as a consequence of an underlying influence of a defective DNA repair process, may lead the way to additional targeted therapies.[86]

Approximately 5% of common cancers, such as colorectal or breast cancer, represent hereditary Mendelian diseases attributable to high-penetrance mutations in single predisposition genes.[93,94] Some 20% to 30% of cancers are familial, i.e., show familial clustering, the reasons for which are diverse and likely to involve both genetic and nongenetic (environmental) factors. The remaining majority of cancer cases are considered sporadic. Twin studies can provide important insights into the relative contributions of inherited and environmental factors to the causation of cancer.[95] A higher concordance for cancer among monozygotic twins, who share all genes, compared to dizygotic twins, who share half of their genes, would point to the importance of genetic effects. Heritability is a term denoting the fraction of phenotypic variability attributable to genetic factors and ranges from 0% (all variability is due to environmental factors) to 100% (all variability is due to genetic factors). Prostate cancer is among cancers showing the highest heritability estimates: 57% in the investigation by Mucci et al.[95] In the same study, heritability estimates for breast cancer and CRC were 31% and 15%, respectively. Mucci et al. also evaluated familial cancer risks and found significant excess familial risk of developing any cancer (37% in dizygotic twins and 46% in monozygotic twins compared to 32% in the whole twin cohort) and for specific types of cancer, including prostate and breast.

Cancer susceptibility genes can be categorized according to the minor allele frequency (MAF) and the relative risk conferred.[94,96] As mentioned earlier, penetrance refers to the proportion of individuals with a given genotype that express the phenotype associated with the genotype. Using breast cancer as a phenotypic example, rare high-penetrance alleles, such as those affecting *BRCA1* and *BRCA2* genes, occur with frequencies below 0.1% in the population and increase cancer risk 10-fold or more. Many genes belonging to this category were identified by genetic linkage analysis in the past, and more recently, by exome or genome sequencing. Rare moderate-penetrance alleles, such as those affecting the *CHEK2* or *PALB2* genes, occur with population frequencies of 1% or below and increase cancer risk 2-fold. Such genes have been discovered by various methods, including candidate gene analysis and exome/genome sequencing. Common low-penetrance alleles, including multiple loci (such as *ESR1*) identified by genome-wide association studies, are common in the population (MAF >10%) and increase cancer risk only 1.1- to 1.5-fold.

To date, more than 100 genes have been identified that confer highly or moderately increased risks of cancer.[97] Most cancer predisposition genes (103/114, 90%) are tumor suppressor genes contributing to cancer through loss-of-function mutations. The remaining 10% represent oncogenes (e.g., *RET*) that predispose to cancer through gain-of-function mutations. In most cases (see Table 1.3 for examples), the risk allele of a cancer predisposition gene

TABLE 1.3: Tumor Suppressor Genes and Oncogenes Involved with Germline Mutation–Associated Cancer Syndromes[32]

Tumor Suppressor Genes

Gene and Pathway	Syndrome	Inheritance	Hereditary Tumor(s)
APC (WNT)	Familial adenomatous polyposis (FAP)	Dominant	Multiple adenomas of the colon; gastric polyps, duodenal and small intestinal adenomas, thyroid tumors, CRC
AXIN2 (WNT)	Attenuated FAP	Dominant	Oligopolyposis syndrome, CRC[87]
RNF43 (WNT via ubiquitin ligase)	Sessile serrated polyposis syndrome	Dominant	Multiple serrated polyps of the colon, CRC[88]
GREM1 (SMAD4, BMP signaling; TGFβ)	Hereditary mixed polyposis syndrome	Dominant	Adenomatous, hyperplastic and mixed polyps of the colon, CRC[89]
E-cadherin, or CDH1 (WNT)	Hereditary diffuse gastric carcinoma	Dominant	Diffuse gastric cancer[90]
EXT1,2 (WNT)	Hereditary multiple exostoses	Dominant	Bone tumors
PTCH (GLI)	Gorlin syndrome	Dominant	Skin and brain tumors (medulloblastoma)
SUFU (HH)	Medulloblastoma	Dominant	Skin and brain tumors
FH (HIF1)	Hereditary leiomyomatosis	Dominant	Leiomyomas and renal cell cancer
SDHA, -B, -C, D, and -AF2 RET, VHL, NF1, MAX, TMEM127	Familial pheochromocytoma and paraganglioma	Dominant	Paragangliomas, pheochromocytomas[91]
VHL (HIF1)	Von Hippel-Lindau syndrome	Dominant	Kidney, etc.
p53 (TP53)	Li-Fraumeni syndrome	Dominant	Breast, sarcomas, adrenal, brain, and others
WT1 (p53)	Familial Wilms tumor	Dominant	Wilms tumor
STK11 (PIK3CA)	Peutz-Jeghers syndrome	Dominant	Hamartomas of the gastrointestinal tract (childhood); adults: cancers of the brain (gliomas), breast, lung, esophagus, stomach, pancreas, small intestine, CRC, ovary, uterus, testes, cervix (adenoma malignum)
PTEN (PIK3CA)	Cowden syndrome; Bannayan-Riley Ruvalcaba syndrome	Dominant	Breast, thyroid, endometrium, CRC, kidney, melanoma
CDKN2A (p16^{ink4A}, p14^{ARF}) (RB)	Familial malignant melanoma	Dominant	Melanoma, pancreas, others
CDK4	Familial malignant melanoma	Dominant	Melanoma
RB1	Hereditary retinoblastoma	Dominant	Eye (retinoblastoma)
NF1	Neurofibromatosis, type 1	Dominant	Neurofibromas
SMAD4, BMPR1A (SMAD4)	Juvenile polyposis	Dominant	CRC, gastric cancer, small intestinal cancers

(Continued)

TABLE 1.3: Tumor Suppressor Genes and Oncogenes Involved with Germline Mutation–Associated Cancer Syndromes[32] (Continued)

MEN1 (MEN1)	Multiple endocrine neoplasia 1 (MEN1)	Dominant	Pituitary, parathyroid, pancreas (islet cell) carcinoids[92]
NF2 (regulates merlin production in neurons)	Neurofibromatosis, type 2	Dominant	Meningioma, acoustic neuroma
BHD (regulates folliculin production)	Birt-Hogg-Dube syndrome	Dominant	Renal, hair follicles

Oncogenes

Gene	Syndrome	Inheritance	Hereditary Tumors
Kit	Familial gastrointestinal stromal tumors (GISTs)	Dominant	GISTs
Met	Hereditary papillary renal cell carcinoma	Dominant	Kidney
PDGFRA	Familial gastrointestinal stromal tumors	Dominant	GISTs
RET	Multiple endocrine neoplasia type II	Dominant	Thyroid, parathyroid, adrenal

(WNT = WNT signaling pathway; BMP = bone morphogenetic protein; TGF-β = tumor growth factor-β; GLI = glioma-associated oncogene; HH = hedgehog; HIF1 = hypoxia inducible factor 1; PIK3CA = phosphatidylinositol-4,5-bisphosphate 3-kinase catalytic subunit alpha; RB = retinoblastoma.

GIST = gastrointestinal stromal tumor; PDGFRA = platelet-derived growth factor receptor-α.

Adapted with permission from Vogelstein B, Kinzler KW. Cancer genes and the pathways they control, Nat Med 2004 Aug;10(8):789–799).

is dominant and capable of producing disease in heterozygotes. Autosomal dominant risk alleles show vertical transmission in pedigrees, with disease phenotype present in successive generations. As mentioned, according to Knudson's two-hit hypothesis, tumor suppressor genes are recessive on a cellular level, since biallelic inactivation is needed for tumor initiation.[1] Less frequently, the risk allele is recessive, producing disease only when both alleles are defective (i.e., in a homozygote). Autosomal recessive alleles display horizontal phenotypes in pedigrees so that disease phenotype may be seen in multiple siblings but not in their parents. A few cancer predisposition genes may cause phenotypes in both monoallelic and biallelic mutation carriers, often with more severe clinical manifestations in the latter. For example, germline heterozygosity for mutations of the MMR genes *MLH1*, *MSH2*, *MSH6*, and PMS2 causes Lynch syndrome with adult-onset cancers, whereas homozygosity for the mutations or compound heterozygosity with two different disease-causing mutations at a locus underlies constitutional mismatch repair deficiency syndrome (CMMRD) with childhood cancers of a distinct spectrum.[66,98]

Sporadic presentation does not exclude hereditary disease, since a cancer-predisposing mutation may arise *de novo* in gametogenesis of one of the parents or in the fertilized egg. By convention, *de novo* mutation refers to a mutation found in all cells of an individual but not detected in that individual's parents. The proportion of *de novo* germline mutations varies according to the predisposing gene. Such mutations have been reported to be rare for *BRCA1/2* genes[99] and Lynch syndrome–associated MMR genes,[100] whereas nearly one-third of *APC*-mutation-positive FAP cases may be attributable to *de novo* germline mutations.[101]

A predisposing mutation may occur in a mosaic pattern, being present in only a proportion of egg or sperm cell precursors (germline mosaicism) or somatic cells (somatic mosaicism). Germline and somatic mosaicism can be present at the same time, depending on the developmental stage at which the mutation occurs. The *APC* gene provides an illustrative example: high-coverage next-generation sequencing of *APC* in leukocyte and colorectal tumor–derived DNA from patients with unexplained sporadic adenomatous polyposis identified low-level mosaicism of a pathogenic *APC* mutation in 25% (5/20) of cases.[102] It is clinically important to diagnose *APC* mosaicism in apparently sporadic polyposis cases, since if primordial germ cells are affected, the recurrence risk in children is up to 50% (depending on the distribution of the mutation in the germ tissues). The parents and siblings are not at risk of being mutation carriers, only the offspring.

EPIGENETICS IN CANCER

In 2001, the Human Genome Project established a reference nucleotide sequence for the human genome.[103] Fourteen years later, the National Institutes of Health (NIH) Roadmap Epigenetics Consortium mapped the important regulatory (epigenetic) marks across the human DNA sequence.[79] While the human genome is generally preserved in all cell types at all times, the epigenome is not. Epigenetic regulation is responsible for the differential gene expression required considering the type of cell and tissue, developmental stage, parental origin (genomic imprinting), environmental conditions, and other circumstances. Differential expression is achieved by DNA methylation, chromatin states (histone modifications and nucleosome remodeling), and noncoding RNAs.[104] Reduced levels of DNA methylation at selected loci in tumor cells compared to normal cells, a phenomenon termed DNA hypomethylation, was one of the earliest observations of epigenetic dysregulation in primary human tumors.[18] An opposite phenomenon, namely coordinated hypermethylation of tumor suppressor gene promoters (CIMP, *CpG Island Methylator Phenotype*), was subsequently defined and linked to sporadic colorectal tumors with mismatch repair deficiency via *MLH1* promoter methylation.[105] Later studies have established disruption of virtually all classes of epigenetic control as a universal feature of cancer cells, and the epigenome provides a fingerprint for the cell type of cancer origin.[79]

An epigenetic alteration is defined as a heritable change in the expression (function) of a gene where the sequence of DNA remains unaltered. Heritability in this context primarily refers to the maintenance of epigenetic patterns from cell to daughter cell when DNA replicates during cell division (mitotic heritability). Identical methylation patterns across cell generations are, however, poorly applicable to cancer cells, in which losses and gains of methylation (hypomethylation and hypermethylation, respectively) are common, both at selected loci and genome-wide.

The presence of unaltered DNA sequences may not be required either, since a cancer-associated epigenetic change (epimutation) can be induced by a genetic change located *in cis* (on the same DNA molecule) or *in trans* (on a different DNA molecule, often on a different chromosome). For example, an SNV in the promoter region of *MLH1* (c.-27C>A) that abolished a transcription factor binding site was shown to induce *MLH1* promoter methylation in a Lynch syndrome family.[106] Such a situation is known as "secondary epimutation" to distinguish it from "primary epimutation" in which no underlying change in DNA sequence is detectable.[107]

Epimutation can be acquired or constitutional. The previously mentioned *MLH1* c.-27C>A–associated epimutation was constitutional and showed dominant transmission in the Lynch syndrome pedigree.[106] The latter aspect—transgenerational heritability—mainly applies to secondary epimutations only. Even so, deviation from regular genetic transmission may occur: the *MLH1* c.-27C>A–associated epimutation was found to be erased in spermatozoa but reinstated in the somatic cells of the offspring later.[106]

Genome-wide investigations have shown that more than 1000 CpG islands can be methylated in individual tumors.[108] The abundance of epigenetic alterations, combined with their dynamic and reversible nature, makes it difficult to distinguish "driver" epigenetic changes from "passenger" alterations. Driver changes are causally related to the neoplastic process and confer a selective advantage, whereas passenger changes are retained by chance during cell proliferation. As epigenetic changes can silence tumor suppressor genes, activate oncogenes, and regulate cell fate transitions, theoretical prerequisites for a "driver" nature exist.[109] Experimental evidence is available to support this notion. Examination of CRC cells with highly impaired DNA methyltransferases (i.e., DKO cells) identified a set of specific genes that maintained methylation even when global DNA methylation was artificially reduced. It was demonstrated that these genes had to be silenced by methylation for cancer cells to survive.[110] The genes represented previously unknown tumor suppressor genes and included many acting as G-protein–coupled receptors. In another investigation, genome-wide profiling identified over 200 genes with promoter hypomethylation in clinical samples of hepatocellular carcinoma. A subsequent study on selected genes (e.g., *RASAL2* and *NENF* and other genes with oncogenic properties) showed that gene activation by hypomethylation was required for continued cancer cell proliferation and invasiveness.[111] Finally, epigenetic mechanisms are key regulators of genomic integrity and often underlie genomic instability, an "enabling" hallmark of cancer.[112] Many DNA repair genes listed in Table 1.2 are sensitive to promoter methylation.[113] As mentioned earlier, the 12% subset of sporadic cancers with MSI-high are attributable to *MLH1* promoter methylation. Global genome hypomethylation is associated with chromosomal instability present in most human tumors.[114] Hypomethylation of *LINE-1*, a prevalent transposon, is frequent in CRC and other cancers and a distinct characteristic of a familial subgroup of colorectal carcinomas without MMR deficiency, termed familial colorectal cancer type X.[115]

▦ GENETIC DIAGNOSTICS: GERMLINE TESTING, DIAGNOSTIC PANELS, AND SOMATIC SEQUENCING

Germline Testing

Much of the accumulated data on the genetic basis of cancer is in active clinical use. At one time, it was necessary to recognize the clinical phenotype, choose one likely genetic culprit, and then find a laboratory that could sequence that gene. The process became commercialized in the early 2000s, and now the situation is quite different. Multiple genetic testing companies offer genetic panels that include sequencing of the genes most likely to be associated with a specific type or group of cancers. For example, when there are familial clusters of breast and ovarian cancers, the panels include the *BRCA1/2* genes, as well as those genes that participate in that DNA repair pathway, such as *CHEK2, PALB2, BARD1, NBN, BRIP1, RAD50, RAD51C/D,* and *ATM*. The lists of genes on each cancer panel are updated as new information emerges. There are familial gastrointestinal gene panels that include the genes for the polyposis syndromes such as *APC, MutYH, SMAD4, BMPR1A, PTEN, CHEK2,* and the four Lynch syndrome genes: *MSH2, MLH1, MSH6,* and *PMS2*. There are also genetic panels specifically focused on familial gynecological cancers (*BRCA1/2, CHEK2, ATM, PALB1, BRIP1, RAC51C, PTEN,* and the Lynch syndrome genes) and prostate cancer (*BRCA1/2, ATM, HOXB13, CHEK2, PALB2, NBN,* etc.). There are panels with 30 to 40 (or more) genes that cover a broad range of cancer risk for families with confusing pedigrees. The costs of diagnostic sequencing have fallen dramatically, and the leading companies will sequence all of the genes known to be related to a familial syndrome for less than the cost of analyzing an individual gene not that long ago. The number of panels and genes on each panel is constantly being updated, as are the techniques used to analyze the genes. Some companies use next-generation exome sequencing platforms, but others perform more extensive analyses for copy number variation and RNA sequencing to be able to properly interpret deletions, duplications, and balanced inversions. Some companies are more complete than others in their ability to interpret sequence variants. Genetic testing leads to a large number of variants of uncertain significance (VUS—discussed earlier), and one must keep in mind that these VUS reports do not indicate a likely pathogenic mutation. When enough data are accumulated, often requiring extensive matching of the sequence variant with cancer development in multiple families, most VUSs are actually benign.

The practitioner must find the optimal resource for genetic testing. Testing can be done on blood or saliva at this time. Insurance coverage is another issue, as some insurance covers genetic testing, but others do not.

Germline Panels

There is a growing appreciation of the relative impact of familiality and germline mutations in the genesis of cancer in the general population. For example, an industry-sponsored study by Yurgelun et al. of a 25-gene panel was evaluated on 1260 patients selected for testing because of a concern about Lynch syndrome in 2012–2013. Germline mutations indicative of Lynch syndrome were found in 9% of the group, and another 5.6% had mutations in other non–Lynch syndrome familial predisposition genes, including *BRCA1* and *BRCA2*. Thus, a nontrivial proportion of these individuals had identifiable relevant germline mutations, but there were unexpected results that were difficult to interpret as well in this highly selected group of patients.[116] This same group performed a study on 1058 unselected consecutive CRC patients using their own 25-gene panel and next-generation sequencing between 2008 and 2014, using most of the previously mentioned genes as well as some additional candidates (*p53, CDKN2A, STK11,* and *CDH1*). In this study, 9.9% had a convincing and relevant germline mutation and 3.1% had a Lynch syndrome mutation. However, some CRC patients unexpectedly had mutations in familial breast cancer genes, challenging the clinical interpretation.[117] It is not obvious what clinical strategy should be used in the family of a CRC patient in which a familial breast or other cancer gene is found. Traditionally, the screening and surveillance strategies followed the family history, and data are not yet available to know how effective screening will be when directed by germline mutations that do not match the clinical cancer phenotypes.

Diagnostic gene panels have also been used to evaluate patients with CRC who are 50 years old or younger. One assumption was that a large proportion of young patients with CRC would have Lynch syndrome, but this was not exactly true. The largest study found germline mutations in about 16% of these young CRC patients, and about half were Lynch syndrome.[118] A second study of early-onset CRC found germline mutations in 20% of the patients,[119] and the family history was of limited help in predicting these mutations. Many of these studies used registries that were highly selected and may have suffered from referral bias. However, it is likely the case that even looking at a relatively young cohort, the proportion with actionable germline mutations will be no more than 20%, and is likely to be in the range of 10% for unselected groups of CRC. The problem is that some of the mutations are in genes that do not match the expectations from the pedigree.

Somatic Genetic Testing of Cancer and Therapeutics

Somatic genetic testing of cancers has two uses at this time. Testing for mutations in cancer is primarily performed to identify genetic targets for chemotherapy. This largely began with the identification of the implications of finding estrogen and progesterone receptor status, as well as expression of the *HER2* gene in breast cancers, which have important therapeutic implications in that disease. There is a growing list of platforms for genetic testing of various tumors, and there will be unique testing panels for each type of cancer.

A mathematical analysis of cancer growth dynamics made an interesting prediction.[120] The net accumulation of new cancer cells is estimated to occur at a rate of about 0.01 per day, since the generation of new cells is about 0.14 per day and the death rate is about 0.13 per day. One would only need to increase the death rate to something over 0.14 per day for the tumor to begin to shrink. We are likely to have drugs now or in the future that can achieve that for each driver mutation. The problem is the rate of mutation may permit the driver oncogene to escape the suppressive effect of the drug. The number of different mutations that would confer resistance for a given oncogene may be large (i.e., 50 to 200), but would not be infinite. If one had more than one drug that could inhibit the driver gene, the chance that a single cell would develop multiple "escape" mutations simultaneously would become very small. The optimism is due to the prediction that it may take only two effective drugs to overcome the problem of mutationally driven resistance.[120]

A second type of somatic testing of cancers is related to specific, meaningful mutational signatures found in some tumors. In the case of CRC, the simultaneous discovery of MSI in 1993 by three groups led to an awareness that dMMR activity was found in >95% of CRCs from Lynch syndrome patients.[34–36] A similar pattern of MSI and abnormal DNA MMR immunohistochemistry was found in endometrial cancers. The enthusiasm for this was tempered by the later understanding that although about 15% of CRCs have dMMR and MSI, most of these (12% of the total group) are caused by the nonfamilial CIMP, as described earlier. When looking for MSI in CRC, older patients tend strongly to have hypermethylation of *MLH1*, and younger patients tend to have Lynch syndrome. So, screening all CRCs for MSI was not entirely efficient.

All of this became immensely more important when it was discovered that all patients with dMMR activity and MSI were candidates for immune checkpoint therapy.[38] In fact, the finding of MSH in a tumor of any organ is a Food and Drug Administration (FDA)–approved indication for the use of immune checkpoint therapy, the first time that a somatic test for any type of cancer was linked to an indication for therapy—regardless of the organ involved.[121]

The details of somatic testing and the implications for therapeutics are covered in each of the specific organ-related cancers in this book.

▥ WHAT IS THE FUTURE?

The future is usually hard to predict, as unexpected disruptive changes will appear on the landscape, but it is a reasonable guess that cancer genetics will be intensely studied for the foreseeable future. For each of the familial genetically driven diseases, we have at least one genetic culprit, but many families do not have the expected germline mutation. It may be required that all of the genes whose proteins work in a serial signaling pathway will need to be on the gene panel for testing. It is perhaps likely that there are many more germline mutations responsible for familial syndromes, but as they are discovered, we may find that ever smaller numbers of families have each of these, and there are likely to be "private" mutations limited to just one kindred. The growing efficiency of DNA sequencing and the use of corroborative techniques such as RNA sequencing to confirm the deleterious effects of mutations will lead to the gradual reduction of the proportion of genetic testing results that come back with a VUS.

Each cancer has its own combination of driver mutations, and we do not have enough potent drugs that target all of the known driver mutations—*KRAS* being one of the chief challenges. It is likely that it will be possible to simultaneously "drug" interacting genetic targets that work in parallel and achieve a much greater degree of clinical success. As mentioned, the problem of mutational-driven drug resistance is a serious one, but perhaps not insurmountable. There is a lot of work to be done, but the prospects for progress are excellent.

References

1. Knudson AGJr. Mutation and cancer: statistical study of retinoblastoma. *Proc Natl Acad Sci U S A.* 1971;68:820–823.

2. Sieber OM, Lamlum H, Crabtree MD, et al. Whole-gene APC deletions cause classical familial adenomatous polyposis, but not attenuated polyposis or "multiple" colorectal adenomas. *Proc Natl Acad Sci U S A.* 2002;99:2954–2958.

3. Nielsen M, Bik E, Hes FJ, et al. Genotype-phenotype correlations in 19 Dutch cases with APC gene deletions and a literature review. *Eur J Human Genet.* 2007;15:1034–1042.

4. Miyaki M, Konishi M, Kikuchi-Yanoshita R, et al. Characteristics of somatic mutation of the adenomatous polyposis coli gene in colorectal tumors. *Cancer Res.* 1994;54:3011–3020.

5. Poffenberger MC, Metcalfe-Roach A, Aguilar E, et al. LKB1 deficiency in T cells promotes the development of gastrointestinal polyposis. *Science.* 2018;361:406–411.

6. Alberici P, Gaspar C, Franken P, et al. Smad4 haploinsufficiency: a matter of dosage. *Pathogenetics.* 2008;1:2.

7. Kim BG, Li C, Qiao W, et al. Smad4 signalling in T cells is required for suppression of gastrointestinal cancer. *Nature.* 2006;441:1015–1019.

8. Kinzler KW, Vogelstein B. Landscaping the cancer terrain. *Science.* 1998;280:1036–1037.

9. Moller P, Seppala T, Bernstein I, et al. Incidence of and survival after subsequent cancers in carriers of pathogenic MMR variants with previous cancer: a report from the prospective Lynch syndrome database. *Gut.* 2017;66:1657–1664.

10. Spirio L, Olschwang S, Groden J, et al. Alleles of the APC gene: an attenuated form of familial polyposis. *Cell.* 1993;75:951–857.

11. Heppner Goss K, Trzepacz C, Tuohy TM, et al. Attenuated APC alleles produce functional protein from internal translation initiation. *Proc Natl Acad Sci U S A.* 2002;99:8161–8166.

12. Giardiello FM, Krush AJ, Petersen GM, et al. Phenotypic variability of familial adenomatous polyposis in 11 unrelated families with identical APC gene mutation. *Gastroenterology.* 1994;106:1542–1547.

13. Joslyn G, Richardson DS, White R, et al. Dimer formation by an N-terminal coiled coil in the APC protein. *Proc Natl Acad Sci U S A.* 1993;90:11109–11113.

14. Boland CR, Goel A. Microsatellite instability in colorectal cancer. *Gastroenterology.* 2010;138:2073–2087 e3.

15. Wood RD. Fifty years since DNA repair was linked to cancer. *Nature.* 2018;557:648–649.

16. Herman JG, Baylin SB. Gene silencing in cancer in association with promoter hypermethylation. *N Engl J Med.* 2003;349:2042–54.

17. Goel A, Boland CR. Epigenetics of colorectal cancer. *Gastroenterology.* 2012;143:1442–1460 e1.

18. Feinberg AP, Vogelstein B. Hypomethylation distinguishes genes of some human cancers from their normal counterparts. *Nature.* 1983;301:89–92.

19. ENCODE Project Consortium. An integrated encyclopedia of DNA elements in the human genome. *Nature.* 2012;489:57–74.

20. Lander ES. Initial impact of the sequencing of the human genome. *Nature.* 2011;470:187–197.

21. Abecasis GR, Altshuler D, Auton A, et al. A map of human genome variation from population-scale sequencing. *Nature.* 2010;467:1061–1073.

22. Boland CR. Non-coding RNA: it's not junk. *Dig Dis Sci.* 2017;62:1107–1109.

23. Abecasis GR, Auton A, Brooks LD, et al. An integrated map of genetic variation from 1,092 human genomes. *Nature.* 2012;491:56–65.

24. Stratton MR. Exploring the genomes of cancer cells: progress and promise. *Science.* 2011;331:1553–1558.

25. Alexandrov LB, Nik-Zainal S, Wedge DC, et al. Signatures of mutational processes in human cancer. *Nature.* 2013;500:415–521.

26. Comprehensive molecular characterization of human colon and rectal cancer. *Nature.* 2012;487:330–337.

27. Bailey MH, Tokheim C, Porta-Pardo E, et al. Comprehensive characterization of cancer driver genes and mutations. *Cell.* 2018;174:1034–1035.

28. Campbell BB, Light N, Fabrizio D, et al. Comprehensive analysis of hypermutation in human cancer. *Cell.* 2017;171:1042–1056 e10.

29. Varmus H, Bishop JM. Biochemical mechanisms of oncogene activity: proteins encoded by oncogenes. Introduction. *Cancer Surv.* 1986;5:153–158.

30. Vogelstein B, Papadopoulos N, Velculescu VE, et al. Cancer genome landscapes. *Science.* 2013;339:1546–1558.

31. Turner KM, Deshpande V, Beyter D, et al. Extrachromosomal oncogene amplification drives tumour evolution and genetic heterogeneity. *Nature.* 2017;543:122–125.

32. Vogelstein B, Kinzler KW. Cancer genes and the pathways they control. *Nat Med.* 2004;10:789–799.

33. Hawn MT, Umar A, Carethers JM, et al. Evidence for a connection between the mismatch repair system and the G2 cell cycle checkpoint. *Cancer Res.* 1995;55:3721–3275.

34. Aaltonen LA, Peltomaki P, Leach FS, et al. Clues to the pathogenesis of familial colorectal cancer. *Science.* 1993;260:812–816.

35. Ionov Y, Peinado MA, Malkhosyan S, et al. Ubiquitous somatic mutations in simple repeated sequences reveal a new mechanism for colonic carcinogenesis. *Nature.* 1993;363:558–561.

36. Thibodeau SN, Bren G, Schaid D. Microsatellite instability in cancer of the proximal colon. *Science.* 1993;260:816–819.

37. Boland CR, Thibodeau SN, Hamilton SR, et al. A National Cancer Institute Workshop on Microsatellite Instability for cancer detection and familial predisposition: development of international criteria for the determination of microsatellite instability in colorectal cancer. *Cancer Res.* 1998;58:5248–5257.

38. Le DT, Uram JN, Wang H, et al. PD-1 blockade in tumors with mismatch-repair deficiency. *N Engl J Med.* 2015;372:2509–2520.

39. Brosens LA, Langeveld D, van Hattem WA, et al. Juvenile polyposis syndrome. *World J Gastroenterol.* 2011;17:4839–4844.

40. Miller DG. On the nature of susceptibility to cancer. The presidential address. *Cancer.* 1980;46:1307–1318.

41. Vogelstein B, Fearon ER, Hamilton SR, et al. Genetic alterations during colorectal-tumor development. *N Engl J Med.* 1988;319:525–532.

42. Bodmer WF, Bailey CJ, Bodmer J, et al. Localization of the gene for familial adenomatous polyposis on chromosome 5. *Nature.* 1987;328:614–616.

43. Solomon E, Voss R, Hall V, et al. Chromosome 5 allele loss in human colorectal carcinomas. *Nature.* 1987;328:616–619.

44. Bos JL, Fearon ER, Hamilton SR, et al. Prevalence of ras gene mutations in human colorectal cancers. *Nature.* 1987;327:293–297.

45. Forrester K, Almoguera C, Han K, et al. Detection of high incidence of K-ras oncogenes during human colon tumorigenesis. *Nature.* 1987;327:298–303.

46. Baker SJ, Fearon ER, Nigro JM, et al. Chromosome 17 deletions and p53 gene mutations in colorectal carcinomas. *Science.* 1989;244:217–221.

47. Groden J, Thliveris A, Samowitz W, et al. Identification and characterization of the familial adenomatous polyposis coli gene. *Cell.* 1991;66:589–600.

48. Kinzler KW, Nilbert MC, Su LK, et al. Identification of FAP locus genes from chromosome 5q21. *Science.* 1991;253:661–665.

49. Fearon ER, Cho KR, Nigro JM, et al. Identification of a chromosome 18q gene that is altered in colorectal cancers. *Science.* 1990;247:49–56.

50. Boland CR, Sato J, Appelman HD, et al. Microallelotyping defines the sequence and tempo of allelic losses at tumour suppressor gene loci during colorectal cancer progression. *Nat Med.* 1995;1:902–909.

51. Otori K, Oda Y, Sugiyama K, et al. High frequency of K-ras mutations in human colorectal hyperplastic polyps. *Gut.* 1997;40:660–663.

52. Rosenberg DW, Yang S, Pleau DC, et al. Mutations in BRAF and KRAS differentially distinguish serrated versus non-serrated hyperplastic aberrant crypt foci in humans. *Cancer Res.* 2007;67:3551–3554.

53. Leggett B, Whitehall V. Role of the serrated pathway in colorectal cancer pathogenesis. *Gastroenterology.* 2010;138:2088–2100.

54. Brosens LA, van Hattem A, Hylind LM, et al. Risk of colorectal cancer in juvenile polyposis. *Gut*. 2007;56:965–967.

55. Omori Y, Ono Y, Tanino M, et al. Pathways of progression from intraductal papillary mucinous neoplasm to pancreatic ductal adenocarcinoma based on molecular features. *Gastroenterology*. 2019;156:647–661 e2.

56. Ribas A, Wolchok JD. Cancer immunotherapy using checkpoint blockade. *Science*. 2018;359:1350–1355.

57. Al-Tassan N, Chmiel NH, Maynard J, et al. Inherited variants of MYH associated with somatic G:C-->T:A mutations in colorectal tumors. *Nat Genet*. 2002;30:227–232.

58. Sampson JR, Dolwani S, Jones S, et al. Autosomal recessive colorectal adenomatous polyposis due to inherited mutations of MYH. *Lancet*. 2003;362:39–41.

59. Sieber OM, Lipton L, Crabtree M, et al. Multiple colorectal adenomas, classic adenomatous polyposis, and germ-line mutations in MYH. *New Engl J Med*. 2003;348:791–799.

60. Nielsen M, Joerink-van de Beld MC, Jones N, et al. Analysis of MUTYH genotypes and colorectal phenotypes in patients with MUTYH-associated polyposis. *Gastroenterology*. 2009;136:471–476.

61. Milholland B, Dong X, Zhang L, et al. Differences between germline and somatic mutation rates in humans and mice. *Nat Commun*. 2017;8:15183.

62. Adam R, Spier I, Zhao B, et al. Exome sequencing identifies biallelic MSH3 germline mutations as a recessive subtype of colorectal adenomatous polyposis. *Am J Hum Genet*. 2016;99:337–351.

63. Olkinuora A, Nieminen TT, Martensson E, et al. Biallelic germline nonsense variant of MLH3 underlies polyposis predisposition. *Genet Med*. 2019 Aug;21(8):1868–1873.

64. Bellido F, Pineda M, Aiza G, et al. POLE and POLD1 mutations in 529 kindred with familial colorectal cancer and/or polyposis: review of reported cases and recommendations for genetic testing and surveillance. *Genet Med*. 2016;18:325–332.

65. Peltomaki P. Lynch syndrome genes. *Fam Cancer*. 2005;4:227–232.

66. Durno C, Boland CR, Cohen S, et al. Recommendations on surveillance and management of biallelic mismatch repair deficiency (BMMRD) Syndrome: a consensus statement by the US Multi-Society Task Force on Colorectal Cancer. *Gastroenterology*. 2017;152:1605–1614.

67. Belhadj S, Mur P, Navarro M, et al. Delineating the phenotypic spectrum of the NTHL1-associated polyposis. *Clin Gastroenterol Hepatol*. 2017;15:461–462.

68. Wallace SS. Base excision repair: a critical player in many games. *DNA Repair (Amst)*. 2014;19:14–26.

69. Kamileri I, Karakasilioti I, Garinis GA. Nucleotide excision repair: new tricks with old bricks. *Trend Genet*. 2012;28:566–573.

70. Jiricny J. Postreplicative mismatch repair. *Cold Spring Harb Perspect Biol*. 2013;5:a012633.

71. Church DN, Briggs SE, Palles C, et al. DNA polymerase epsilon and delta exonuclease domain mutations in endometrial cancer. *Hum Mol Genet*. 2013;22:2820–2828.

72. Loeb LA. Mutator phenotype may be required for multistage carcinogenesis. *Cancer Res*. 1991;51:3075–3079.

73. Kass EM, Jasin M. Collaboration and competition between DNA double-strand break repair pathways. *FEBS Lett*. 2010;584:3703–3708.

74. Prakash R, Zhang Y, Feng W, et al. Homologous recombination and human health: the roles of BRCA1, BRCA2, and associated proteins. *Cold Spring Harb Perspect Biol*. 2015;7:a016600.

75. Woodbine L, Gennery AR, Jeggo PA. The clinical impact of deficiency in DNA non-homologous end-joining. *DNA Repair (Amst)*. 2014;16:84–96.

76. Jeggo PA, Pearl LH, Carr AM. DNA repair, genome stability and cancer: a historical perspective. *Nat Rev Cancer*. 2016;16:35–42.

77. Cleaver JE. Xeroderma pigmentosum: a human disease in which an initial stage of DNA repair is defective. *Proc Natl Acad Sci U S A*. 1969;63:428–435.

78. Moriwaki S. Human DNA repair disorders in dermatology: a historical perspective, current concepts and new insight. *J Dermatol Sci*. 2016;81:77–84.

79. Romanoski CE, Glass CK, Stunnenberg HG, et al. Epigenomics: roadmap for regulation. *Nature*. 2015;518:314–316.

80. Kandoth C, Schultz N, Cherniack AD, et al. Integrated genomic characterization of endometrial carcinoma. *Nature*. 2013;497:67–73.

81. Chen CC, Feng W, Lim PX, et al. Homology-directed repair and the role of BRCA1, BRCA2, and related proteins in genome integrity and cancer. *Annu Rev Cancer Biol*. 2018;2:313–336.

82. Rashid M, Fischer A, Wilson CH, et al. Adenoma development in familial adenomatous polyposis and MUTYH-associated polyposis: somatic landscape and driver genes. *J Pathol*. 2016;238:98–108.

83. Grolleman JE, de Voer RM, Elsayed FA, et al. Mutational signature analysis reveals NTHL1 deficiency to cause a multi-tumor phenotype. *Cancer Cell*. 2019;35:256–266 e5.

84. Barault L, Amatu A, Bleeker FE, et al. Digital PCR quantification of MGMT methylation refines prediction of clinical benefit from alkylating agents in glioblastoma and metastatic colorectal cancer. *Ann Oncol*. 2015;26:1994–1999.

85. Cerrato A, Morra F, Celetti A. Use of poly ADP-ribose polymerase [PARP] inhibitors in cancer cells bearing DDR defects: the rationale for their inclusion in the clinic. *J Exp Clin Cancer Res*. 2016;35:179.

86. Deihimi S, Lev A, Slifker M, et al. BRCA2, EGFR, and NTRK mutations in mismatch repair-deficient colorectal cancers with MSH2 or MLH1 mutations. *Oncotarget*. 2017;8:39945–39962.

87. Rivera B, Perea J, Sanchez E, et al. A novel AXIN2 germline variant associated with attenuated FAP without signs of oligodontia or ectodermal dysplasia. *Eur J Hum Genet*. 2014;22:423–426.

88. Taupin D, Lam W, Rangiah D, et al. A deleterious RNF43 germline mutation in a severely affected serrated polyposis kindred. *Hum Genome Var*. 2015;2:15013.

89. Jaeger E, Leedham S, Lewis A, et al. Hereditary mixed polyposis syndrome is caused by a 40-kb upstream duplication that leads to increased and ectopic expression of the BMP antagonist GREM1. *Nat Genet*. 2012;44:699–703.

90. van der Post RS, Vogelaar IP, Carneiro F, et al. Hereditary diffuse gastric cancer: updated clinical guidelines with an emphasis on germline CDH1 mutation carriers. *J Med Genet*. 2015;52:361–374.

91. Neumann HPH, Young WF Jr., Eng C. Pheochromocytoma and paraganglioma. *New Engl J Med*. 2019;381:552–565.

92. Thakker RV, Newey PJ, Walls GV, et al. Clinical practice guidelines for multiple endocrine neoplasia type 1 (MEN1). *J Clin Endocrinol Metab*. 2012;97:2990–3011.

93. Lynch HT, Lynch PM, Lanspa SJ, et al. Review of the Lynch syndrome: history, molecular genetics, screening, differential diagnosis, and medicolegal ramifications. *Clin Genet*. 2009;76:1–18.

94. Foulkes WD. Inherited susceptibility to common cancers. *New Engl J Med*. 2008;359:2143–2153.

95. Mucci LA, Hjelmborg JB, Harris JR, et al. Familial risk and heritability of cancer among twins in Nordic countries. *JAMA*. 2016;315:68–76.

96. Fletcher O, Houlston RS. Architecture of inherited susceptibility to common cancer. *Nat Rev Cancer*. 2010;10:353–361.

97. Rahman N. Realizing the promise of cancer predisposition genes. *Nature*. 2014;505:302–308.

98. Bodo S, Colas C, Buhard O, et al. Diagnosis of constitutional mismatch repair-deficiency syndrome based on microsatellite instability and lymphocyte tolerance to methylating agents. *Gastroenterology*. 2015;149:1017–1029 e3.

99. Golmard L, Delnatte C, Lauge A, et al. Breast and ovarian cancer predisposition due to de novo BRCA1 and BRCA2 mutations. *Oncogene*. 2016;35:1324–1327.

100. Morak M, Laner A, Scholz M, et al. Report on de-novo mutation in the MSH2 gene as a rare event in hereditary nonpolyposis colorectal cancer. *Eur J Gastroenterol Hepatol*. 2008;20:1101–1105.

101. Aretz S, Uhlhaas S, Caspari R, et al. Frequency and parental origin of de novo APC mutations in familial adenomatous polyposis. *Eur J Hum Genet*. 2004;12:52–58.

102. Spier I, Drichel D, Kerick M, et al. Low-level APC mutational mosaicism is the underlying cause in a substantial fraction of unexplained colorectal adenomatous polyposis cases. *J Med Genet*. 2016;53:172–179.

103. Lander ES, Linton LM, Birren B, et al. Initial sequencing and analysis of the human genome. *Nature*. 2001;409:860–921.

104. Allis CD, Jenuwein T. The molecular hallmarks of epigenetic control. *Nat Rev Genet*. 2016;17:487–500.

105. Toyota M, Ahuja N, Ohe-Toyota M, et al. CpG island methylator phenotype in colorectal cancer. *Proc Natl Acad Sci U S A*. 1999;96:8681–8686.

106. Hitchins MP, Rapkins RW, Kwok CT, et al. Dominantly inherited constitutional epigenetic silencing of MLH1 in a cancer-affected family is linked to a single nucleotide variant within the 5'UTR. *Cancer Cell*. 2011;20:200–213.

107. Oey H, Whitelaw E. On the meaning of the word 'epimutation'. *Trend Genet*. 2014;30:519–520.

108. Sanchez-Vega F, Gotea V, Margolin G, et al. Pan-cancer stratification of solid human epithelial tumors and cancer cell lines reveals commonalities and tissue-specific features of the CpG island methylator phenotype. *Epigenetics Chromatin*. 2015;8:14.

109. Shen H, Laird PW. Interplay between the cancer genome and epigenome. *Cell*. 2013;153:38–55.

110. De Carvalho DD, Sharma S, You JS, et al. DNA methylation screening identifies driver epigenetic events of cancer cell survival. *Cancer Cell*. 2012;21:655–667.

111. Stefanska B, Cheishvili D, Suderman M, et al. Genome-wide study of hypomethylated and induced genes in patients with liver cancer unravels novel anticancer targets. *Clin Cancer Res*. 2014;20:3118–3132.

112. Hanahan D, Weinberg RA. Hallmarks of cancer: the next generation. *Cell*. 2011;144:646–674.

113. Gao D, Herman JG, Guo M. The clinical value of aberrant epigenetic changes of DNA damage repair genes in human cancer. *Oncotarget*. 2016;7:37331–37346.

114. Eden A, Gaudet F, Waghmare A, et al. Chromosomal instability and tumors promoted by DNA hypomethylation. *Science*. 2003;300:455.

115. Goel A, Xicola RM, Nguyen TP, et al. Aberrant DNA methylation in hereditary nonpolyposis colorectal cancer without mismatch repair deficiency. *Gastroenterology*. 2010;138:1854–1862.

116. Yurgelun MB, Allen B, Kaldate RR, et al. Identification of a variety of mutations in cancer predisposition genes in patients with suspected Lynch syndrome. *Gastroenterology*. 2015;149:604–613 e20.

117. Yurgelun MB, Kulke MH, Fuchs CS, et al. Cancer susceptibility gene mutations in individuals with colorectal cancer. *J Clin Oncol*. 2017;35:1086–1095.

118. Pearlman R, Frankel WL, Swanson B, et al. Prevalence and spectrum of germline cancer susceptibility gene mutations among patients with early-onset colorectal cancer. *JAMA Oncol*. 2017;3:464–471.

119. Stoffel EM, Koeppe E, Everett J, et al. Germline genetic features of young individuals with colorectal cancer. *Gastroenterology*. 2018;154:897–905 e1.

120. Bozic I, Reiter JG, Allen B, et al. Evolutionary dynamics of cancer in response to targeted combination therapy. *Elife*. 2013;2:e00747.

121. Lemery S, Keegan P, Pazdur R. First FDA approval agnostic of cancer site - when a biomarker defines the indication. *New Engl J Med*. 2017;377:1409–1412.

Risk Assessment in the Primary Care Office: Identification of Patients for Referral

Hayley Cassingham and Heather Hampel

▧ IMPORTANCE OF REFERRAL TO CANCER GENETICS

For primary care physicians, genetics is quickly becoming an integral part of patient care. Many patients are becoming more aware of genetic contributions to common diseases like cancer (Table 2.1) and may ask for guidance regarding the possibility of genetic testing or a better understanding of their risks of developing cancer. Primary care physicians must recognize which of their patients need cancer genetics services to provide a detailed risk assessment and/or coordinate genetic testing for inherited cancer gene variants, as this may have implications for both the patient and their family members. Specifically, identifying hereditary risk factors for cancer could inform treatment decisions for individuals with cancer, direct surveillance and management for the prevention or early detection of future cancers, and identify at-risk relatives that could benefit from genetic testing and, if positive, increased surveillance. Additionally, referring patients to a cancer genetics specialist can help identify the most appropriate individual in a family to undergo genetic testing, as it may not always be the patient who is initially referred.

In this chapter we will identify the most common and most important indications for referral to a cancer genetics specialist and how to connect patients to these services.

There are a multitude of highly detailed genetic evaluation and testing guidelines for hereditary cancer syndromes. These guidelines can change frequently, and statements released by different professional organizations may be discordant, adding to the difficulty of identifying the most appropriate patients for referral. For example, the Amsterdam criteria and Bethesda guidelines aim to assess who is likely to have a pathogenic variant in a Lynch syndrome gene (the most common inherited form of colorectal and endometrial cancers) and who should undergo microsatellite instability (MSI) testing (a screening test for Lynch syndrome) on their colorectal cancer tumors, respectively. Both guidelines have undergone revisions, include different lists of Lynch syndrome–associated tumors, and have been shown to be

TABLE 2.1: Benign and Malignant Tumors and the Criteria That Warrant Assessment for Cancer Predisposition Regardless of Family History

Cancer/Feature (Proband or FDR)	Syndrome(s) to Consider
Adrenocortical carcinoma	LFS, OMIM: 151623
Breast cancer (male)	HBOC, OMIM: 604370, 612555
Breast cancer (female) diagnosed ≤45 yr, triple negative ≤60 yr, or metastatic	HBOC, OMIM: 604370, 612555; LFS, OMIM: 151623
Cervix (adenoma malignum)	PJS, OMIM: 175200
Colorectal cancer diagnosed <50 yr or at any age with abnormal IHC or microsatellite instability	LS, OMIM: 120435, 120436
Desmoid tumor	FAP, OMIM: 175100
Endolymphatic sac tumor	VHL, OMIM: 193300
Endometrial cancer diagnosed <50 yr or at any age with abnormal IHC or microsatellite instability	LS, OMIM: 120435, 120436
Gastrinoma	MEN1, OMIM: 131100
Hemangioblastoma (CNS or retinal)	VHL, OMIM: 193300
Ovarian/fallopian tube/primary peritoneal cancer	HBOC, OMIM: 604370, 612555; LS, OMIM: 120435, 120436
Ovarian sex cord tumor with annular tubules	PJS, OMIM: 175200
Ovarian small cell carcinoma, hypercalcemic type	RPS, OMIM: 613325
Pancreatic adenocarcinoma	HBOC, OMIM: 604370, 612555; FPC, OMIM: 260350
Paraganglioma/pheochromocytoma	HPPS, OMIM: 115310, 168000, 605373, 601650, 154950, 613403; VHL OMIM: 193300; MEN2, OMIM: 171400, 155240, 162300
Primary pigmented nodular adrenocortical dysplasia	Carney, OMIM: 160980
Prostate (metastatic)	HBOC, OMIM: 604370, 612555
Retinoblastoma	Hereditary RB, OMIM: 180200
Rhabdoid tumors	RP, OMIM: 609322, 613325
Sertoli cell tumor	PJS, OMIM: 175200
Skin (oral or ocular neuromas on the lip, tongue, eyelid, or sclera)	MEN2, OMIM: 171400, 155240, 162300
Skin (cutaneous leiomyoma)	HLRCC, OMIM: 605839, 150800
Thyroid (medullary thyroid cancer)	MEN2, OMIM: 171400, 155240, 162300

Abbreviations: FAP = familial adenomatous polyposis; FPC = familial pancreatic cancer; HBOC = hereditary breast ovarian cancer syndrome; HLRCC = hereditary leiomyomatosis and renal cell carcinoma; HPPS= hereditary paraganglioma pheochromocytoma syndrome; LFS = Li-Fraumeni syndrome; LS = Lynch syndrome; MEN1 = Multiple endocrine neoplasia type 1; MEN2 = multiple endocrine neoplasia type 2; PJS = Peutz-Jeghers syndrome; RB = retinoblastoma; RP = rhabdoid predisposition; VHL = Von Hippel-Lindau syndrome

sensitive but not specific in the identification of patients with Lynch syndrome. Primary care physicians often maintain busy patient schedules and have limited time to devote to evaluation and discussion regarding the possible hereditary implications of each patient's medical and family history. This makes it difficult for providers to do an in-depth risk assessment. To assist with this process, this chapter includes simplified versions of the referral criteria focusing on common cancers (Figure 2.1) that will be encountered in practice.

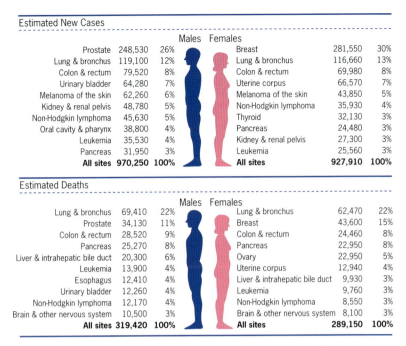

Estimated New Cases

Males			Females		
Prostate	248,530	26%	Breast	281,550	30%
Lung & bronchus	119,100	12%	Lung & bronchus	116,660	13%
Colon & rectum	79,520	8%	Colon & rectum	69,980	8%
Urinary bladder	64,280	7%	Uterine corpus	66,570	7%
Melanoma of the skin	62,260	6%	Melanoma of the skin	43,850	5%
Kidney & renal pelvis	48,780	5%	Non-Hodgkin lymphoma	35,930	4%
Non-Hodgkin lymphoma	45,630	5%	Thyroid	32,130	3%
Oral cavity & pharynx	38,800	4%	Pancreas	24,480	3%
Leukemia	35,530	4%	Kidney & renal pelvis	27,300	3%
Pancreas	31,950	3%	Leukemia	25,560	3%
All sites	**970,250**	**100%**	**All sites**	**927,910**	**100%**

Estimated Deaths

Males			Females		
Lung & bronchus	69,410	22%	Lung & bronchus	62,470	22%
Prostate	34,130	11%	Breast	43,600	15%
Colon & rectum	28,520	9%	Colon & rectum	24,460	8%
Pancreas	25,270	8%	Pancreas	22,950	8%
Liver & intrahepatic bile duct	20,300	6%	Ovary	22,950	5%
Leukemia	13,900	4%	Uterine corpus	12,940	4%
Esophagus	12,410	4%	Liver & intrahepatic bile duct	9,930	3%
Urinary bladder	12,260	4%	Leukemia	9,760	3%
Non-Hodgkin lymphoma	12,170	4%	Non-Hodgkin lymphoma	8,550	3%
Brain & other nervous system	10,500	3%	Brain & other nervous system	8,100	3%
All sites	**319,420**	**100%**	**All sites**	**289,150**	**100%**

FIGURE 2.1: American Cancer Society leading sites of new cancer cases and deaths – 2021 estimates (Reproduced with permission from Siegel RL, Miller KD, Fuchs HE, Jemal A. Cancer Statistics, 2021, CA Cancer J Clin 2021 Jan;71(1):7–33).

▨ MOST COMMON INDICATIONS FOR REFERRAL TO CANCER GENETICS

Patients with a personal history or family history (particularly first-degree relatives, which include parents, siblings, and children; or second-degree relatives, which include aunts and uncles, nieces and nephews, grandparents, and grandchildren) of any of the following common cancers should be referred to cancer genetics:

- Breast cancer diagnosed ≤ 45 years of age
- Triple-negative breast cancer diagnosed ≤ 60 years of age
- Male breast cancer diagnosed at any age
- Metastatic breast cancer diagnosed at any age
- Metastatic prostate cancer diagnosed at any age
- Colorectal cancer diagnosed < 50 years of age regardless of immunohistochemical (IHC) staining or MSI test results
- Colorectal cancer diagnosed ≥ 50 years of age with abnormal IHC (absence of MLH1, MSH2, MSH6, or PMS2 proteins) or MSI
- Endometrial cancer diagnosed < 50 years of age regardless of IHC staining or MSI test results
- Endometrial cancer diagnosed ≥ 50 years of age with abnormal IHC (absence of MLH1, MSH2, MSH6, or PMS2 proteins) or MSI
- Ovarian, fallopian tube, or primary peritoneal cancer diagnosed at any age
- Pancreatic cancer diagnosed at any age

TABLE 2.2: Prevalence of Pathogenic or Suspect Pathogenic Variants in Patients with Various Cancer Types

Cohort	Prevalence of Pathogenic or Likely Pathogenic Germline Cancer Susceptibility Gene Variants	References
Epithelial ovarian/fallopian tube cancer	18.1%–23.6%	[21,22]
Breast cancer	9.3%	[1]
Breast cancer (stage I–III)	10.7%	[24]
Breast cancer (triple negative)	14.1%–24.9%	[1,4,25]
Colorectal cancer	9.9%	[13]
Colorectal cancer (age <50 yr)	16.0%–18.3%	[26,27]
Pancreatic cancer	3.8%–8.2%	[23,28–30]
Prostate cancer (metastatic)	11.8%	[19]
Endometrial cancer	9.2%	[16]

This is not a comprehensive list of referral indications, even within these cancer types; however, it does incorporate the easiest list of common cancers warranting a cancer genetics referral based on a single case in the patient or their close relatives. Table 2.2 summarizes the prevalence of pathogenic or suspected pathogenic variants in different tumor types.

▦ DETAILED REFERRAL INDICATIONS FOR THE MOST COMMON CANCER TYPES

Breast Cancer

Breast cancer is the most common cancer type in women in the United States, with one in every eight women (12.8%) affected in their lifetime (https://seer.cancer.gov/statfacts/html/breast.html). As with most cancers, the majority of breast cancers that develop are not associated with any hereditary risk factor and generally occur at later ages. For this reason, early-onset breast cancers could indicate a higher likelihood that an individual carries a genetic mutation. The most common hereditary cause for breast cancer is hereditary breast and ovarian cancer (HBOC) syndrome, which is due to pathogenic variants (previously known as deleterious mutations) in the *BRCA1* or *BRCA2* genes. However, there are other high-risk genes (e.g., *TP53*, *PTEN*) and moderate-risk genes (e.g., *PALB2*, *CHEK2*, *ATM*) that can also cause an increased risk for breast and other cancers. Multigene panel testing for 25 cancer susceptibility genes among 35,000 breast cancer patients found that 9.3% have a pathogenic variant in one of these genes.[1]

Aside from women who are diagnosed with breast cancer at age 45 or younger, other women with a breast cancer history could benefit from a cancer genetics consultation. Women with a triple-negative breast cancer (negative for estrogen and progesterone receptors and for Her-2) at or before age 60 are eligible for genetic testing, as a significant proportion of them are attributable to mutations in the *BRCA1/2* or *PALB2* gene. While 12% to 15% of all breast cancers are triple negative, 80% of breast cancers among women with *BRCA1* mutations are triple negative.[2,3] Because of this, a greater proportion of women with triple-negative breast cancer (24.9%) will be found to carry a pathogenic variant compared to those whose breast cancers are not triple negative.[4] Male breast cancer is significantly less common than female breast cancer, with only 0.12% of men developing breast cancer in their lifetime. A recent study found that 18.1% of male breast cancer patients have a pathogenic variant in a cancer susceptibility gene (mainly *BRCA2* followed by *CHEK2*).[5] As a result, a man with breast cancer diagnosed at any age should be referred to cancer genetics. Additionally, women with more than one primary breast cancer (in the contralateral or ipsilateral breast) should be referred to cancer genetics. It is also known that individuals of Ashkenazi Jewish ancestry have a higher likelihood of carrying a pathogenic *BRCA* mutation; 1 in 40 Ashkenazi Jews has a *BRCA* mutation, compared to 1 in 300 to 1 in 800 non-Jewish individuals in the general population.[6-8] Therefore, a patient with breast cancer at any age that is of Ashkenazi Jewish descent should be referred to cancer genetics. Finally, patients with metastatic breast cancer could also potentially benefit from genetic testing, since a recent study (OlympiAD) has shown an increased progression-free survival (2.8 months) and 42% lower risk of disease progression or death for metastatic breast cancer patients with a germline *BRCA* mutation treated with a poly-ADP ribose polymerase (PARP) inhibitor versus standard therapy.[9]

Recently, the American Society of Breast Surgeons (ASBrS) released a recommendation that any woman with breast cancer diagnosed at any age be offered genetic testing (https://www.breastsurgeons.org/docs/statements/Consensus-Guideline-on-Genetic-Testing-for-Hereditary-Breast-Cancer.pdf). This recommendation was based on a study finding that a similar number of breast cancer patients tested positive for pathogenic variants in cancer genes among patients who met National Comprehensive Cancer Network (NCCN) guidelines (9.39%) and those who did not meet guidelines (7.9%).[10] The recommendation has yet to be supported by other professional organizations such as the NCCN and has not yet been widely adopted. However, having a discussion with all breast cancer patients about whether they would like to consider pursuing genetic testing or further risk assessment may be warranted.

Some patients with a cancer diagnosis may undergo genetic testing of their tumor to assist in determining the most appropriate treatment for that individual's cancer. While most of the variants identified on these tests are somatic (acquired and unique to the tumor), occasionally germline (inherited) variants are found. Primary care providers likely are not ordering this type of testing, but they may still encounter these test reports in their patients' medical records. Any patient who has a pathogenic variant in the *BRCA1* or *BRCA2* gene identified on tumor testing should be referred to cancer genetics, as a large proportion of these variants are in fact germline and therefore heritable.[11,12]

Colorectal Cancer

Colorectal cancer is the third most common cancer in the United States with around a 4.2% lifetime risk (https://seer.cancer.gov/statfacts/html/colorect.html). Multigene panel testing among 1058 colorectal cancer patients found that 9.9% have a pathogenic variant in a cancer susceptibility gene.[13] The most common hereditary cause of colorectal cancer is Lynch syndrome, accounting for 3% to 5% of all cases. Lynch syndrome cancers are characterized by microsatellite instability (found in 15% of all colorectal cancers but 87% of Lynch syndrome colorectal cancers) due to defective mismatch repair. It has been recommended that all colorectal cancers be screened for Lynch syndrome at the time of diagnosis by performing either MSI testing or IHC staining for the four mismatch repair proteins (*MLH1, MSH2, MSH6,* and *PMS2*; the absence of any of the four proteins indicates that the tumor is likely microsatellite unstable). Given that Lynch syndrome is more common among microsatellite-unstable cancers, any patients with abnormal MSI testing (or abnormal IHC) should be referred to cancer genetics for further evaluation. As with most cancers, patients diagnosed with colorectal cancer at an earlier age are more likely to have a hereditary cancer syndrome. Studies using multigene panel testing among colorectal cancer patients diagnosed under age 50 have found that 16% to 18% have a mutation in a cancer susceptibility gene.[14,15] For this reason, patients diagnosed with colorectal cancer under age 50 should be referred to cancer genetics.

Endometrial Cancer

Endometrial cancer is the fourth most common cancer among women, with a 3.1% lifetime risk (https://seer.cancer.gov/statfacts/html/corp.html). Multigene panel testing among unselected endometrial cancer patients found that 9.2% have a pathogenic variant in a cancer susceptibility gene.[16] Lynch syndrome is the most common hereditary cause of endometrial cancer, accounting for 2.3% to 5.9% of cases.[16–18] Similar to colorectal cancer, MSI is a characteristic of Lynch syndrome in endometrial cancers (25% of endometrial cancers are microsatellite unstable), and this can be determined either by MSI testing or IHC of the mismatch repair proteins. Any endometrial cancer patients with MSI (or abnormal IHC) should be referred for cancer genetics evaluation. In addition, early-onset endometrial cancer patients are more likely to have a hereditary cancer syndrome (24%) and should be referred to cancer genetics.[16]

Prostate Cancer

Prostate cancer is the most common cancer type to occur men, with approximately one in nine (11.6%) men diagnosed in their lifetime (https://seer.cancer.gov/statfacts/html/prost.html). Multigene panel testing among 692 men with metastatic prostate cancer found that 11.8% had a pathogenic variant in a cancer susceptibility gene.[19] A study of 3607 men with prostate cancer who underwent genetic testing at a commercial laboratory found that 17.2% had a pathogenic variant in a cancer susceptibility gene; however, these patients may have had strong family histories of cancer that warranted cancer genetic testing.[20] At this time, all men with metastatic prostate cancer should be referred for cancer genetics evaluation.

Ovarian Cancer

Unlike breast cancer, ovarian cancer is a relatively rare diagnosis for women in the United States. Only about 1.3% (1 in 79) women in the general population will be diagnosed with an ovarian cancer in her lifetime (https://seer.cancer.gov/statfacts/html/ovary.html). The majority of ovarian cancers that develop are epithelial and arise in the fallopian tube or ovary itself, or sometimes the peritoneum. A larger proportion of ovarian cancers are attributable to hereditary risk factors (approximately 18% to 24%), though most still occur at later ages.[21,22] As a result, all women with ovarian, fallopian tube, or primary peritoneal cancer warrant referral to cancer genetics. Pathogenic variants in the *BRCA1/2* genes account for most hereditary ovarian cancers.[21,22]

Pancreatic Cancer

Pancreatic cancer is another cancer type that is relatively rare in the general population, with only approximately 1 in 64 individuals (1.6%) diagnosed in their lifetime (https://seer.cancer.gov/statfacts/html/pancreas.html). The majority of these cancers are pancreatic adenocarcinomas, which develop in the exocrine cells of the pancreas. Multigene panel testing in 3030 unselected pancreatic cancer patients found that 8.2% had a mutation in a cancer susceptibility gene, and five genes in particular were determined to have caused the pancreatic cancers (*CDKN2A*, *TP53*, *MLH1*, *BRCA2*, and *ATM*).[23] Given the poor prognosis for pancreatic cancer patients and the fact that some germline genetic mutations are actionable therapeutic targets for treatment, it is now recommended that all pancreatic cancer patients be offered germline genetic testing.

Indications for Referral Based on Family History

It is equally important to be able to identify whether a patient's family history of cancer is potentially indicative of a hereditary cancer predisposition syndrome. Any individual with a first- or second-degree relative meeting any of the criteria listed at the beginning of this chapter should be referred to cancer genetics. It is possible that a patient's family member was never referred to genetics themselves or that a family member is no longer available for genetic risk assessment and testing. While an unaffected patient with a family history of cancer may not be the most informative individual to undergo testing, it may still be appropriate for them to do so or to help communicate with other relatives who need to be tested. In many cases, cancer diagnoses in a family may not appear suspicious for a hereditary cancer syndrome by themselves, but in combination with several other cases of related cancers in a family, a cancer genetics referral may still be warranted. For example, any individual with three or more cases of breast, ovarian, prostate (with a Gleason score of >7), or pancreatic cancer on the same side of the family at any age should be referred for a genetics consultation, as this could be indicative of HBOC syndrome. Similarly, families with three or more cases of colon, endometrial, ovarian, gastric, or other Lynch syndrome–associated cancer warrant a referral. A 2014 American College of Genetics and Genomics (ACMG) and National Society of Genetic Counselors (NSGC) practice guideline for indications for cancer genetics referral by Hampel et al. is a much more comprehensive resource for those cancer types and referral indications that are not included here.[31] These include indications for skin cancer, polyposis, brain tumors, stomach cancer, and other less common or rare tumors.

Indications for Referral for Less Common Cancers or Tumors

There are a myriad of other cancer or tumor diagnoses that could raise suspicion for a hereditary cancer condition. Many of these may be encountered very rarely in a primary care practice or in general. Table 2.1 includes a list of cancer or tumor types that should generate a referral to cancer genetics if there is a single case in an individual or close blood relative, regardless of any other family history or syndromic features.[31]

▦ HOW TO REFER PATIENTS TO A CANCER GENETIC COUNSELOR

Providers can refer their patients to cancer genetics either in person at a nearby cancer genetics program or to a telegenetic counseling company if there are no clinics nearby or if it is easier for their patient.

Referral to a Local Cancer Genetics Program

There are generally cancer genetic counselors in every large city in the United States. Depending on the state, most patients should not have to drive more than two hours to receive services. To find a nearby cancer genetic counselor, visit the NSCG Find a Counselor page at www.findageneticcounselor.com. Genetic counselors can be searched for by ZIP code using a 5- to 100-mile radius. Select "Cancer" from the Types of Specialization list, then hit Search.

A local cancer genetic counselor can also be found through the National Cancer Institute Cancer Genetics Services directory at http://www.cancer.gov/cancertopics/genetics/directory. At that site, cancer genetics providers can be found by cancer type, syndrome name, city, state, or country. All of the providers listed specialize in cancer genetics.

Using a Telephone-Based Genetic Counseling Service for Patients

If there is no nearby cancer genetic counselor or if your patient's schedule does not allow them to attend a cancer genetics appointment during usual working hours, several companies will provide telephone genetic counseling for patients who would not otherwise have access (often with video as well). Examples of these companies include InformedDNA (www.informeddna.com), Genome Medical (www.genomemedical.com), Advanced Tele-Genetic Counseling (www.at-gc.com), and DNA Direct (www.dnadirect.com), among others. They can either develop partnerships with hospitals to provide their genetic counseling services or they can work directly with patients, billing their insurance for the service. Hospital systems that would like to speak to a representative about adding genetic counseling to their hospital system should contact representatives from these companies directly. Other genetic counselors that provide telemedicine services can also be found on NSGC's Find a Genetic Counselor page (cited earlier) by selecting the "By Telephone" option instead of the "In Person" option.

CONCLUSION

Identifying patients at hereditary risk for cancer can be very valuable for the patient and their family members. This information can determine what cancers an individual is at risk for so they can benefit from intensive surveillance and prevention options in an attempt to prevent the cancers or diagnose them early when they are most treatable. In addition, this information is increasingly driving treatment decisions for cancer patients, with PARP inhibitors being used for individuals with mutations in the *BRCA* pathway, and immunotherapy being used for individuals with mismatch repair–deficient tumors (including most tumors in individuals with Lynch syndrome). It is likely that in the next 5 to 10 years, all cancer patients will be offered germline genetic testing (and, when appropriate, tumor genetic testing) at the time of diagnosis. Then, genetic counseling and testing can be offered to those who test positive and their at-risk relatives. However, we are not quite there yet, so there is still a need to refer patients who have a cancer diagnosis with a reasonable likelihood of being hereditary and unaffected patients who have a family history of cancer that is possibly hereditary. It is hoped that the criteria presented in this chapter, which are based on the NCCN guidelines but are simplified, will help clinicians more easily identify patients who can benefit from a referral to cancer genetics.

References

1. Buys SS, Sandbach JF, Gammon A, et al. A study of over 35,000 women with breast cancer tested with a 25-gene panel of hereditary cancer genes. *Cancer*. 2017;123(10):1721–1730.
2. Foulkes WD, Smith IE, Reis-Filho JS. Triple-negative breast cancer. *N Engl J Med*. 2010;363(20):1938–1948.

3. Domagala P, Huzarski T, Lubinski J, et al. Immunophenotypic predictive profiling of BRCA1-associated breast cancer. *Virchows Arch*. 2011;458(1):55–64.

4. Hoyer J, Vasileiou G, Uebe S, et al. Addition of triple negativity of breast cancer as an indicator for germline mutations in predisposing genes increases sensitivity of clinical selection criteria. *BMC Cancer*. 2018;18(1):926.

5. Pritzlaff M, Summeror P, McFarland R, et al. Male breast cancer in a multi-gene panel testing cohort: insights and unexpected results. *Breast Cancer Res Treat*. 2017;161(3):575–586.

6. Roa BB, Boyd AA, Volcik K, Richards CS. Ashkenazi Jewish population frequencies for common mutations in BRCA1 and BRCA2. *Nat Genet*. 1996;14(2):185–187.

7. Whittemore AS. Risk of breast cancer in carriers of BRCA gene mutations. *N Engl J Med*. 1997;337(11):788–789.

8. American College of Obstetrics and Gynecologists, et al. ACOG Practice Bulletin No. 103: hereditary breast and ovarian cancer syndrome. *Obstet Gynecol*. 2009;113(4):957–966.

9. Robson M, Im SA, Senkus E, et al. Olaparib for metastatic breast cancer in patients with a germline BRCA mutation. *N Engl J Med*. 2017;377(6):523–533.

10. Beitsch PD, Whitworth PW, Hughes K, et al. Underdiagnosis of hereditary breast cancer: are genetic testing guidelines a tool or an obstacle? *J Clin Oncol*. 2019;37(6):453–460.

11. Meric-Bernstam F, Brusco L, Daniels M, et al. Incidental germline variants in 1000 advanced cancers on a prospective somatic genomic profiling protocol. *Ann Oncol*. 2016;27(5):795–800.

12. Schrader KA, Cheng DT, Joseph V, et al. Germline variants in targeted tumor sequencing using matched normal DNA. *JAMA Oncol*. 2016;2(1):104–111.

13. Yurgelun MB, Kulke MH, Fuchs CS, et al. Cancer susceptibility gene mutations in individuals with colorectal cancer. *J Clin Oncol*. 2017;35(10):1086–1095.

14. Pearlman R, Frankel WL, Swanson B, et al. Prevalence and spectrum of germline cancer susceptibility gene mutations among patients with early-onset colorectal cancer. *JAMA Oncol*. 2017;3(4):464–471.

15. Stoffel EM, Koeppe E, Everett J, et al. Germline genetic features of young individuals with colorectal cancer. *Gastroenterology*. 2018;154(4):897–905 e1.

16. Ring KL, Bruegl AS, Allen BA, et al. Germline multi-gene hereditary cancer panel testing in an unselected endometrial cancer cohort. *Mod Pathol*. 2016;29(11):1381–1389.

17. Hampel H, Frankel W, Panescu J, et al. Screening for Lynch syndrome (hereditary nonpolyposis colorectal cancer) among endometrial cancer patients. *Cancer Res*. 2006;66(15):7810–7817.

18. Hampe, H, Panescu J, Lockman J, et al. Comment on: screening for Lynch syndrome (hereditary nonpolyposis colorectal cancer) among endometrial cancer patients. *Cancer Res*. 2007;67(19):9603.

19. Pritchard CC, Mateo J, Walsh MF, et al. Inherited DNA-repair gene mutations in men with metastatic prostate cancer. *N Engl J Med*. 2016;375(5):443–453.

20. Nicolosi P, Ledet E, Yang S, et al. Prevalence of germline variants in prostate cancer and implications for current genetic testing guidelines. *JAMA Oncol*. 2019;5(4):523–528.

21. Norquist BM, Harrell MI, Brady MF, et al. Inherited mutations in women with ovarian carcinoma. *JAMA Oncol*. 2016;2(4):482–490.

22. Walsh T, Casadei S, Lee MK, et al. Mutations in 12 genes for inherited ovarian, fallopian tube, and peritoneal carcinoma identified by massively parallel sequencing. *Proc Natl Acad Sci U S A*. 2011;108(44):18032–18037.

23. Hu C, Hart SN, Polley EC, et al. Association between inherited germline mutations in cancer predisposition genes and risk of pancreatic cancer. *JAMA*. 2018;319(23):2401–2409.

24. Tung N, Lin NU, Kidd J, et al. Frequency of germline mutations in 25 cancer susceptibility genes in a sequential series of patients with breast cancer. *J Clin Oncol*. 2016;34(13):1460–1468.

25. Couch FJ, Hart, SN, Sharma P, et al. Inherited mutations in 17 breast cancer susceptibility genes among a large triple-negative breast cancer cohort unselected for family history of breast cancer. *J Clin Oncol*. 2015;33(4):304–311.

26. Pearlman R, Frankel WL, Swanson B, et al. Prevalence and spectrum of germline cancer susceptibility gene mutations among patients with early-onset colorectal cancer. *JAMA Oncol*. 2017;3(4):464–471.

27. Stoffel EM, Koeppe E, Everett J, et al. Germline genetic features of young individuals with colorectal cancer. *Gastroenterology*. 2017;154(4):897–905.

28. Cancer Genome Atlas Research Network. Integrated genomic characterization of pancreatic ductal adenocarcinoma. *Cancer Cell.* 2017;32(2):185–203 e13.

29. Grant RC, Selander I, Connor AA, et al. Prevalence of germline mutations in cancer predisposition genes in patients with pancreatic cancer. *Gastroenterology.* 2015;148(3):556–564.

30. Shindo K, Yu J, Suenaga M, et al. Deleterious germline mutations in patients with apparently sporadic pancreatic adenocarcinoma. *J Clin Oncol.* 2017;35(30):3382–3390.

31. Hampel H, Bennett RL, Buchanan A, et al. A practice guideline from the American College of Medical Genetics and Genomics and the National Society of Genetic Counselors: referral indications for cancer predisposition assessment. *Genet Med.* 2015;17(1):70–87.

CHAPTER 3

Principles of Cancer Risk Assessment and Genetic Counseling

Amy Killie, Jonica Richards, Camille Varin-Tremblay, and Karina L. Brierley

INTRODUCTION

It is estimated that ~5% to 10% of all cancers are hereditary, meaning that they developed largely as a result of a germline mutation in a cancer predisposition gene. Rapidly evolving genetic technology is increasingly allowing for tailored cancer therapy, screening, and risk reduction for individuals with an inherited cancer predisposition. Essential steps in ensuring the realization of the promise of personalized medicine include appropriate risk assessment, development of a management plan, patient education, and facilitation of patient coping. This chapter describes the essential elements of the traditional process of cancer genetic counseling and risk assessment, including the intake and collection of personal and family medical history, risk assessment, informed consent, genetic testing, and psychosocial assessment. However, the field of hereditary cancer genetic counseling and testing has changed significantly over the past decade with rapidly increasing demand and concerns about access to genetic counseling and testing. This changing landscape has led to the proposal and implementation of various alternative care delivery models which often preserve at least some of the elements of the traditional process yet may utilize a differing order, importance, delivery method, and providers of these elements. Identified barriers to access, as well as some alternative care delivery models, will also be introduced in this chapter.

SPORADIC, FAMILIAL, AND HEREDITARY CANCER

All cancer is considered to be a genetic process, as it is due to genetic changes that accumulate in the deoxyribonucleic acid (DNA) of an individual throughout their lifetime and alter the way the cells grow and divide. However, genetic changes causing an increased risk for certain cancers can also be inherited from parent to child if these changes are present in the germ cells (i.e., egg and sperm) of a parent. When an individual inherits a nonfunctioning (also known as "mutated") copy of a gene related to hereditary cancer, that individual is at an increased risk throughout their lifetime for developing cancer. It is estimated that 5% to 10% of cancer is due to a specific inherited genetic cause.[1] In general, cancer falls into three specific categories: sporadic cancer, familial cancer, and hereditary cancer.

The majority of cancer occurs sporadically. Sporadic cancer occurs when there are genetic mutations that accumulate in the DNA of an individual over time. This occurs due to random chance, lifestyle choices, and certain environmental factors and is not due to an inherited genetic mutation. Families with sporadic cancer will generally have cancers at the typical age of onset with no apparent pattern of inheritance. For these individuals, it is very unlikely that genetic testing will reveal a genetic mutation that will explain the personal and/or family history of cancer. Sporadic cancer occurs due to a combination of both modifiable and nonmodifiable risk factors. Examples of nonmodifiable risk factors include aging, ethnicity, and gender; examples of modifiable risk factors include alcohol and tobacco use, physical inactivity, and occupational exposures.[2]

When there are multiple relatives with the same or related types of cancer but the cancer in the family does not appear to follow a clear inheritance pattern and is not necessarily at an earlier than expected age, this is considered to be familial cancer. In familial cancer, we are unable to identify an inherited genetic mutation, although there appears to be more cancer in the family than we would expect by chance alone. Families that fall into this category could be explained by a combination of environmental and lifestyle factors, generally in combination with small genetic factors that are shared among family members.

Hereditary cancer occurs when a specific genetic change or mutation is passed down through the family from parent to child and causes an increased risk for certain types of cancer. Some of the most common examples of hereditary cancer include hereditary breast and ovarian cancer syndrome (HBOCS) and Lynch syndrome. When evaluating a family for a hereditary cancer syndrome, it is important to evaluate for certain risk factors (or "red flags") in the family history that can increase the suspicion for a hereditary form of cancer. Some examples of red flags for hereditary cancers include early-onset cancer (under the age of 50); multiple individuals on the same side of the family with the same or related types of cancer; multiple cases of cancer in the same individual; rare cancer diagnoses in a family (such as pancreatic or ovarian cancer, which may raise the suspicion for hereditary breast and ovarian cancer, or medullary thyroid cancer, which raises the suspicion for multiple endocrine neoplasia type 2 [MEN type 1]); unusual presentations of cancer (such as male breast cancer); and certain ethnic groups with higher incidences of hereditary cancer, such as the Ashkenazi Jewish population.

▓ KEY COMPONENTS OF THE CANCER GENETIC COUNSELING PROCESS

The first major component during a standard genetic counseling session is the patient's own medical history. During a cancer risk assessment, the first obvious determination would be if the patient has a personal history of cancer and, if so, what type of cancer and at what age were they diagnosed. Pathology records confirming the cancer diagnosis are critical, as the cancer type, as well as any specifics in cancer pathology, may significantly alter the risk assessment as well as the differential diagnosis. For example, "triple-negative breast cancer," which refers to invasive breast cancers that are estrogen receptor (ER), progesterone receptor (PR), and HER-2 negative, can be associated with *BRCA1* mutations.[3]

A patient's cancer screening practices are also essential to obtain during a medical history intake. These might include the patient's current breast cancer screening practices, the frequency of their colonoscopies, annual dermatological exams, and so forth. Biopsies or findings on such screenings may also be relevant even if they are not cancerous, especially the finding of polyps on colonoscopies.[4] The pathology and the number of colon polyps, for example, can not only alter the risk assessment but also the differential.[3]

In a similar vein, patients should be directly asked about nonmalignant features that can be associated with certain hereditary cancer syndromes, especially if the syndrome in question is high on the differential. For example, individuals with Cowden syndrome (caused by pathogenic mutations in the *PTEN* gene) can present with skin findings called trichilemmomas, as well as macrocephaly or autism. Therefore, asking a patient about any skin findings or biopsies from dermatological exams in addition to obtaining a head circumference can add information that may be essential to the final risk assessment.[3]

After the medical history is obtained, a detailed family history is necessary to complete the assessment process.[5] Family histories should be obtained up through three generations, which include first-degree relatives (children, siblings, parents), second-degree relatives (uncles, aunts, grandparents, half-siblings), and third-degree relatives (first cousins, great aunts, great uncles, great-grandparents). This three-generation strategy should be used for both the maternal and paternal sides of the family. This can be easily drawn in the form of diagram called a pedigree (also sometimes referred to as a "family tree"), which illustrates affected individuals and their biological relatives.[6] Figure 3.1 shows an example pedigree tracking cancer history specifically. A pedigree makes it easy to visualize cancer histories in

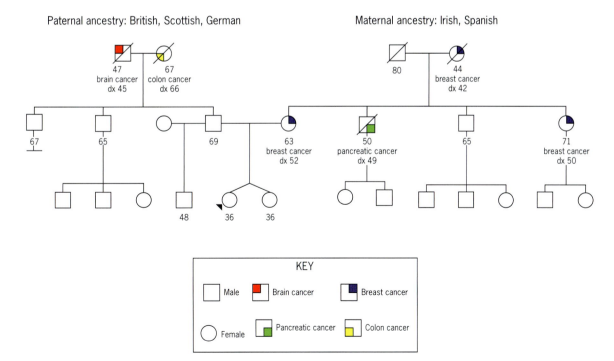

FIGURE 3.1: Example pedigree of a 36-year-old female proband.

families, helping to aid in the risk assessment as well as the patient's own understanding and clarifying any misunderstandings.[7] Tracing the family tree beginning with the most recent generations and ending with the older generations, as well as obtaining the information first from the maternal or paternal side before switching to the other side of the family, makes it easier for a patient to follow and provide clear information.

The most standard questions for both sides of the family, regardless of medical history, include the number of relatives ("How many sisters did your mother have?", "How many relatives are still living and what are their current ages?", and "How many relatives are deceased and what was the age and cause of their death?"). The number of relatives and their ages of death can become important when the final risk assessment is being performed. Additionally, ethnicity and ancestry should be ascertained from both sides of the family, as certain ethnicities are at higher risk of having a hereditary cancer syndrome due to a "founder effect."[5] One major example of this is individuals of Ashkenazi Jewish ancestry, who are at a higher risk of having HBOCS due to the increased frequency of *BRCA* mutations within the Ashkenazi Jewish population.

The single most important health history question is whether or not a relative has been diagnosed with cancer. The age of diagnosis is critical, as this can increase or decrease suspicion of a hereditary cancer syndrome. Pathology confirming the type of cancer can be extremely helpful, as the type of cancer can add more suspicion for a hereditary cancer syndrome.[3,4] For example, medullary thyroid cancer is associated with MEN2, whereas other types of thyroid cancer (such as papillary or follicular) are not. However, obtaining a pathology may be impossible given difficulties obtaining medical records, a relative being deceased, strained familial relationships, etc. Therefore, as much as possible, the type of cancer that the patient is reporting in a family member should be taken at face value.

When pathology is not available, determining the primary site of a cancer diagnosis is also critical. For example, some patients may report a family history of "bone cancer" or "brain cancer" when they may actually mean that the bones or brain were sites of metastasis. Attempting to clarify this with the patient through questioning ("Do you think your uncle's cancer began in his bones or do you think it started somewhere else and spread to his bones?") is extremely useful, as it could affect the risk assessment. Additionally, knowing whether or not a relative had multiple primary cancers would be an important factor to distinguish from a metastatic cancer.[2]

Depending upon the type of cancer, appropriate follow-up questions should be asked in regard to environmental exposures. Certain nongenetic risk factors may increase the risk of certain cancers, and the presence of these risk factors may reduce suspicion of a hereditary component, while the absence of these risk factors may increase suspicion of a hereditary component. For example, tobacco use, while a risk factor for multiple types of cancers, is strongly associated with risks for lung, bladder, kidney, throat, and stomach cancer. As another example, nulliparous women and women who have their first child over the age of 30 are at higher risks of uterine cancer and breast cancer, respectively.

While cancer diagnoses in the family and specific information regarding these cancer diagnoses may be the most essential material obtained from a family history intake, it is also important to ask follow-up questions for affected as well as unaffected relatives. It is just as important to confirm how many relatives in the family have no history of cancer as it is to confirm the number of relatives with personal histories of cancer. A large family size with multiple unaffected relatives may reduce the risk of a hereditary cancer syndrome.[2] As a specific example, having multiple unaffected women in the family whose ovaries are still intact could reduce the risk of HBOCS.

Some surgeries may reduce the risk of cancer and therefore act as limitations in a risk assessment. For example, women who have undergone bilateral salpingo-oophorectomy (BSO) have significantly reduced their risk of ovarian cancer, and women who have undergone BSO prior to menopause have reduced their risk of breast cancer.[3] With patients who have a personal history of breast cancer, the absence of any family history of breast and ovarian cancer could be potentially explained by such a surgery. Cancer screening practices of relatives may also be necessary to ascertain. For example, if a patient is being seen based on their history of multiple colon polyps, it would be important to get details on the results of close relatives' colonoscopy screening.[3] Additionally, as previously described, questions about noncancerous-related findings of family members would also be essential if there is concern for a hereditary cancer syndrome with associated nonmalignant features.

Finally, general limitations to the family tree can make a seemingly straightforward risk assessment more complicated. A few limitations have been described earlier (including surgeries that can reduce cancer risk, unclear cancer diagnoses, and cancer diagnoses not confirmed with pathology reports). However, another major limitation is family size. Small family sizes or family members dying at a young age could possibly explain the absence of a significant family history of cancer, while large families with relatives living to older ages may reduce suspicion of a hereditary predisposition to cancer.[5] Family dynamics can also play a role in limitations. Patients may have large families and yet have no information regarding their health histories due to familial issues that resulted in estrangement, one parent moving away, or a parent dying when the patient was young. Patients who are adopted may have a complete absence of information regarding their biological relatives. These limitations may make a risk assessment less clear-cut; however, it is incorporating nuances like this that make the overall risk assessment more meaningful.

After the medical and family history have been completed, the final risk assessment can be performed. The following features are general to hereditary cancer syndromes; however, specific hereditary cancer predispositions may have specific features that are unique to that predisposition. Please see the chapters on specific risk assessments for individual cancer syndromes.

Providing information on genetics and basic genetic concepts can help aid in a patient's understanding of hereditary cancer. Every patient will have a different level of base knowledge of genetics and may even bring common misconceptions about genetics to an appointment, such as the idea that individuals with a hereditary risk of cancer have "the gene" for that particular type of cancer ("I want to see if I have the breast cancer gene"). A discussion of the Knudson "two-hit hypothesis," illustrated in Figure 3.2, can be helpful to some patients, as it illustrates why families with a hereditary risk of cancer may have cancer diagnosed at younger ages, more cancers in the family, and more rare or unusual presentation of cancers.[3]

This discussion can also be a good segue to the discussion on inheritance, as it illustrates that individuals with a hereditary cancer syndrome have one "working" and one "nonworking" copy of a gene. The majority of hereditary cancer syndromes are inherited in an autosomal dominant manner, meaning that a single mutation is sufficient to cause the associated risk of cancer. This means that an individual with a mutation has a 50% chance with each

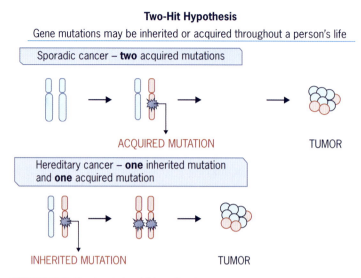

Two-Hit Hypothesis

Gene mutations may be inherited or acquired throughout a person's life

Sporadic cancer – **two** acquired mutations

ACQUIRED MUTATION   TUMOR

Hereditary cancer – **one** inherited mutation
and **one** acquired mutation

INHERITED MUTATION   TUMOR

FIGURE 3.2: Knudson's two-hit hypothesis.

pregnancy (one in two) of passing that same mutations on to future children. This would also mean that siblings of an individual identified to have a mutation would also be at a 50% risk of having that same mutation.

Because genetic testing has implications not just for a patient's own healthcare and future management but also for other family members, informed consent is a critical component of all pretest counseling. Informed consent confirms that a patient is aware of the risks, benefits, and limitations of genetic testing and feels comfortable with proceeding with testing at this time. The American Society of Clinical Oncology (ASCO) has outlined the basic components that should be included in the informed consent process for patients interested in pursuing genetic testing for hereditary cancer predispositions as follows:[8]

1. Information on the specific genetic mutation(s) or genomic variant(s) being tested, including whether the range of risk associated with the variant will affect medical care
2. Implications of a positive and negative result
3. Possibility that the test will not be informative
4. Options for risk estimation without genetic or genomic testing
5. Risk of passing a genetic variant to children
6. Technical accuracy of the test, including, where required by law, licensure of the testing laboratory
7. Fees involved in testing and counseling and, for direct to consumer (DTC) testing, whether the counselor is employed by the testing company
8. Psychological implications of the test results (benefits and risks)
9. Risks and protections against genetic discrimination by employers or insurers
10. Confidentiality issues, including for DTC testing companies, policies related to privacy and data security
11. Possible use of DNA testing samples in future research

12. Options and limitations of medical surveillance and strategies for prevention after genetic and genomic testing

13. Importance of sharing genetic and genomic test results with at-risk relatives so that they may benefit from this information

14. Plans for follow-up after testing

In particular, patients commonly have questions about the possibility of being discriminated against by health insurance companies or other types of insurance if they were identified to have a mutation. The Genetic Information Nondiscrimination Act (GINA) is a law that was passed in 2008 that protects individuals from genetic discrimination in health insurance and employment. This means that it is illegal for a person's genetic information to be used in determination of health insurance coverage or premiums.[9] It also means that a person's genetic information cannot be used in any employment decisions, including hiring or firing.

This law applies to most health insurance companies and most employers. Discrimination protection from GINA does not apply to individuals who are members of the U.S. military who receive their health insurance through Tricare, veterans who receive their healthcare through the Veterans Association, individuals who receive their healthcare through the Indian Health Service, and federal employees who receive care through the Federal Employees Health Benefits Program. Additionally, individuals who are employed by companies with fewer than 15 employees and individuals who are employed by the U.S. military or the federal government are not protected by GINA.[9] It is important to note that GINA does not provide protection from discrimination based on a person's medical history, including any current symptoms or other medical issues. For example, a person's cancer diagnosis could be used as a determining factor for health insurance coverage or premiums regardless of any genetic test results.[10]

While health insurance and employment are protected under GINA, GINA does not protect against discrimination by life, disability, and long-term care insurances. Therefore, these types of policies could potentially use a person's genetic information in their determination process for coverage.[10] Any life, disability, or long-term care insurance policy that is in place prior to genetic testing cannot be revoked retroactively regardless of the results. Therefore, individuals with no personal history of cancer or other significant health conditions without one of these policies in place may wish to consider setting a policy in place prior to testing if they have particular concerns about potential discrimination.

▦ IDEAL TESTING CANDIDATE

After contracting with the patient, obtaining information regarding the personal and family history, and conducting a risk assessment, the next step is to determine who in the family is the most informative person (if anyone) to undergo genetic testing for hereditary cancer syndromes. Within a given family, the ideal first person to test is the individual with the highest risk of testing positive for a hereditary cancer predisposition syndrome. This will be the individual, or one of the individuals, who makes the family suspicious for a hereditary predisposition to cancer. Generally, this will be an individual with a personal diagnosis of cancer. For example, if a family is suspicious for HBOCS, it would be best to test someone in the family with a personal history of early-onset breast cancer, ovarian cancer, or pancreatic cancer (or another cancer related to HBOCS). Beginning testing with this individual allows for the most informative test results in the family. If a hereditary predisposition to cancer is identified in an affected family member, it allows for subsequent cascade testing of other members within the family who are at risk of inheriting the genetic mutation. On the other hand, if a hereditary predisposition to cancer is not identified in the most informative testing candidates within the family, this significantly decreases the risk for a hereditary predisposition to cancer within the family, and genetic testing may not be indicated for other family members.

In the case that the ideal candidate or candidates for genetic testing are unavailable, genetic testing should be offered to unaffected family members, although it is important to keep in mind the limitations of testing an unaffected individual. In this situation, it is best to start by testing the next best candidate for testing (for example, a first-degree relative of an affected individual). In the event that the test is negative, the interpretation of the negative result is more difficult and the results are uninformative for other family members. Genetic testing should therefore be offered to other unaffected family members, even if a hereditary predisposition to cancer has not yet been identified in the family.

CIRCUMSTANCES TO CONSIDER GENETIC TESTING

There are several important circumstances in which genetic testing for hereditary cancer syndromes can be considered. The circumstance in which testing is being considered could have an impact on the timing of testing, the type of testing offered to the patient, and the chosen laboratory.

Individuals who have a personal diagnosis of cancer may consider genetic testing if they are affected with cancer or another malignancy that is suspicious for a hereditary cause. In these cases, there are many factors that may affect the timing of genetic testing. It is important to consider the patient's situation and where they are in the treatment process, as the timing of genetic testing has the potential to affect surgical or treatment decisions. Certain laboratories offer "urgent" testing for *BRCA1* and *BRCA2*, which may be appropriate in these situations. For example, genetic testing for individuals with a diagnosis of breast cancer and a personal and/or family history suggestive of HBOCS may consider genetic testing prior to undergoing surgery, as women with a genetic mutation in the *BRCA1* or *BRCA2* gene may consider different surgery (i.e., double mastectomy vs. lumpectomy) given the high risk for breast cancer and the increased risk for a second primary breast cancer. Therefore, it is important to discuss the potential outcomes of testing with patients prior to proceeding with genetic testing to get a sense of the need for urgent testing. Furthermore, women with *BRCA1* and *BRCA2* mutations with metastatic breast cancer, ovarian cancer, and possibly other *BRCA*-related cancers could be considered for treatment with targeted therapy (such as a poly-ADP ribose polymerase [PARP] inhibitor).[11] Therefore, the results of genetic testing can have an impact on not only surgical decision-making but also treatment decisions.

The second situation in which to consider testing for a hereditary predisposition to cancer is when a familial pathogenic variant has been identified. In this situation, cascade genetic testing is recommended for at-risk family members. There are many different factors to take into consideration when discussing testing for a familial mutation. First, it is important to consider the age of the individual. For the majority of hereditary cancer syndromes, professional guidelines recommend against testing minors, as recommendations for screening and surgery typically do not begin in childhood and will therefore not alter childhood management.[12] This differs with several hereditary cancer predisposition syndromes, such as familial adenomatous polyposis syndrome, which can present with childhood cancers and polyps and therefore would change medical management in childhood. Generally, the accepted recommendation is to begin screening for individuals with classical familial adenomatous polyposis between the ages of 10 and 12 years,[13,14] which is important to consider when coordinating genetic testing for minors in this case.

Another common situation in which to consider genetic testing for a hereditary cancer predisposition syndrome is when a patient is unaffected with a concerning family history or a patient with a personal history of cancer who is not currently under treatment. Although these are often not urgent situations, many of the same considerations should be made in regards to the timing of testing, including considerations for the age of the patient, life insurance and other insurances,[9] and availability of more informative members of the family for testing depending on the situation.

CONSIDERATIONS IN SELECTING A LABORATORY AND THE APPROPRIATE TEST

There are several considerations to make in terms of both the laboratory to use and the test to select for the patient. First, it is important to consider insurance coverage of genetic testing and the associated out-of-pocket costs that the patient may accrue. When meeting with a patient, it is important to assess whether their personal and family history meets national guidelines for genetic testing. Additionally, it is important to consider whether their personal and family history meets their insurance guidelines for genetic testing, as many insurances have written guidelines for when they will cover specific testing. Occasionally, it is possible that the patient could meet national guidelines for genetic testing but not meet their insurance criteria for genetic testing. If the client does not meet their insurance guidelines for genetic testing, certain laboratories offer self-pay options. The cost of testing, meeting insurance criteria, and billing policies of the laboratories should all be taken into consideration when deciding which laboratory to select for testing.

It is also important to take into consideration certain other factors of the laboratory, such as the test menu selection, the approximate turnaround time of the test, and whether other family members have had positive genetic testing. For example, if a patient's mother had positive genetic testing through a specific laboratory, it is often recommended to send your patient's specimen to the same laboratory for testing. This is so that the laboratory will have a positive control for testing and to ensure that the laboratory has seen the familial mutation before and it is in their detectable range. In the event that sending the specimen to the same laboratory as a family member is not feasible, it is possible to call another laboratory for confirmation that the familial mutation is in their detectable range. Additionally, some laboratories will request or require a positive control from the family member with the known mutation for comparison.

To determine the appropriate test selection for a patient, it is important for genetic counselors to consider several factors. For certain patients, the personal and/or family history could be suggestive of more than one hereditary cancer predisposition syndrome. For example, a patient could have a personal history of early-onset breast cancer (suggestive of HBOCS) and a family history of colon and uterine cancer, suggestive of Lynch syndrome. Additionally, advances in the knowledge of hereditary cancer predisposition syndromes have led to the identification of additional genes related to hereditary cancers such as breast cancer, for which we can now test for additional genes (*ATM, PALB2,* and *CHEK2,* for example). When this is the case, the genetic counselor should discuss the option of multigene panel testing. See the section on multigene panel testing later for additional information.

▨ GENETIC TESTING FOR AT-RISK FAMILY MEMBERS

Depending on the results of genetic testing, there will be different implications for family members. If a genetic mutation is identified, all at-risk family members should be offered genetic counseling and testing. Depending on the degree of relation, family members will be at different risks of inheriting the familial mutation. For example, for the majority of hereditary cancer predisposition syndromes that are autosomal dominant, first-degree relatives are at a 50% risk to inherit the familial mutation, second-degree relatives are at a 25% risk, and so on. In the event that the parents of an individual who tests positive for a genetic mutation are available for testing, they should be offered testing to determine from whom the mutation was inherited. In the event that parents are not available for testing, members from both sides of the family should be offered genetic testing until it is determined from which side of the family the genetic mutation was inherited. There is also a possibility of a "*de novo*" mutation in an individual, in which neither parent carried the mutation, but it was a new event in the individual. This is common in the case of Li-Fraumeni syndrome (*TP53* gene) and hereditary hemorrhagic telangiectasia syndrome and juvenile polyposis syndrome (*SMAD4* gene).[15,16] In this event, family members (other than offspring) are generally not considered to be at risk for the mutation. However, the possibility of gonadal mosaicism in one of the parents cannot be ruled out, and thus siblings may wish to have testing to clarify their risks.

Although the majority of hereditary cancer predisposition syndromes are inherited in an autosomal dominant fashion, there are several examples of hereditary predisposition syndromes that display autosomal recessive inheritance patterns. An example of this includes *MUTYH*-associated polyposis syndrome (MAP). MAP is caused by homozygous mutations in the *MUTYH* gene and causes a significantly increased risk for adenomatous colon polyps and colon cancer. Homozygotes generally present with 10 to 100 colon adenomatous polyps by the age of 50.[17] On the other hand, *MUTYH* heterozygotes do not have MAP and do not have the same increased risk for colorectal cancer as do homozygotes. Research has indicated that *MUTYH* heterozygotes may have a slightly increased risk for colon cancer; however, additional research is needed in this area.[18]

▨ POSSIBLE GENETIC TEST RESULTS

When a patient is undergoing genetic testing for a hereditary predisposition to cancer, there are several possible test results. It is important to talk through these possible results while consenting the patients to testing.

The first possible test result is a positive result, meaning that a pathogenic variant was identified in a gene related to hereditary cancer. This means that the individual has an increased risk for certain types of cancers. A positive test result now allows for recommendations to be made for the screening and management of the individual. Additionally, cascade testing should now be offered for other family members, including (but not limited to) children, parents, and siblings.

The second possible test result is an uninformative negative result. This occurs when no prior genetic testing has taken place in the family and the individual tests negative for any pathogenic variants in the hereditary cancer genes that were tested. Uninformative genetic test results can have several different interpretations, including the following:

1. The cancers in the individual or family are not due to a hereditary predisposition.
2. There is a mutation in a gene that was examined that was not detectable by the current technology.
3. There is a mutation in another gene that has not been analyzed or has not yet been discovered.
4. Other family members who have had cancer have a hereditary predisposition to cancer, which was not inherited by the patient who has been tested. If the family history remains suspicious, genetic counseling and testing may be recommended to other family members.

In the event of an uninformative negative result, it is important to examine the rest of the family history and to recommend testing other family members if necessary. Consider if the most informative person in the family has had testing or if genetic testing would be indicated for other family members. If the most informative candidate is deceased, recommend testing for other individuals in the family. Encourage patients to keep you updated on the results of other testing that takes place within the family, as this could change management recommendations for your patient. Additionally, patients should be encouraged to update the clinic on any new cancers in the family. For individuals with uninformative negative results, screening and management recommendations should be based on the patient's personal and family history.

The third possible test result is a "true negative" result. This means that a pathogenic mutation has previously been identified in the family and an individual tests negative for the same pathogenic mutation. With a true negative result, the individual is considered to be back down to the population risk for the cancers associated with the pathogenic mutation previously identified in the family. Assuming that the genetic mutation previously identified in the family explains the family history of cancer, these individuals can follow population risk screening recommendations. However, it is important to remember that for several moderate-risk cancer genes, a familial mutation may not explain the entire family history. For example, a *CHEK2* mutation in a family with a significant history of breast cancer may not provide the entire explanation for the breast cancer in the family. In this case, it is also important to take into consideration any family history that is not explained by the familial pathogenic mutation when making management recommendations.

The last possible test result is a variant of uncertain significance (VUS). This is an inconclusive result in which a genetic variant was identified in a gene but the laboratory does not have enough data to classify this variant as a pathogenic variant or a benign variant that does not affect the gene. The significance and function of the variant are currently unknown. In most situations, genetic testing for unaffected family members for VUSs is not recommended, although in some cases genetic testing for affected family members can help clarify the meaning of a variant. As the laboratory gathers more evidence and data over time regarding the variant, it will be reclassified into either a pathogenic variant or a benign variant. VUSs are not used to make recommendations for screening or management changes. In cases in which a variant is identified, as is the case with an uninformative negative result, management and screening recommendations should be based on the personal and family history.

▓ MULTIGENE PANEL TESTING

Genetic testing in the cancer setting has evolved greatly over the last decades. Traditionally, single-gene testing in families suspicious for a genetic predisposition to cancer was time consuming and costly. This was a step-wise process, in which the most common genetic factors, such as HBOCS (*BRCA1* and *BRCA2*) were tested first, followed by testing the less common genetic factors, such as *PALB2* and *ATM,* for a family suspicious for a hereditary predisposition to breast cancer. Multigene panel testing via next-generation sequencing (NGS) has more recently become clinically available. The U.S. Supreme Court invalidated Myriad Genetics' patent on the *BRCA1* and *BRCA2* genes in June 2013, which allowed greater access to genetic testing.[19] Other genetic testing companies were able to include the *BRCA1* and *BRCA2* genes in their multigene panels. Due to competition between genetic testing companies and new technologies, the price of genetic testing ultimately dropped over the years. This new technology has proven to be cost- and time-effective, but often the cancer risks and potential screening and management recommendations associated with newly identified genes are not yet fully defined.[20]

Multigene panel testing improves the mutation detection rate in families who do not follow the classic hereditary cancer syndromes presentation.[21,22] For example, some families with a number of individuals affected with breast cancer who tested negative for the *BRCA1* and *BRCA2* mutations in the past were found to have a mutation in one of the lower-penetrance genes associated with an increased risk for breast cancer, such as *ATM* and *CHEK2*.[23] Couch et al. have shown that these moderate-penetrance genes are the most commonly mutated genes among white women with breast cancer after *BRCA1* and *BRCA2* genes.[24] In most cases, clinicians can use this information to personalize the screening management for these individuals and family members, such as adding breast magnetic resonance imaging (MRI) to the annual screening for breast cancer,[25] although clinical decision-making with these genes is not as straightforward when compared to mutations in *BRCA1* and *BRCA2*, which have been studied for a longer period.

As more genes are included on these tests and more individuals are being tested for a genetic predisposition to cancer, our knowledge of these genes and their usefulness in the clinical setting improves tremendously. Although multigene panel testing allows us to gather more information to better understand the hereditary contribution to cancer in some families, there are still many unknowns and limitations associated with multigene panel testing.

The available technology seems to have surpassed our knowledge with regard to cancer genetics, clinical recommendations, and management. As the size of the test offered to patients increases, the rate of VUSs ultimately increases.[21,22] As previously reviewed in this chapter, it is unclear whether these variants increase the risk for cancer or whether they are a normal genetic variation. Because most of these variants are reclassified as normal variation by the genetic laboratories over the years, we do not take any clinical actions based on VUSs unless reclassified as disease-causing variants. Genetic data sharing between laboratories is important to reduce the number of patients who receive uncertain results.[26]

There are many options for genetic testing. One of the roles of genetic counselors is to help patients navigate between these options for them to make the best decision with regard to their personal preferences. Clinically available multigene panels include genes of varying risks for a wide spectrum of cancers.[27] High-penetrance genes confer more than a four-fold lifetime risk for one or more cancers. Guidelines for screening and prevention are established by national or expert opinion. Examples of high-risk genes include *BRCA1, BRCA2, CDH1, TP53, MLH1, MSH2,* and more. Moderate-risk genes confer approximately a two- to four-fold risk of developing one or more cancers. There are limited guidelines for screening and recommendations. Examples of moderate-risk genes include *ATM, BRIP1, CHEK2, PALB2,* and many more. Because studies that support clinical utility of these genes is lacking,[20] clinicians may adjust their screening and management recommendations based on the patient's personal and family history of cancer. Every year, there are discoveries of new genes that may confer an increased risk for cancer. These genes have not been studied for a long time, and the lack of knowledge presents significant challenges in making recommendations for management.

The option of multigene panel testing also increases the risk of incidental findings.[28] For an example, consider the following situation: A patient with a family history of colon cancer is referred to genetic counseling. This patient decides to pursue multigene panel testing, which includes genes associated with other types of cancers. The patient is found to have a *CDH1* mutation, which confers substantial risks for lobular breast cancer and diffuse gastric cancer.[29] We consider this as an incidental finding because the patient has no personal or family history suggestive of a *CDH1* mutation. How should we manage identified genetic mutations inconsistent with the family history? Recommendations associated with a *CDH1* mutation include risk-reducing gastrectomy between the age of 18 and 40; high-risk breast cancer screening, which includes an annual mammogram and an annual breast MRI; or the consideration of a bilateral mastectomy.[29] Should a patient with a *CDH1* mutation and no family history of gastric or breast cancer undergo a prophylactic mastectomy and gastrectomy? This example illustrates the complexity of multigene testing and the need to obtain better data.

Whole-exome sequencing (WES) and whole-genome sequencing (WGS) have also become more accessible in the clinical setting over the last decade, and these testing methodologies add even more complexity to genetic testing than the multigene panel. Genetic laboratories can use WES and WGS as opposed to multigene panels but focus their analysis on genes associated with hereditary cancers. The use of WES and WGS is of great value, especially in the setting of rare diseases, but there is an important risk of incidental or secondary findings in genes unrelated to the primary indication for genetic testing. Some of these findings may be of medical value for the care of these patients and should indeed be reported to the patient. The American College of Medical Genetics and Genomics (ACMG) made recommendations for clinical laboratories to disclose certain classes or types of mutations in predetermined genes.[30] Most of these genes are related to hereditary cancer predisposition or inherited cardiac conditions. If testing is performed through exome or genome sequencing, it is important for genetic counselors or physicians to discuss the risk of incidental findings with patients. It is also common for genetic counselors in the cancer setting to see patients who had genetic testing ordered by a different specialty (e.g., cardiology) and were found to have a mutation in a gene associated with hereditary cancers. In this case, the counselor offers posttesting genetic counseling and reviews the cancer risks, management, and implications for family members associated with the specific incidental finding. These results may come as a shock for patients, especially if the pretest counseling did not include incidental finding risks.

The increased rate of VUSs, the variety in penetrance of cancer-associated genes, the lack of recommended guidelines, and the risk for incidental findings may be a source of anxiety for patients.[28] It is important for patients to be aware of these risks prior to pursuing genetic testing. This information may have an impact on whether the patient wants to pursue genetic testing or on the selection of the genetic test. It is also important for clinicians to understand these risks and limitations to avoid the adoption of inappropriate screening or risk-reducing surgeries.

Multigene panel testing can be useful in determining an individual's risk for cancer and to adjust the screening recommendations for these individuals, but it is important to keep in mind the risks and limitations of these multigene panels.

PSYCHOSOCIAL ASSESSMENT

Another key component of the traditional cancer genetic counseling and risk assessment process is psychosocial assessment and support. We will briefly introduce this topic as an element of the cancer genetic counseling process, but ethical, legal, and psychosocial issues in cancer genetic counseling will also be covered in more detail in Chapter 16.

Psychosocial assessment and support are generally woven through other elements of the cancer genetic counseling visit. At the start of the visit, the provider often briefly contracts with the client to assess their goals for the session and their motivations for seeking genetic counseling. This can help the provider tailor the information to the client. During the collection of personal and family medical history, important aspects of psychosocial assessment are often elicited, which could include the patient's experiences with cancers, experiences with loss due to cancer, health behaviors (including cancer screening), psychological history, beliefs about the causes of cancer, concerns and fears related to cancer, and reasons for pursuing cancer genetic risk assessment and testing.[31,32] In addition, family dynamics, communication patterns, and support systems often come to light during the collection of the family medical history (e.g., patients may indicate that they are not in contact with particular family members and thus do not know their medical history or may indicate whether or not certain relatives have been open to discussing genetic testing).[3,32] During the risk assessment, education, and informed consent aspects of the cancer genetic counseling process, practitioners can also gather information about the patient's perceived risk, reaction to risk assessment, readiness for testing, and anticipated reactions to possible test results.[3,32] For example, a young woman with a recent diagnosis of breast cancer may indicate that if she tests positive at least it will explain why she developed breast cancer and confirm her decision to consider bilateral mastectomy. The information collected during this assessment can then be applied by the practitioner to help patients adjust to new information, correct misconceptions, facilitate informed decision-making, provide support and anticipatory guidance, assess patient readiness for testing, prepare patients for potential test results, and personalize the discussion of benefits and risks of genetic testing.[31] Gathering psychosocial information may also help the practitioner identify patients at risk for adverse psychosocial outcomes who may benefit from consultation with a mental health provider and more in-depth consideration of readiness for genetic testing. In addition, assessment of family communication patterns may help identify barriers to dissemination of information and patient needs for further support to facilitate this dissemination of information to relatives.

LIMITATIONS AND BARRIERS OF TRADITIONAL CANCER GENETIC COUNSELING AND ALTERNATIVE CARE DELIVERY MODELS

The field of hereditary cancer genetic counseling and testing has changed significantly over the past 5 to 10 years, with several important developments leading to rapidly increasing demand. Some key events driving demand have included faster and less expensive genetic testing techniques, Angelina Jolie's opinion editorial piece, and the Supreme Court decision to overturn exclusive *BRCA1/2* patents.[33] Initiatives to increase awareness and availability of testing, broader acceptance of genetic testing (including DTC testing), patients returning for "updated testing" in the era of multigene panels, and Food and Drug Administration (FDA) approval of targeted therapies (such as PARP inhibitors) for *BRCA*-associated cancers have also contributed to growing demand.[33] A recent survey of genetic counselors showed that these changes in the field are already affecting components of counseling in the "traditional model," including counselors trading depth for breadth and spending more of their time counseling about uncertainty.[34]

As demand increases, a variety of barriers to access and efficacy of hereditary cancer genetic counseling have been raised by experts in the field. The most frequently cited barriers are those related to the availability of an adequate workforce, including a limited supply of providers with appropriate training in cancer genetics, particularly culturally and linguistically diverse providers and those accessible to patients in rural areas.[35,36] Other barriers are related to the failure of healthcare providers to identify and refer patients appropriately, including time constraints, not obtaining and updating an adequate family history, lack of awareness of who to refer and/or how to refer, and misconceptions that may discourage referrals (e.g., concerns about discrimination and/or cost).[35] Cost and lack of or insufficient insurance coverage may also be barriers for some patients.[35,36]

The bulk of this chapter has reviewed the key elements of the traditional cancer genetic counseling process. These traditional models and tenets of cancer genetic counseling were based on testing in the setting of research protocols and traditional pediatric/prenatal/Huntington disease counseling and testing models at academic medical centers.[36] They also arose in the era of more limited, expensive genetic testing options, which necessitated the collection of detailed information in order to generate a differential diagnosis and request the necessary stepwise testing.[36] However, decreasing costs and more widespread availability and use of broader testing options (e.g., multigene panels, WES) have led to less emphasis and need for pretest generation of extensive differential diagnosis and stepwise testing.[36] These shifts along with recognition of barriers of traditional genetic counseling models have led to the proposal and implementation of various alternative care delivery models. Many elements of the "traditional cancer genetic counseling process" described in this chapter remain key in alternative service delivery models, yet order, importance, delivery method, and by whom these elements are performed, as well as method of identification and referral of patients, vary.[37]

Several models for delivering care still directly involve genetic counselors in the pretest counseling process but leverage alternative methods of delivering genetic counseling. These models include use of telephone, telemedicine/telegenetics (video conference), web-based, and group counseling.[33] Models utilizing telephone, telemedicine, and group genetic counseling have been studied and shown to be equivalent to traditional in-person, one-on-one genetic counseling with respect to an increase in patient knowledge, patient satisfaction, and psychosocial measures. Some studies have also demonstrated cost-effectiveness and/or time savings of these alternative models.[33] However, in some cases, a significant number of patients declined phone or group counseling, preferring in-person, individual counseling.[33]

Models without direct pretest involvement of a genetic counselor have been less well-studied. These models are usually "testing first" models with broad consent to comprehensive testing coordinated by nongenetics professionals.[38] These models may be in the context of collaborative partnerships between nongenetics providers who are providing direct care and ordering testing and genetic providers who serve as a hub of education, information and resources, and/or case review and consultation.[38] Collection of additional information and referral to a genetics professional for further counseling after test results are available may be performed either for all patients or for select patients (for example, those with variant and/or positive results or strong family histories).[33] These models almost certainly improve patient access to genetic testing with the opportunity for patients to stay within their local community, and some studies have shown high levels of patient satisfaction and acceptability.

Some significant barriers to implementation of these alternative models and/or improved access to genetics services remain. Revision of reimbursement strategies will almost certainly be critical to allow institutions providing genetic professional services to recoup the costs of these services, particularly when provided outside of traditional in-person, one-on-one models of care.[38] Despite the existence of GINA, lack of awareness of its protections and limitations of its protections (e.g., military healthcare [Tricare], life insurance, disability insurance) likely also still serve as barriers to patients pursuing genetic counseling and testing services.[38] Therefore, efforts to increase public awareness of GINA, as well as efforts to address gaps in protection provided by GINA, may be necessary to further enhance access and uptake of genetic testing.[38]

▓ CONCLUSION

Genetic testing for hereditary cancer has grown more widespread and essential for treatment, screening, and prevention decision-making for a number of cancers. Traditional approaches to cancer genetic counseling and risk assessment include detailed pretest collection of personal and family medical history, risk assessment, informed consent, and psychosocial assessment, as described in this chapter. However, with rapidly increasing demand for genetic testing and concerns about access to genetic counseling and testing, various alternative care delivery models have been proposed and are starting to be implemented. These may differ in the order, importance, delivery method, and providers of the essential elements of the traditional cancer genetic counseling and risk assessment process described in this chapter. Although the exact delivery models for hereditary cancer risk assessment and genetic counseling will likely continue to evolve, many of the key elements described in this chapter will remain important for genetic test result interpretation, risk assessment, appropriate medical management, and facilitation of patient adjustment, and thus ultimately ensure the realization of the promise of personalized medicine.

References

1. National Cancer Institute. The Genetics of Cancer. https://www.cancer.gov/about-cancer/causes-prevention/genetics. Updated October 12, 2017. Accessed August 12, 2020.

2. Scheneider KA. *Counseling about Cancer: Strategies for Genetic Counseling.* 3rd ed. Hoboken, NJ: John Wiley & Sons; 2011.

3. Shannon KM, Patel D. Principles of cancer genetic counseling and genetic testing. In *Principles of Clinical Cancer Genetics: A Handbook from the Massachusetts General Hospital.* Boston, MA: Springer US; 2010: 23–40.

4. Lewis KM. Identifying hereditary cancer: genetic counseling and cancer risk assessment. *Curr Probl Cancer.* 2014;38(6):216–225.

5. PDQ Cancer Genetics Editorial Board. Cancer Genetics Risk Assessment and Counseling (PDQ˚): Health Professional Version. 2019 Sep 27. In: PDQ Cancer Information Summaries [Internet]. Bethesda (MD): National Cancer Institute (US); 2002-. https://www.ncbi.nlm.nih.gov/books/NBK65817/. Access date October 2019.

6. Bennett RL, French KS, Resta RG, et al. Standardized human pedigree nomenclature: update and assessment of the recommendations of the National Society of Genetic Counselors. *J Genet Couns.* 2008;17(5):424–433.

7. Veach PMC, LeRoy B, Callanan NP. *Facilitating the Genetic Counseling Process: Practice-Based Skills.* Cham, Switzerland: Springer; 2018.

8. Robson ME, Storm CD, Weitzel J, et al. American Society of Clinical Oncology Policy Statement Update: genetic and genomic testing for cancer susceptibility. *I Clin Oncol.* 2010;28(5):893–901.

9. Genetic Alliance, Genetics and Public Policy Center at Johns Hopkins University, & National Coalition for Health Professional Education in Genetics. Genetic. http://www.ginahelp.org/GINAhelp.pdf. Published May 2010. Accessed October 2019.

10. Hudson KL, Holohan M, Collins FS. Keeping pace with the times—The Genetic Information Nondiscrimination Act of 2008. *New Engl J Med.* 2008;358(25):2661–2663.

11. Munroe M, Kolesar J. Olaparib for the treatment of BRCA-mutated advanced ovarian cancer. *Am J Health Syst Pharm.* 2016;73(14):1037–1041.

12. National Society of Genetic Counselors. Genetic Testing of Minors for Adult-Onset Conditions. www.nsgc.org/p/bl/et/blogaid=860. Published February 15, 2017. Updated April 12, 2018. Accessed August 12, 2020.

13. Vasen HFA, Moslein G, Alonso A, et al. Guidelines for the clinical management of familial adenomatous polyposis (FAP). *Gut.* 2008;57(5):704–713.

14. Syngal S, Brand RE, Church JM, et al. ACG Clinical Guideline: genetic testing and management of hereditary gastrointestinal cancer syndromes. *Am J Gastroenterol.* 2015;110(2):223–263.

15. Larsen Haidle J, Howe JR. Juvenile Polyposis Syndrome. GeneReviews. https://www.ncbi.nlm.nih.gov/books/NBK1469/. Published May 13, 2003. Updated March 9, 2017. Accessed August 12, 2020.

16. Schneider K, Zelley K, Nichols KE, et al. Li-Fraumeni Syndrome. GeneReviews. https://www.ncbi.nlm.nih.gov/books/NBK1311/. Published January 19, 1999. Updated November 21, 2019. Accessed August 12, 2020.

17. Nielsen M, Infante E, Brand R. MUTYH Polyposis. GeneReviews. https://www.ncbi.nlm.nih.gov/books/NBK107219/. Published October 4, 2012. Updated October 10, 2019. Accessed August 12, 2020.

18. Jones N, Vogt S, Nielsen M, et al. Increased colorectal cancer incidence in obligate carriers of heterozygous mutations in MUTYH. *Gastroenterology.* 2009;137(2):489–494.

19. *Association for Molecular Pathology v. Myriad Genetics, Inc.* 569 I.S. (2013). United States Supreme Court.

20. Tung N, Domchek SM, Stadler Z, et al. Counselling framework for moderate-penetrance cancer-susceptibility mutations. *Nat Rev Clin Oncol.* 2016;13:581–588.

21. Lincoln SE, Kobayashi Y, Anderson M, et al. A systematic comparison of traditional and multigene panel testing for hereditary breast and ovarian cancer genes in more than 1000 patients. *J Mol Diagn.* 2015;17(5):533–544.

22. Ricker C, Culver JO, Lowstuter K, et al. Increased yield of actionable mutations using multi-gene panels to assess hereditary cancer susceptibility in an ethnically diverse clinical cohort. *Cancer Genet.* 2016;209:130–137.

23. Slavin TP, Maxwell KN, Lilyquist J, et al. The contribution of pathogenic variants in breast cancer susceptibility genes to familial breast cancer risk. *NPJ Breast Cancer.* 2017;3:22.

24. Couch F, Shimelis H, Hu C, et al. Associations between cancer predisposition testing panel genes and breast cancer. *JAMA Oncol.* 2017;3(9):1190–1196.

25. National Comprehensive Cancer Network. Genetic/Familial High-Risk Assessment: Breast, Ovarian, and Pancreatic (Version 1.2020).

26. Raza S, Hall A. Genomic medicine and data sharing. *Br Med Bull.* 2017:123(1):35–45.

27. Easton DF, Pharoah PDP, Antoniou AC, et al. Gene-panel sequencing and the prediction of breast-cancer risk. *New Engl J Med.* 2015;372:2243–2257.

28. Hall MJ, Forman AD, Pilarksi R, et al. Gene panel testing for inherited cancer risk. *J Natl Compr Canc Netw.* 2014;12(9).

29. National Comprehensive Cancer Network. Gastric Cancer (Version 3.2019).

30. Kalia S, Adelman K, Bale S, et al. Recommendations for reporting of secondary findings in clinical exome and genome sequencing, 2016 update (ACMG SF v2.0): a Policy statement of the American College of Medical Genetics and Genomics. *Genet Med.* 2017;19:249–255.

31. Trepanier A, Ahrens M, McKinnon W, et al. Genetic cancer risk assessment and counseling: recommendations of the National Society of Genetic Counselors. *J Genet Counsel.* 2004;13:83–114.

32. Riley BD, Culver JO, Skrzynia C, et al. Essential elements of genetic cancer risk assessment, counseling, and testing: updated recommendations of the National Society of Genetic Counselors. *J Genet Counsel.* 2012;21:151–161.

33. McCuaig J, Armel S, Care M, et al. Next-generation service delivery: a scoping review of patient outcomes associated with alternative models of genetic counseling and genetic testing for hereditary cancer. *Cancers.* 2018;10(11):435.

34. Hooker GW, Clemens KR, Quillin J, et al. Cancer genetic counseling and testing in an era of rapid change. *J Genet Counsel.* 2017;26:1244–1253.

35. Weitzel JN, Blazer KR, MacDonald DJ, et al. Genetics, genomics, and cancer risk assessment. *CA.* 2011;61:327–359.

36. Trepanier AM, Allain DC. Models of service delivery for cancer genetic risk assessment and counseling. *J Genet Counsel.* 2014;23:239–253.

37. Cohen SA, Gustafson SL, Marvin ML, et al. Report from the National Society of Genetic Counselors Service Delivery Model Task Force: a proposal to define models, components, and modes of referral. *J Genet Counsel.* 2012;21:645–651.

38. Radford C, Prince A, Lewis K, et al. Factors which impact the delivery of genetic risk assessment services focused on inherited cancer genomics: expanding the role and reach of certified genetics professionals. *J Genet Counsel.* 2014;23:522–530.

CHAPTER 4

Laboratory Methods in Cancer Genetics Testing

Rosa M. Xicola and Allen Bale

As technology advances, the identification of genetic factors that trigger cancer development in the hereditary setting is advancing as well. New conditions are being established, and genetic testing companies are offering an increasing catalog of genes associated with hereditary syndromes.

Cancer develops due to defects in genes involved in essential cellular processes. Hereditary cancer syndromes can be grouped based on defects in two overarching cellular processes:

- DNA repair pathways; examples include hereditary breast and ovarian cancer syndrome 22(*BRCA1/2*, *PALB2*), Lynch syndrome (*MLH1*, *MSH2*, *MSH6*, *PMS2*), polyposis syndromes (*MUTYH*, *NTHL1*), Li-Fraumeni syndrome (*TP53*), Ataxia-telangiectasia (*ATM*), Fanconi anemia (*FANCD*), and DICER syndrome (*DICER*).
- Cell proliferation and signaling pathways; examples include familial adenomatous polyposis (*APC*), neurofibromatosis type 1 (*NF1*), familial retinoblastoma (*RB*), multiple endocrine neoplasia type 1/2 (*MEN1/2*), Cowden syndrome (*PTEN*), Peutz-Jeghers syndrome (*STK11*), hereditary diffuse gastric cancer syndrome (*CDH1*), Carney syndrome (*PRKAR1A*), and juvenile polyposis (*BMPR1A*, *SMAD4*).

In the following sections we will discuss the types of germline defects that cause these syndromes and the most up-to-date methodology to identify those defects.

■ TYPES OF GENETIC ALTERATIONS AFFECTING CANCER PREDISPOSITION GENES

Small-Scale Alterations

At the single-gene level, there are two main types of variants that affect nucleotide sequence: single-base nucleotide variants and small insertions or deletions. Single-base nucleotide variants that are most likely to affect the protein encoded by a gene include missense (change in amino acid), nonsense (introduction of a premature termination codon), loss of the normal initiation codon, loss of the normal stop codon, and alteration of the splice sites in

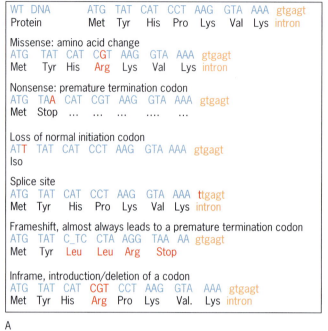

A

B

FIGURE 4.1: A. Nucleotide variants. B. Chromosomal variant.

the intronic bases that flank the exons (Figure 4.1A). Occasionally synonymous variants, which do not alter an encoded amino acid, can affect gene function through effects on splicing. Splice sites are located at the boundary of an exon and an intron. Splicing variants in these sequences can disrupt ribonucleic acid (RNA) splicing, resulting in the loss of exons or the inclusion of introns. Insertion or deletions of small nucleotide sequences can result in frameshift variants or in-frame alterations. Frameshift variants almost always lead to a premature termination codon and act similarly to nonsense variants.

Large-Scale Alterations

Structural variants include deletions, duplications, inversions, and translocations (Figure 4.1B) and can occur between chromosomal sequences affecting several exons of the same gene or several genes and bigger chromosomal regions.

◼ LABORATORY METHODS TO TEST GENETIC ALTERATIONS

Next-Generation Sequencing

Next-generation sequencing (NGS) has revolutionized molecular testing and is now the gold-standard technique used in cancer genetic testing. Hereditary cancer predisposition is typically diagnosed by sequencing germline deoxyribonucleic acid (DNA) extracted from blood leukocytes or saliva. The DNA in saliva, while minimally contaminated with mouth flora, contains mainly leukocyte DNA with a smaller amount of buccal cell DNA. For patients undergoing genetic testing who have leukemia or other malignancies of blood-forming tissues, cultured fibroblasts from a skin biopsy are a reliable source of germline DNA, uncontaminated with malignant clones that may confound germline testing due to the presence of somatic cancer-related variants. Likewise, patients who have undergone bone marrow transplantation from a donor must be tested from a source of DNA other than blood or saliva.

RNA sequencing is sometimes used as an adjunct to DNA sequencing, mainly for its ability to detect aberrant splice forms that may indicate intronic DNA variants that interfere with normal RNA splicing and decrease or eliminate production of protein from one allele of a gene.

Targeted vs. Global Sequencing Next-generation sequencers are designed to sequence whole genomes and originally were used largely for that purpose. Although the cost of DNA and RNA sequencing continues to plummet, the technology remains at a stage in which clinical whole-genome sequencing stretches the financial limitations of healthcare systems. In addition, most of the clinically relevant information in the human genome is confined to the coding regions and regulatory regions of genes—only 1% to 2% of the whole genome—so it is cost-effective to select regions that will be sequenced.

A commonly used method for sequencing only the relevant portions of the genome is whole-exome sequencing (WES). Prior to sequencing, human DNA is hybridized to an array containing exons, and only those DNA fragments that bind the array undergo sequencing. This captured DNA includes exons, flanking exon–intron boundaries, and flanking upstream and downstream sequences that may contain regulatory elements.

More restricted, custom capture libraries can be used to target specific portions of the genome of interest, such as a set of candidate genes for a particular disease. Many such gene panels have been devised for hereditary cancer syndromes, and the custom capture approach is commonly used for multigene panel testing (MGPT) offered by clinical laboratories.

Sequencing Methodology There are two basic strategies for high-throughput sequencing: sequencing by synthesis and nanopore sequencing. Sequencing by synthesis is similar to traditional Sanger sequencing but performed on a highly miniaturized, massively parallel scale. For example, a state-of-the-art Sanger sequencing instrument can analyze 96 DNA sequences simultaneously and read 2.75 million bases per day. State-of-the-art high-throughput instruments can sequence 20 billion DNA molecules simultaneously and read over 1 trillion bases per day.

The basic methodology is for a DNA polymerase molecule to replicate a single-stranded nucleic acid template. As the template is replicated, the sequencing machine detects each nucleotide that is added. Two commonly used platforms—Illumina and Ion Torrent—use clones of amplified DNA molecules as a template and provide short-sequence reads in the range of 200 bases. One platform, Pacific Biosciences, sequences single DNA molecules in real time and provides reads thousands of bases long. Because the polymerase used by Pacific Biosciences pauses slightly at the sites of methylated bases, this technology has some capacity to evaluate both DNA sequence and DNA methylation simultaneously.

Nanopore sequencing is based on translocation of nucleotides through a nanopore, which results in a characteristic current change that is converted into a base-pair read. An enzyme attached to the nanopore binds to a single strand of DNA and unzips the DNA one base pair at a time. Nanopore DNA sequencing offers the possibility of a label-free, single-molecule approach that can be performed without the need for sample amplification. The advantages of nanopore sequencing are the very long read lengths that can be achieved and the ability of the nanopores to distinguish and correctly interpret modified bases from unmodified bases. Detection of 5-methylcytosine allows for global methylation analysis simultaneously with sequence analysis.

Bioinformatics Once the sequencers generate a file for each sample being sequenced, a significant bioinformatics effort takes place to identify variants.

A standard bioinformatics pipeline to identify single nucleotide changes and small insertion/deletions is structured in three main sequential processes[1]: base calling, alignment, and variant calling. Each step results in three NGS files: FASTQ, BAM (binary sequence alignment file), and VCF, respectively (Figure 4.2).

FASTQ files are text files containing the sequence of the reads with a quality score for each base, represented as an ASCII character.[2] BAM files are the binary version of SAM files. A Sequence Alignment Map (SAM) file is a text file that contains the read sequences aligned to a reference genome sequence.[3] NGS data can be visualized using the BAM files (Figure 4.3).

The end result of NGS is the generation of a Variant Call Format file (VCF file). VCF files are text files that contain a header describing the fields in the body of the file followed by eight mandatory columns of information. Each row of the file represents one variant identified in the analysis. For each variant there is a description of chromosome, genomic position, reference nucleotide, alternate nucleotide, and sequencing quality metrics.[4]

NGS can also identify structural variants when sequencing reads do not align properly to the reference genome. There are four types of methods: read-count, read-pair, split-read, and *de novo* assembly. Specialized algorithms have been developed for each method.[5]

Read-count methods are based on depth of coverage. Depth of coverage is the number of unique reads that include a given nucleotide in the reconstructed sequence. Assuming the

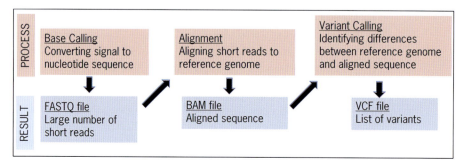

FIGURE 4.2: Schematic NGS bioinformatics pipeline.

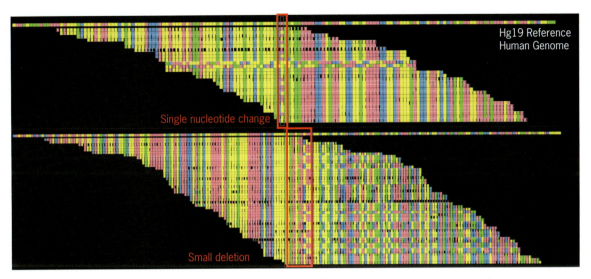

FIGURE 4.3: Sequencing reads are visualized using the aligned BAM file.

sequencing process is uniform, the number of reads aligning to a region follows a Poisson distribution and is expected to be proportional to the number of times the region appears in the DNA sample: a genomic region that has been deleted will have fewer reads aligning to it than the same region in normal DNA. Likewise, duplicated regions will have more reads than the same region in normal DNA.[6]

Read-pair methods identify structural variants by locating groups of the discordant read pairs described earlier. This method compares the average insert size between the actual sequenced read pairs with the expected size based on a reference genome. In paired-end sequencing, the DNA fragments are expected to have a specific distribution around the insert size. This method detects deviations from expected library insert size (reads the map at inconsistent distances).[7]

Split-read methods take advantage of paired-end sequencing. Split reads contain the breakpoint of the structural variant. The identification of a pair, one end of which is anchored to the reference genome and the other end maps imprecisely, could be explained by the presence of a structural variant or indel breakpoint.[8]

De novo assembly is based on directly mapping structural variant breakpoints at the nucleotide level without relying on the discordant mapping of paired-end reads, if the reads are long and accurate enough. Direct comparison of individual genomes by *de novo* assembly is performed rather than comparing to a reference genome.[9]

Other Methods Used in DNA-Based Diagnostics

Other traditional methods used for deletions and duplications detection include Multiple Ligation Probe Amplification (MLPA) and microarray-based comparative genomic hybridization (aCGH). These technologies are not based on NGS but are still widely used.

MLPA, a registered trademark of MRC-Holland, is used to determine the copy number of all exons in a gene or multiple genes, thus identifying any copy-number variation present.

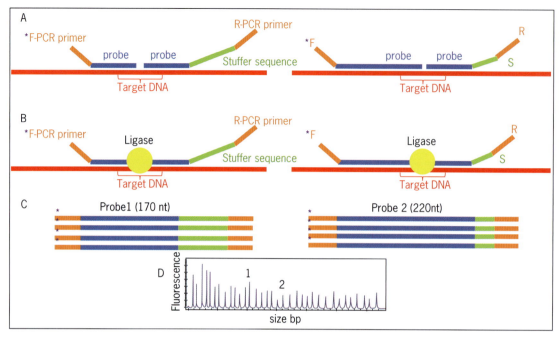

FIGURE 4.4: MLPA steps. A. Hybridization. B. Ligation. C. Amplification. D. Capillary gel electrophoresis.

Each probe is complementary to the DNA target region, and all probes have the same poly-merase chain reaction (PCR) primer binding sequences. One of the probe pair contains the fluorescent forward PCR primer, and the other probe the reverse PCR primer and a stuffer. The size of the stuffer varies between probes, and therefore each amplification has a unique length (Figure 4.4A). In the next step, the enzyme ligase will ligate both probes for further amplification. However, if there is any type of mismatch, the enzyme will not be able to ligate both probes and there will be no amplification (Figure 4.4B and C). The number of probe ligation products is a measure for the number of target sequences in the sample. Lastly, after amplification, capillary electrophoresis will separate by fragment size and the fluorescence signal will be recorded (Figure 4.4D). By comparing each sample to a reference, you can obtain a ratio signal for each peak. When the ratio is <0.5, you have identified a deletion, but if the ratio >1.5, that indicates duplication.

Microarray-aCGH[10] is a technique based on the hybridization of labeled DNA from the patient and a reference DNA to a set of probes designed based on the reference genome. Each DNA is labeled with different fluorophores, and the relative hybridization intensity of the patient and reference signals at a given location are proportional to the relative copy number of those sequences in the test and reference genomes. aCGH has some detection limitations, as it can only identify unbalanced structural variants that affect copy number but not balanced variants such as inversions or translocations.

Single-site testing is used to test a known mutation already identified in a family member. The same type of germline DNA sample is used, and the identification of a specific muta-tion is performed by Sanger sequencing. However, Sanger sequencing is becoming less used nowadays, as it can miss mutations identified by NGS.

VARIANT CLASSIFICATION

Once a variant report is generated, a bioinformatics pipeline is used to annotate the variants. The output of the pipeline typically includes such parameters as population frequency, which human phenotype is associated with variants in the affected gene (e.g., associated disease in the OMIM database), whether the specific variant has been reported in people with a disease, and *in silico* predictions of pathogenicity (e.g., conservation score, Polyphen, SIFT, and others). Allele frequency is typically derived from the Genome Aggregation Database (https://gnomad.broadinstitute.org/), which includes over 100,000 individuals and has incorporated data from several older databases. Information about previous reports of a particular variant among people with disease is mainly derived from ClinVar,[14] a National Institutes of Health (NIH)–supported archival database that aggregates information about genomic variation and its relationship to human health. ClinGen[11] is a related NIH-supported project that contributes expert curation to entries in ClinVar. The Human Gene Mutation Database is a commercial source (Qiagen) of large amounts of curated data similar to ClinVar.

The detailed annotation provided by bioinformatics pipelines[11,14] is useful in determining the likelihood that a variant is causing a patient's phenotype. For example, cancer predisposition syndromes are almost always rare conditions with a low frequency in the general population. A variant with an allele frequency in a control population that is greater than a few percentage points is inconsistent with a disease-causing mutation. An allele frequency over 5% in population databases is considered strong support for a benign interpretation.[12] In contrast, a variant with a frequency lower than 1/100,000 in the general population that has been reported as pathogenic in the ClinVar database is almost certainly causing disease.

Rare variants in cancer-predisposing genes are considered potential disease-related candidates. One hundred and fourteen cancer-predisposing genes have been described. Mutations in these confer high or moderate risks of cancer (>two-fold relative risks), and at least 5% of individuals with relevant mutations develop cancer.[13]

This variety of resources provides a wide body of knowledge, and the incorporation of NGS as a routine test in clinical laboratories is resulting in the identification of new variants never reported before. Thus, there is a need for proper evaluation and classification of variants

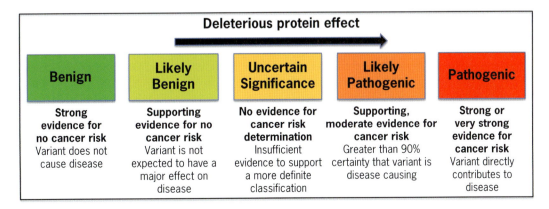

FIGURE 4.5: Five-tier variant classification system.

based on their potential effect on protein function and association with disease. For that reason, clinical laboratories are developing robust programs that properly classify new genetic variants. In order to help harmonize this process, the American College of Medical Genetics and Genomics (ACMG) and the Association for Molecular Pathology (AMP) published a set of standards and guidelines for the interpretation of sequence variants.[12] The guidelines recommend classification of variants based on the strength of the association of the variant and the development of the disease and based on the certainty of that classification. This recommendation has been translated for the clinical laboratories in a five-tier classification, from benign to pathogenic (Figure 4.5).

UNDERSTANDING A GENETIC TESTING RESULT REPORT

Genetic testing reports have four main sections: a summary result section, an interpretation and description of the mutations identified, a section with information regarding the assay performed, and a clinical management section based on the findings.

The results summary section will explain the findings identified and state the results. These can include:

1. Pathogenic variants: Meets strict criteria based on scientific and medical evidence as a disease-causing variant. Nevertheless, genetic testing should be used in conjunction with other clinical information when possible.

2. Likely pathogenic variants: Sufficient evidence exists to justify using the genetic test result in clinical decision-making when combined with other evidence for the disease in question (e.g., supporting biochemical findings, imaging studies, or physical findings).

3. Variant of uncertain significance (VUS): Variant for which current information is insufficient to determine pathogenicity. A substantial proportion of VUSs prove to be benign as more data become available. A VUS should not be used in clinical decision-making. Efforts to resolve the classification of the variant as pathogenic or benign should be undertaken.

4. No variants reported: No differences from the standard human genome reference sequence were found, or only genetic variants known to be benign polymorphisms were found, or only silent variants or deep intronic variants not known to affect gene function were found.

5. Incidental findings: In addition to variants related to the patient's indication for testing, incidental findings of unsuspected, disease-related mutations may be discovered when whole-exome or whole-genome sequencing is the methodology used to query cancer genes. The American College of Medical Genetics and Genomics has issued a set of guidelines that establish the standard of care for reporting incidental findings.[16] Among 60 genes considered "actionable" and therefore reportable—that is, underlie a serious or life-threatening disease for which there is established curative or preventive treatment—nearly half fall into the category of cancer predisposition. Most of the remaining genes are related to cardiac disease. The ACMG has issued conflicting statements regarding informed consent for whole-genome sequencing or WES analysis, but in the most recent publication suggested that patients should be able to "opt out" of receiving secondary findings.[14] However, it should be pointed out that informed consent for clinical laboratory testing is not the standard of care in medical practice, and "genetic

exceptionalism" is not universally accepted by practitioners of genetics.[15] Highly consequential incidental findings are much more common in radiologic studies, such as computed tomography (CT) scans and magnetic resonance imaging (MRI), than in exome or genome sequencing, and case law sets clear precedents for the radiologist's responsibility to report incidental findings with no patient consent.[16]

The interpretation and description of the findings identified would summarize the evidence that allows the clinical laboratory to classify the variant in one of the tiers mentioned earlier. In this section, clinical laboratories would reference any resource they use to perform their classification.

The assay information section will include a detailed explanation of the assay performed and what specific methodology was used for analysis. This section will describe the genes analyzed with their sequence IDs, and it will mention which techniques were used in the assay.

Lastly, every report will conclude with a clinical section describing the clinical phenotype associated with alterations in the gene identified. This section will also describe the gene-related cancer risks and a description of clinical management to be considered.

GENETIC TESTING REGULATIONS

As the field of genomics advances, genetic and genomic tests are becoming more common, yet most genetic tests today are not directly regulated under the Food and Drug Administration (FDA).

The Centers for Medicare & Medicaid Services (CMS) regulates all laboratories that test (including genetic testing) humans in the United States through the Clinical Laboratory Improvement Amendments (CLIA). The objective of the CLIA program is to ensure good laboratory practices, including proper labeling of samples entering the laboratory, tracking of samples throughout the laboratory process to avoid sample mix-ups, quality control of reagents and equipment, appropriate standard operating procedures, proper training and certification of laboratory personnel, and proper methods to validate new tests and monitor the performance of existing tests. CLIA does not specifically monitor analytical validity or clinical utility of genetic tests.

Most genetic testing for cancer predisposition falls under the category of complex, laboratory-developed tests (LDTs), where the test is developed by a CLIA-approved laboratory and does not rely on commercial FDA-approved kits. To date, the FDA has practiced enforcement discretion for LDTs. This means that LDTs are being used in the clinic without the FDA's assessment of their analytical and clinical validity. However, the FDA has drafted new guidance to describe how it intends to regulate NGS genetic tests and verify their analytical and clinical validity. Since they are still in draft form, they are not being implemented yet (https://www.genome.gov/10002335/regulation-of-genetic-tests/). Indeed, there is a need for newer types of regulations as the landscape of genetic testing is starting to change.

DIRECT-TO-CONSUMER GENETIC TESTING

A new wave of tests is emerging in the form of direct-to-consumer genetic testing. There is a clear public interest in acquiring personal genetic information.[17] Genetic companies are moving from ancestry markers and genealogic relationships to actual genetic testing of actionable genes.[18] As a clear, new turn on direct-to-consumer testing, recently the FDA granted permission to 23andMe to report the presence of any of the three common Ashkenazi Jew mutations in *BRCA1/2* (https://www.fda.gov/NewsEvents/Newsroom/PressAnnouncements/ucm599560.htm). However, the test does not analyze the whole gene, and the mutations tested are seen almost exclusively in a specific ethnicity. In the Ashkenazi Jew population, 2.5% of individuals carry one of these three mutations.[19] However, the overall frequency of any type of mutation in *BRCA1/2* is about 0.25% for the rest of the population.[20] Therefore, testing those three mutations outside the Ashkenazi Jewish population does not provide meaningful information.

A hybrid model where consumers purchase the test but a physician orders it on behalf of the customer is gaining market acceptance. This model allows the consumer's own clinician to order the test, or the testing laboratory provides an independent physician. This physician reviews every case before placing the order. However, there is usually no interaction between consumer and physician, which is viewed as a drawback by some experts in the field. Veritas, Helix, and Color Genomics use this model. These companies offer testing for ancestry, disease-risk assessment, or medication response based on the individual's genetic makeup. Veritas also offers whole-genome sequencing.

The application of NGS to clinical use has transitioned from a technique limited to academic and research institutions to a widely utilized tool in private industry. The FDA has opened the door to application of this technology in direct-to-consumer testing that bypasses the traditional medical infrastructure for pretest counseling and posttest medical interpretation of data. With the plummeting cost and wide availability of comprehensive cancer testing, new scalable models of genetic counseling are being developed, and the benefits and risks of direct-to-consumer medical testing are being explored.

▨ SOMATIC TISSUE TESTING

Testing for inherited conditions focuses on analyzing germline DNA. However, genetic analysis for somatic mutations in tumor tissue is also offered in the context of precision medicine and targeted therapy. Often somatic mutations are detected via paired germline and tumor testing, which can identify inherited germline pathogenic variants as well as somatic variants. It is not uncommon for somatic tumor testing to uncover an unsuspected, inherited predisposition because many cancer syndromes are not 100% penetrant (gene carriers may show no disease), and particularly in small families there may be no obvious family history of cancer. Genetic counseling is not typically pursued prior to somatic tumor testing, but patients should be informed that this testing could uncover a genetic disorder.

In the setting of mismatch repair deficiency, tumor analysis can identify (1) microsatellite instability, which indicates response to immunotherapy treatment[21,22]; (2) *BRAF* V600E mutation, which is associated with poorer prognosis and different therapeutic response[23]; (3) *MLH1* methylation, which indicates that the tumor is sporadic and not due to Lynch syndrome; and (4) a mismatch repair gene mutation confirming Lynch syndrome when the analysis includes germline testing of paired samples. Recently, the identification of somatic-only mutations in the mismatch repair genes has been associated with a subtype of cancer called Lynch-like syndrome.[24,25] Some of these Lynch-like syndrome tumors have been associated with germline variants in other DNA repair genes.[26–29]

Finally, paired testing would identify germline and somatic mutations in homologous recombination repair genes, which would identify (1) patients that are at an increased risk of developing breast, ovarian, and other cancers and (2) and tumors that would benefit from poly-ADP ribose polymerase (PARP) inhibitors.[30–32]

References

1. Roy S, Coldren C, Karunamurthy A, et al. Standards and guidelines for validating next-generation sequencing bioinformatics pipelines: a joint recommendation of the Association for Molecular Pathology and the College of American Pathologists. *J Mol Diagn*. 2018;20(1):4–27.

2. Cock PJ, Fields CJ, Goto N, et al. The Sanger FASTQ file format for sequences with quality scores, and the Solexa/Illumina FASTQ variants. *Nucleic Acids Res*. 2010;38(6):1767–1771.

3. Li H, Handsaker B, Wysoker A, et al. The Sequence Alignment/Map format and SAM tools. *Bioinformatics*. 2009;25(16):2078–2079.

4. Danecek P, Auton A, Abecasis G, et al. The variant call format and VCF tools. *Bioinformatics*. 2011;27(15):2156–2158.

5. Tattini L, D'Aurizio R, Magi A. Detection of genomic structural variants from next-generation sequencing data. *Front Bioeng Biotechnol*. 2015;3:92.

6. Magi A, Tattini L, Pippucci T, et al. Read count approach for DNA copy number variants detection. *Bioinformatics*. 2012;28(4):470–478.

7. Korbel JO, Urban AE, Affourtit JP, et al. Paired-end mapping reveals extensive structural variation in the human genome. *Science*. 2007;318(5849):420–426.

8. Karakoc E, Alkan C, O'Roak BJ, et al. Detection of structural variants and indels within exome data. *Nat Methods*. 2011;9(2):176–178.

9. Nijkamp JF, van den Broek MA, Geertman JM, et al. De novo detection of copy number variation by co-assembly. *Bioinformatics*. 2012;28(24):3195–3202.

10. Pinkel D, Albertson DG. Comparative genomic hybridization. *Annu Rev Genomics Hum Genet*. 2005; 6:331–354.

11. Rehm HL, Berg JS, Brooks LD, et al. ClinGen–the Clinical Genome Resource. *N Engl J Med*. 2015;372(23):2235–2242.

12. Richards S, Aziz N, Bale S, et al. Standards and guidelines for the interpretation of sequence variants: a joint consensus recommendation of the American College of Medical Genetics and Genomics and the Association for Molecular Pathology. *Genet Med*. 2015;17(5):405–424.

13. Rahman N. Realizing the promise of cancer predisposition genes. *Nature*. 2014;505(7483):302–308.

14. Kalia SS, Adelman K, Bale SJ, et al. Recommendations for reporting of secondary findings in clinical exome and genome sequencing, 2016 update (ACMG SF v2.0): a policy statement of the American College of Medical Genetics and Genomics. *Genet Med*. 2017;19(2):249–255.

15. Evans JP, Burke W. Genetic exceptionalism. Too much of a good thing? *Genet Med*. 2008;10(7):500–501.

16. Clayton EW, Haga S, Kuszler P, et al. Managing incidental genomic findings: legal obligations of clinicians. *Genet Med*. 2013;15(8):624–629.

17. Roberts JS, Gornick MC, Carere DA, et al. Direct-to-consumer genetic testing: user motivations, decision making, and perceived utility of results. *Public Health Genomics*. 2017;20(1):36–45.

18. Check Hayden E. The rise and fall and rise again of 23andMe. *Nature*. 2017;550(7675):174–177.

19. Roa BB, Boyd AA, Volcik K, et al. Ashkenazi Jewish population frequencies for common mutations in BRCA1 and BRCA2. *Nat Genet*. 1996;14(2):185–187.

20. McClain MR, Palomaki GE, Nathanson KL, et al. Adjusting the estimated proportion of breast cancer cases associated with BRCA1 and BRCA2 mutations: public health implications. *Genet Med*. 2005;7(1):28–33.

21. Le DT, Uram JN, Wang H, et al. PD-1 Blockade in tumors with mismatch-repair deficiency. *N Engl J Med*. 2015;372(26):2509–2520.

22. Le DT, Durham JN, Smith KN, et al. Mismatch repair deficiency predicts response of solid tumors to PD-1 blockade. *Science*. 2017;357(6349):409–413.

23. Caputo F, Santini C, Bardasi C, et al. BRAF-mutated colorectal cancer: clinical and molecular insights. *Int J Mol Sci*. 2019;20(21):5369.

24. Mensenkamp AR, Vogelaar IP, van Zelst-Stams WA, et al. Somatic mutations in MLH1 and MSH2 are a frequent cause of mismatch-repair deficiency in Lynch syndrome-like tumors. *Gastroenterology*. 2014;146(3):643–646.e8.

25. Geurts-Giele WR, Leenen CH, Dubbink HJ, et al. Somatic aberrations of mismatch repair genes as a cause of microsatellite-unstable cancers. *J Pathol*. 2014;234(4):548–559.

26. Xicola RM, Clark JR, Carroll T, et al. Implication of DNA repair genes in Lynch-like syndrome. *Familial Cancer*. 2019;18(3):331–342.

27. Xavier A, Olsen MF, Lavik LA, et al. Comprehensive mismatch repair gene panel identifies variants in patients with Lynch-like syndrome. *Mol Genet Genomic Med*. 2019;7(8):e850.

28. Castillejo A, Vargas G, Castillejo MI, et al. Prevalence of germline MUTYH mutations among Lynch-like syndrome patients. *Eur J Cancer*. 2014;50(13):2241–2250.

29. Jansen AM, van Wezel T, van den Akker BE, et al. Combined mismatch repair and POLE/POLD1 defects explain unresolved suspected Lynch syndrome cancers. *Eur J Hum Genet*. 2016;24(7):1089–1092.

30. Fong PC, Boss DS, Yap TA, et al. Inhibition of poly(ADP-ribose) polymerase in tumors from BRCA mutation carriers. *N Engl J Med*. 2009;361(2):123–134.

31. Mateo J, Carreira S, Sandhu S, et al. DNA-repair defects and olaparib in metastatic prostate cancer. *N Engl J Med*. 2015;373(18):1697–1708.

32. Mirza MR, Monk BJ, Herrstedt J, et al. Niraparib maintenance therapy in platinum-sensitive, recurrent ovarian cancer. *N Engl J Med*. 2016;375(22):2154–2164.

CHAPTER 5

Breast Cancer

Juliana Costa, Mariya Rozenblit, Julia Foldi, and Erin W. Hofstatter

■ INTRODUCTION

Breast cancer is the most commonly diagnosed cancer among American women, with nearly 276,500 invasive diagnoses expected in 2020 in the United States alone.[1] Over the past three decades, treatment for breast cancer has improved dramatically, including new systemic treatments, surgical and radiation techniques, molecular profiling, and imaging modalities. Despite these advances, breast cancer remains the second-leading cause of female cancer deaths in the United States, with over 42,000 deaths estimated to occur in 2020.[1]

If breast cancer morbidity and mortality rates are to improve, more must be done to increase early detection and prevention rates by identifying the women at highest risk for breast cancer. Effective breast cancer screening and prevention strategies have been developed, such as genetic testing, use of breast magnetic resonance imaging (MRI), preventive medications, and risk-reducing surgeries. However, broad implementation of these measures has been limited to date, in part due to lack of available training for providers who directly care for patients at increased risk.

As such, the aim of this chapter is to provide a practical, clinical approach to breast cancer risk assessment, genetic testing, and risk management for patients deemed to be at increased risk of breast cancer. Specific topics include breast cancer risk factors, family history risk modeling, referral criteria for genetic testing and interpretation of testing results, clinical management of high-risk patients with either a specific hereditary breast cancer syndrome or increased risk based on family history, and discussion on how these syndromes might specifically affect breast cancer treatment.

■ BREAST CANCER RISK ASSESSMENT

The purpose of formal breast cancer risk assessment should be to identify those women at highest risk based on personal or family history and, in particular, those who require referral for genetic counseling and testing. Identifying high-risk patients allows an opportunity for providers to counsel their patients on potential breast cancer risk reduction options, such as enhanced screening, surgical interventions, and/or risk-reducing medications. Moreover, breast cancer risk assessments can be used to counsel both genetic mutation carriers and noncarriers on how best to lower their risk of breast cancer, as well as other cancers, through appropriate screening and healthy lifestyle modifications.

Breast Cancer Risk Factors

Risk factors for breast cancer have traditionally been grouped into six major categories, namely demographic, familial/genetic, reproductive/hormonal, lifestyle, personal history, and other causes of risk. Each of these groups are discussed in detail here and are summarized in Table 5.1.

It is important to recognize that breast cancer risk factors vary in terms of strength of association with breast cancer risk. Major "do-not-miss" risk factors for breast cancer include age, female gender, highly penetrant genetic mutations, strong family history of breast cancer, chest irradiation exposure, prior history of breast cancer, and breast atypia.[2] It is crucial that these specific factors be queried as part of formal breast cancer risk assessment.

It should also be noted that any specific risk factor in an individual patient does not in and of itself directly explain a cancer diagnosis; rather, cancer development in a given patient is typically felt to be the result of several additive or synergistic elements, including the interaction of a person's underlying genetics, with the given collection of lifetime exposures/habits, and—ultimately—the random chance that a specific deoxyribonucleic acid (DNA) replication error occurs in a given cell that crosses a threshold to cancer development.[2] Breast cancer development is complex, and there is typically not a single "reason" why a person may go on to develop a cancer. Instead, breast cancer is thought to result from the accumulation of damaging events over time, layered upon the background of a given individual's baseline genetic makeup.

Finally, in counseling a patient about breast cancer risk, it should be recognized that some risk factors are modifiable, while others are not.[2] For example, demographics such as age and gender are fixed, whereas lifestyle choices and weight are potentially modifiable.[3] Ironically, it is the strongest of the known breast cancer risk factors that are, unfortunately, nonmodifiable. However, given that breast cancer development is ultimately the result of a number of factors, it is important to counsel patients around those risk factors that *can* be changed in order to maximize breast cancer risk reduction.[3]

TABLE 5.1: Breast Cancer Risk Factors

Demographic	Familial/genetic	Reproductive/ hormonal	Lifestyle	Personal History	Others
*Gender *Age **Ethnicity**	**Family history** *Genetic **predisposition**	Age at menarche Age of first full-term pregnancy Breastfeeding Oral contraceptives Menopause Use of hormone replacement therapy	Obesity Weight gain Physical activity Diet Alcohol use Tobacco use	***Prior history of breast cancer** ***Breast density** ***Breast atypia** ***Chest radiation exposure**	DES use Long-term night shift work

*Major/strong risk factor (relative risk >3)

Demographic Factors

Gender and age Gender and age are the two strongest risk factors for breast cancer, with breast cancer affecting females at 150× the rate of males.[1] The estimated number of new breast cancer cases in the United States in 2020 is 271,000, of which about 2620 are men.[1] As in most epithelial malignancies, breast cancer incidence increases with age. The median age at the time of breast cancer diagnosis is approximately 62 years.[1] A woman living in the United States has a 12.4% lifetime risk of being diagnosed with breast cancer, which equates to about one in every eight women.[1] This incidence rate has slowly increased since the 1970s, at which time the lifetime risk was 1 in 11.[1] This increase has been attributed to a number of factors, including longer life expectancy, changes in reproductive pattern, post-menopausal hormone use, the rising prevalence of obesity, and increased detection through mammographic screening.[4]

Breast cancer in men accounts for less than 1% of the total number of breast cancer cases in the United States, with lifetime risks for men estimated to be roughly 1 in 1000.[5] Compared to women, men typically present with more advanced-stage disease at diagnosis due to decreased awareness of the possibility of developing breast cancer and, consequently, delayed diagnosis. Similar to women, the incidence in men increases with age, with cases most commonly diagnosed between the ages of 60 and 70.[5] Several other factors have been identified that contribute to the risk of developing breast cancer in men, including radiation exposure, *BRCA1/2* mutations, family history of breast cancer, and hyperestrogenic states, which can result from disorders such as Klinefelter syndrome, gynecomastia, alcohol use, liver cirrhosis, and obesity.[5]

Ethnicity There are differences in breast cancer incidence and death rates by race and ethnicity, with non-Hispanic white and non-Hispanic black women having a higher incidence than other racial and ethnic groups.[6] Of note, while non-Hispanic white women are known to have a higher breast cancer incidence rate in the age 65 to 84 group, non-Hispanic black women have a higher incidence before age 40 and are more likely to die from breast cancer at every age.[6] Explanations for these outcome disparities are a topic of intense research and have been attributed to both biological and social factors.

Familial/Genetic Factorvs

Family history Family history of breast cancer is associated with an increased risk of breast cancer in both men and women.[7] The increase in risk is the highest when a first-degree relative (i.e., a parent, child, or sibling) has breast cancer.[7] Compared to women without a family history, risk of breast cancer is about 2 times higher for women with one affected first-degree female relative, and 3 to 4 times higher if more than one first-degree relative is affected.[7] The risk is even higher for women whose first-degree relative was diagnosed at a younger age or if breast cancer was diagnosed in both breasts. It is important to note that most women who develop breast cancer do not have a family history of the disease; in fact, only ~15% to 20% of breast cancers are associated with a family history of breast cancer.[7]

Genetic predisposition Genetic predisposition and inherited cancer syndromes are among the strongest of breast cancer risk factors, though account for only ~10% of all breast cancer.[7] Genetic mutations vary in terms of their associated cancer risks, with high penetrant mutations such as *BRCA1/2*, *TP53*, and *PALB2* carrying lifetime risks approaching 50% to 85%.[7] Other known hereditary breast cancer mutations have more moderate or low penetrance risk, such as *ATM* and *CHEK2*, with lifetime risks ranging closer to 20% to 40%.[7] These and other known mutations are discussed in more detail in Section III of this chapter.

Reproductive/Hormonal Factors Overall, it is thought to be the length of menstrual life—particularly the fraction of it occurring prior to the first full-term pregnancy—that has a major effect on the lifetime risk of breast cancer in women. As such, there are three events in a woman's life that have a major impact on her risk of developing breast cancer, namely age at menarche, age at first parity, and age at menopause.[8] Other lifetime exposures that affect hormone levels, such as hormone replacement therapy, birth control pills, and breastfeeding, also play a role in breast cancer risk.[9]

Age at menarche or first menstruation The average age of menarche in the United States is age 12 to 13. Women who started their menstruation prior to age 12 are felt to have a slight increased lifetime risk of breast cancer, whereas those women with later menarche appear to have decreased risk.[10]

Age at first full-term pregnancy Women who give birth to their first child at age 35 or younger appear to have a lower lifetime risk of breast cancer compared to those women who give birth at an older age or who are nulliparous.[11] For example, one study showed that women who give birth over the age of 35 have been found to have a 40% higher risk of breast cancer compared to those women who give birth before age 20.[11] Having a greater number of children also appears to decrease breast cancer risk.[11] It is important to note, however, that there appears to be a small and transient increase in breast cancer risk in the first 10 years following a full-term pregnancy, particularly in women who are older at the time of first birth, which then dissipates over time.[11]

Age at menopause The average age of menopause in the United States is approximately age 52. Menopause that occurs late (i.e., after age 55) has been shown to increase risk of breast cancer.[12] Conversely, menopause that occurs early can be protective; one such study showed that menopause onset 10 years prior to the median (52 years) reduced the lifetime risk of breast cancer by about 35%.[12]

Breastfeeding There is a substantial body of research suggesting that breastfeeding for a year or longer slightly reduces a woman's lifetime risk of breast cancer, with longer duration of breastfeeding associated with greater risk reduction.[13] This risk reduction is estimated to be ~4% for every 12 months of breastfeeding, perhaps because breastfeeding inhibits menstruation or perhaps structural changes occur in the breast during lactation; the exact mechanism remains unknown.[13]

Oral contraceptives The use of birth control pills has previously been linked to increased breast cancer risk, although many recent studies report conflicting results.[14] A recently published, large observational cohort study assessing the association between hormonal contraceptive use and the risk of breast cancer found a statistically greater risk of breast cancer among women using contemporary hormonal contraceptives than among women who had never used hormonal contraceptives.[14] Increased risk was also seen among women who used a progestin-only intrauterine device (IUD).[14] However, it is important to note that the overall absolute increase in breast cancers diagnosed among current and recent users of any hormonal contraceptive was approximately 13 per 100,000 person-years, or approximately 1 extra breast cancer for every 7690 women using hormonal contraception for 1 year.[14] Importantly, the increased risk of breast cancer disappeared 5 years following discontinuation of contraceptives, even among women with the longest cumulative contraceptive use. Other studies have not shown evidence of persisting risk after discontinuation of hormonal contraceptives. As such, while it is reasonable to initially consider nonhormonal methods of contraception for women at increased risk of breast cancer, use of oral contraceptives is not contraindicated and should be used if clinically indicated.

Hormone replacement therapy Combined postmenopausal hormone replacement therapy (HRT; estrogen and progestin) is known to be associated with an increased risk of developing breast cancer, though observed absolute increases remain small. Risk appears to persist after discontinuation of therapy, albeit at a decreased rate. However, estrogen-only hormone replacement does not appear to carry the increased risk of breast cancer seen with combined HRT and, in fact, some studies suggest it may even lower breast cancer risk in women.[15,16] It is important to remember that postmenopausal estrogen-only HRT has been associated with an increased incidence of endometrial cancers, and this formulation is therefore safest in those women who have had a hysterectomy.[2]

Lifestyle Factors Modifiable risk factors such as obesity, diet, and physical activity have gained more attention in breast cancer epidemiology in recent years as risk factors for the development of breast cancer.

Obesity Postmenopausal risk of breast cancer is about 1.5 times higher in overweight women and 2 times higher in obese women when compared with lean women, most likely due at least in part to higher levels of estrogen, which is primarily produced in fat tissue in postmenopausal women.[17] Furthermore, obesity is linked to type 2 diabetes, which has recently been associated with postmenopausal breast cancer development.[18] In contrast, obesity seems to be protective against premenopausal breast cancer in women ages 40 to 49, the mechanism of which remains unclear but appears to be limited to hormone receptor–positive breast cancers.[19]

Weight gain Weight gain alone is also linked with breast cancer. In a large meta-analysis, researchers found that each 5 kg (about 11 pounds) gained during adulthood increases the risk of postmenopausal breast cancer by about 11%.[20] Weight loss has not been similarly associated with a decrease in breast cancer risk; this is more difficult to examine given that weight loss is often not sustained, and studies have so far shown inconsistent results.

Physical activity Regular physical activity has been shown to reduce the risk of multiple types of cancer, including breast cancer, and the protective effect is independent of body mass index (BMI). Recommended physical activity from the American Cancer Society includes at least 150 minutes per week of moderate-intensity exercise, such as brisk walking.[21]

Diet The relationship between diet and breast cancer risk remains controversial and is an active area of research. There is some evidence that high levels of fruit and/or vegetable consumption may reduce the risk of hormone receptor–negative breast cancers, which might be due to higher levels of carotenoids, micronutrients found in fruit and vegetables.[22] Other specific dietary recommendations from the American Cancer Society include adoption of a largely plant-based diet, limitation of red meat and processed meats, and increased intake of whole grains.[21] Portion control is additionally recommended. Though it is commonly held among the lay-public that soy intake increases breast cancer risk, studies are mixed and no definitive link between soy and breast cancer risk has been identified to date.[23]

Alcohol Numerous studies have shown that alcohol consumption increases the risk of breast cancer in women by about 7% to 10% for each 10 g of alcohol (about one standard alcoholic beverage) consumed per day on average.[21] Recommendations regarding alcohol intake vary in regard to breast cancer risk, but generally advise a limitation of an average of one serving per day for women.[24]

Tobacco use Though studies are mixed, some research suggests an increased risk of breast cancer in women who smoke, particularly long-term and heavy smokers who started smoking prior to their first pregnancy.[25] Given the common dual use of tobacco concurrently with alcohol, specific association of tobacco with breast cancer risk has been difficult to define to date.

Personal History

Prior history of breast cancer Personal history of prior breast cancer also affects breast cancer risk. Women diagnosed with breast cancer, particularly prior to age 40, have an increased risk of developing breast cancer in the opposite breast. Ductal carcinoma in situ (DCIS) is considered a potential precursor lesion to invasive breast cancer and is associated with an increased risk of developing a new invasive breast cancer. Compared to women with no history of DCIS, those with DCIS are about 10 times more likely to develop an invasive breast cancer.[25] Risks for a second primary breast cancer following a first breast cancer diagnosis are typically estimated to range from ~0.5% to 1% per year, cumulative over time.[26]

Breast atypia Lobular carcinoma in situ (LCIS) is not considered a direct precursor lesion to invasive breast cancer, but is rather a strong risk factor for breast cancer development.[27] Women with LCIS are 7 to 12 times more likely to develop invasive breast cancer in either breast than those without LCIS,[26] where women with LCIS are estimated to have a 1% to 2% annual risk of invasive breast cancer diagnosis.[26] Lesions with atypia such as atypical ductal hyperplasia (ADH) and atypical lobular hyperplasia (ALH), are associated with a 4- to 5-fold increased risk,[28] and exact risks conferred by ADH and ALH can be estimated using the Breast Cancer Risk Assessment Tool (BCRAT), also known as the Gail model,[29] discussed later in the chapter. Proliferative lesions without atypia and nonproliferative lesions such as fibroadenomas and fibrocystic changes are not strongly associated with increased risk of breast cancer.

Breast density Women with dense breast tissue on mammography also have a higher lifetime risk of developing breast cancer.[29,30] Dense breast tissue can only be determined by undergoing a mammogram.[30] Breast tissue is considered dense when >50% of the mammographic field appears to have fibrous or glandular, rather than fatty, tissue. For women between the ages of 40 and 74, approximately 43% of women have dense breasts.[31] Women with dense breasts are grouped into categories of either "heterogenous" or "extremely" dense tissue, with 40% and 10% of all women falling into each category, respectively.[31] In terms of breast cancer risk, it is primarily those women with extremely dense breast tissue that appear to have up to a 4-fold increase in risk compared to women with fatty, nondense breasts.[31] Though the exact etiology of risk related to breast density remains to be understood, it is known to be an independent risk factor for breast cancer and not entirely due to impaired ability of mammography to detect small cancers.[32]

Many different factors can influence breast density. A few include oral contraceptive pills (OCPs) and HRT, which can increase density, and age and chemoprevention therapy, which can lower it.[33]

Radiation exposure Women treated with high-dose radiation therapy to the chest between ages 10 and 30, such as for Hodgkin lymphoma, are known to have a 2-fold increase in lifetime breast cancer risk.[29] The risk appears to be largest when exposure occurs at a younger age, when breast tissue is starting to develop during puberty.[29] Increased breast cancer risk appears to begin about 8 years after radiation exposure and remains elevated for more than 3 decades of life.[29]

Other Breast Cancer Risk Factors

DES Diethylstilbestrol (DES) was given to some pregnant women in the 1940s through 1960s and was thought to lower the risk of miscarriage. It is now recognized that these women have an approximately 30% increased risk of developing breast cancer compared to women who have never taken DES.[34] Furthermore, some studies suggest that women whose mothers took DES during pregnancy might also have a slightly higher risk of breast cancer.[34]

Long-term night shift work Long-term night shifts, particularly during early adulthood, may be associated with a slightly increased risk of breast cancer.[35] This is thought to be related to disruption of melatonin production by exposure to light at night; experimental evidence suggests that melatonin, in addition to regulating sleep, may also inhibit the growth of small tumors and prevent formation of new tumors.[35] More research is needed to clarify this association.

Factors Not Known to Be Associated with Breast Cancer
There are persistent claims that certain factors are associated with an increased risk of breast cancer, which may or may not have been based on earlier studies that have since been deemed invalid. For example, abortion has been linked to an increased risk of breast cancer in an early study, which has since been disproven by a large body of solid scientific.[36] There is also no evidence of a valid association between breast implants and the risk of breast cancer.[37] Finally, there has been no convincing increased risk of breast cancer found from hair dyes, antiperspirants, cell phone use, bras, and sugar intake.[38]

Practical Breast Cancer Risk Assessment

For risk assessment to be useful and applicable to the patient, the collection of risk factor information should be translated into individual risk estimates whenever possible. This can be accomplished either by (1) the recognition and diagnosis of a hereditary cancer syndrome, where breast cancer lifetime risk estimates are known, or (2) the use of a validated breast cancer risk model, such as the IBIS Risk Model, in those patients in whom no hereditary syndrome can be found.

Recognition of Hereditary Breast Cancer Syndromes and Indications for Genetic Testing
The National Comprehensive Cancer Network (NCCN) has developed comprehensive guidelines to aid in identifying those patients who may be affected by a hereditary breast cancer syndrome. In addition to performing a thorough medical history, surgical history, and physical exam with special attention to developmental anomalies or skin lesions, evaluation of the patient requires collection of a detailed family history, which should include a three-generation pedigree of both maternal and paternal sides of the family and documentation of ethnicity on each side.[29] Information regarding type of cancer, bilaterality, and age at diagnosis for each family member should be included.[29] In addition, it should be determined if anyone in the family has undergone genetic testing and when that test was performed.[29]

It is important to recognize that, on occasion, family history can be misleading and can lead to overestimation or underestimation of risk.[29] For example, information regarding whether any family members underwent chemoprevention or risk-reducing surgery is important. Individuals with an unknown family history or who have fewer than two female first- or

TABLE 5.2: Hereditary Breast Cancer "Red Flags"		
Known Mutation in Family	**Individuals with a blood relative with a known pathogenic cancer susceptibility gene**	
Outdated Testing	Individuals who meet any other criteria but had limited/single-gene testing (i.e., before 2013)	
Personal History of Breast Cancer **PLUS** **a Personal or Family History**	Breast cancer diagnosed before the age of 45	Breast cancer diagnosed before the age of 60 with triple-negative breast cancer
	Breast cancer diagnosed between ages 46 and 50 with either: a) Unknown family history b) Second breast cancer diagnosis any age c) ≥1 blood relatives with breast, ovarian, pancreatic, or high-grade prostate cancer	Breast cancer diagnosed at any age with: a) Ashkenazi Jewish ancestry b) ≥1 blood relative ≤50 with ovarian, pancreatic, or prostate cancer at any age c) ≥3 diagnoses of breast cancer in patient d) Close blood relatives
	Male breast cancer at any age	Epithelial ovarian cancer at any age
	Endocrine pancreatic cancer at any age	Metastatic or intraductal prostate cancer at any age
	High grade (≥7 Gleason) prostate cancer with: a) Ashkenazi Jewish Ancestry b) ≥1 blood relative ≤50 with ovarian, pancreatic, or prostate cancer at any age c) ≥2 close relatives with breast or prostate cancer any grade, any age	Metastatic breast cancer to aid in systematic therapy decision-making (e.g., PARP inhibitors)
Family History of Cancer	An affected or unaffected individual with a first- or second-degree blood relative meeting any of the relevant criteria earlier	An affected or unaffected individual who does not meet the criteria listed earlier but has a probability of ≥5% of a *BRCA1/2* pathogenic variant based upon probability models (Tyrer-Cuzick, BRCAPro, etc.)

second-degree relatives may have an underestimated risk of having a familial pathogenic variant.[7] Conversely, some families appear to have many cancers, but which may in fact be related to shared cancer risk factors such as smoking, alcohol use, or obesity, rather than a hereditary cancer-causing gene.[27]

Hereditary Breast Cancer Syndrome "Red Flags": Indications for Genetic Testing
Practitioners must recognize a number of factors that warrant referral to a genetic counselor. The NCCN and others have outlined these "red flags" in detail,[7] which are summarized in Table 5.2. In general, the most significant red flags for referral for genetic counseling and testing include a personal or family history of:

- A known genetic pathogenic variant in a patient or family member
- Ashkenazi Jewish ethnicity, in combination with a personal or family history of breast, ovarian, pancreatic, or aggressive prostate cancer

- Early onset breast cancer diagnosed prior to age 50
- Multiple individuals (two or more) affected with breast cancer on the same side of the family, particularly if diagnosed prior to age 50
- More than one cancer diagnosis within a single individual, such as two breast cancers or the combination of breast and ovarian cancer
- Specific cancer types, such as "triple negative" (estrogen-, progesterone-, and Her2-negative) breast cancer diagnosed before age 60
- Ovarian cancer at any age
- Male breast cancer at any age
- Pancreatic cancer at any age
- High grade (Gleason 7 or higher) or metastatic prostate cancer
- Outdated testing (i.e., genetic testing performed prior to 2013 should prompt a new referral, given recent updates)

Identification of one or more of these "red flags" should prompt a referral to a genetic counselor.

Genetic Testing: Practical Considerations All patients who choose to pursue genetic testing should receive specific education *prior to testing* about what genetic testing entails, what information may or may not be learned from testing, and possible benefits and risks. Essential elements of genetic counseling and testing are described elsewhere in this book; please refer to Chapter 4 for details. Briefly, patients should understand several key features of genetic testing, including types of testing, possible results, and actions to take prior to testing. Specific counseling regarding test results should also occur following test completion so that results can be accurately interpreted and applied. A few key elements of genetic counseling and testing are highlighted next.

Panel testing Next-generation sequencing technology now makes it possible to simultaneously test multiple sets of genes that are associated with multiple cancer phenotypes, often referred to as "panel testing" or "multigene testing." Most patients undergoing genetic testing will have a panel test performed, as this is the most cost-effective and efficient way to diagnose a hereditary syndrome. Panels range in size from a small number of syndrome-specific genes to over 100 different genes or more. Patients should understand that many genes included on genetic testing panels do not have known cancer risks to date and remain poorly understood.

Variants of uncertain significance With modern-day genetic testing, particularly where multiple genes are being concurrently tested, there is an increased likelihood of finding a variant of unknown significance (VUS).[7] In fact, VUSs are quite common and are seen in up to 30% to 40% of all multigene genetic test results.[39] VUSs are not known to be associated with cancer risk and should be ignored clinically.[7] However, this can sometimes be confusing to patients, and patients should be counseled in advance of the test about this possible result.

Interpretation of negative testing results Depending on the results of the test, the family history of cancer may or may not be explained. In other words, a negative genetic test result does not necessarily negate the risk of having a family history of breast cancer; in fact, most women undergoing genetic testing receive benign testing results.[7] Thus, pretest and posttest genetic counseling is very important to aid in the interpretation and application of genetic testing results to help a patient understand her risk in the face of negative testing.[7]

Discrimination and privacy protection Patients should be aware that there is federal legislation, called the Genetic Information Nondiscrimination Act (GINA 2008) that protects against health insurance and employment discrimination.[40] However, there is currently no legal protection against denial of life insurance or long-term-care insurance; patients should ideally have these policies in place *prior to* undergoing genetic testing if applicable.

Direct-to-consumer testing Direct-to-consumer (DTC) genetic testing has gained popularity in the last two decades. It is important to note that, for diagnostic intent, all testing should be done in a laboratory that is certified by the Clinical Laboratory Improvement Amendments (CLIA). Results received from commercial entities, such as 23andMe or ancestry.com, are usually acquired through microarray-based single-nucleotide polymorphism (SNP) testing, have not always been validated by clinical studies, and the error rate may be high.[41,42] However, there are important instances in which DTC results are shown to hold a degree of accuracy. One specific example includes the 23andMe results for the three Ashkenazi Jewish *BRCA 1* and *2* mutations.[41] While this specific testing is reliable, receiving cancer genetic testing results from DTC companies such as 23andMe can be confusing to patients and providers, since there are hundreds of known *BRCA* mutations and several other hereditary cancer genes that are not included in this commercial DTC testing panel. Thus, providers should always approach patients based on standard risk-assessment guidelines to determine whether personal and family history warrant genetic counseling or testing.[42] All DTC results, positive or negative, should be confirmed by a genetic counselor if a patient is suspected to be of increased risk based on traditional criteria.

Tumor sequencing Some patients affected by breast or other cancers may undergo genetic sequencing of their tumor to identify therapeutic targets. It is important to understand that tumor sequencing typically examines and reports only on somatic, rather than germline, mutations.[43] In other words, most tumor sequencing tests may miss or underreport mutations that may be germline in origin.[43] Conversely, some commonly reported somatic mutations—such as *TP53*—may be unique to the tumor itself and may not be present in the germline.[44] Thus, tumor profiling does not replace germline testing and should not be a substitute for traditional comprehensive germline testing when identifiable risk factors are present.[44]

Risk Models for Familial Breast Cancer All patients who present with a strong family history of breast cancer should initially be referred for genetic testing, as described earlier. However, in most circumstances, genetic testing will not identify any hereditary cancer genetic syndrome. In these cases, application of a risk assessment model specifically designed to capture familial risk is the next best step. Several models have been developed which aim to assess an individual's breast cancer risk based on family history, including the IBIS risk model, the Claus model, and BOADICEA. These, and other common risk assessment models, are discussed in detail next.

IBIS risk model The IBIS Risk Model, also known as the Tyrer-Cuzick model, was originally created for high-risk patients and is now considered a more comprehensive model for assessing the risk of breast cancer in all patients with a suggestive family history.[2] Among available familial risk models, the IBIS model is one of the most commonly used for clinical purposes. The IBIS risk model can be accessed free online via various web links; the link to the most updated, original version of the model can be found at http://www.ems-trials.org/riskevaluator/.

a) Sample data entry

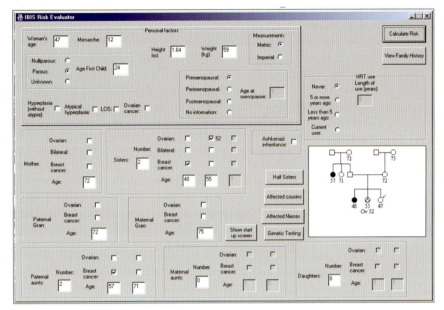

b) Sample output

After pressing the "calculate risk" button   After pressing the "print preview" button

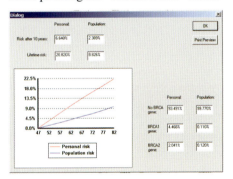
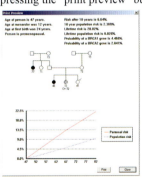

FIGURE 5.1: IBIS risk model sample data entry and output. a) Sample data entry. b) Sample output. (Data from Kurian AW, Hughes E, Bernhisel R, et al. Performance of the IBIS/Tyrer-Cuzick(TC) Model by race/ethnicity in the Women's Health Iniative, J Clin Oncol. 2020;May20;38(15 Suppl):1503.).

Designed to estimate a 5- to 10-year risk of breast cancer, as well as the lifetime risk of breast cancer until the age of 85, the IBIS model was one of the first models to incorporate both genetic risk factors and nonhereditary risk factors.[45,46] The model allows for the creation of a simple three-generation pedigree and includes information regarding known breast and ovarian cancer history, Ashkenazi Jewish ethnicity, and *BRCA1/2* genetic testing results within the patient and family.[45,46] Nonhereditary risk factors included in the model for the individual patient are current age, age at menarche, age at menopause, age at first live birth, height/weight (BMI), history of HRT, and personal history of atypical hyperplasia or LCIS.[46] Breast density has recently been added to the IBIS model as well. A representative, completed example of the IBIS risk model and its output can be seen in Figure 5.1.[46]

It is important to recognize that no risk model is perfectly accurate for an individual patient, and calculated risk may vary substantially depending on the information included in the model. It should be noted that while the estimations are intended to provide guidance for recommendations, clinical judgement is required to interpret risk and to apply results to individual patients, because overestimation of risk can lead to unnecessary testing and treatment. The IBIS model is known to overestimate risk in some cases, particularly in Hispanic patients, in patients with dense breast tissue, and in those patients with LCIS or breast atypia.[47] Model results should be interpreted with caution in these circumstances, and consideration of alternative models should be used, particularly for women with breast atypia.

It is also important to note that risk changes over time based on age and other factors. The lifetime risk of a younger patient will always be greater than for older patients because the span of time between their current age and life expectancy by definition is greater.[46] Therefore, risk scores should be updated every few years as the patient ages and as risk factors change.

Claus model The Claus model was one of the first models developed to assess the risk of familial breast cancer. While the Claus model takes into account the number and degree of relatives on both the paternal and maternal sides of the family, as well as their ages at breast cancer diagnosis,[2] this model does not take into account any other risk factors. Furthermore, the model risk derivations are based on data from the 1980s, prior to when *BRCA1/2* were discovered, and therefore the data may overestimate familial risk in settings of negative genetic testing. Though the Claus model is commonly cited for use in various breast cancer screening guidelines, other models such as IBIS provide a more accurate and tailored clinical assessment of breast cancer risk.

BOADICEA The BOADICEA model was originally designed to predict the probability of *BRCA1* or *BRCA2* mutation but is now commonly used for familial-based breast cancer risk assessment.[2] This model takes into account the patient's extended family history, including breast and ovarian cancer history, and therefore is more likely to account for a polygenic component as compared to other models.[48–50] BOADICEA also includes other lifestyle and hormonal risk factors for breast cancer. This model is free for use and can be found online at https://ccge.medschl.cam.ac.uk/boadicea/.

BRCAPRO The BRCAPRO model was also designed to predict the risk of being a *BRCA1* or *BRCA2* carrier. BRCAPRO incorporates *BRCA1* and *BRCA2* mutation frequencies, cancer penetrance in mutation carriers, and age of first-degree and second-degree relatives at breast cancer diagnosis.[2] Unlike IBIS and BOADICEA, this model does not take into account non-hereditary risk factors or any other genetic information.[2] Therefore, it may underestimate risk in individuals with other breast cancer pathogenic variants or polygenic components or other breast cancer risk factors.[2]

Breast Cancer Risk Assessment Tool (BCRAT/Gail model) The BCRAT, also known as the modified Gail model, was originally developed by the National Cancer Institute and is designed to estimate the 5-year and lifetime risk of developing breast cancer for individual women older than 35 years of age.[2] The BCRAT includes specific breast cancer risk factors such as current age, age at menarche, age at first live birth, number of first-degree relatives with breast cancer, number of previous benign biopsies, presence of atypical hyperplasia on biopsy, and race.[51] The model is free for use and can be found online at http://www.cancer.gov/bcrisktool.

Though the BCRAT is felt to be a useful risk assessment tool for women with breast atypia, it is known to significantly underestimate breast cancer risk in women with *BRCA1/2* or other genetic mutations, women with a strong family history of breast cancer, and women who received thoracic radiation.[52] The BCRAT may also overestimate or underestimate risk in nonwhite women.[52] Thus, while research is ongoing to improve the accuracy of the BCRAT, the model should be used primarily as a general assessment in patients *without* a strong family history and/or for those women with ADH or ALH.

MANAGEMENT OF PATIENTS WITH HEREDITARY BREAST CANCER SYNDROMES

Specific elements of breast cancer risk management for patients with genetic predisposition, as well as for those patients with strong family history, should include discussion of both screening and prevention options. To this end, the NCCN has developed a detailed set of management guidelines for each major hereditary cancer syndrome, and clinicians should refer back frequently to these guidelines, as they are subject to change each year. The most recent NCCN guidelines can be found at nccn.org and are summarized in Table 5.3.[7]

Breast cancer screening recommendations typically include a selection of screening modality and frequency of testing, including mammograms, ultrasounds, breast MRI, and/or clinical breast exams, tailored to the patient's level of risk.[29] Screening recommendations should also include consideration of screenings for other organ systems, depending on the genetic syndrome or family history.[7] It is important for patients to understand that cancer screening, while essential for early detection of cancer, does not serve to *prevent* cancer development.

Major risk-reduction and prevention options that should be reviewed with patients will vary based on the specific genetic syndrome and family history, but should include discussion of three essential elements, namely (1) surgical options, (2) risk-reducing medications, and (3) lifestyle modifications.[2] Patients should also receive psychosocial support as needed and information on implications for children and other family members.

It is crucial to recognize that management of hereditary breast cancer is not a "one-size-fits-all" phenomenon. First, different genetic syndromes carry different breast cancer risks; for example, high-penetrance mutations such as *BRCA1/2* have substantial lifetime risks of breast cancer, whereas moderate-penetrance genes carry less risk (Figure 5.2).

Furthermore, individual cancer risks vary within and among families, even with the same genetic mutation.[7] Several considerations should play into the creation of a risk management plan, including the patient's age, specific gene mutation, family history, competing health risks, patient understanding of cancer risks, and short- and long-term goals. Note that a patient's goals and values may change over time; for example, a wish to breastfeed or carry a pregnancy may be very relevant to a *BRCA* carrier in her twenties or thirties but may no longer be relevant for a carrier in her forties or fifties. As such, decisions around the pursuit and timing of prophylactic mastectomy and oophorectomy will, by definition, vary among patients; patient preferences should be accommodated whenever possible. Ultimately, there is no single "right" way to manage patients with hereditary breast cancer syndromes; instead, it is a delicate balance of maximizing potential benefits versus risks and working with individual patients to find what is "right" for them at that given moment of their life.

TABLE 5.3: Hereditary Cancer Risk Management			
	Breast Cancer Risk and Management	**Ovarian Cancer Risk and Management**	**Other Cancer Risks and Management**	**Notes#**
ATM	Risk: Moderate increase Mammo: Annual, starting age 40 MRI: Consider annual, starting age 40 RRM: Evidence insufficient, manage based on FH	Risk: Possible increase RRSO: Evidence insufficient, manage based on FH	Pancreatic: Possible increase; consider screening based on FH	• c.7271T>G variant may carry higher risk of breast cancer • Counsel for risk of autosomal recessive condition in offspring • No need to avoid therapeutic radiation if clinically indicated
BARD1	Risk: Possible increase; manage based on FH	Risk: Insufficient evidence of increased risk	Insufficient evidence for other cancer risks	
BRCA1	Risk: High increase Mammo: Annual, starting age 30 MRI: Annual, starting age 25 RRM: Discuss option	Risk: Increased RRSO: Consider at age 35–40	Pancreatic: Possible increase; consider screening based on FH Prostate: Consider screening starting age 49 Melanoma: Consider annual derm and eye exams	
BRCA2	Risk: High increase Mammo: Annual, starting age 30 MRI: Annual, starting age 25 RRM: Discuss option	Risk: Increased RRSO: Consider at age 40–45	Pancreatic: Possible increase; consider screening based on FH Prostate: Screening starting age 40 Melanoma: Consider annual derm and eye exams	• Counsel for risk of autosomal recessive condition in offspring
BRIP1	Risk: Possible increase; manage based on FH	Risk: Increased RRSO: Consider at age 45–50	Insufficient evidence for other cancer risks	• Counsel for risk of autosomal recessive condition in offspring
CDH1	Risk: High increase Mammo: Annual, starting age 30 MRI: Consider annual, starting age 30 RRM: Evidence insufficient, manage based on FH	No increased risk	Diffuse gastric cancer: High increase; Risk reducing gastrectomy recommended age 18-40	• Gastrectomy for those without FH gastric cancer is controversial, but should be considered vs aggressive screening and periodic biopsies
CHEK2	Risk: Moderate increase Mammo: Annual, starting age 40 MRI: Consider annual, starting age 40 RRM: Evidence insufficient, manage based on FH	No increased risk	Colon: Possible increase; considered screening colonoscopy starting age 40, with 5-year intervals	• c.I157T variant may carry lower risk of breast cancer

TABLE 5.3:	Hereditary Cancer Risk Management (*Continued*)			
	Breast Cancer Risk and Management	**Ovarian Cancer Risk and Management**	**Other Cancer Risks and Management**	**Notes#**
NBN	Risk: Increased ONLY for 657del5 variant Mammo: Annual, starting age 40 MRI: Consider annual, starting age 40 RRM: Evidence insufficient, manage based on FH	Risk: Possible increase RRSO: Evidence insufficient, manage based on FH	Insufficient evidence for other cancer risks	• Counsel for risk of autosomal recessive condition in offspring
NF1	Risk: Increased ONLY until age 50 Mammo: Annual, starting age 30 MRI: Consider annual, from ages 30–50 RRM: Evidence insufficient, manage based on FH	No increased risk	Malignant peripheral nerve sheath tumors, GIST, others	• Recommend referral to NF1 specialist for management
PALB2	Risk: Moderate to high increase, based on FH Mammo: Annual, starting age 30 MRI: Consider annual, starting age 30 RRM: Evidence insufficient, manage based on FH	Risk: Possible increase RRSO: Evidence insufficient, manage based on FH	Pancreatic: Increased risk; consider screening based on FH	• Counsel for risk of autosomal recessive condition in offspring
PTEN	Risk: High increase Mammo: Annual, starting age 30 MRI: Consider annual, starting age 30 RRM: Discuss option	No increased risk	Endometrial: Consider screening by age 35; consider hysterectomy after childbearing complete Thyroid: Annual ultrasound starting age 7 Colon: Screening by age 35, 5-year intervals Renal cell: Ultrasound every 1–2 years starting age 40 Melanoma: Annual derm exam Brain tumors: No routine screening, unless symptoms	
RAD51C/D	Risk: Possible increase; manage based on FH	Risk: Increased RRSO: Consider at age 45–50	Insufficient evidence for other cancer risks	• Counsel for risk of autosomal recessive condition in offspring (RAD51C)

(Continued)

TABLE 5.3: Hereditary Cancer Risk Management *(Continued)*

	Breast Cancer Risk and Management	Ovarian Cancer Risk and Management	Other Cancer Risks and Management	Notes#
STK11	Risk: High increase Mammo: Annual, starting age 30 MRI: Annual, starting age 25 RRM: Evidence insufficient, manage based on FH	Risk: Increased RRSO: Evidence insufficient, manage based on FH	Gastrointestinal: Colonoscopy and upper endoscopy every 2–3 years starting in teenage; small bowel evaluation at age 8 (baseline) and then resume at age 18, every 2–3 years Pancreatic: Screening starting age 30–35 GYN: Annual PAP starting age 18; consider ovarian and endometrial screening age 30 Benign GU: Evaluate for early puberty; annual testicular exam starting age 10 Lung: Tobacco counseling	
TP53	Risk: High increase Mammo: Annual, starting age 30 MRI: Annual, starting age 20 RRM: Discuss option	No increased risk	Multiple tumor risks: Soft tissue sarcoma, osteosarcoma, colon, gastric, CNS tumors, adrenocortical carcinomas, leukemia, others Toronto/NCCN screening recommendations: • CPE every 6–12 months including neuro exam • Colonoscopy and upper endoscopy every 2–5 years starting age 25 • Annual derm exam starting age 18 • Annual whole body MRI • Annual brain MRI • Consider annual abdominal and pelvic ultrasound (Toronto)	

#Age by which to begin screenings may be modified based on family history (typically beginning 5–10 years earlier than the youngest diagnosis in the family but not later than stated in the table) or specific gene variant

RRM: Risk reducing mastectomy

RRSO: Risk reducing salpingo-oophorectomy

FH: Family history

CPE: Complete physical exam

Data from Daly MB, Pilarski R, Yurgelun MB, et al: NCCN Guidelines Insights: Genetic/Familial High-Risk Assessment: Breast, Ovarian, and Pancreatic, Version 1.2020, J Natl Compr Canc Netw 2020 Apr;18(4):380-391.

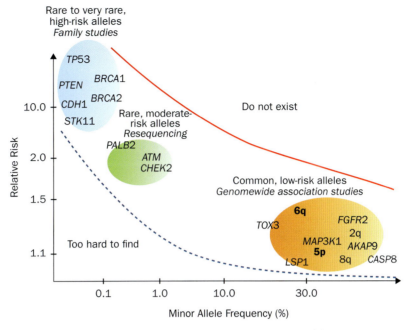

FIGURE 5.2: Breast cancer susceptibility genes and loci, according to relative risk.

High-Penetrance Genetic Syndromes

BRCA1/2 Among patients with hereditary breast cancer, it is estimated that approximately 50% are caused by mutations in the *BRCA1/2* genes. *BRCA1* and *BRCA2* are autosomal dominant genes and encode for proteins involved in tumor suppression. *BRCA1* is located on chromosome 17 and is involved in DNA repair and regulation of the cell cycle checkpoints in response to DNA damage.[53] *BRCA2* is located on chromosome 13 and is involved in repair of replication-mediated double-stranded DNA breaks.[54]

Hundreds of pathogenic or likely pathogenic variants have been identified in each of these genes. *BRCA1/2* mutations can be found in about 1 in every 200 people in the general population, distributed equally between males and females.[7] Among Ashkenazi Jews, the prevalence is much higher, at approximately 1 in 40, due to periods of social and geographic isolation over time.[7]

While *BRCA* pathogenic variants are considered to be highly penetrant, the probability of developing breast cancer can vary, even within families with the same variant. Lifetime risk of breast cancer varies from 40% to 85%, with 15% to 60% risk of ovarian cancer.[7,55] Among those women who develop *BRCA*-associated breast cancer, *BRCA1* carriers are more likely to develop triple-negative breast cancer (~60% to 70%),[53] whereas *BRCA2* carriers tend to develop hormone-positive breast cancers.[54] *BRCA* mutations, more so with *BRCA2* than *BRCA1*, also carry increased risk for pancreatic cancer (~5% lifetime risk), male breast cancer (<10%), prostate cancer (~30%), and possibly melanoma (~5% lifetime risk).[7,55] These risks are summarized in Table 5.4.

A key aspect of risk assessment in *BRCA1/2* carriers, as well as in other hereditary cancer syndromes, is that both short- and long-term risks vary by age,[56] as shown in Table 5.5. In

TABLE 5.4: *BRCA1/2* Related Lifetime Cancer Risks

	General Population	*BRCA1*	*BRCA2*
Breast Cancer	12%–13%	50%–85%	40%–70%
Second Primary Breast Cancer	3.5% within 5 years Up to 11%	Up to 40%–65% at 20 years	Up to 40%–50% at 20 years
Ovarian Cancer	1%–2%	15%–60%	15%–40%
Male Breast Cancer	0.1%	1%–2%	5%–10%
Prostate Cancer	15%–20%	<30%	<39%
Pancreatic Cancer	0.5%	1%–3%	2%–7%
Melanoma	1.6%	N.S.	Up to 5%

N.S. Not significant

Data from Adam MP, Ardinger HH, Pagon RA, et al: GeneReviews. Seattle, WA: University of Washington; 1993.

terms of lifetime risk, the commonly quoted risk of up to 50% to 85% with a *BRCA* mutation specifically refers to the total lifetime chance that a 30-year-old woman might develop breast cancer from the time she is 30 until she reaches the age of 80. However, *remaining* lifetime risk will *decline* over time, such that the lifetime risk for an unaffected 65- or 70-year-old *BRCA* carrier is much smaller by comparison, having lived through several decades of her life without having had breast cancer, and would be estimated to be only about 15%. Similarly, with short-term risks, risk can vary by age. Specifically, the 10-year risk of developing breast cancer in a 20-year-old *BRCA1* carrier is only 1.8% by age 30, whereas the 10-year risk for a 40-year-old with a *BRCA1* mutation is much higher, at 20% by age 50. Thus, when making decisions about if and when to intervene with prophylactic surgeries, it is helpful to become oriented with a given patient's specific short- and long-term risks.

Management of patients with a *BRCA1/2* mutation should include a plan for breast cancer screening and prevention, as well as consideration for other cancer risks, including ovarian, pancreatic, melanoma, and prostate cancers as applicable.

Breast Cancer Risk Management
Screening: In general, breast cancer screening for women who have tested positive for a *BRCA* pathogenic or likely pathogenic variant begins at age 25 but can start earlier if needed based on family history.[29] Patients of all ages are encouraged to do periodic breast self-exams and to report any changes to their health care provider. For women older than 25, a clinical breast exam is specifically recommended to occur every 6 to 12 months.[6,29]

For women age 25 to 29, an annual breast MRI with contrast is recommended, ideally performed on days 7 to 15 of the menstrual cycle.[57] MRI is preferred in this age range due to the theoretical risk of radiation exposure from mammography in this young population.[57] Women age 30 to 75 should undergo an annual mammogram in addition to annual breast MRI screening.[6,29] Often, these two screening modalities are staggered by 6 months to allow for multiple imaging opportunities during a single calendar year, though data around absolute benefits from this approach are mixed.[58] The addition of screening ultrasound to a regimen of mammogram and MRI is controversial, though it may be useful in those patients

TABLE 5.5: Predicted Mean Cancer Risk to Currently Unaffected *BRCA1/2* Mutation Carriers										
	Risk (%) of Developing Cancer by Age									
	30 Years		**40 Years**		**50 Years**		**60 Years**		**70 Years**	
Current Age	**Mean**	**95% CI**	**Mean**	**95% CI**	**Mean**	**95% CI**	**Mean**	**95% CI**	**Mean**	**95% CI**
Breast cancer: *BRCA1*										
20 years	1.8	1.4 to 2.2	12	9.5 to 14	29	24 to 35	44	37 to 52	54	46 to 63
30 years	—		10	8.2 to 13	28	23 to 24	44	36 to 52	54	45 to 63
40 years	—		—		20	16 to 25	38	31 to 45	49	41 to 58
50 years	—		—		—		22	18 to 27	37	30 to 44
60 years	—		—		—		—		19	15 to 24
Breast Cancer: *BRCA2*										
20 years	1	0.78 to 1.4	7.5	5.8 to 9.8	21	17 to 26	35	28 to 42	45	38 to 53
30 years	—		6.6	5.1 to 8.6	20	16 to 26	35	28 to 42	45	38 to 53
40 years	—		—		15	12 to 19	30	24 to 36	42	34 to 49
50 years	—		—		—		18	15 to 22	32	26 to 38
60 years	—		—		—		—		17	14 to 20
Ovarian cancer: *BRCA1*										
20 years	1	0.68 to 1.8	3.2	2.3 to 5.1	9.5	7.3 to 13	23	18 to 28	39	34 to 44
30 years	—		2.2	1.6 to 3.4	8.7	6.7 to 12	22	18 to 27	39	34 to 43
40 years	—		—		6.7	5.2 to 8.9	20	17 to 24	38	33 to 41
50 years	—		—		—		15	12 to 17	34	29 to 36
60 years	—		—		—		—		22	20 to 23
Ovarian cancer: *BRCA2*										
20 years	0.19	0.09 to 0.47	0.7	0.37 to 1.5	2.6	1.5 to 4.5	7.5	5.1 to 11	16	12 to 20
30 years	—		0.52	0.28 to 1	2.4	1.5 to 4.2	7.4	5.1 to 11	16	12 to 20
40 years	—		—		1.9	1.2 to 3.2	7	4.8 to 10	16	12 to 20
50 years	—		—		—		5.2	3.7 to 7.2	14	11 to 17
60 years	—		—		—		—		9.8	7.8 to 11

Note: The CI is provided for the mean risk, not the risk itself.
Reproduced with permission from Chen S, Parmigiani G: Meta-analysis of BRCA1 and BRCA2 penetrance, J Clin Oncol 2007 Apr 10;25(11):1329-1333.

with extremely dense tissue in whom mammogram is less sensitive.[6] Screening management for women older than 75 should be made on an individual basis; commonly, women in this age group will discontinue MRI but will continue with annual mammograms until life expectancy is less than 5 to 10 years and she remains in reasonably good health.[29]

Risk-reducing surgery: Counseling should include discussion of the option of risk-reducing mastectomy (RRM), though RRM may not be appropriate for every patient.[2] Several studies have shown that RRM substantially reduces the risk of breast cancer development to lifetime risks of <5%.[59,60] However, it is important to recognize that while RRM is the most effective way to prevent breast cancer development, it has not definitively been shown to reduce mortality.[2] This is likely due to the fact that *BRCA* carriers are typically undergoing aggressive screening; it has been shown that with a regimen of annual mammogram and MRI, breast cancers are typically caught at stage 0 (DCIS) or stage I nearly 95% of the time, when breast cancer is highly curable.[2] Thus, counseling regarding RRM should be anchored to the potential benefits of improved quality of life, omission of frequent screenings, and avoidance of the risk of having to potentially undergo future breast cancer treatment, rather than a goal of prolonged life expectancy.[2] Counseling should take also into account a given patient's expected short-term and lifetime risks in order to weigh risks and benefits. The most notable risks of RRM include surgical risks of a major procedure, a 4- to 6-week recovery time if breast reconstruction is pursued, loss of skin and nipple sensation, inability to breastfeed, and potential impact on sexuality and body image.[2]

Patients should additionally be cautioned that breast reconstruction techniques, while excellent, can sometimes be disappointing if patient expectations are not set appropriately.[2,61] Patients should expect that breast reconstruction is a lengthy process, which can sometimes take up to 6 to 12 months to complete.[2] The reconstructed breast, whether by implant or by autologous tissue reconstruction, will likely have visible scars. However, nipple-sparing procedures are considered to be safe for most patients and can help preserve a natural appearance of the breast reconstruction.[61]

An important cohort of *BRCA* patients who may be considering RRM include those carriers who have been diagnosed with ovarian cancer. However, these patients generally should be dissuaded from immediate RRM for two reasons, namely (1) lower-than-expected risk of breast cancer and (2) high risk of ovarian cancer recurrence within the first 5 years from diagnosis.[7] Interestingly, recent studies have shown that risk of subsequent breast cancer in women who have undergone treatment for ovarian cancer is significantly lower than their unaffected peers and rests at only ~5% over the next 10 years.[62] Though the exact reasons for this reduced risk remain undetermined, it may be related to the receipt of platinum-based and other chemotherapy agents for ovarian cancer treatment, which are also known to be effective in treating breast cancer; this chemotherapy may eliminate breast cancer stem cells that otherwise would have become clinically evident in future years. It is also important for patients and providers to understand that risk of ovarian cancer recurrence within the first 5 years of diagnosis unfortunately remains quite high.[7] Undergoing RRM in the midst of ovarian cancer treatment and potential recurrence would not serve the best interests of most patients. As such, patients should prioritize the treatment and recovery from ovarian cancer in the first 5 years from diagnosis, after which time consideration of RRM becomes more feasible and beneficial.

Medications: Several medications have been shown to reduce the risk of breast cancer, including tamoxifen, raloxifene, and aromatase inhibitors. These medications have been shown to reduce the relative risk of hormone-positive breast cancer by ~50% in women at increased risk, based on family history and other risk factors.[2] Details regarding the use of risk-reducing medications are discussed in more detail later in the chapter. However, data regarding the benefit of these medications in *BRCA* carriers is quite sparse. Limited retrospective studies have shown a potential similar benefit of tamoxifen in *BRCA2* carriers, but numbers of patients in these studies are small.[63] There are no prevention data available regarding raloxifene or aromatase inhibitors in this population. Further, given the propensity of *BRCA1* carriers to develop hormone-negative breast cancer, the use of tamoxifen may not have substantial benefit. Thus, given the high risk of breast cancer in *BRCA* patients, it is reasonable to discuss the use of preventive medications such as tamoxifen,[64] but patients should be cautioned that data are limited. The benefits of OCP use and HRT use in *BRCA* carriers should also be considered; these agents are recommended for ovarian cancer risk reduction and relief from premature menopausal symptoms and cannot be used concurrently with tamoxifen. Further discussion of OCP and HRT can be found later.

Lifestyle: As with any patient at increased risk of breast cancer, *BRCA* carriers should be counseled about healthy lifestyle modifications, though data are admittedly scarce to define precise risk-reduction impact specifically in hereditary cancer syndromes.[65] Patients should be counseled about diet, exercise, achieving a healthy weight, limiting alcohol, and avoidance of tobacco.[65]

Ovarian Cancer Risk Management Management of hereditary ovarian cancer risk is discussed in detail in Chapter 9.

Screening: Unfortunately, efficacy of ovarian cancer screening is known to be poor in terms of its ability to catch disease early in order to improve cancer outcomes. However, *BRCA* carriers may wish to pursue ovarian cancer screening starting at age 30 after discussion of benefits and risks.[7] Screening typically entails a transvaginal pelvic ultrasound every 6 to 12 months and a CA-125 tumor marker blood test every 6 to 12 months.[7] Screening remains controversial, however, and should be pursued at the discretion of the patient and provider.

Surgery: Risk-reducing salpingo-oophorectomy (RRSO) is the most effective way to prevent ovarian and fallopian tube cancer, particularly due to the lack of reliable methods for early detection. A large prospective study of women with *BRCA1/2* mutations showed that surgery reduced the risk of gynecological tumors by 85% compared to observation over 3 years (HR 0.15 CI 0.04 to 0.56).[66] It also reduced all-cause mortality by 77%[67] and reduced the risk of breast cancer by 43% to 56% due to decreased estrogen from the removal of the ovaries.[68]

In *BRCA1* carriers, RRSO is typically recommended by age 35 to 40 and upon completion of child-bearing. In *BRCA2* carriers, RRSO is recommended by age 40 to 45 and upon completion of child-bearing. It is possible to delay this surgery in *BRCA2* carriers, since these women appear to develop ovarian cancer 8 to 10 years later than *BRCA1* carriers.[67]

There may also be an increased risk of serous uterine cancer in *BRCA1* carriers, although there are limited data and absolute risks appear low.[69] Risks and benefits of concurrent hysterectomy should be discussed for *BRCA1* carriers, but more data are needed, and hysterectomy has yet to become a firm recommendation by the NCCN. A potential advantage for premenopausal *BRCA* carriers to undergo hysterectomy at the time of RRSO is the potential reduced cancer risk from estrogen-only HRT compared to combined HRT.[2]

Medications: OCPs have been shown to reduce the risk of ovarian cancer in *BRCA* carriers.[70] With 5 years of OCP use, risk of ovarian cancer is reduced by up to 60%, whereas risk reduction approaches 80% with 8 or more years of OCP use.[70] Meanwhile, OCP use has not been shown to substantially affect breast cancer risk in *BRCA* carriers, though data are mixed.[70] Given the proven benefit for ovarian cancer risk reduction, on balance, OCPs should be considered for use.

Patients undergoing early menopause via RRSO should be placed on HRT, given the multiple significant short- and long-term health and quality-of-life effects of surgical menopause. Studies have shown that HRT does not negate the potential risk-reducing benefit for breast cancer and does not increase the risk of breast cancer.[71]

Other Cancer Risk Management

Melanoma: There is a possible small increased risk of melanoma in male and female *BRCA* carriers.[7,72] Patients can consider an annual skin exam and annual eye exam to screen for melanoma. Patients should be counseled about skin cancer prevention options, such as use of sunscreen and avoiding sunburns.[7]

Pancreatic cancer: There is a possible small increased risk of pancreatic cancer in male and female *BRCA* carriers, particularly if there is a family history of pancreatic cancer.[7] Though there are no NCCN screening guidelines that are overtly recommended at this time, patients with a strong family history of pancreatic cancer can consider screening abdominal MRI and endoscopic ultrasound. Ideally, consideration of enrollment in a clinical trial, such as the CAPS5 screening study, would be an alternative approach.[73] Patients should be counseled about lifestyle modifications to reduce the risk of pancreatic cancer, such as avoidance of alcohol and tobacco.

Prostate cancer: Prostate cancer screening is recommended for *BRCA2* carriers starting at age 40 and can be considered in *BRCA1* carriers.[7] Digital rectal exams and annual prostate specific antigen (PSA) should be discussed.

Male breast cancer: Men who test positive for *BRCA1/2* should be educated about breast self-exams starting at age 35.[7] They should also undergo an annual clinical breast exam.[7] There is no data to support annual mammographic screening at this time.[7]

Other Considerations In addition to specific cancer screening and prevention recommendations, it is important to provide information on the following issues for *BRCA* and other hereditary cancer syndrome patients. All of these issues are addressed in detail elsewhere in this book:

- Psychosocial support: Many patients who learn of a hereditary cancer syndrome experience significant distress and fear. It is important to recognize and normalize this possibility with patients and offer support and referrals as needed.

- Family planning: Patients of childbearing age may wish to pursue in vitro fertilization (IVF) with genetic testing of embryos, commonly referred to as preimplantation genetic diagnosis. This process enables the couple to select an embryo that does not carry the known deleterious mutation and therefore will not be passed down to the child. Though this process has significant potential legal and ethical implications and is not universally covered by insurance, patients should be aware of the option if they wish to pursue it.

- Individuals of childbearing age with a known *BRCA2* mutation should consider prenatal genetic counseling and a discussion of reproductive options, as there may be an increased risk for Fanconi anemia for offspring. Children with Fanconi anemia are at increased risk of developing bone marrow failure, leukemia, and other cancers, as well as physical differences such as changes in the thumb, small skull size, and short stature. For this reason, individuals with a *BRCA2* mutation who are of reproductive age may wish to consider having their partners tested for mutations in the *BRCA2* gene before becoming pregnant. If both parents have a *BRCA2* mutation, then there is a 25% risk their children will have Fanconi anemia.

- Informing family members: Patients should be reminded that close relatives should undergo genetic testing for the known genetic mutation. If it is unknown whether inheritance is maternal or paternal, members on both sides of the family should undergo testing.

LI-FRAUMENI (TP53) Li-Fraumeni syndrome (LFS) is a rare autosomal dominant disorder, estimated to be involved in about 1% of hereditary breast cancers,[7,74] Germline *TP53* mutations are highly penetrant and are associated with 100% lifetime cancer incidence.[7,75] LFS is classically associated with an increased risk of soft tissue sarcomas, osteosarcomas, breast cancer, colon cancer, gastric cancer, central nervous system (CNS) tumors, and adrenocortical carcinomas.[7]

In addition to the "red flag" testing criteria described earlier in the chapter, specific consideration for LFS should be considered for individuals who have a personal or family history of soft tissue sarcoma, osteosarcoma, CNS tumor, and breast cancer, particularly if onset occurs at an early age.[7] Adrenocortical carcinoma, choroid plexus carcinoma, or rhabdomyosarcoma of embryonal anaplastic subtype at any age should also prompt testing.[7,76] Though historically the classic LFS and Chompret criteria have been used to guide testing for LFS,[7,76] recent advances in technology have allowed for panel testing to include *TP53* alongside other hereditary cancer syndromes.[77]

Patients diagnosed with LFS should ideally be referred to a hereditary cancer specialty program, given the exceedingly high cancer risks. Surveillance and management guidelines for LFS have been described by NCCN (see Table 5.3). The recently updated Toronto guidelines have also been shown to be highly effective for this population, which are outlined later.[78]

Breast Cancer Risk Management Periodic breast self-exams are recommended for women who test positive for LFS starting at age 18.[7] Clinical breast exams are recommended every 6 to 12 months starting at age 20, along with an annual breast MRI with contrast.[7] From age 30 to 75 annual breast MRI and mammogram are recommended.[7]

Risk-reducing mastectomy should also be discussed, with similar considerations as for *BRCA* carriers described earlier.[7] There are no data which specifically address the use of preventive medications in LFS. When it is possible, therapeutic radiation should be avoided and minimal use of computed tomography (CT) scan.[7]

As with any patient at increased risk of breast cancer, *TP53* carriers should be counseled about healthy lifestyle modifications, though data are admittedly scarce to define precise risk-reduction impact specifically in hereditary cancer syndromes.[79] Patients should be counseled about diet, exercise, achieving a healthy weight, limiting alcohol, and avoiding tobacco.

Other Cancer Risk Management As described earlier, LFS patients are also at high risk for soft tissue sarcomas, osteosarcomas, colon cancer, gastric cancer, CNS tumors, and adrenocortical carcinomas, in addition to second malignancies and other rare cancers. Therefore, several screening interventions are recommended by the NCCN for adults older than age 18 including:[7]

- Comprehensive physical exam, including a neurological exam, is recommended every 6 to 12 months.
- Colonoscopy and upper endoscopy is recommended every 2 to 5 years starting at age 25 or 5 years before the earliest colon cancer in the family (whichever comes first).
- Annual whole-body skin exam by a dermatologist is recommended starting at age 18.
- Annual whole-body MRI. A prospective observational trial of *TP53* mutation carriers that incorporated annual whole-body MRI showed that at 11-year follow-up, 84% of patients who underwent surveillance were alive compared to 49% of patients who opted out.[78]
- Annual brain MRI (can be included as part of the whole-body MRI).

The Toronto protocol additionally recommends consideration of annual abdominal and pelvic ultrasound.[78] For children with LFS, the Toronto protocol recommends that active screening start at birth, including abdominal and pelvic ultrasounds every 3 to 4 months, annual brain and body MRI, and regular physical exams.[78]

PTEN Mutations in the *PTEN* gene can cause at least two overlapping hereditary cancer syndromes called Cowden syndrome and Bannayan-Riley-Ruvalcaba syndrome (BRRS) that together are sometimes collectively called *PTEN*-hamartoma tumor syndrome (PHTS).

PHTS is a rare autosomal dominant disorder typically characterized by hamartomas; developmental disorders; macrocephaly; and increased risk of several cancers, including breast, thyroid, endometrial, colorectal, skin (particularly melanoma), and renal cell carcinoma.[7,80] The *PTEN* mutation has a high penetrance for cancer susceptibility, estimated at 80%.[7,81] Lifetime risk of breast cancer for these women is estimated at 25% to 50% with average age at diagnosis of 38 to 50 years old.[7,82] Benign (noncancerous) tumors may also be seen within PHTS families, namely of the breast, thyroid, uterus, colon, skin, mucous membranes (lining of the mouth and nose), and sometimes the brain.[7,80]

Cowden syndrome and BRRS can present, in a single family and between families, with a wide spectrum of physical and developmental findings.[7,80] For this reason it is impossible to predict which findings any one affected family member may have, even within the same family. In addition to classic "red flag" criteria for hereditary breast cancer syndromes (Table 5.3), further considerations for PHTS include a personal or family history of any of the PTEN cancers listed earlier, particularly if the history also includes one or more of the following benign conditions: cerebellar tumors, autism spectrum disorder, macrocephaly, trichilemmomas, multiple gastrointestinal (GI) hamartomas or ganglioneuromas, macular pigmentation of the glans penis, mucocutaneous lesions (trichilemmomas, palmoplantar keratosis, oral papillomatosis, verrucous facial papules), esophageal glycogenic acanthuses, lipomas, benign thyroid lesions, testicular lipomatosis, and vascular anomalies.[83]

Breast Cancer Risk Management Periodic breast self-exams are recommended for women who test positive for a *PTEN* mutation starting at age 18.[7] Clinical breast exams are recommended every 6 to 12 months starting at age 25.[7] Annual mammograms and breast MRI screening with contrast is recommended starting at age 30 to 35 or 5 to 10 years before the earliest known breast cancer in the family (whichever comes first).[7]

Risk-reducing mastectomy should also be discussed, with similar considerations as for *BRCA* carriers described earlier.[7] There are no data that specifically address the use of preventive medications in PHTS. Healthy lifestyle modifications should be discussed, though data are admittedly scarce to define precise risk-reduction impact specifically in hereditary cancer syndromes. Patients should be counseled about diet, exercise, achieving a healthy weight, limiting alcohol, and avoiding tobacco.[65]

Other Cancer Risk Management
Endometrial cancer: Screening with annual endometrial biopsy with or without annual ultrasound can be considered. It is important to note that transvaginal ultrasound in premenopausal women is controversial due to the wide range in endometrial thickness throughout the normal menstrual cycle, and transvaginal ultrasound in postmenopausal women has not been shown to be sensitive or specific.[7] Women with *PTEN* should pay close attention

to any abnormal vaginal bleeding or irregularities in the menstrual cycle.[7] The option of hysterectomy should be discussed when childbearing is complete.[7]

Thyroid cancer: An annual comprehensive physical exam is recommended starting at age 18 with particular attention to the thyroid. In addition, an annual thyroid ultrasound is recommended, including in childhood if *PTEN* is known.[7]

Colon cancer: Colonoscopy is recommended starting at age 35 or 5 to 10 years prior to the earliest known colon cancer in the family and should be repeated at least every 5 years, if not more frequently, depending on findings.[7]

Renal cell carcinoma: Renal ultrasound can be considered starting at age 40 and repeated every 1 to 2 years.[7]

Skin cancer/melanoma: Annual dermatology exams are recommended.[7]

Brain tumors: No routine screening is recommended for brain tumors, but a brain MRI should be pursued if symptoms are present.[7] Consideration of psychomotor assessment in children with a *PTEN* mutation is advised.[7]

CDH1 Hereditary diffuse gastric cancer syndrome (HDGC) is caused by mutations in the *CDH1* gene, which is associated with significantly increased risks of diffuse gastric cancer and breast cancer.[7,84,85] *CDH1* mutations are inherited in an autosomal dominant manner but are rare among the general population. The *CDH1* gene is located on chromosome 17 and is responsible for the production of the cell adhesion protein E-cadherin, which is found in epithelial cells.[86] The disruption of cell binding leads to the formation of abnormal tissue growth in affected organs.[87]

The lifetime risk of diffuse gastric cancer (DGC) with a *CDH1* mutation is 56% to 70%, with men having a greater risk than women.[7] Instead of developing as a distinct mass, DGC (also referred to as signet ring carcinoma or isolated cell-type carcinoma) classically forms underneath the surface of the stomach and can oftentimes be found in multiple areas. The majority of DGC in individuals with *CDH1* mutations occur before age 40.[7]

Women with a *CDH1* mutation also have a 39% to 52% lifetime risk for breast cancer,[88] specifically lobular-type breast cancer (LBC). LBCs comprise ~10% to 15% of all breast cancers and can be difficult to detect on mammogram due to their typical "spider-like" growth pattern.[88] Importantly, an increasing body of work has found *CDH1* mutations in LBC patients with no family history of gastric cancer through widespread panel testing in recent years.[88] Thus, it is unclear whether the penetrance of *CDH1* may vary from mutation to mutation as it relates to gastric cancer and breast cancer, and further research must be done to clarify risks and management recommendations.

Individuals with a *CDH1* mutation may also have an increased risk of developing colon cancer, but the exact risk is currently unknown. Additional study is needed to confirm this association.

In addition to classic "red flag" criteria for hereditary breast cancer syndromes (Table 5.3), further considerations for testing for *CDH1* mutations include:[7]

- Two or more family members diagnosed with DGC at any age, with at least one confirmed DGC

- A DGC diagnosis before the age of 40
- A family history of both DGC and LBC, especially if one or more is diagnosed before the age of 50
- Bilateral LBC

Breast Cancer Risk Management Periodic self-breast exams are recommended for women who test positive for a *CDH1* mutation starting at age 18.[7] Clinical breast exams are recommended every 6 to 12 months starting at age 25.[7] Annual mammograms and breast MRI screening with contrast are recommended starting at age 30 or 5 to 10 years before the earliest known breast cancer in the family (whichever comes first).[7] Addition of a breast ultrasound can be considered, especially if breast tissue is mammographically dense, given the challenges of detecting LBC on mammogram.[7]

RRM should also be discussed, with similar considerations as for *BRCA* carriers described earlier. A number of specific considerations may lead to mastectomy as a prophylactic solution in *CDH1* carriers. Among these considerations are the development of precursive atypical breast lesions, which can increase the risk of LBC by up to 5-fold. Other considerations include a family history of LBC and the preference of the patient.[87]

There are no data that specifically address the use of preventive medications in *CDH1* carriers. As with any patient at increased risk of breast cancer, healthy lifestyle modifications should be reviewed, though data are admittedly scarce to define precise risk-reduction impact specifically in hereditary cancer syndromes. Patients should be counseled about diet, exercise, achieving a healthy weight, limiting alcohol, and avoiding tobacco.[65]

Other Cancer Risk Management
Gastric cancer: Screening for diffuse gastric cancer through stomach biopsies has not been shown to detect diffuse-type gastric cancer at an early, treatable stage. For this reason, risk-reducing gastrectomy (removal of the stomach) is recommended between ages 18 and 40, particularly if other family members have had gastric cancer. There is controversy over how to manage gastric cancer risk in *CDH1* carriers without a family history of DGC. However, recent studies have shown that at the time of gastrectomy, most individuals with a *CDH1* mutation have a number of precancerous lesions in their stomach, which were not detected using endoscopy screening.[89]

Endoscopy with random biopsies is used to look for evidence of clinically significant lesions in the stomach and is an option for those who decline or postpone gastrectomy. However, early gastric cancer, or precancerous lesions, including signet ring cells, may or may not be detected by endoscopy, and patients should be aware of this limitation in sensitivity. This procedure, if pursued, should be performed in a center with expertise in *CDH1*.

STK11 *STK11* mutations occur in 30% to 70% of cases of Peutz-Jeghers syndrome (PJS), which is a rare, autosomal dominant genetic disease that is characterized by the formation of hamartomatous polyps in the GI tract.[7,90] *STK11* is located on chromosome 19 and holds instructions for a tumor-suppressing enzyme called serine/threonine kinase 1.[90] Serine/threonine kinase 1 aids in cell polarization and apoptosis, as well as regulating energy use in the cell.[90]

Most individuals with PJS have an increased risk of developing multiple GI polyps, specifically Peutz-Jeghers–type hamartomatous polyps, which are considered noncancerous growths.[91] These polyps are most common in the small intestine, but can also develop in the stomach, colon, rectum, and other places in the body. These polyps can become quite large and cause health problems, including abdominal pain, intussusception, obstruction, rectal bleeding, and anemia.[91]

The majority of individuals with PJS develop hyperpigmented macules (dark blue to brown spots that look like freckles) inside and around the mouth, eyes, nostrils, and anus; on the lips and fingers; and on the genitalia.[91] These typically develop in childhood and can fade over time, especially in adults.[91]

Individuals with PJS also have an increased lifetime risk of developing cancer. Breast cancer risks for women approach 54% lifetime risk.[7] Other cancer risks include colorectal cancer (39% lifetime risk), stomach cancer (29%), pancreatic cancer (11% to 36%), small intestinal cancer (13%), and lung cancer (7% to 17%). Women with PJS have an elevated risk of developing ovarian (21% lifetime risk), endometrial (9%), and cervical cancer (10%, specifically for a rare, aggressive type of cervical cancer called adenoma malignum).[91] Men and women with PJS have an increased chance to develop benign (noncancerous) tumors of the ovaries and testes.[91]

In addition to classic "red flag" criteria for hereditary breast cancer syndromes (Table 5.3), and assessment for the cancers listed earlier, further considerations for testing for *STK11* mutations include a personal or family history of individuals with more than two hamartomatous polyps and mucocutaneous pigmentation.[7]

Breast Cancer Risk Management Periodic breast self-exams are recommended for women who test positive for a *STK11* mutation starting at age 18.[7] Clinical breast exams are recommended every 6 to 12 months starting at age 25.[7] Annual MRI screening generally starts at age 25, with addition of annual mammograms starting at age 30.

RRM and lifestyle modifications should also be discussed, with similar considerations as for *BRCA* carriers described earlier. There are no data that specifically address the use of preventive medications in *STK11* carriers.

Other Cancer Risk Management Individuals diagnosed with PJS should be monitored closely for all cancer types and should be referred to a specialized team.

Gastrointestinal cancers: Colonoscopy and upper endoscopy screening are recommended every 2 to 3 years starting in the late teenage years. Small intestinal visualization is recommended with CT or MRI enterography or video capsule endoscopy at age 8. Then, it should be repeated again by age 18 and every 2 to 3 years thereafter. Repeat visualization exams should also occur if prompted by reported symptoms.

Pancreatic cancer: Though screening remains controversial, patients with *STK11* can consider either magnetic resonance cholangiopancreatography (MRCP) with contrast or endoscopic ultrasound every 1 to 2 years starting at age 30 to 35. Pancreatic cancer screening should ideally be performed at a center with an experienced gastroenterologist.

Gynecologic cancers: For women with PJS, there are options for cervical, ovarian, and endometrial cancer screening. Cervical cancer screening would include annual Pap smear and physical exam beginning by age 18. Though screening has not yet been shown to be effective, endometrial and ovarian cancer screening can be considered by age 30 and would include transvaginal ultrasound, CA-125 blood marker screen, consideration of endometrial biopsy, and physical exam in an attempt to detect endometrial and ovarian cancer at an early stage. Women with PJS should be aware of the signs and symptoms of uterine and ovarian cancer, such as postmenopausal bleeding, pelvic or abdominal pain, bloating, increase in abdominal girth, and feelings of fullness or frequent urination. There are no guidelines that currently recommend prophylactic salpingo-oophorectomy or hysterectomy.

Benign ovarian and testicular tumors: Patients should be regularly screened for signs of precocious puberty, starting at age 8. In males, annual testicular exam should begin at age 10 with observation for any signs of abnormal feminization.

Lung cancer: There are no lung cancer screening guidelines at this time, but PJS patients should be counseled against the use of tobacco.

PALB2 PALB2 (partner and localizer of *BRCA2*) works in conjunction with *BRCA2* to repair DNA by acting as a localizing agent. *PALB2* mutations are present in 1% to 3% of women with breast cancer.[7]

Although *PALB2* has historically been considered a moderate-penetrance gene, it is increasingly viewed to be more appropriately categorized among other high-penetrance genes because, when coupled with a family history, its penetrance appears to approach that of *BRCA2*.[92]

Specifically, lifetime breast cancer risk for an individual with a *PALB2* mutation with no first-degree relatives with breast cancer is 35%.[92] However, this risk increases to 58% for an individual with two first-degree relatives with breast cancer.[92] The risk for a second primary breast cancer in women with *PALB2* mutation may be higher than in the general population, but additional study is needed to confirm this risk.[92]

Individuals with *PALB2* may also have an increased risk of pancreatic cancer,[7] speculated to be as high as *BRCA1/2* carriers, particularly in the presence of a family history. However, additional study is needed to confirm this risk.[93] Risk for ovarian cancer with *PALB2* remains indeterminant, and risk-reducing salpingo-oophorectomy is not recommended for PALB2 carriers.[94] Similarly, for men, there may be increased risk for prostate cancer, but risks remain unclear at this time.[7]

Individuals of childbearing age with a known *PALB2* mutation should consider prenatal genetic counseling and a discussion of reproductive options, as there may be an increased risk for Fanconi anemia type N for offspring.[7] Children with Fanconi anemia are at increased risk of developing bone marrow failure, leukemia, and other cancers, as well as physical differences such as changes in the thumb, small skull size, and short stature.[95] For this reason, individuals with a *PALB2* mutation who are of reproductive age may wish to consider having their partners tested for mutations in the *PALB2* gene before becoming pregnant.[7] If both parents have a *PALB2* mutation, then there is a 25% risk their children will have Fanconi anemia type N.[96]

Breast Cancer Risk Management Annual mammograms and annual breast MRIs are recommended for women with *PALB2* mutations starting at the age of 30, as the risk for breast cancer increases by more than 1% each year starting at this age.[7]

RRM and lifestyle modifications should also be discussed, with similar considerations as for *BRCA* carriers described earlier.[7] There are no data that specifically address the use of preventive medications in *PALB2* carriers.

Other Cancer Risk Management

Pancreatic cancer: There is a possible small increased risk of pancreatic cancer in male and female *PALB2* carriers, particularly if there is a family history of pancreatic cancer. Though there are no NCCN screening guidelines that are overtly recommended at this time, patients with a strong family history of pancreatic cancer can consider screening abdominal MRI and endoscopic ultrasound. Ideally, consideration of enrollment in a clinical trial, such as the CAPS5 screening study, would be an alternative approach. Patients should be counseled about lifestyle modifications to reduce the risk of pancreatic cancer, such as avoidance of alcohol and tobacco.

Ovarian cancer: RRSO is not yet specifically recommended at this time, as there remains insufficient evidence regarding a causal relationship between *PALB2* and ovarian cancer. However, management considerations and RRSO options should be based on family history of ovarian cancer.

Moderate-Penetrance Genetic Syndromes

Due to the expansion of multigene testing, moderate-penetrance gene mutations are increasingly being identified and are found in approximately 2% to 5% of patients who undergo genetic testing.[97] Whereas high-penetrance gene mutations typically carry lifetime risks of breast cancer of 50% or higher, lifetime risks with moderate-penetrance mutations are lower and more commonly range from ~25% to 40%,[7] keeping in mind that the average risk of breast cancer is ~12% to 13% (Figure 5.2). As such, recommendations for the management of these mutations often differ from high-penetrance genes.

There are two important caveats in managing moderate-penetrance gene mutations, namely the avoidance of either overestimation or underestimation of risk. In regard to overestimation of risk, treating moderate-penetrance genes with guidelines meant for high-penetrance genes can ultimately lead to patient harm. Aggressive preventive measures, such as prophylactic mastectomy or prophylactic oophorectomy, are typically unnecessary for moderate-penetrance mutations and are disproportionate to the level of risk conferred by these genes. These procedures cause distress and have a major impact on quality of life. Moreover, many genes that are considered to be potentially moderate risk do not yet have defined risk parameters and lack specific management guidelines. As such, it is important that patients receive appropriate education and guidance from a provider experienced in genetic counseling before undergoing testing and prior to significant management decisions.

In regard to underestimation of risk, in cases where there is a strong family history of breast cancer and a known moderate-penetrance mutation in the family (such as *ATM* or *CHEK2*), individuals within the family that test *negative* for the known moderate-penetrance gene do *not* necessarily have a reduced risk of breast cancer.[39] Unlike the "true negative" concept in high-penetrance genes, absence of a known familial moderate-penetrance gene does not preclude an individual from increased risk based on family history, and risk should be managed based on the family history of breast cancer. One explanation for this observation is that with moderate-penetrance genes like *ATM* and *CHEK2,* the risk of breast cancer seen within a family is not solely related to the gene mutation alone but is also influenced by other modifier genes, shared exposures, and environmental factors.[39]

Risk estimates and management guidelines for both high- and moderate-penetrance genes will continue to evolve over time. It is essential for clinicians who counsel patients with hereditary breast cancer syndromes to remain up to date on recent guidelines year to year. Many resources exist to aid in this process, such as the NCCN Genetic/Familial High Risk Assessment guidelines (nccn.org) and ASCO guidelines (asco.org).

ATM   *ATM* (ataxia-telangiectasia mutated) encodes a serine/threonine kinase that is activated by DNA double-strand breaks and is involved in activating DNA damage checkpoints such as cell cycle arrest, DNA repair, and apoptosis.[98] A meta-analysis of 19 studies has shown that cumulative lifetime risk of breast cancer in *ATM* carriers is 6% by age 50 and 33% by age 80.[99] Prevalence of *ATM* mutations among breast cancer patients is approximately 1%, but may be more common among young breast cancer patients.[7] Of note, specific *ATM* mutations, such as the c.7271T>G missense mutation, may confer up to a 69% lifetime risk of breast cancer.[100] Other cancer risks for *ATM* are not well-defined, but may include pancreatic cancer, ovarian cancer, and prostate cancer.[7]

In addition, individuals of childbearing age with a known *ATM* mutation should consider prenatal genetic counseling and a discussion of reproductive options, as there may be an increased risk for the autosomal recessive condition ataxia telangiectasia (AT) for offspring.[101] AT is a rare childhood syndrome characterized by progressive lack of coordination and muscle movements with onset between ages 1 and 4 years old, as well as dilated blood vessels of the eye (called telangiectases), immune defects, and increased risks for leukemia and lymphoma.[101] For this reason, individuals with an *ATM* mutation who are of reproductive age may wish to consider having their partners tested for mutations in the *ATM* gene before becoming pregnant.

Breast Cancer Risk Management   Annual mammograms and consideration of an annual breast MRI are recommended for women with *ATM* mutations starting at the age of 40, or potentially earlier if needed based on the family history.[7] Clinical breast exam should be performed every 6 to 12 months.[7]

There are no data on the benefit of RRM, but this could be considered in the context of a strong family history with similar considerations as for *BRCA* carriers described earlier.[7] There are no data that specifically address the use of preventive medications in *ATM* carriers. As with other patients at increased risk of breast cancer, lifestyle modifications should also be discussed.

Of note, for those women with an *ATM*-associated breast cancer, there is currently no strong evidence to suggest therapeutic radiation treatment should be avoided.[7]

Other Cancer Risk Management

Pancreatic cancer: There is a possible small increased risk of pancreatic cancer in male and female *ATM* carriers, particularly if there is a family history of pancreatic cancer. Though there are no NCCN screening guidelines that are overtly recommended at this time, patients with a strong family history of pancreatic cancer can consider screening abdominal MRI and endoscopic ultrasound. Ideally, consideration of enrollment in a clinical trial, such as the CAPS5 screening study, would be an alternative approach. Patients should be counseled about lifestyle modifications to reduce the risk of pancreatic cancer, such as avoidance of alcohol and tobacco.

Ovarian cancer: RRSO is not yet specifically recommended at this time, as there remains insufficient evidence regarding a causal relationship between *ATM* and ovarian cancer. However, management considerations and RRSO options should be based on family history of ovarian cancer.

CHEK2 CHEK2 (cell cycle checkpoint kinase 2) is a tumor suppressor gene that is involved in DNA repair, cell cycle arrest, and apoptosis in response to DNA damage.[7,102] Mutations in *CHEK2* have been linked to a moderate risk of developing breast cancer, with lifetime risks ranging from 20% in patients with no family history of breast cancer up to 44% in those patients with a strong family history.[103] Prevalence of *CHEK2* mutations among breast cancer patients is ~1%, and is more commonly seen among Northern and Eastern Europeans.[7,104,105] Most of what is known about *CHEK2* cancer risks have primarily been based on the specific common variant 1100delC.[7,104,105] However, other *CHEK2* mutations exist that appear to carry less cancer risk, such as the missense mutation I157T.[104] Thus, when counseling patients, it is important to know the specific *CHEK2* mutation to avoid overestimation of risk. Other cancer risks with *CHEK2* mutations include a possible increased risk of colon cancer.[103]

Breast Cancer Risk Management Annual mammograms and consideration of an annual breast MRI are recommended for women with *CHEK2* mutations starting at the age of 40, or potentially earlier if needed based on the family history.[7] Given its lower associated risks, breast MRI may not be necessary for those patients with the *CHEK2* I157T variant. Clinical breast exam should be performed every 6 to 12 months.[7]

There are no data on the benefit of RRM, and risk should be managed based on family history.[7] There are no data that specifically address the use of preventive medications in *CHEK2* carriers. As with other patients at increased risk of breast cancer, lifestyle modifications should also be discussed.

Other Cancer Risk Management Given the slightly elevated risks for colon cancer associated with a *CHEK2* mutation, the NCCN guidelines recommend colonoscopy screening beginning at age 40 with the interval of time between screenings not to exceed 5 years.[7]

Other Moderate-Penetrance Genes Several additional gene mutations are currently under study for possible associated risks of breast cancer, which include *BARD1, BRIP1, NBN, RAD51C* and *D, NBN, NF1,* and Lynch syndrome genes (*MLH1, MSH2, MSH6, PMS2, EPCAM*).[7] Currently, there is insufficient evidence for specific gene-related breast cancer risk management recommendations for any of these genes; patients with deleterious mutations should be therefore followed for increased breast cancer risk based on their family history[7] (Table 5.3). As breast cancer risk estimates are expected to evolve over time, it is important for clinicians to remain up to date with specific management guidelines, as they may change from year to year.

It is important to recognize, however, that increased cancer risks other than breast cancer have been well-established in some of these genes. For example, women with Lynch syndrome are at increased risk for colon, endometrial, ovarian, and other cancers.[106] *BRIP1, RAD51C,* and *RAD51D* have been shown to be associated with increased risk for ovarian cancer.[107] Specific cancer risk management for these and other genetic syndromes can be found elsewhere in this book and are summarized in Table 5.3.

Low-Penetrance Genetic Syndromes

Low-penetrance genetic syndromes are thought to be characterized by a collection of several weak genetic alterations, commonly referred to as SNPs.[108] Any single SNP alteration does not individually confer significantly increased risk for breast cancer. However, current research is investigating whether the inheritance of many SNPs, particularly at key genome points, may predict higher rates of breast cancer.[108]

These patterns of SNP alterations for breast cancer risk determination are often referred to as polygenic risk scores.[109] To date, genome-wide association studies (GWAS) have identified around 170 SNPs of interest. Though polygenic risk scores are currently marketed for use by some genetic testing companies in order to help define a woman's risk of developing breast cancer, no polygenic risk model has been broadly validated for clinical use and should be interpreted with extreme caution. There has been serious concern about the applicability of SNP-derived polygenic risk scores in women of non-European descent; to date, most of the testing has been centered around European populations, which do not share the same genetic profile of women from African, Asian, or Indigenous descent.[110] Though the development of polygenic risk scores holds promise, the NCCN does not currently recommend the use of SNPs and polygenic risk scores to define breast cancer risk in a clinical setting.[108]

■ MANAGEMENT OF PATIENTS WITH A FAMILY HISTORY OF BREAST CANCER

When patients with a family history of breast cancer present for genetic testing, in a vast majority of cases, testing will return negative for any deleterious mutations. However, as described earlier in this chapter, it is well understood that patients with a strong family history of breast cancer are at increased risk despite negative testing. Risk assessment for patients with familial breast cancer, in the absence of an identifiable hereditary cancer syndrome, should be performed using the IBIS risk model or other family-based risk model. Increased risk is typically quantified as a lifetime risk of greater than 20% to 25%, as defined by models that strongly consider family history.[2] Defining breast cancer risk as accurately as possible should always serve as a next step following negative genetic testing in order to provide guidance for risk management options. Risk estimations should be repeated periodically over time to account for change in age and other risk factors, including any change in family history, over time.

Specific elements of breast cancer risk management for patients with a strong family history should include discussion of both screening and prevention options. To this end, the NCCN has developed a detailed set of management guidelines for breast cancer risk reduction,[2] which can be found at nccn.org.

As for hereditary breast cancer syndromes, breast cancer screening recommendations typically include a selection of screening modality and frequency of testing, including mammograms, ultrasounds, breast MRI, and/or clinical breast exams, tailored to the patient's level of risk.[2] It is important for patients to understand that breast cancer screening, while essential for early detection of cancer, does not serve to *prevent* cancer development.

Major risk-reduction and prevention options that should be reviewed with patients will vary based on the strength of the family history, but should include discussion of three essential elements, namely (1) surgical options, (2) risk-reducing medications, and (3) lifestyle modifications. Patients should also receive psychosocial support as needed, as many patients find themselves distressed by their worry over developing future breast cancer based on their family history.

Screening

Mammograms For patients who are at an increased risk based on family history, the American College of Radiology recommends beginning annual mammograms 5 to 10 years earlier than the earliest age of diagnosis in a close relative and no earlier than the age of 30.[6] Generally, mammograms before the age of 30 are not recommended because breast tissue continues to develop until this age; therefore, limiting radiation to developing tissue generally takes precedence over screening until this age. Annual mammograms should continue until life expectancy is less than 5 to 7 years, as evaluated by age or health conditions.[6] Currently, 3D tomosynthesis is the best option available for improving mortality outcomes, and this technology is increasingly becoming a standard of care.[29] It should be noted that the optimal time for any type of breast screening is day 7 to 15 of the menstrual cycle.[29]

Breast MRI The NCCN guidelines recommend annual MRIs as an addition to mammogram screenings for two categories of patients:[29]

1. An untested patient whose relative is a known genetic mutation carrier
2. A patient whose lifetime risk is equal to or greater than 20% to 25%, as defined by models that rely on family history, such as the IBIS risk model

In both situations, genetic testing should be suggested, first and foremost, either for the patient directly or for first-degree relatives. If a high-risk patient declines testing or does not test positive for relevant genetic mutations, annual breast MRIs may be appropriate.[6] MRI screening can also be considered if risk factors suggest an increased susceptibility for LCIS and ALH/ADH, though guidelines are mixed and should be based on the individual patient's needs.[6,29]

Breast MRI screening is known to have high sensitivity and increases detection rates for populations deemed high risk by models such as IBIS.[6] However, MRI has also been shown to have less specificity than mammogram and can often lead to false-positive results and unnecessary biopsy.[29] Some have additional concerns over repeated exposures to gadolinium-based contrast, though clinical detriment has yet to be proven.[29] Thus, it is important to balance the benefits and risks of MRI screening when considering its use.

To avoid overuse, some guidelines recommend MRI screening when the patient is evaluated as having a lifetime risk threshold greater or equal to 25%, rather than a lower threshold of 20%.[31] From a clinical standpoint, using the higher end of the 20% to 25% range is appropriate, as risk models such as IBIS tend to be highly sensitive to factors that naturally increase with age. It should be noted that consideration of breast MRI in the context of lifetime risk should not be assessed until the time when mammogram screening is deemed to be appropriate (i.e., 5 to 10 years prior to the earliest diagnosis in the family).[29]

Breast MRI may also be used as an alternative to mammograms in order to limit radiation exposure to a patient under 30 who would otherwise qualify for mammogram screening due to family history.[29] As with mammogram, the optimal time for breast MRI screening is day 7 to 15 of the menstrual cycle.[29,111]

Ultrasound There are no guidelines that specifically recommend the use of breast ultrasound as a modality for screening women at increased risk, though ultrasound has been shown to improve cancer detection in women at increased risk over mammogram alone.[6] Women with dense breast tissue should certainly consider having an ultrasound if they do not otherwise qualify for MRI or choose not to pursue it.[6]

Special Considerations: Pregnancy and Nursing. During pregnancy, radiographic mammographic and MRI screening should be paused for the duration of the pregnancy.[112] Patients can resume screening ~3 to 6 months after delivery, even if they are currently nursing. Patients should pump or nurse before any type of screening.[113]

With a mammogram, it should be noted that nursing tissue is quite dense and glandular, and these patients may benefit from a 3D mammogram and same-day ultrasound.[112]

While it is appropriate to screen nursing mothers using breast MRI as far as gadolinium exposure is concerned, it may be beneficial to recommence 3 months after breastfeeding has stopped.[113] However, this is contraindicated if the patient is at severe risk for breast cancer or plans to nurse for an above-average amount of time (over 6 months).[112]

Prevention

Surgical Options Surgical prevention, in the form of RRM, is not overtly recommended for women at increased risk based on family history alone.[2] Generally, recommendations for RRM are reserved for patients who test positive for a high-penetrance gene mutation and are therefore known to be at significantly increased risk.[7] However, patients with a strong family history of breast cancer who test negative for genetic mutations may still elect to undergo prophylactic breast tissue removal.[2]

Bilateral salpingo-oophorectomy (BSO) is also not overtly recommended for women with a family history of breast cancer. While some gene mutations, such as *BRCA1/2,*[113] are related to an increased risk of both breast and ovarian cancer, there is no clear increased risk of ovarian cancer in a woman with a family history of breast cancer in the absence of an identified genetic mutation.[114]

BSO is an invasive procedure that causes chemical menopause and a host of short- and long-term effects, including increased risk for osteoporosis, cardiovascular disease, and potential cognitive changes and menopausal symptoms.[2] As such, BSO is only recommended for patients with a known genetic mutation and can be considered in those who have a specific family history of ovarian cancer.[2]

Chemoprevention Preventive medications, commonly referred to as "chemoprevention," should be considered in women with a family history of breast cancer.[2] These medications can lower breast cancer risk by up to 50% or more in women at increased risk of breast cancer,[2] defined by models such as the IBIS risk model or by the BCRAT.[2] "Increased risk" for the consideration of preventive medications is defined as a 5-year risk of 1.7% or higher.[2]

For those patients who meet the risk threshold, four medication options can be considered. Two medications, namely tamoxifen and raloxifene, fit into the category of selective estrogen receptor modulators (SERMs), whereas exemestane and anastrozole are categorized as aromatase inhibitors (AI). Though all of these medications have been shown to significantly decrease breast cancer incidence, none have been shown to improve mortality. The NCCN has outlined specific recommendations to aid in selection of a chemoprevention agent.[2]

Tamoxifen Since 1992, tamoxifen has been studied for breast cancer risk reduction in pre-menopausal and postmenopausal women in several randomized trials.[115-117] Evidence has demonstrated that a daily 20-mg dose administered over 5 years nearly halved the risk of breast cancer in all age groups.[116] Moreover, this preventive effect appears to last up to 10 years after the last dose is administered, offering 15 years or more of total protection.[117]

Tamoxifen is the only chemopreventive medication that can be prescribed to both post-menopausal and premenopausal women.[2] In addition to breast cancer risk reduction, a further benefit of tamoxifen for postmenopausal women is the potential for improved bone density.[2] However, patients also frequently exhibit bothersome side effects like hot flashes, leg cramps, and irritability.[2] In rarer cases, side effects such as blood clots, pulmonary embolism, stroke, and uterine cancer can occur and warrant caution when prescribing, particularly to older patients.[2] Monitoring for cataracts is also recommended.

Given the known benefits and risks of tamoxifen, research is currently underway examining the possibility of a lower effective dose. Initial results from the TAM-001 study, where patients with DCIS and breast atypia received 5-mg daily doses of tamoxifen versus placebo for 3 years, demonstrated that a lower dose and duration of tamoxifen may be just as effective as the current recommended dosage.[118] Though longer-term follow-up is needed, the NCCN supports use of a lower dose of tamoxifen in patients who otherwise qualify for chemoprevention but who cannot tolerate other doses or preparations.[2]

Raloxifene Raloxifene is a SERM approved in postmenopausal women for both the treatment of osteoporosis and for breast cancer risk reduction.[2] Although the STAR trial found it to be slightly less effective than tamoxifen,[119] it may be recommended as an alternative depending on patient tolerance and other risk factors. Raloxifene is prescribed as a 60-mg daily dose for 5 years for the purposes of breast cancer risk reduction, though patients may opt to continue beyond 5 years if helpful for bone health.[2] It should be noted that raloxifene protection decreases over time after the medication is discontinued.[120] Raloxifene studies have shown that after the initial 5 years of treatment, in follow-up covering an additional 21 months, raloxifene is only 76% as effective as tamoxifen over the same period.[120]

In general, raloxifene side effects tend to be better tolerated than tamoxifen in terms of vasomotor symptoms.[2] However, patients taking raloxifene may report more vaginal dryness.[2] In rarer cases, side effects such as blood clots, pulmonary embolism, and stroke may occur, though with less frequency than tamoxifen. Unlike tamoxifen, raloxifene is not associated with an increase in uterine cancer[2] and thus may be prescribed safely to postmenopausal women.

Aromatase inhibitors (exemestane and anastrozole) The second category of chemoprevention includes two medications: exemestane and anastrozole. Both AIs have comparable outcomes and side effects and have been shown to reduce the risk of invasive breast cancer by 50% to 65% when taken daily for 5 years.[121,122] Exemestane and anastrozole are not yet Food and Drug Administration (FDA) approved for breast cancer risk reduction, but are common in clinical use.

Like raloxifene, AIs are only indicated for use in postmenopausal women.[2] There is not yet sufficient data to conclude on the protective advantages of AIs after medication is discontinued.

While AIs produce more favorable outcomes in terms of breast cancer reduction, the most cited reason for discontinuation is due to side effects, including hot flashes, night sweats, vaginal dryness, muscle aches and pains, and mild bone loss.[2] Bone marrow density should be monitored alongside any AI prescription. However, AI use is not associated with uterine cancer risk or increased risk of thromboembolic disease, and thus may be preferred based on a patient's tolerance for side effects.[2]

Deciding among chemopreventive therapies[2] For patients who qualify for chemopreventive therapy, the following factors should guide decision-making:

- Is the patient premenopausal or postmenopausal?
- Will an increase or decrease in bone density affect this patient?
- Is this patient at risk for uterine cancer?
- How well does the patient tolerate side effects, such as vasomotor symptoms or muscle/joint pain?

In general, it is advised that patients who qualify for chemoprevention should at least trial a medication; if poorly tolerated, it can be switched to an alternative agent or stopped altogether. It should be noted that patients undergoing chemoprevention with tamoxifen, raloxifene, or either aromatase inhibitor should not undergo concurrent OCP use or hormone replacement therapy.

Lifestyle Recommendations

As mentioned earlier in the chapter, several lifestyle modifications can limit or reduce the risk of breast cancer. The American Cancer Society recommends the following:[21,123]

1. Achieve and maintain a healthy weight. Women who gain 25 kg or more after the age of 18 are at a higher risk for breast cancer.
2. Get adequate exercise, typically defined as 75 to 150 minutes of moderate to vigorous activity per week. Several large studies indicate that women who exercise at least 60 minutes per day show decreased risk for breast cancer.
3. Eat healthily at all ages. This is indicated not only because a healthy BMI is associated with decreased risk but also because diets that include a high intake of fruits and vegetables may be associated with decreased risk, even in patients with a sedentary lifestyle.
4. Limit alcohol consumption. Although an alcohol-free lifestyle is best, the NCCN recommends limiting consumption to a maximum of one drink per day.

Other lifestyle considerations include avoidance of tobacco and limiting use of HRT when possible.[2,124,125] However, in patients where quality of life is poor due to the impact of menopause, HRT can and should be used if needed, for the shortest duration possible.

BREAST CANCER MANAGEMENT IN THE SETTING OF HEREDITARY BREAST CANCER SYNDROMES

There are several misconceptions surrounding breast cancer treatment in patients who test positive for a hereditary breast cancer genetic mutation. Some common misconceptions include:

- Treatment requires substantially different approaches than other breast cancer patients
- The breast cancer itself is more aggressive, with worse outcomes, than in patients without a genetic mutation

- A double mastectomy is required or recommended in all cases
- Radiation must be avoided in all cases
- Systemic therapy, including choice of chemotherapy, should differ from standard of care

Other misconceptions may circulate, making it pivotal that patient options are discussed in detail, with a strong regard for risks and outcomes. In general, a breast cancer diagnosis in a patient with a genetic mutation requires similar standards of care as a diagnosis in a patient without a breast cancer mutation. Nuances of breast cancer management in the context of a hereditary breast cancer syndrome will be discussed next.

Breast Cancer Outcomes

While the likelihood of specific breast cancer incidence is known to be higher among patients with genetic mutations as compared to other patients, breast cancer outcomes are the same, stage for stage, for any given breast cancer diagnosis. In addition, while specific mutations such as *BRCA1* are associated with a greater likelihood of aggressive subtypes (i.e., triple-negative breast cancer),[104] each breast cancer subtype progresses the same way in a carrier as it would a noncarrier with the same diagnosis and same stage of disease.[126] Long-term cure rates and survival rates from breast cancer are similar among genetic carriers and noncarriers.[126]

Misconceptions over poorer outcomes among mutation carriers have stemmed from the fact that mutation status may be unknown to the carrier; as such, these individuals at high risk may not be undergoing the recommended aggressive surveillance guidelines, and therefore may present with breast cancer at a more advanced stage.[127]

Though patients with *BRCA1/2* mutations are known to carry a higher risk of contralateral breast cancers, several studies have shown no difference in overall survival of these patients.[128]

In one small study, Kirova et al. compared tumors in patients with *BRCA1* and *BRCA2* germline mutations and a family history of breast cancer with noncarriers and controls.[127] They found that although germline carriers were more likely to have stage III tumors, they did not demonstrate higher risk for ipsilateral tumors, even after 13.4 years.[128] However, germline carriers with a family history had double the rates of contralateral tumors. Nevertheless, the overall survival of germline carriers versus noncarriers showed no significant difference.[129,130] Similarly, a meta-analysis by Valachis et al. compared breast cancer diagnoses in 526 patients with *BRCA1* and *BRCA2* germline mutations to 2320 patients with no germline mutations.[131] Although the risk of contralateral breast cancer was greater in patients with germline mutations, no significant difference in overall survival rate was found.[131]

Surgical Options

Several surgical options are available to women with a hereditary breast cancer diagnosis, including lumpectomy with radiation or single mastectomy, with or without contralateral RRM.[2] In regard to definitive treatment for a given breast cancer, lumpectomy with radiation is considered to be equally effective as mastectomy in mutation carriers.[132] Consideration for prophylactic RRM should turn on several factors, including the patient's risk of recurrence from their given breast cancer, current age and comorbidities, and estimated risks of developing a second primary breast cancer.[2,131]

Breast-Conserving Therapy Breast-conserving therapy (BCT; i.e., lumpectomy plus radiation) is sometimes overlooked in favor of mastectomy in genetic mutation carriers. However, even in mutation carriers, BCT provides similar treatment outcomes as mastectomy in terms of overall survival.[133] Specifically, BCT shows similar prognosis outcomes and recurrence rates for genetic carriers as it does for noncarriers.[134]

Regarding the use of radiation, therapeutic breast cancer radiation treatment has not been associated with a significantly increased risk of ipsilateral cancers in *BRCA1/2, ATM,* or other mutation carriers,[130] with the sole exception of *TP53,* where any therapeutic radiation should be avoided.[104] According to both the American Society of Clinical Oncology (ASCO) and NCCN, the same standards of care in regard to the use of radiation that is applied to noncarriers should be followed for patients with genetic mutations.[2] As such, BCT is a viable treatment option for any patient diagnosed with breast cancer, regardless of whether they are a gene mutation carrier. Patients should receive counseling that considers their preferences, expected aesthetic outcomes, and comorbidities.[130,132.133]

Mastectomy and RRM Many women with a known hereditary genetic mutation will opt to pursue double mastectomies when faced with a breast cancer diagnosis. As discussed earlier, mastectomy for the definitive treatment of the known breast cancer is certainly a reasonable option and carries a potential advantage of not having to undergo radiation treatment, especially when the cancer is small and node negative.[132] As compared to lumpectomy, single mastectomy is a larger, more involved procedure, but may still be appropriate even in women at older ages.[132] However, it is important for patients to understand that mastectomy offers an equivalent cure rate and survival rate to BCT,[132] as many patients erroneously believe that "more surgery" is "better surgery."

Contralateral RRM aims to prevent the occurrence of a future second primary breast cancer and thus should be considered as a prophylactic treatment for the unaffected contralateral breast. As with BCT, it is important for patients to understand that while contralateral RRM can reduce the risk of developing a new breast cancer, it has not been shown to improve life expectancy.[132] Consideration for prophylactic RRM should therefore turn on factors other than improved survival, such as the patient's risk of recurrence from their given breast cancer, their current age and comorbidities, and the estimated risks of developing a second primary breast cancer during their expected remaining lifetime.[134] For example, risks for future contralateral breast cancer is known to be higher among young *BRCA* carriers and can approach risks as high as 30%.[135] However, risks of contralateral breast cancer in older *BRCA* patients may be surprisingly low, especially for women in their 60s or 70s.[135]

For those women with no known genetic mutation but with a strong family history of breast cancer, it should be noted that these women also carry an elevated risk of contralateral breast cancer, slightly less than that of mutation carriers. For example, in a study of 1521 contralateral breast cancer cases, Reiner et al. found that women with no known genetic mutation and a first-degree relative with breast cancer had a 10-year absolute risk for contralateral breast cancer of 8.1%. If the first-degree relative was diagnosed before age 40, this risk approached rates similar to that of *BRCA1/2* carriers (14.1% vs. 18.4% for carriers).[129] Thus, while double mastectomies in this cohort are not overtly recommended by any guidelines, RRM can nonetheless be considered in these cases.

Systemic Therapy

At this time, ASCO- and NCCN-recommended best practice in regard to systemic therapy is to implement the same standards of care for mutation carriers as would be applied to noncarriers. However, promising research indicates that there may soon be viable options for more refined, targeted treatment for genetic mutation carriers.

Platinum-Based Chemotherapy Data are conflicting regarding an enhanced response of *BRCA* carriers to platinum-based chemotherapy for the treatment of breast cancer. In one small trial, *BRCA1* carriers diagnosed with breast cancer were treated with 75 mg/m^2 of cisplatin every 3 weeks for four cycles, and 61% exhibited a pathologic complete response.[136] However, the recent INFORM trial compared the use of neoadjuvant single-agent cisplatin with a standard-of-care combination of doxorubicin/cyclophosphamide in *BRCA* carriers, and no significant advantage to platinum therapy was observed.[137] Thus, further research is needed before platinum-based chemotherapy can be applied as a universal standard of care to patients with *BRCA1/2*-associated breast cancer in the curative setting.

Data regarding use of platinum agents in the metastatic setting are also mixed.[138,139] However, the NCCN does include both cisplatin and carboplatin as standard-of-care options for patients with *BRCA*-related metastatic breast cancer.[139]

PARP Inhibitors Poly-ADP ribose polymerase (PARP) inhibitors, namely olaparib and talazoparib, have been recently FDA-approved for the treatment of metastatic Her-2–negative breast cancer in patients with *BRCA* mutations.[140,141] In the landmark OlympiAD trial, Robson et al. found that olaparib improved progression-free survival by 2.8 months longer on average in *BRCA* carriers with metastatic breast cancer as compared to standard chemotherapy.[142] In a similar randomized trial of over 400 *BRCA* carriers with metastatic breast cancer, called the EMBRACA trial, talazoparib was shown to improve progression-free survival by 3 months compared to traditional chemotherapy.[143] Thus, use of PARP inhibition is now recommended as part of standard-of-care therapy in the metastatic breast cancer setting for patients with *BRCA* mutations.

Other PARP inhibitors are under study for use in *BRCA*-associated breast cancer, including veliparib and niraparib. Further research is underway to demonstrate the role of PARP inhibition in both the adjuvant and neoadjuvant settings and in genetic mutations other than *BRCA*.

References

1. U.S. Breast Cancer Statistics. Breast Cancer.org. https://www.breastcancer.org/symptoms/understand_bc/statistics. Published June 25, 2020. Accessed September 11, 2020.

2. National Comprehensive Cancer Network. Breast Cancer Risk Reduction (Version 1.2020). NCCN.org. August 18, 2020.

3. Bevers TB, Helvie M, Bonaccio E, et al. Breast Cancer Screening and Diagnosis, Version 3.2018, NCCN Clinical Practice Guidelines in Oncology. *J Natl Compr Canc Netw*. 2018;16(11):1362–1389.

4. Fuller MS, Lee CI, Elmore JG. Breast cancer screening: an evidence-based update. *Med Clin North Am*. 2015;99(3):451–468.

5. Gucalp A, Traina TA, Eisner JR, et al. Male breast cancer: a disease distinct from female breast cancer. *Breast Cancer Res Treat*. 2019;173(1):37–48.

6. Monticciolo DL, Newell MS, Moy L, Niell B, Monsees B, Sickles EA. Breast cancer screening in women at higher-than-average risk: recommendations from the ACR. *J Am Coll Radiol*. 2018;15(3 Pt A):408–414.

7. National Comprehensive Cancer Network. Genetic/Familial High-Risk Assessment: Breast, Ovarian, and Pancreatic (Version 1.2020). https://doi.org/10.6004/jnccn.2020.0017. Accessed August 18, 2020.

8. Kelsey JL, Gammon MD, John EM. Reproductive factors and breast cancer. *Epidemiol Rev*. 1993;15(1):36–47.

9. Colditz GA, Rosner B. Cumulative risk of breast cancer to age 70 years according to risk factor status: data from the Nurses' Health Study. *Am J Epidemiol*. 2000;152(10):950–964.

10. Ritte R, Lukanova A, Tjønneland A, et al. Height, age at menarche and risk of hormone receptor-positive and -negative breast cancer: a cohort study. *Int J Cancer*. 2013;132(11):2619–2629.

11. Ewertz M, Duffy SW, Adami HO, et al. Age at first birth, parity and risk of breast cancer: a meta-analysis of 8 studies from the Nordic countries. *Int J Cancer*. 1990;46(4):597–603.

12. Hsieh CC, Trichopoulos D, Katsouyanni K, Yuasa S. Age at menarche, age at menopause, height and obesity as risk factors for breast cancer: associations and interactions in an international case-control study. *Int J Cancer*. 1990;46(5):796–800.

13. Collaborative Group on Hormonal Factors in Breast Cancer. Breast cancer and breastfeeding: collaborative reanalysis of individual data from 47 epidemiological studies in 30 countries, including 50302 women with breast cancer and 96973 women without the disease. *Lancet*. 2002;360(9328):187–195.

14. Mørch LS, Skovlund CW, Hannaford PC, et al. Contemporary hormonal contraception and the risk of breast cancer. *N Engl J Med*. 2017;377(2017):2228–2239.

15. Nelson HD, Walker M, Zakher B, Mitchell J. Menopausal hormone therapy for the primary prevention of chronic conditions: a systematic review to update the U.S. Preventive Services Task Force recommendations. *Ann Intern Med*. 2012;157:104–113.

16. Bakken K, Fournier A, Lund E, et al. Menopausal hormone therapy and breast cancer risk: impact of different treatments. The European Prospective Investigation into Cancer and Nutrition. *Int J Cancer*. 2011;128:144–156.

17. The Premenopausal Breast Cancer Collaborative Group. Association of body mass index and age with subsequent breast cancer risk in premenopausal women. *JAMA Oncol*. 2018;4(11):e181771.

18. Kang C, LeRoith D, Gallagher EJ. Diabetes, obesity, and breast cancer. *Endocrinology*. 2018;159(11):3801–3812.

19. Picon-Ruiz M, Morata-Tarifa C, Valle-Goffin JJ, et al. Obesity and adverse breast cancer risk and outcome: mechanistic insights and strategies for intervention. *CA Cancer J Clin*. 2017;67(5):378–397.

20. Keum N, Greenwood DC, Lee DH, et al. Adult weight gain and adiposity-related cancers: a dose-response meta-analysis of prospective observational studies. *J Natl Cancer Inst*. 2015;107:107–121.

21. Kushi LH, Doyle C, McCullough, et al. American Cancer Society guidelines on nutrition and physical activity for cancer prevention. *CA: A Cancer Journal for Clinicians*. 2012;62:30–67.

22. De Cicco P, Catani MV, Gasperi V, et al. Nutrition and breast cancer: a literature review on prevention, treatment and recurrence. *Nutrients*. 2019;11(7):1514.

23. Wei Y, Lv J, Guo Y, et al. Soy intake and breast cancer risk: a prospective study of 300,000 Chinese women and a dose-response meta-analysis. *Eur J Epidemiol*. 2020;35(6):567–578.

24. Chen WY, Rosner B, Hankinson SE, et al. Moderate alcohol consumption during adult life, drinking patterns, and breast cancer risk. *JAMA*. 2011;306(17):1884–1890.

25. Jones ME, Schoemaker MJ, Wright LB, et al. Smoking and risk of breast cancer in the Generations Study cohort. *Breast Cancer Res*. 2017;19(1):118.

26. Lopez-Garcia MA, Geyer FC, Lacroix-Triki M, et al. Breast cancer precursors revisited: molecular features and progression pathways. *Histopathology*. 2010;57:171–192.

27. King TA, Pilewskie M, Muhsen S, et al. Lobular carcinoma in situ: a 29-year longitudinal experience evaluating clinicopathologic features and breast cancer risk. *J Clin Oncol*. 2015;33:3945–3952.

28. Morrow M, Schnitt SJ, Norton L. Current management of lesions associated with an increased risk of breast cancer. *Nat Rev Clin Oncol*. 2015;12:227–238.

29. National Comprehensive Cancer Network. Breast Cancer Screening and Diagnosis (Version 1.2019). NCCN. org. Accessed August 18, 2020.

30. Freer PE, Slanetz PJ. Breast density and screening for breast cancer. UpToDate. https://www.uptodate.com/contents/breast-density-and-screening-for-breast-cancer?sectionName=Average%20or%20low%20risk%20(%3C15%20percent%20lifetime%20risk)&topicRef=7564&anchor=H16928812&source=see_link#H16928812 Accessed August 30, 2020.

31. Vourtsis A, Berg WA. Breast density implications and supplemental screening. *Eur Radiol*. 2019; 29(4):1762–1777.

32. Seely JM, Alhassan T. Screening for breast cancer in 2018-what should we be doing today? *Curr Oncol*. 2018;25(Suppl 1):S115–S124.

33. Lee CI, Chen LE, Elmore JG. Risk-based breast cancer screening: implications of breast density. *Med Clin North Am*. 2017;101(4):725–741.

34. Troisi R, Hatch EE, Titus L, et al. Prenatal diethylstilbestrol exposure and cancer risk in women. *Environ Mol Mutagen*. 2019;60(5):395–403.

35. Pham TT, Lee ES, Kong SY, et al. Night-shift work, circadian and melatonin pathway related genes and their interaction on breast cancer risk: evidence from a case-control study in Korean women. *Sci Rep*. 2019;9(1):10982.

36. Deng Y, Xu H, Zeng X. Induced abortion and breast cancer: An updated meta-analysis. *Medicine (Baltimore)*. 2018;97(3):e9613.

37. Noels EC, Lapid O, Lindeman JH, et al. Breast implants and the risk of breast cancer: a meta-analysis of cohort studies. *Aesthet Surg J*. 2015;35(1):55–62.

38. Factors That Do Not Increase Breast Cancer Risk. https://ww5.komen.org/BreastCancer/FactorsThatDoNotIncreaseRisk.html. Updated February 14, 2020. Accessed September 13, 2020.

39. Richards S, Aziz N, Bale S, et al. Standards and guidelines for the interpretation of sequence variants: a joint consensus recommendation of the American College of Medical Genetics and Genomics and the Association for Molecular Pathology. *Genet Med*. 2015;17:405–423.

40. Prince AE, Roche MI. Genetic information, non-discrimination, and privacy protections in genetic counseling practice. *J Genet Couns*. 2014;23(6):891–902.

41. Oh B. Direct-to-consumer genetic testing: advantages and pitfalls. *Genomics Inform*. 2019;17(3):e33.

42. Covolo L, Rubinelli S, Ceretti E, et al. Internet-based direct-to-consumer genetic testing: a systematic review. *J Med Internet Res*. 2015;17(12):e279.

43. Frey MK, Kim SH, Bassett RY, et al. Rescreening for genetic mutations using multi-gene panel testing in patients who previously underwent non-informative genetic screening. *Gynecol Oncol*. 2015;139(2):211–215.

44. Tischler J, Crew KD, Chung WK. Cases in precision medicine: the role of tumor and germline genetic testing in breast cancer management. *Ann Intern Med*. 2019;171(12):925–930.

45. Tyrer J. Duffy SW, Cuzick J. A breast cancer prediction model incorporating familial and personal risk factors. *Stat Med*. 2004;23:1111–1130.

46. Cuzick J, Brentnall A. Models for assessment of breast cancer risk. *DI Europe*. 2016;32(5):54–55.

47. Kurian, AW, Hughes, E., Bernhisel R, et al. Performance of the IBIS/Tyrer-Cuzick (TC) Model by race/ethnicity in the Women's Health Initative. *J Clin Oncol*. 2020;38(Suppl):abstr 1503.

48. Evans DG, Howell A. Breast cancer risk-assessment. *Breast Cancer Res*. 2007;9:213–221.

49. Parmigiani G, Berry D, Aguiliar O. Determining carrier probabilities for breast cancer-susceptibility genes BRCA1 and BRCA2. *Am J Hum Genet*. 1998;62(1):145–158.

50. Antoniou AC, Pharoah PP, Smith P et al. THE BOADICEA model of genetic susceptibility to breast and ovarian cancer. *Br J Cancer*. 2004;91:1580–1590.

51. Pankratz VS, Hartmann LC, Degnim AC, et al. Assessment of the accuracy of the Gail model in women with atypical hyperplasia. *J Clin Oncol*. 2008;26:5374–5379.

52. Spiegelman D, Colditz GA, Hunter D, et al. Validation of the Gail et al. model for predicting individual breast cancer risk. *J Natl Cancer Inst*. 1994;86:600–607.

53. Yun MH, Hiom K. Understanding the functions of BRCA1 in the DNA-damage response. *Biochem Soc Trans*. 2009;37:597–604.

54. Cipak L, Watanbe N, Bessho T. The role of BRCA2 in replication-coupled DNA interstrand cross-link repair in vitro. *Nat Struct Mol Biol*. 2006;13:729–733

55. Petrucelli N, Daly MB, Feldman GL. BRCA1 and BRCA2 hereditary breast and ovarian cancer. In: Adam MP, Ardinger HH, Pagon RA, et al. (eds.). GeneReviews. Seattle, WA: University of Washington; 1993-2021.

56. Chen S, Parmigiani G. Meta-analysis of BRCA1 and BRCA2 penetrance. *J Clin Oncol*. 2007;25:1329–1333.

57. American College of Radiology. ACR Practice Parameter for The Performance of Contrast-Enhanced Magnetic Resonance Imaging (MRI) Of The Breast. https://www.acr.org/-/media/ACR/Files/Practice-Parameters/mr-contrast-breast.pdf. Published 2018. Accessed August 30, 2020.

58. Elmore JG. UpToDate. https://www.uptodate.com/contents/screening-for-breast-cancer-strategies-and-recommendations?csi=19b23d56-fcaa-4471-9ad4-8d6fa8156ae5&source=contentShare#topicContent. Published July 17, 2020. Accessed August 28, 2020.

59. Li X, You R, Wang X, et al. Effectiveness of prophylactic surgeries in BRCA1 and BRCA2 mutation carriers: a meta-analysis and systematic review. *Clin Cancer Res.* 2016;22:3971–3981.

60. Hartmann LC, Schaid DJ, Woods JE, et al. Efficacy of bilateral prophylactic mastectomy in women with a family history of breast cancer. *N Engl J Med.* 1999;340:77–84.

61. Chiesa F, Sacchini VS. Risk-reducing mastectomy. *Minerva Ginecol.* 2016;68(5):544–547.

62. Domchek SM, Jhaveri K, Patil S, et al. Risk of metachronous breast cancer after BRCA mutation–associated ovarian cancer. *Cancer.* 2013;119:1344–1348.

63. Fisher B, Costantino JP, Wickerham DL, et al. Tamoxifen for prevention of breast cancer: report of the National Surgical Adjuvant Breast and Bowel Project P-1 Study. *J Natl Cancer Inst.* 1998;90(18):1371–1388.

64. Cuzick J, Sestak I, Forbes JF, et al. Anastrozole for prevention of breast cancer in high-risk postmeno-pausal women (IBIS-II): an international, double-blind, randomized placebo-controlled trial. *Lancet.* 2014;383:1041–1048.

65. Kiechle M, Engel C, Berling A, et al. Lifestyle intervention in BRCA1/2 mutation carriers: study protocol for a prospective, randomized, controlled clinical feasibility trial (LIBRE-1 study). *Pilot Feasibility Stud.* 2016;2:74.

66. Kauff ND, Domchek SM, Friebal TM et al. Risk-reducing salpingo-oophorectomy for the prevention of BRCA1 and BRCA2 associated breast and gynecological cancer: a multicenter prospective study. *J Clin Oncol.* 2008;26:1331–1337.

67. Finch AP, Lubinski J, Moller P, et al. Impact of oophorectomy on cancer incidence and mortality in women with a BRCA1 or BRCA2 mutation. *J Clin Oncol.* 2014;32:1547–1553.

68. Rebbeck TR, Lynch HT, Neuhausen SL, et al. Prophylactic oophorectomy in carriers of BRCA1 or BRCA2 mutations. *N Engl J Med.* 2002;346:1616–1622.

69. Shu CA, Pike MC, Jotwani AR, et al. Uterine cancer after risk-reducing salpingo-oophorectomy without hys-terectomy in women with BRCA mutations. *JAMA Oncol.* 2016;2(11):1434–1440.

70. Schrijver LH, Olsson H, Phillips KA, et al. Oral contraceptive use and breast cancer risk: retrospective and prospective analyses from a BRCA1 and BRCA2 mutation carrier cohort study [published correction appears in JNCI Cancer Spectr. 2018 Aug 17;2(3):pky041]. *JNCI Cancer Spectr.* 2018;2(2):pky023.

71. Marchetti C, De Felice F, Boccia S, et al. Hormone replacement therapy after prophylactic risk-reducing salp-ingo-oophorectomy and breast cancer risk in BRCA1 and BRCA2 mutation carriers: a meta-analysis. *Crit Rev Oncol Hematol.* 2018;132:111–115.

72. Moran A, O'Hara C, Khan S, et al. Risk of cancer other than breast or ovarian in individuals with BRCA1 and BRCA2 mutations. *Fam Cancer.* 2012;11(2):235–242.

73. https://clinicaltrials.gov/ct2/show/NCT02000089. Updated June 22, 2020. Accessed September 12, 2020.

74. Sidransky D, Tokino T, Helzlsouer K, et al. Inherited p53 gene mutations in breast cancer. *Cancer Res.* 1992;52(10):2984–2986.

75. Mai PL, Best AF, Peters JA, et al. Risks of first and subsequent cancers among TP53 mutation carriers in the National Cancer Institute Li-Fraumeni syndrome cohort. *Cancer.* 2016;122(23):3673–3681.

76. Chompret A, Abel A, Stoppa-Lyonnet D, et al. Sensitivity and predictive value of criteria for p53 germline mutation screening. *J Med Genet.* 2001;38(1):43–47.

77. Gonzalez KD, Noltner KA, Buzin CH, et al. Beyond Li Fraumeni syndrome: clinical characteristics of families with p53 germline mutations. *J Clin Oncol.* 2009;27:1250–1256.

78. Villani A, Shore A, Wasserman JD, et al. Biochemical and imaging surveillance in germline TP53 mutation carriers with Li-Fraumeni syndrome: 11 year follow-up of a prospective observational study. *Lancet Oncol.* 2016;17(9):1295–305.

79. Schneider K, Zelley K, Nichols K, et al. Li-Fraumeni syndrome. In Adam MP, Ardinger HH, Pagon RA et al., eds. *GeneReviews.* Seattle, WA: University of Washington; 1993–2021.

80. Pilarski R. PTEN Hamartoma tumor syndrome: a clinical overview. *Cancers (Basel).* 2019;11(6):844.

81. Hobert JA, Eng C. PTEN hamartoma tumor syndrome: an overview. *Genet Med.* 2009;11(10):687–694.

82. Pilarski R, Burt R, Kohlman W, et al. Cowden syndrome and the PTEN hamartoma tumor syndrome: system-atic review and revised diagnostic criteria. *J Natl Cancer Inst.* 2013;105:1607–1616.

83. Eng C. Will the real Cowden syndrome please stand up: revised diagnostic criteria. *J Med Genet.* 2000;37:828–830.

84. Kaurah P, MacMillan A, Boyd N, et al. Founder and recurrent CDH1 mutations in families with hereditary diffuse gastric cancer. *JAMA.* 2007;297(21):2360–2372.

85. Pharoah PD, Guilford P, Caldas C; International Gastric Cancer Linkage Consortium. Incidence of gastric cancer and breast cancer in CDH1 (E-cadherin) mutation carriers from hereditary diffuse gastric cancer families. *Gastroenterology.* 2001;121(6):1348–1353.

86. CHD1 Gene. MedlinePlus. https://medlineplus.gov/genetics/gene/cdh1/#conditions. Updated August 18, 2020. Accessed October 16, 2020.

87. Mirandola S, Pellini F, Granuzzo E, et al. Multidisciplinary management of CDH1 germinal mutation and prophylactic management hereditary lobular breast cancer: a case report. *Int J Surg Case Rep.* 2019;58:92–95.

88. Corso G, Intra M, Trentin C, et al. CDH1 germline mutations and hereditary lobular breast cancer. *Fam Cancer.* 2016;15(2):215–219.

89. Jacobs MF, Dust H, Koeppe E, et al. Outcomes of endoscopic surveillance in individuals with genetic predisposition to hereditary diffuse gastric cancer. *Gastroenterology.* 2019;157(1):87–96.

90. STK11 Gene. MedlinePlus. https://medlineplus.gov/genetics/gene/stk11/#conditions. Updated August 18, 2020. Accessed October 16, 2020.

91. McGarrity TJ, Amos CI, Baker MJ. Peutz-Jeghers syndrome. In Adam MP, Ardinger HH, Pagon RA, et al., eds. *GeneReviews.* Seattle, WA: University of Washington; 2001.

92. Antoniou AC, Casadei S, Heikkinen T, et al. Breast-cancer risk in families with mutations in PALB2. *N Engl J Med.* 2014;371(6):497–506.

93. Ngamruengphong S, Canto MI. Screening for pancreatic cancer. *Surg Clin North Am.* 2016;96(6):1223–1233.

94. National Comprehensive Cancer Network. Genetic/Familial High-Risk Assessment: Breast and Ovarian. (Version 3.2019). NCCN.org. 2020.

95. Nepal M, Che R, Zhang J, et al. Fanconi anemia signaling and cancer. *Trends Cancer.* 2017;3(12):840–856.

96. Mehta PA, Tolar J. Fanconi anemia. In Adam MP, Ardinger HH, Pagon RA, et al. eds. GeneReviews. Seattle, WA: University of Washington; 1993–2020.

97. Tung N, Domchek SM, Stadler Z, et al. Counselling framework for moderate-penetrance cancer-susceptibility mutations. *Nat Rev Clin Oncol.* 2016;13(9):581–588.

98. Heikkinen K, Rapakko K, Karppinen SM, et al. Association of common ATM polymorphism with bilateral breast cancer. *Int J Cancer.* 2005;116(1):69–72.

99. Marabelli M, Cheng SC, Parmigiani G. Penetrance of ATM gene mutations in breast cancer: a meta-analysis of different measures of risk. *Genet Epidemiol.* 2016;40:425–431.

100. Southey MC, Goldgar DE, Winqvist R, et al. PALB2, CHEK2 and ATM rare variants and cancer risk: data from COGS. *J Med Genet.* 2016;53(12):800–811.

101. Taylor AM, Lam Z, Last JI, Byrd PJ. Ataxia telangiectasia: more variation at clinical and cellular levels. *Clin Genet.* 2015;87(3):199–208.

102. CHEK2 Breast Cancer Case-Control Consortium. CHEK2*1100delC and susceptibility to breast cancer: a collaborative analysis involving 10,860 breast cancer cases and 9,065 controls from 10 studies. *Am J Hum Genet.* 2004;74(6):1175–1182.

103. Cybulski C, Wokołorczyk D, Jakubowska A, et al. Risk of breast cancer in women with a CHEK2 mutation with and without a family history of breast cancer. *J Clin Oncol.* 2011;29(28):3747–3752.

104. Apostolou P, Fostira F. Hereditary breast cancer: the era of new susceptibility genes. *Biomed Res Int.* 2013;2013:747318.

105. Iniesta MD, Gorin MA, Chien LC, et al. Absence of CHEK2*1100delC mutation in families with hereditary breast cancer in North America. *Cancer Genet Cytogenet.* 2010;202(2):136–140.

106. Watson P, Vasen HF, Mecklin JP, et al. The risk of extra-colonic, extra-endometrial cancer in the Lynch syndrome. *Int J Cancer.* 2008;123:444–449.

107. Loveday C, Turnbull C, Ruark E, et al. Germline RAD51C mutations confer susceptibility to ovarian cancer. *Nat Genet.* 2012;44:475–476.

108. Deng N, Zhou H, Fan H, Yuan Y. Single nucleotide polymorphisms and cancer susceptibility. *Oncotarget.* 2017;8(66):110635–110649.

109. Mavaddat N, Michailidou K, Dennis J, et al. Polygenic risk scores for prediction of breast cancer and breast cancer subtypes. *Am J Hum Genet.* 2019;104(1):21–34.

110. Shieh Y, Fejerman L, Lott PC, et al. A polygenic risk score for breast cancer in US Latinas and Latin American women. *J Natl Cancer Inst.* 2020;112(6):590–598.

111. ACR Practice Parameter for the Performance of Contrast-Enhanced Magnetic Resonance Imaging (MRI) of the Breast. American Academy of Radiology. https://www.acr.org/-/media/ACR/Files/Practice-Parameters/mr-contrast-breast.pdf. Updated 2018. Accessed September 12, 2020.

112. diFlorio-Alexander RM, Slanetz, PJ, Vincoff NS, et al. ACR Appropriateness criteria breast imaging of pregnant and lactating women. *J Am Coll Rad.* 2018;15(11)S263–S274.

113. Metcalfe K, Lynch HT, Foulkes WD, et al. Effect of oophorectomy on survival after breast cancer in BRCA1 and BRCA2 mutation carriers. *JAMA Oncol.* 2015;1(3):306–313.

114. Sherman ME, Piedmonte M, Mai PL, et al. Pathologic findings at risk-reducing salpingo-oophorectomy: primary results from Gynecologic Oncology Group Trial GOG-0199. *J Clin Oncol.* 2014;32(29):3275–3283.

115. Fisher B, Costantino JP, Wickerham DL, et al. Tamoxifen for prevention of breast cancer: report of the National Surgical Adjuvant Breast and Bowel Project P-1 Study. *J Natl Cancer Inst.* 1998;90(18):1371–1388.

116. Cuzick J, Powles T, Veronesi U, et al. Overview of the main outcomes in breast-cancer prevention trials. *Lancet.* 2003;361(9354):296–300.

117. Cuzick J, Forbes J, Edwards R, et al. First results from the International Breast Cancer Intervention Study (IBIS-I): a randomized prevention trial. *Lancet.* 2002;360(9336):817–824.

118. San Antonio Breast Cancer Symposium. Low-Dose Tamoxifen Was Safe and Effective at Reducing Recurrence and New Breast Disease for Patients With DCIS, LCIS, and ADH. https://www.sabcs.org/sabcs/2018/pressreleases/3_74ytz7j4nvug_Low-Dose%20Tamoxifen%20Was%20Safe%20and%20Effective%20at%20Reducing%20Recurrence%20and%20New%20Breast%20Disease%20for%20Patients%20With%20DCIS,%20LCIS,%20and%20ADH.pdf. Published December 6, 2018. Accessed September 2, 2020.

119. Wickerham DL, Costantino JP, Vogel VG, et al. The use of tamoxifen and raloxifene for the prevention of breast cancer. *Recent Results Cancer Res.* 2009;181:113–119.

120. Vogel VG, Costantino JP, Wickerham DL, et al. Update of the National Surgical Adjuvant Breast and Bowel Project Study of Tamoxifen and Raloxifene (STAR) P-2 Trial: preventing breast cancer. *Cancer Prev Res (Phila).* 2010;3(6):696–706.

121. Goss PE, Ingle JN, Alés-Martínez JE, et al. Exemestane for breast-cancer prevention in postmenopausal women [published correction appears in N Engl J Med. 2011 Oct 6;365(14):1361]. *N Engl J Med.* 2011;364(25):2381–2391.

122. Cuzick J, Sestak I, Forbes JF, et al. Use of anastrozole for breast cancer prevention (IBIS-II): long-term results of a randomized controlled trial [published correction appears in Lancet. 2020 Feb 15;395(10223):496]. *Lancet.* 2020;395(10218):117–122.

123. Runowicz CD, Leach CR, Henry NL, et al. American Cancer Society/American Society of Clinical Oncology Breast Cancer Survivorship Care Guideline. *CA Cancer J Clin.* 2016;66(1):43–73.

124. Jones ME, Schoemaker MJ, Wright LB, et al. Smoking and risk of breast cancer in the Generations Study cohort. *Breast Cancer Res.* 2017;19(1):118.

125. Johnson KC, Hu J, Mao Y. Passive and active smoking and breast cancer risk in Canada, 1994–97. *Cancer Causes Control.* 2000;11:211–221.

126. Chen H, Wu J, Zhang Z, et al. Association between BRCA status and triple-negative breast cancer: a meta-analysis. *Front Pharmacol.* 2018;9:909.

127. Kirova YM, Savignoni A, Sigal-Zafrani B, et al. Is the breast-conserving treatment with radiotherapy appropriate in BRCA1/2 mutation carriers? Long-term results and review of the literature. *Breast Cancer Res Treat.* 2010;120(1):119–126.

128. Graeser MK, Engel C, Rhiem K, et al. Contralateral breast cancer risk in BRCA1 and BRCA2 mutation carriers. *J Clin Oncol.* 2009;27(35):5887–5892.

129. Reiner AS, Sisti J, John EM, et al. Breast cancer family history and contralateral breast cancer risk in young women: an update from the Women's Environmental Cancer and Radiation Epidemiology Study. *J Clin Oncol.* 2018;36(15):1513–1520.

130. Lee A, Moon BI, Kim TH. BRCA1/BRCA2 pathogenic variant breast cancer: treatment and prevention strategies. *Ann Lab Med.* 2020;40(2):114–121.

131. Valachis A, Nearchou AD, Lind P. Surgical management of breast cancer in BRCA-mutation carriers: a systematic review and meta-analysis. *Breast Cancer Res Treat.* 2014;144(3):443–455.

132. Moo TA, Sanford R, Dang C, et al. Overview of breast cancer therapy. *PET Clin.* 2018;13(3):339–354.

133. Yamauchi H, Takei J. Management of hereditary breast and ovarian cancer. *Intl J Clin Oncol.* 2018;23(1):45–51.

134. Warrier S, Tapia G, Goltsman D, et al. An update in breast cancer screening and management. *Womens Health (Lond).* 2016;12(2):229–239.

135. Franceschini G, Di Leone A, Terribile D, et al. Bilateral prophylactic mastectomy in BRCA mutation carriers: what surgeons need to know. *Ann Ital Chir.* 2019;90:1–2.

136. Byrski T, Huzarski T, Dent R, et al. Pathologic complete response to neoadjuvant cisplatin in BRCA1-positive breast cancer patients. *Breast Cancer Res Treat.* 2014;147(2):401–405.

137. Tung N, Arun B, Hacker MR, et al. TBCRC 031: randomized phase ii study of neoadjuvant cisplatin versus doxorubicin-cyclophosphamide in germline BRCA carriers with HER2-negative breast cancer (the INFORM trial). *J Clin Oncol.* 2020;38(14):1539–1548.

138. Tutt A, Tovey H, Cheang MCU, et al. Carboplatin in BRCA1/2-mutated and triple-negative breast cancer BRCAness subgroups: the TNT Trial. *Nat Med.* 2018;24(5):628–637.

139. Gradishar WJ, Anderson BO, Abraham J, et al. Breast Cancer. Version 3.2020, NCCN Clinical Practice Guidelines in Oncology. *J Natl Compr Canc Netw.* 2020;18(4):452–478.

140. FDA Approves Olaparib for Germline BRCA-Mutated Metastatic Breast Cancer. FDA. https://www.fda.gov/drugs/resources-information-approved-drugs/fda-approves-olaparib-germline-brca-mutated-metastatic-breast-cancer. Updated January 12, 2020. Accessed September 30, 2020.

141. FDA Approves Talazoparib for gBRCAm HER2-Negative Locally Advanced or Metastatic Breast Cancer. FDA. https://www.fda.gov/drugs/drug-approvals-and-databases/fda-approves-talazoparib-gbrcam-her2-negative-locally-advanced-or-metastatic-breast-cancer. Updated December 14, 2018. Accessed September 30, 2020.

142. Robson M, Im SA, Senkus E, et al. Olaparib for metastatic breast cancer in patients with a germline BRCA mutation [published correction appears in N Engl J Med. 2017 Oct 26;377(17):1700]. *N Engl J Med.* 2017;377(6):523–533.

143. Litton JK, Rugo HS, Ettl J, et al. Talazoparib in patients with advanced breast cancer and a germline BRCA mutation. *N Engl J Med.* 2018;379(8):753–763.

CHAPTER 6

Gastrointestinal Polyposis Syndromes

Marcia Cruz-Correa and Veroushka Ballester

Gastrointestinal (GI) polyposis syndromes are a group of conditions that are associated with an increased lifetime risk of colorectal adenocarcinoma and extraintestinal malignancies. The polyposis syndromes have traditionally been categorized according to polyp histology (adenomatous, hamartomatous, and serrated) and clinical phenotype. Criteria to be considered in differentiating the various polyposis conditions include polyp distribution throughout the GI tract, polyp number, the presence of extraintestinal manifestations or malignancy, and family history. Identification of relevant causative genes has improved our understanding of specific polyposis conditions, including phenotypic characteristics and associated cancer risks. The most common feature for when to consider a polyposis diagnosis and germline genetic testing is the finding of 10 or more colonic polyps, polyposis in other parts of the GI tract, and polyps in young individuals with a family history of a polyposis diagnosis. The clinical importance of these syndromes relates to their inheritance. Mutation-specific genetic testing offers the opportunity to test family members for the pathogenic mutation found in an index case, allowing a more personalized approach for cancer prevention with tailored screening and surveillance interventions.

ADENOMATOUS POLYPOSIS SYNDROMES

Familial Adenomatous Polyposis

Familial adenomatous polyposis (FAP) is one of the most clearly defined polyposis syndromes. It is an autosomal dominant adenomatous polyposis condition caused by a germline mutation in the *APC* gene on chromosome 5q21, with nearly complete penetrance. *APC* is a tumor suppressor gene, and the loss of *APC* is among the earliest events in the chromosomal instability colorectal tumor pathway. Reported incidence varies from 1 in 7000 to 1 in 22,000 births.[1] Up to one-third of newly diagnosed cases not belonging to previously identified families appear to represent either *de novo* germline mutations or mosaicism.

The classic form of FAP is characterized by hundreds to thousands of colonic adenomatous polyps that typically begin to emerge after the first decade of life. An attenuated version

TABLE 6.1: Cancer Risks of Extracolonic Tumors in Familial Adenomatous Polyposis		
Malignancy	**Relative Risk**	**Absolute Lifetime Risk (%)**
Desmoid	852.0	15.0
Duodenal tumors and cancer	330.8	5.0–12.0
Thyroid cancer	7.6	2.0
Brain cancer	7.0	2.0
Ampullary cancer	123.7	1.7
Pancreas cancer	4.5	1.7
Hepatoblastoma	847.0	1.6
Gastric caner	Not defined	0.6

Reproduced with permission from Galiatsatos P, Foulkes WD. Familial adenomatous polyposis, Am J Gastroenterol 2006 Feb;101(2):385-398.

(AFAP), also caused by a mutation in *APC,* typically causes fewer than 100 polyps. The risk for colorectal cancer in FAP approaches 100% by age 50, and the recommended intervention is annual sigmoidoscopies or colonoscopies in adolescence and prophylactic colectomy in young adulthood or when the polyp burden becomes too high to be managed endoscopically.

In addition to a high risk of colon adenomas in FAP patients, various extracolonic manifestations have been described, including upper gastrointestinal tract adenomas and adenocarcinomas; fundic gland stomach polyps; nonepithelial benign tumors (osteomas, epidermal cysts, dental abnormalities); desmoid tumors; congenital hypertrophy of retinal pigment epithelium; and malignant tumors (thyroid, medulloblastoma, and hepatoblastoma) (Table 6.1). Gardner syndrome was previously the diagnosis for FAP patients who manifested with colorectal polyposis, osteomas, and soft tissue tumors. However, Gardner syndrome has been shown genetically to be a variant of FAP, and thus the term *Gardner syndrome* is essentially no longer used in clinical practice.[1]

Clinical Phenotype

Colon Adenomas and Colorectal Cancer The estimated risk of developing colonic adenomas in individuals who inherit a pathogenic variant in the *APC* gene has been estimated to be more than 90%.[4,5] By age 10 years, 15% of carriers of the *APC* germline variant have adenomas; by age 20 years, the probability increases to 75%; and by age 30 years, 90% will have presented with FAP.[3-6] The age of symptom presentation, as well as the colonic polyp density, correlates with the location of the mutation in the *APC* gene. Fewer adenomas, which are predominantly in the right colon, are seen in individuals with AFAP (see the section "Attenuated Familial Adenomatous Polyposis), which correlates with mutations at the far proximal and distal portions of the *APC* gene. Studies suggest the presence of other contributing factors to the onset and frequency of polyp formation, which explains the discrepancy between disease manifestations among individuals with the same *APC* pathogenic variant. A study by Dejea et al. evaluated the role of the microbiome on carcinogenesis in individuals with FAP. They studied the colonic mucosa of patients with FAP who developed polyps early in life and identified patchy bacterial biofilms composed predominately of *Escherichia coli* and *Bacteroides fragilis.* These data suggest a link between early neoplasia of the colon and tumorigenic bacteria.[7]

Colonic adenocarcinoma is the inevitable consequence of FAP without any intervention. Most individuals with FAP will develop colorectal cancer (CRC) by the fourth decade of life.[3-5] Consequently, screening and surveillance guidelines recommend annual colonoscopy beginning at puberty.

Extracolonic Manifestations

Stomach Tumors The most common gastric polyps associated with FAP are fundic gland polyps. Their incidence has been estimated to be up to 60% in patients with FAP.[8-10] These polyps histologically consist of distorted fundic glands with microcysts lined with fundic-type epithelial cells or foveolar mucous cells.[11,12] Although fundic gland polyps are considered nonneoplastic, focal dysplasia has been reported in fundic gland polyps of FAP patients.[12]

Adenomatous polyps occur in the stomach of about 10% of patients with FAP. They are most often confined to the antrum but are occasionally found in the body and fundus. If a polyp with high-grade dysplasia is identified, the recommendation is polypectomy with subsequent surveillance endoscopy in 3 to 6 months.[13]

Duodenum and Small Bowel Tumors Duodenal adenocarcinoma is one of the leading causes of death in FAP patients who have had prophylactic colectomy. Duodenal adenomas are found in up to 90% of FAP patients. Most are located in the first and second portions of the duodenum, particularly in the periampullary region.[14,15] There is a 4% to 12% lifetime incidence of duodenal adenocarcinoma in FAP patients.[16-18] Although polyps in the duodenum can be difficult to treat, they can be managed successfully with endoscopy, but with potential complications, primarily pancreatitis, bleeding, and duodenal perforation.[19,20] Given that the risk of duodenal adenocarcinoma correlates with the size, number, and severity of dysplasia, a scoring system known as the Spigelman Classification has been developed to identify individuals with FAP at highest risk of developing duodenal adenocarcinoma[21] (see Table 6.2). Based on this classification system, the risk for duodenal adenocarcinoma increases to 36% for Spigelman stage IV patients.[18]

Desmoid Tumors Desmoid tumors are locally infiltrating fibromatous tumors that may arise in the musculoaponeurotic tissues. Desmoids occur rarely in the general population but have been found in approximately 10% of individuals affected with FAP.[22] They are most common in the mesentery and abdominal wall in patients with FAP. The incidence of desmoids varies with the location of the pathogenic variant in the *APC* gene. *APC* pathogenic variants occurring between codons 1445 and 1578 have been associated with an increased incidence of desmoid tumors.[22,23] Individuals with *APC* genotypes predisposing to desmoid tumors, including *APC* mutation at the 3' end or codon 1445, are at higher risk of developing desmoids after

TABLE 6.2: Spigelman Classification[21]			
Polyps	**1 Point**	**2 Points**	**3 Points**
Number	1–4	5–20	>20
Size	1–4 mm	5–10 mm	>10 mm
Histology	Tubular	Tubulovillous	Villous
Dysplasia	Mild	Moderate	Severe

Stage I, 1–4 points; Stage II, 5–6 points; Stage III, 7–8 points; Stage IV, 9–12 points

surgery.[24,25] Desmoid tumors are one of the most common causes of morbidity and mortality in FAP patients who have had prophylactic colectomy. A desmoid risk factor scale, which includes gender, presence of extracolonic manifestations, family history of desmoids, and genotype, is available to identify patients who are likely to develop desmoid tumors.[26]

Desmoids do not metastasize, but may infiltrate adjacent structures and can lead to intestinal obstruction, infarction, and ureteral obstruction.[27] The natural history of desmoids is variable. About 10% of desmoid tumors may grow rapidly, and about 10% may resolve.[24] Although the most common symptom is abdominal pain, only about one-third of abdominal desmoids cause pain. Desmoid tumors may be the first manifestation of FAP in some patients and families. Furthermore, some families with *APC* mutations exhibit desmoids as their only disease manifestation.

Congenital Hypertrophy of the Retinal Pigment Epithelium Multiple and bilateral patches of congenital hypertrophy of the retinal pigment epithelium (CHRPE), also called *pigmented ocular fundus lesions*, have been described as a common manifestation of FAP and are present in approximately 75% of FAP patients.[28,29] These lesions are discrete, darkly pigmented, round, oval, or kidney shaped and are often present at birth or in early childhood. The presence of CHRPE correlates closely with mutations in specific areas of the *APC* gene. The presence of CHRPE in association with colon polyps is highly specific (92%) but only moderately sensitive (76%) for FAP.[28] It is important to acknowledge the existence of benign variants of CHRPE (classic CHRPE and grouped pigmentation of the retina), since their similarity has often led to misdiagnosis and therefore unnecessary screening. The identification of CHRPE associated with FAP is crucial, since it is a common early finding, and its association with de novo APC mutations has a high probability of invasive adenocarcinoma.[30]

Osteomas Multiple osteomas were the first extracolonic lesion to be associated with FAP. These lesions are benign bone growths found most commonly on the skull and mandible but may occur on any bone of the body. They are often evident on panoramic dental radiographs. Osteomas may occur in children who are at risk for FAP before the onset of colonic polyposis, but they can continue to occur throughout life. They have no malignant potential and are not a clinical problem except for occasional cosmetic concern.

Other Tumors

Adrenal Adenomas Adrenal adenomas have been reported in individuals with FAP. Two studies found their occurrence to be significantly higher than in the general population, 7% and 13%, respectively, compared with a prevalence of 0.6% to 3.4% in non-FAP patients.[31,32] Several cases of functioning adrenal adenomas and adrenal carcinomas have also been noted in these same series, but association of these more advanced lesions with FAP is uncertain.

Papillary Thyroid Cancer Up to 1% to 2% of FAP patients have papillary thyroid cancer.[33] The mean age of diagnosis of thyroid cancer is 28 years. A female predominance is observed, and the histology is predominantly papillary, commonly with a cribriform pattern. Familial aggregation has been observed, and mutation analysis has revealed that most mutations in FAP patients with thyroid cancer are identified outside the mutation cluster region.[28]

Hepatoblastoma Hepatoblastoma is a fatal malignancy that occurs in the first 5 years of life. If confined to the liver, it can be cured by radical surgical resection. Multiple cases have been described in patients with an *APC* pathogenic variant. Up to 10% of children with hepatoblastoma will be found to have FAP.[34–36]

Brain Tumors Turcot syndrome was previously the diagnosis for FAP patients who manifested with colorectal and brain tumors. Studies have shown that colon polyposis and medulloblastomas are associated with *APC* pathogenic variants and therefore FAP. Medulloblastoma occurs primarily in children and accounts for approximately 80% of tumors in individuals with FAP.[37]

Gallbladder, Bile Ducts, and Pancreas Both adenomatous changes and cancer have been reported in the gallbladder, bile ducts, and pancreas of individuals with FAP. Biliary and pancreatic duct obstructions have arisen from both benign and malignant lesions.

Attenuated Familial Adenomatous Polyposis

Attenuated FAP (AFAP) is associated with particular *APC* pathogenic variants, including pathogenic variants at the 5' end of the *APC* gene and exon 4 in which patients can present with 2 to >500 adenomas, pathogenic variants at the 3' region in which patients have <50 adenomas, and exon 9–associated phenotypes in which patients may have 1 to 150 adenomas without upper gastrointestinal manifestations.[38,39] Patients with AFAP have fewer colonic adenomas than those with classic FAP and are predominantly located in the proximal colon. The emergence of adenomas is believed to be around the age of mid-to-late twenties.[40] The average age at diagnosis is older than classic FAP at age 56 years.[38,41,42] Patients with AFAP present with extracolonic manifestations similar to those in classic FAP, including fundic gland polyps, duodenal adenomas, duodenal adenocarcinoma, osteomas, epidermoid cysts, and desmoid tumors. AFAP may be challenging to diagnose without genetic testing. *APC* testing is pivotal in the evaluation of these patients, since the differential diagnosis is broad and includes *MUTYH*, Lynch syndrome, biallelic mismatch repair deficiency (BMMRD), and polymerase proofreading-associated polyposis (*POLD1* and *POLE*).

Genetic Testing for FAP

Individuals with a phenotype suggestive of FAP are candidates for genetic testing. Multigene panel testing is a reasonable option, since it has the advantage of detecting germline mutations that would not have been discovered based on the patient's clinical phenotype and family history. In addition, it can increase the yield of identifying germline mutations for syndromes with genetic heterogeneity and overlapping phenotypes.

Cascade genetic testing in which at-risk family members are tested for a known pathogenic variant is important to help tailor screening and surveillance strategies and determine which at-risk relatives need to undergo more aggressive screening. The families of most patients diagnosed with FAP have an autosomal dominant inheritance. However, approximately 25% of patients with FAP have a *de novo* pathogenic variant in *APC*.[43] The recommendation to start screening at puberty is challenging, given that genetic testing of minors is not endorsed unless the benefits justify genetic testing, as is the case of a pedigree with a known *APC* pathogenic variant.[44] If at-risk minors are not tested, the recommendation is to perform a sigmoidoscopy beginning at ages 10 to 15 years.[45]

Screening and Surveillance

The primary goal of screening and surveillance is to prevent cancer. In view of the high risk of developing colon cancer and extracolonic cancers in FAP, empiric screening guidelines have been suggested on the basis of these risks and the likely ages of cancer development (Table 6.3).

TABLE 6.3: Screening Recommendations in Familial Adenomatous Polyposis

Cancer	Age to Begin Screening (years)	Screening Interval (years)	Screening Procedures
Colon	10–12, late teens if AFAP	1	Sigmoidoscopy or colonoscopy if AFAP
Duodenal or periampullary	20–25	1–3	EGD also with "side-viewing" exam of the duodenal papilla
Pancreatic	–	–	None given
Thyroid	10–12	1	Physical examination, possibly ultrasound
Gastric	20–25	1–3	Same as for duodenal
Desmoids	–	–	CT/MRI*
Central nervous system, usually cerebellar medulloblastoma (Turcot syndrome)	First decade	1	Annual physical examination, possibly periodic MRI scan of head in affected families
Hepatoblastoma	6 months	3–6 months	Possibly liver palpation, hepatic ultrasound, α-fetoprotein during first decade of life

*If family history or symptoms. Periodicity is not well established.[46]

AFAP, Attenuated familial adenomatous polyposis.

Colon Screening Colon screening should be performed in those individuals at risk of FAP or in those with a known pathogenic variant in *APC*. Screening guidelines for classic FAP recommend evaluation for the onset of polyposis by sigmoidoscopy or colonoscopy annually, beginning at 10 to 15 years of age.[45] However, colonoscopy is the screening tool of choice, particularly given recognition of AFAP, which presents with proximal polyp distribution. Once polyps are present, prophylactic surgery has been shown to improve survival.[47] Nevertheless, in patients with AFAP with advanced age and low polyp burden, surgery may be deferred if there is no evidence of dysplasia and polyp burden can be managed endoscopically. Recommendations for screening in individuals with AFAP can be delayed until the late teens to mid-twenties and be performed every 1 to 2 years. Individuals who have tested negative for a known family pathogenic variant do not need to follow FAP-intensive endoscopic surveillance. The recommendation is that they undergo average-risk screening.[45]

Upper Gastrointestinal Screening Upper gastrointestinal (GI) screening recommendations include a baseline endoscopy with side-viewing endoscope to visualize the duodenal papilla, starting at ages 25 to 30 years,[48] although some recommend an initial examination at the time of diagnosis and earlier screening if other family members have exhibited advanced duodenal disease at an earlier age. Recommended intervals for surveillance vary according to endoscopic findings and are based on the Spigelman classification. The recommended interval is as follows: (1) every 4 years for Spigelman stage 0; (2) every 2 to 3 years for stage I; (3) every 1 to 3 years for stage II disease; (4) every 6 to 12 months for stage III disease; and (5) for stage IV, consider surgical evaluation (see Table 6.2). Recommended intervals are based on expert opinion, although for stages 0 to 2 interval recommendations are based on data generated by a Dutch/Scandinavian duodenal surveillance trial.[49] The stomach should be examined during endoscopy, and any polyps thought to be of concern because of size or gross appearance should be biopsied. The management of gastric adenomas should be individualized based on size and degree of dysplasia.

Screening for Other Malignancies and Desmoids Patients who carry *APC* germline pathogenic variants are at increased risk of other types of malignancies, including thyroid cancer, desmoids, hepatoblastoma, and medulloblastoma. Consensus opinion recommends thyroid examination by palpation annually, starting at age 10 to 12 years, in view of risk and ease of examination. Annual thyroid ultrasound has also been recommended. Screening is not done for desmoids, but evaluation is done for palpable masses or symptoms. Periodic abdominal imaging is not generally recommended but may be considered if desmoids have been an issue in family members. Surveillance for medulloblastomas with regular imaging in asymptomatic patients is not recommended. Careful evaluation should be done for individuals with central nervous system (CNS) symptoms even in those who have not presented with polyps because brain tumors may present before the diagnosis of polyps in more than half of patients with FAP.[37] Evaluation is also important among individuals with a family member with a history of CNS malignancy, given that familial clustering may occur. Since evidence is lacking, the value of screening for hepatoblastoma is debatable. Consensus opinion recommends liver palpation, liver ultrasound, and serum α-fetoprotein every 3 to 6 months in children until the age of 7 years. Specific biliary evaluation is done only for abnormal laboratory tests or symptoms.

Ileal Pouch and Rectal Screening After Colectomy Adenomas may develop in the ileal pouch after total proctocolectomy with ileal pouch anal anastomosis (IPAA) surgery, or they may develop in the anal transition zone. Therefore, lifelong endoscopic surveillance is required. Screening of the pouch and anal transition zone should be done yearly. When colectomy with ileorectal anastomosis (IRA) is performed, rectal cancer risk still remains, and yearly proctoscopy is warranted. Conversion from IRA to IPAA may occasionally be needed because of the development of numerous or advanced rectal adenomas.

Clinical Management

Colorectal Surgery Risk-reducing surgery is the standard of care to prevent CRC once polyps are histologically advanced or polyp burden cannot be managed endoscopically. An appropriately timed colectomy remains the foundation of colon cancer prevention in FAP. Timing of risk-reducing surgery usually depends on number of polyps, size, histology, and symptoms.[50] Surgical options for patients with FAP include proctocolectomy with IPAA, total colectomy with IRA, or total proctocolectomy with ileostomy (TPC). Rectal polyp burden at the time of surgical evaluation may dictate which surgical intervention should be done, either proctocolectomy with IPAA or IRA. Colectomy with IRA is a single-stage procedure with slightly less morbidity than the IPAA surgery, but rectal cancer risk remains and yearly surveillance is warranted. Rectum-sparing surgery is an alternative to proctocolectomy with IPAA in those patients with relative rectal sparing of polyps (fewer than 20 polyps), who are compliant with surveillance, and who understand the risk of rectal cancer despite periodic surveillance.[51] Conversion from IRA to IPAA may occasionally be needed due to development of numerous or advanced rectal adenomas. Possible complications from surgery include increased bowel frequency, incontinence, some loss of fertility in women, and some loss of sexual function in men. *APC* mutation location, allowing prediction of severity of rectal polyposis and likelihood of future proctectomy completion, has been suggested as a factor to consider in determining which procedure should be done. Pathogenic variants reported to increase rectal cancer risk and eventual proctectomy completion after IRA include variants in exon 15 codon 1250, exon 15 codons 1309 and 1328, and exon 15 variants between codons 1250 and 1464.[52-54] A laparoscopic approach is now used most often for both surgical approaches. Patients who undergo an IPAA should continue yearly surveillance of the pouch because of the cumulative risk of developing adenomas in the pouch. Although rare, carcinoma of the anal transition zone after proctocolectomy has been reported in FAP patients.[55]

Patients with AFAP are usually managed with colonoscopic polypectomy and may possibly never need to undergo surgery. If surgical management is indicated because of the development of numerous or advanced adenomas, these patients almost always undergo a colectomy and IRA. Proctocolectomy with IPAA is almost never needed for individuals with AFAP because of rectal sparing of polyps.

Upper Gastrointestinal Tract FAP patients with Spigelman stage I and II disease have a low risk of cancer and can be managed with regular surveillance and selected endoscopic treatment. Individuals with advanced disease—Spigelman stage III or IV—require endoscopic or surgical management. Based on Spigelman classification, the risk for duodenal adenocarcinoma increases to 36% for stage IV disease; therefore these patients require more aggressive therapies.[18] Multiple factors play a role in selecting endoscopic or surgical treatment approaches for duodenal adenoma management. These factors include patient comorbidities, evidence of advanced dysplasia, and availability of trained physicians. Possible therapies include endoscopic resection or ablation, local surgical resection, or definitive surgical resection, which includes pancreaticoduodenectomy (Whipple procedure), pancreas-sparing duodenectomy, or segmental duodenectomy. Individuals with FAP managed with endoscopic resection remain at high risk of developing recurrent duodenal adenomas.[56] Complications from endoscopic resection include perforation, hemorrhage, and pancreatitis. Typically for ampullary lesions, an endoscopic ultrasound should be performed to evaluate for pancreatic or biliary duct involvement, and stenting may be required to prevent possible pancreatitis and strictures. Surgical ampullectomy, surgical resection of duodenal polyps, or mucosectomy can be performed,[57] but they are also associated with a high risk of local recurrence. Pancreaticoduodenectomy, pancreas-sparing duodenectomy, and segmental duodenectomy significantly reduce the risk of developing periampullary adenocarcinoma and offer the best chance for polyp eradication.[57-60] A study by Johnson et al. that evaluated the outcome of FAP patients with Spigelman stage III and IV disease showed that FAP patients who underwent definitive surgical treatment had a local recurrence rate of 9% after a mean follow-up for 44 months, which was significantly lower compared to endoscopic or local resection.[56] Treatment approaches must be carefully weighed, considering complications and prevention of cancer. Referral to a Center of Excellence is recommended, especially for patients with advanced Spigelman stages. Management of gastric adenomas should be individualized based on the degree of dysplasia and the size of the adenomas.

Desmoid Tumors Evaluation and treatment for desmoids is undertaken for symptoms, functional disruption, or imminent risk to adjacent structures. Multiple treatments, including antiestrogens, nonsteroidal antiinflammatory drugs (NSAIDs), chemotherapy, and radiation therapy have been generally unsuccessful in the management of desmoids. Surgery is often challenging in cases of intraabdominal desmoids because of high rates of morbidity and recurrence. Although pharmacologic treatment is favored by surgical intervention, surgery remains an important option in selected cases. Because intraabdominal desmoids often involve the mesentery or encase vessels or organs, medical therapies are usually first attempted. Abdominal wall desmoids can be treated with surgical resection, but recurrence rates are high.

Several studies have evaluated the response of raloxifene, tamoxifen, or the combination of raloxifene and sulindac.[61,62] A small study of 13 patients with intraabdominal desmoids by Tonelli et al. that evaluated the effects of 120 mg daily of raloxifene on progression of desmoid tumors and mesenteric fibromatosis showed that raloxifene decreases desmoid tumor and mesenteric fibromatosis size and symptoms without side effects.[61] Another study by Hansmann et al. that evaluated 13 patients with FAP-associated desmoids who received tamoxifen 120 mg daily or a combination of raloxifene 120 mg daily and sulindac 300 mg daily suggested that the combination of these treatments may be effective in slowing the growth of desmoids.[62] There are also reports using pirfenidone and imatinib mesylate with some success in disease regression.[63,64] A multidisciplinary and multimodality approach to desmoids treatment is encouraged.

Chemoprevention Much attention and effort have been given to examining chemoprevention for colonic and duodenal polyps in FAP. Currently, there are no Food and Drug Administration (FDA)–approved drugs for chemoprevention in FAP. Celecoxib (a specific cyclooxygenase 2 [COX-2] inhibitor) and sulindac (a nonspecific COX-2 inhibitor) have been associated with regression in the size and number of polyps. In view of the uncertainty of cancer prevention with sulindac, it is not considered a substitute for colectomy but has shown utility in rectal surveillance by substantially decreasing the number of adenomas needing removal at periodic examination. Celecoxib appears to have a more modest effect in the colon and rectum, but some effect in duodenal adenoma regression. Celecoxib was approved for use in the United States for several years for FAP, but this indication has now been removed. Concern over cardiovascular side effects of long-term COX-2 inhibitors has dampened enthusiasm for their use in FAP. Chemoprevention studies examining NSAIDs and other agents continue in the hopes that colectomy might be delayed.

New studies with low-dose aspirin have also been conducted in patients with FAP and Lynch syndrome, which show evidence of a positive effect on the development and progression of adenomas of the colon.[65] The role of other agents such as curcumin, difluoromethylornithine (DFMO), and XAV939 (pharmacological selective inhibitor of tankyrase)[66] have also been the focus of recent studies.

Curcumin has been proposed as an alternative chemopreventive agent to other antiinflammatory drugs since it inhibits COX activity. However, a randomized placebo-controlled clinical trial failed to demonstrate efficacy of oral curcumin in decreasing or preventing colorectal/ileal adenomas among FAP patients.[67] The combination of curcumin with conventional chemotherapy such as 5-floururacil, the mainstay chemotherapeutic agent for CRC, is also being studied to evaluate its ability to enhance the chemotherapeutic effects or decrease resistance to treatment.[68]

DFMO is a potent enzyme-activated irreversible inhibitor of ornithine decarboxylase (ODC), the first enzyme in the polyamine synthesis that has been proven to be significantly elevated in presymptomatic patients with germline APC mutations.[69] Studies show that DFMO has anti-CRC activity arising from thymidine synthesis. However, there are certain limitations to the clinical use of this compound, such as its side effect profile when used at high doses. These include hearing loss, diarrhea, abdominal pain, emesis, anemia, leukopenia, and thrombocytopenia.

Other Non-*APC* Gene–Related Adenomatous Polyposis Conditions

MUTYH-Associated Polyposis MUTYH-associated polyposis (MAP) is an autosomal recessive attenuated polyposis syndrome caused by biallelic germline variants in *MUTYH,* a gene involved in deoxyribonucleic acid (DNA) oxidative damage repair. *MUTYH* is located on chromosome 1p34.3-32.1.[70] MAP is characterized by an increased risk for CRC (35% to 75%) and multiple adenomatous polyps (20 to 100, occasionally more).[71,72] Full gene sequencing of *MUTYH* is recommended in individuals with polyposis without a pathogenic variant in the *APC* gene. Given the autosomal recessive inheritance of MAP, siblings of an affected patient have a 25% chance of carrying biallelic MUTYH pathogenic variants and should be offered testing. In Caucasians of Northern European descent, two variants, Y179C and G396D, account for 70% of biallelic pathogenic variants in MAP patients.[73] However, the prevalence of these variants varies by ethnicity and race, and additional pathogenic variants have been reported. Biallelic *MUTYH* pathogenic variants are found in 7% (95% CI, 6% to 8%) of patients with 20 to 99 adenomas and 7% (CI, 6% to 8%) of patients with 100 to 999 adenomas.[74]

Monoallelic pathogenic variants in *MUTYH* are commonly detected. Approximately 1% to 2% of the general population carries a pathogenic variant in *MUTYH*.[75] Monoallelic *MUTYH* pathogenic variants do not have much effect on CRC risk (odds ratio 1.15; 95% CI, 0.98 to 1.36) in the absence of family history of CRC.[76] The risk of CRC in monoallelic *MUTYH* carriers with a family history of the disease is approximately 2-fold compared to the general population.[72] Similar to individuals with a family history of a first-degree relative with CRC diagnosed before the age of 50 years, *MUTYH* heterozygotes with a first-degree relative with CRC warrant more intensive surveillance compared to the general population.[72,77]

Clinical Presentation and Natural History

Colonic Phenotype The colonic phenotype of MAP is difficult to distinguish from patients with multiple adenomas, AFAP, or FAP. MAP is usually more similar to AFAP in presenting with fewer adenomas. Although the predominant polyp type is adenoma, serrated adenomas and hyperplastic polyps may also be seen in MAP patients.[78] The CRC associated with MAP is predominantly right-sided, may present with synchronous lesions at presentation, and have a better prognosis compared to sporadic CRC.[70] Recommendations for colonic surveillance range between yearly and every 3 years beginning at age 18 to 30 years.[45,71]

Extracolonic Phenotype Extracolonic manifestations in MAP occur less frequently than in FAP and AFAP.[79,80] The lifetime risk of extracolonic tumors in MAP is not as well defined as the colorectal phenotype. Multiple extracolonic cancers have been reported in patients with MAP, including gastric, small intestinal, endometrial, liver, ovarian, bladder, thyroid, skin cancers (melanoma, squamous, and basal cell carcinoma), and breast cancer in females.[81–83] Although rare, other findings seen in patients with MAP include sebaceous gland adenomas, epitheliomas, lipomas, CHRPE, osteomas, desmoid tumors, epidermoid cysts, and pilomatrixomas.

Individuals with MAP often develop duodenal adenomas and are at risk of developing duodenal cancer. However, the incidence of duodenal polyps and the risk of duodenal cancer is less well defined in MAP compared to FAP. The lifetime risk of duodenal cancer in MAP has been estimated to be 4%.[82] Although gastric lesions have been found in patients with MAP, data are currently lacking to support an increased risk of gastric cancer. Compared to FAP, duodenal polyps in MAP appear to be less prevalent with a later age of onset. Consequently, upper endoscopic screening should be started at age 25 to 30 years.[45]

Clinical Management

Guidelines for the management of the colon in MAP recommend colonoscopy surveillance between once a year and every 3 years beginning at age 25 to 30 years.[71,83] If polyp burden cannot be managed endoscopically or if evidence of advanced histology is present, total colectomy with ileorectal anastomosis or subtotal colectomy should be considered, depending on polyp burden.[71,84] Similar to AFAP and FAP, subtotal colectomy with close surveillance would seem to be the best option for those with relative rectal sparing. Restorative proctocolectomy is indicated if the rectum is substantially involved. Given the risk of duodenal cancer in MAP, upper GI endoscopy should be considered starting around age 25 to 30 years and repeated at intervals based on the burden of involvement according to the Spigelman criteria.[83]

Other Polyposis-Related Syndromes

The phenotype of AFAP or *MUTYH*-associated polyposis is also associated with *POLE* and *POLD1* genes. Germline mutations that affect the proofreading domains of *POLE* and *POLD1* genes give rise to a phenotype of multiple adenomas and early-onset CRC collectively known as polymerase proofreading-associated polyposis (PPAP).[85] The *POLD1* variant has also been associated with endometrial tumors. The frequency, extracolonic phenotype, and genetic testing guidelines for this dominantly inherited condition are still to be determined. There is a paucity of data on the optimal surveillance approach for individuals with a germline pathogenic variant in *POLE* and *POLD1*. Some guidelines are endorsing early and frequent colonoscopy screening. Consensus is lacking with regard to surveillance; thus, patients with PPAP should be managed clinically.

Hereditary mixed polyposis syndrome (HMPS) is a rare syndrome caused by pathogenic variants in the *GREM1* gene, a bone morphogenetic protein antagonist. This syndrome has been associated with *GREM1* pathogenic variants among Ashkenazi Jews. The phenotype of HMPS is characterized by oligopolyposis, which includes a variety of histology including adenomas, serrated adenomas, atypical juvenile polyps, and hyperplastic polyps. It is also characterized by early-onset CRC. There is a high degree of variability in polyp number, histology, and age of onset. Extracolonic malignancies have been described in a small number of pathogenic carriers.

The *NTHL1* gene is associated with an autosomal recessive adenomatous polyposis phenotype with an increased risk of CRC. Carriers of biallelic germline *NTHL1* pathogenic variants have extracolonic malignancies, including endometrial cancer.[86] Currently, there is no known risk of cancer for individuals with a single monoallelic germline pathogenic variant in *NTHL1*. Cumulative cancer risk is uncertain, and there are minimal data on the optimal surveillance approach.

Serrated polyposis syndrome (SPS), previously referred to as hyperplastic polyposis syndrome (HPS), is characterized by a predisposition to sessile serrated polyps. SPS is diagnosed based on clinical criteria, as the genetic etiology remains elusive. Rarely, families with SPS can be identified as harboring a germline pathogenic variant in the *RNF43* gene.[87,88] The World Health Organization (WHO) diagnostic criteria for SPS traditionally included any one of the following: (1) at least 5 serrated polyps proximal to the sigmoid colon with 2 or more of them larger than 10 mm in diameter; (2) any number of serrated polyps proximal to the sigmoid colon in an individual who has a first-degree relative with SPS; or (3) more than 20 serrated polyps of any size distributed throughout the colon. In 2019, the WHO updated the diagnostic criteria, dropping criteria (2), and updating the other two criteria to (1) at least 5 serrated polyps proximal to the rectum, all being $\geq$5 mm in size, with at least 2 being $\geq$10 mm and (2) more than 20 serrated polyps of any size distributed throughout the colon, with at least 5 being proximal to the rectum. Approximately half of SPS cases have a positive family history of CRC.[89] The prevalence of CRC in patients who meet criteria for SPS is 50% or more.[89] Very limited data exist as to whether extracolonic polyps or cancers are associated with SPS. Management of patients with known SPS includes colonoscopy with polypectomy. Clearance of all polyps is preferred, but not always feasible. Colonoscopy should be repeated every 1 to 3 years, depending on the number and size of serrated and adenomatous polyps. Subtotal colectomy with ileorectal anastomosis should be considered if polyposis cannot be controlled endoscopically or if there is evidence of histologically advanced polyps or colon cancer. Data do not support extracolonic cancer screening at this time. The frequency and age of initiation of colonoscopy screening in at-risk family members of patients with SPS is less clear. The National Comprehensive Cancer Network recommends that first-degree relatives should have colonoscopy at the earliest of the following: (1) age 40; (2) same age as the youngest SPS diagnosis in the family; (3) 10 years prior to CRC in the family in a patient with SPS.[45] Further work is ongoing to better define the cancer risks in probands and their relatives so that more accurate risk stratification and screening recommendations can be made.

Constitutional Mismatch Repair Deficiency Syndrome

Constitutional mismatch repair deficiency syndrome (CMMRDS) is a rare autosomal recessive syndrome caused by homozygous pathogenic variants in mismatch repair (MMR) genes.[90] The *PMS2* gene is markedly overrepresented in cases of CMMRD. This syndrome is characterized by early childhood onset of malignancies, including hematologic, brain, small bowel, colorectal, and ureter; sarcoma malignancies; and features of neurofibromatosis *NF1*, most notably café-au-lait macules.[91] GI manifestations include colonic polyposis, predominantly adenomas and CRC, which typically present before the age of 20 years.[90] The likelihood of CMMRD involving homozygous MMR gene pathogenic variants is higher among consanguineous unions. No consensus has been reached regarding surveillance guidelines for CMMRDS. Annual colonoscopy, esophagogastroduodenoscopy (EGD), and capsule endoscopy starting in the first decade of life is recommended by the International BMMRD Consortium and the European Consortium for the Care of CMMRD.[9,92] Others have recommended that GI screening start at age 6 to 8 years old.[90] Screening for other Lynch syndrome tumors, such as endometrial, starting in adulthood has been recommended.[92]

▓ HAMARTOMATOUS POLYPOSIS SYNDROMES

Peutz–Jeghers Syndrome

Definition, Epidemiology, and Clinical Characteristics Peutz–Jeghers syndrome (PJS) is an autosomal dominant inherited syndrome that includes histologically distinctive hamartomatous polyps of the GI tract and characteristic melanocytic macules on the lips, perioral region, and buccal region, which fade with age.[93,94] The mucocutaneous melanin pigment spots are seen in more than 95% of cases. Germline pathogenic variants in the *STK11* gene at chromosome 19p13.3 have been identified in patients with PJS.[21,33,95,96] A high risk for GI and non-GI cancers is integral to this condition, including malignancies in the colon, stomach, pancreas, breast, and ovary. The cumulative risk for breast cancer is estimated to be 32% to 54% and 21% for ovarian cancer.[97] For pancreatic cancer, the risk has been estimated to be more than 100-fold higher than for the general population.[97] Individual risks by tumor site are shown in Table 6.4. Distinctive tumors in women include cervical adenoma malignum, a rare and aggressive adenocarcinoma of the cervix,[98] and ovarian sex-cord tumors with annular tubules, which is a benign tumor but can cause symptoms related to increased estrogen production. Males with PJS are predisposed to developing Sertoli-cell testicular tumors.[99] Some individuals would consider prophylactic mastectomies, as well as prophylactic hysterectomies with bilateral salpingo-oophorectomy, after childbearing age.

GI polyps occur in 88% to 100% of patients. Their frequency by segment is stomach, 24%; small bowel, 96%; colon, 27%; and rectum, 24%.[100,101] Polyp growth begins in the first decade of life, but patients typically do not develop symptoms until the second or third decade.[102,103] Symptoms arise from larger polyps, which may infarct, ulcerate, bleed, and cause intestinal

TABLE 6.4: Cancer Risks and Surveillance Recommendations for Peutz-Jeghers Syndrome
Data from references[104,105]

Cancer	Cancer Risk to Age 64 Years	Mean Age of Diagnosis (years)	Age to Begin Surveillance (years)	Surveillance Interval (years)	Surveillance Procedures and Comments
Colon	39%	46	8, 18[a]	3	Colonoscopy[a]
Stomach	29%	30	8, 18[a]	3	Esophagogastroduodenoscopy[a]
Small bowel	13%	42	8, 18[a]	3	Video capsule endoscopy[a]
Pancreas	36%	41	30	1–2	Endoscopic ultrasound, validity of screening uncertain
Breast	54%	37	25	1	Annual self-exam starting age 18, annual MRI and/or mammogram starting at age 25
Ovarian	21%	28	25	1	Pelvic exam and pelvic or transvaginal ultrasound, CA-125 probably not helpful
Uterus	9%	37	25	1	Pelvic exam and pelvic or transvaginal ultrasound
Cervix (adenoma malignum)	10%	34	25	1	Pap smear
SCTAT	20%	40	25	1	Same as uterine and ovarian; Almost all women develop SCTAT, but 20% become malignant
Testicular (Sertoli cell tumor)	9%	9	Birth to teenage years	1	Testicular exam, ultrasound if abnormalities palpated or if feminization occurs; 10%–20% of benign Sertoli-cell tumors become malignant
Lung	15%	51	–	–	No screening recommendations given

[a]Start at age 8. If polyps present, repeat every 3 years; if no polyps, repeat at age 18, then every 3 years, or earlier if symptoms occur.
SCTAT, Sex cord tumors with annular tubules.

obstruction and intussusception. PJS polyps are histologically distinct. They are nondysplastic, have normal overlying epithelium specific to the GI segment in which they are found, and exhibit an arborizing pattern of growth with muscularis mucosae extending into branching fronds of the polyp. Epithelial infolding may result in what is termed pseudo-invasion, which can lead to an incorrect diagnosis of cancer. Adenoma and cancer may occur in PJS polyps.[101] The progression has been referred to as the hamartoma–adenoma–carcinoma sequence.

Diagnosis, Surveillance, and Treatment Diagnosis is made based on evaluating for the presence of any one of the following: (1) two or more histologically confirmed PJS polyps, (2) any number of PJS polyps detected in one individual who has a family history of PJS in a close relative(s), (3) characteristic mucocutaneous pigmentation in an individual who has a family history of PJS in close relatives(s); and (4) any number of PJS polyps in an individual who also has characteristic mucocutaneous pigmentation.[105] In addition to these criteria, genetic testing is commercially available and a standard part of clinical practice. Genetic testing should be provided for asymptomatic children of affected parents from the age of 3 and started earlier if the child is symptomatic.[105]

Management first involves surveillance, as outlined in Table 6.4. Surveillance guidelines for PJS are empiric and based on the risk for GI complications and cancer. A consortium review group has recommended that upper GI endoscopy (EGD) and colonoscopy be done starting at age 8.[104] If polyps are found, both examinations should be repeated every 3 years. If none are found, a second baseline examination should be done at age 18 and every 3 years thereafter. Similarly, surveillance for the small bowel by video capsule endoscopy (VCE) should start at age 8 and subsequently every 3 years if polyps are present.

Treatment involves endoscopic removal of polyps. Colectomy is sometimes necessary if colonic polyp burden cannot be controlled endoscopically or if histology shows neoplastic changes. Intussusception is the primary complication of small bowel polyps, starting at a young age, and continuing throughout life. Surveillance and treatment of the small bowel are based in large part on prevention of this complication. When small bowel intussusception occurs, surgery is often necessary and should include careful examination of the entire small bowel. Intraoperative enteroscopy should be done to clear the small bowel of other PJS polyps.[105] Chemoprevention approaches to decrease polyp burden in PJS are currently under study. PJS polyps exhibit overexpression of COX-2, suggesting that COX-2 inhibitors may have chemopreventive potential in decreasing polyp burden in patients with PJS.[106] To date, no chemoprevention or pharmacological agents are recommended for the management of PJS.

Juvenile Polyposis Syndrome

Definition, Epidemiology, and Clinical Characteristics Juvenile polyposis syndrome (JPS) is a rare autosomal dominant inherited condition characterized by hamartomatous polyposis throughout the GI tract with childhood to early adult onset. JPS is caused by germline pathogenic variants in the *SMAD4* gene (also called the *MADH4/DPC4*) in approximately 15% to 60% of cases[107] and pathogenic variants in the gene encoding bone morphogenic protein receptor 1A, *BMPR1A,* in approximately 25% to 40% of cases.[108,109] A clinical diagnosis of JPS is done when individuals fulfill one or more of the following criteria: (1) more than five juvenile polyps in the colon or rectum; (2) juvenile polyps in other parts of the GI tract; and (3) any number of juvenile polyps in a person with a known family history of juvenile polyps.[110] Inherited syndromes that exhibit the GI phenotype of JPS must also be ruled out, including Cowden syndrome (CS), Bannayan-Riley-Ruvalcaba (BRR) syndrome, and Gorlin syndrome. Approximately 25% of newly diagnosed cases are sporadic and thus represent new or *de novo* mutations, while 75% will have a family history.[100]

Multiple juvenile polyps are found in the colorectum (98%), stomach (14%), jejunum and ileum (7%), and duodenum (7%).[100,107,111,112] Polyps begin to appear in the first decade of life. Rectal bleeding with anemia is the most common presenting symptom. The lifetime risk of CRC in JPS is 39%.[113] There is also an increased risk for gastric cancer, which is up to 29% in individuals who have gastric polyps.[100,107] Severe gastric polyposis and a risk of gastric cancer occur in those with pathogenic variants in *SMAD4*, but rarely in those with *BMPR1A* pathogenic variants.[107,114] Pancreatic and periampullary cancers have also been reported.[111]

A rare and often lethal form of the disease can develop in the first years of life and is referred to as JPS of infancy. Clinical manifestations include GI bleeding, diarrhea, protein-losing enteropathy, and associated developmental delay. This condition can arise from heterozygous mutation of two contiguous genes, *PTEN* and *BMPR1A*, probably explaining the severity of the presentation.[115] JPS patients with *SMAD4* pathogenic variants may present with signs and symptoms of hereditary hemorrhagic telangiectasia (HHT) such as aortic aneurysm, mucocutaneous telangiectasias, arteriovenous malformations, and digital clubbing.[116] In patients found to have features of JPS and HHT, the pathogenic variant is found in the *SMAD4* gene. HHT may also be caused by mutations in other genes besides *SMAD4*, including *ENG* and *ACVRL1*.

Diagnosis, Screening, and Treatment Colorectal screening consists of colonoscopy starting at age 12 and repeated every 1 to 3 years depending on polyp burden.[107] Similarly, upper GI endoscopy should be done every 1 to 3 years beginning at age 12, or earlier if symptoms present. The small bowel should be examined if duodenal polyposis is present or if there is unexplained anemia, protein-losing enteropathy, or other small bowel symptom. Screening should also include annual complete blood count, cardiovascular examination, and HHT protocol evaluation if *SMAD4* mutation is present.[107]

Patients with a large burden of colonic polyps, anemia and/or protein-losing enteropathy, polyps with advanced dysplasia, or the presence of invasive adenocarcinoma, colectomy with IRA or total restorative proctocolectomy is indicated, depending on the number of rectal polyps.[100,107] Complete or partial gastrectomy may also be necessary for patients with advanced dysplasia, gastric cancer, or even massive gastric polyposis that cannot be effectively controlled endoscopically.[100,111]

PTEN Hamartoma Tumor Syndrome

Definition, Epidemiology, and Clinical Characteristics PTEN hamartoma tumor syndrome (PHTS) includes several autosomal dominant disorders that arise from mutations of the *PTEN* gene. The clinical phenotypes overlap considerably, and the conditions appear to be a spectrum of a single disease. The disorders include CS, BRRS, and adult-onset dysplastic gangliocytoma of the cerebellum (Lhermitte-Duclos disease). Approximately 85% of patients diagnosed with CS and approximately 60% of patients with BRRS have a pathogenic variant in the *PTEN* gene.[117] Primary features include multiple hamartomas of the skin, mucous membranes, GI tract, and other organs, as well as an increased risk of cancers of a number of sites. The lifetime risks of associated malignancies from a large database include breast, 85%; thyroid, 35%; endometrium, 28%; colon, 9%; kidney, 34%; and melanoma, 6%, with substantially elevated age-adjusted standardized incidence ratios (95% CI) for breast,

25.4 (19.8 to 32.0); thyroid, 51.1(38.1 to 67.1); endometrium, 42.9 (28.1 to 62.8); colon, 10.3 (5.6 to 17.4); kidney 30.6 (17.8 to 49.4); and melanoma, 8.5 (4.1 to 15.6).[118,119] Individuals with variants in the 5' end or within the phosphate core of *PTEN* usually present with more organ system involvement.[120]

Updated testing criteria have been recently outlined as part of NCCN guidelines.[121] Referral for genetics consultation should be considered for individuals with a personal history of or first-degree relative with (1) adult-onset Lhermitte-Duclos disease or (2) any three of the major or minor criteria that have been established for the diagnosis of CS.[122] The hallmark of the syndrome is the presence of multiple facial trichilemmomas, which are verrucous skin lesions of the face and limbs, and cobblestone-like hyperkeratotic papules of the gingiva, tongue, and buccal mucosa. Other frequent manifestations of the disease include macrocephaly, macular pigmentation of the glans penis, autism spectrum disorder, diffuse esophageal glycogenic acanthosis, multiple cutaneous lipomas, thyroid adenoma and multinodular goiter, renal cell carcinoma, testicular lipomatosis, and vascular anomalies including multiple intracranial developmental venous anomalies.

Colonic polyps are found in up to 93% of individuals with *PTEN* pathogenic variants.[118] Hyperplastic polyps are the most common histological type.[118] However, adenomas and hyperplastic, hamartomatous, and sessile serrated polyps have also been observed. Recent studies have shown an increased risk for early-onset CRC. One multicenter study found 13% of *PTEN* mutation carriers to have colon cancer, all younger than 50 years of age.[123] Data now indicate a 9% to 16% lifetime risk for large bowel cancer.[118,124,125] Recommendations for the age at which to start screening and subsequent surveillance may vary. These recommendations are based on expert opinion and derived from screening guidelines of the relevant cancers in other settings but adjusted for the malignancy risks observed in PHTS.

NCCN Guidelines for Genetic Testing Criteria for PTEN Hamartoma Tumor Syndrome

Individual from a family with a known *PTEN* mutation

Individual meeting clinical diagnostic criteria for CS

Individual with a personal history of any of the following:

BRRS

Adult Lhermitte–Duclos disease

Autism spectrum disorder and macrocephaly

Two or more biopsy-proven trichilemmomas

Two or more major criteria (one must be macrocephaly)

Three major criteria, without macrocephaly

One major and three or more minor criteria

Four or more minor criteria

At-risk individual with one major or two minor criteria and a relative with a clinical diagnosis of CS or BRRS for whom testing has not been performed

Major Criteria

Breast cancer

Endometrial cancer

Follicular thyroid cancer

Multiple GI hamartomas or ganglioneuromas

Macrocephaly (megalocephaly, ≥97th percentile)

Macular pigmentation of glans penis

Mucocutaneous lesions alone if:

One biopsy proven trichilemmoma, or

Multiple palmoplantar keratoses, or

Multifocal or extensive oral mucosal papillomatosis, or

Multiple cutaneous facial papules (often verrucous)

Minor Criteria

Autism spectrum disorder

Colon cancer

Esophageal glycogenic acanthosis (≥3)

Lipomas

Mental retardation (i.e., IQ ≤ 75)

Papillary or follicular variant of papillary thyroid cancer

Thyroid structural lesions (e.g., adenoma, nodule[s], goiter)

Renal cell carcinoma

Single GI hamartoma or ganglioneuroma

Testicular lipomatosis

Vascular anomalies (including multiple intracranial developmental venous anomalies)

[a]If an individual has two or more major criteria, such as breast cancer and nonmedullary thyroid cancer but does not have macrocephaly, one of the major criteria may be included as one of the three minor criteria to meet testing criteria.

Source: Adapted from Ref.[121]

Related Syndromes

Lhermitte–Duclos Disease The rare occurrence of a benign hamartomatous overgrowth of ganglion cells in the cerebellar cortex (called *dysplastic gangliocytoma of the cerebellum*) is called Lhermitte-Duclos disease (LDD). The large majority of adult cases of LDD occur as a part of PHTS.[126]

Bannayan-Riley-Ruvalcaba Syndrome BRRS is a rare congenital disorder characterized by macrocephaly, intestinal hamartomatous polyps, delayed psychomotor development, lipomatosis, hemangiomatosis, and pigmented macules of the glans penis.[43] BRRS is thus now considered a part of PHTS.[44]

▦ MISCELLANEOUS RARE POLYPOSIS SYNDROMES

Cronkhite-Canada syndrome

Cronkhite-Canada syndrome (CCS) is an acquired condition characterized by generalized GI polyposis, cutaneous hyperpigmentation, hair loss, and nail atrophy.[127–129] The average

age at symptom onset is 59 years, with a range of 31 to 86 years. No familial occurrences have been observed, and the etiology of CCS remains unknown.

Polyposis in CCS is present throughout the GI tract except for the esophagus.[130] Microscopically, the polyps are almost identical to juvenile polyps. In contrast to JPS, however, the mucosa between polyps is also histologically abnormal, with edema, congestion, and inflammation of the lamina propria and focal glandular ectasia. Adenomatous polyps can be seen in up to 71% of cases and colon cancer in as high as 25%.[127] Carcinoma of the stomach is also reported as a consequence of CCS.

A number of extraintestinal ectodermal manifestations are observed in almost all patients with CCS. Fingernails and toenails exhibit various degrees of dystrophy, comprising thinning, splitting, and partial separation from the nail bed (i.e., onycholysis). Hair loss also occurs on the scalp, eyebrows, face, axillae, pubic area, and extremities. Hyperpigmentation, appearing as dark, brownish macules, occurs over the upper extremities, lower extremities, face, palms, soles, neck, back, chest, and scalp. The nail, hair, and pigmentation abnormalities are all reversible on remission of the disease. The disease often exhibits a fairly acute onset and a rapidly progressive course. Diarrhea and protein-losing enteropathy may be extremely severe, resulting in profound malnutrition. Complications resulting from malnutrition are a major cause of morbidity and mortality in this syndrome.

The disease may be fatal within a few months, although a more protracted course is also possible, especially if the patient responds to therapy or remits spontaneously. A number of spontaneous remissions have been reported in CCS, and partial or complete remissions have resulted from several different interventions. Therapies have included corticosteroids, immunosuppressants, antibiotics, colectomy, parenteral nutrition, and combinations of these, each with variable success. Periodic examination of the colon and stomach is indicated in long-term survivors with persistent polyps to screen for adenomatous changes and colon cancer.

References

1. Campbell WJ, Spence RA, Parks TG. Familial adenomatous polyposis. *Br J Surg.* 1994;81(12):1722–1733.
2. Galiatsatos P, Foulkes WD. Familial adenomatous polyposis. *Am J Gastroenterol.* 2006;101(2):385–398.
3. Herrera L. Familial Adenomatous Polyposis. New York, NY: A.R. Liss; 1990.
4. Bulow S. Familial polyposis coli. *Dan Med Bull.* 1987;34(1):1–15.
5. Bussey H. *Familial Polyposis Coli. Family Studies, Histopathology, Differential Diagnosis, and Results of Treatment.* Baltimore, MD: The Johns Hopkins University Press; 1975.
6. Berk T, Cohen Z, Bapat B, Gallinger S. Negative genetic test result in familial adenomatous polyposis: clinical screening implications. *Dis Colon Rectum.* 1999;42(3):307–310; discussion 310–302.
7. Dejea CM, Fathi P, Craig JM, et al. Patients with familial adenomatous polyposis harbor colonic biofilms containing tumorigenic bacteria. *Science.* 2018;359(6375):592–597.
8. Watanabe H, Enjoji M, Yao T, Ohsato K. Gastric lesions in familial adenomatosis coli: their incidence and histologic analysis. *Hum Pathol.* 1978;9(3):269–283.
9. Weston BR, Helper DJ, Rex DK. Positive predictive value of endoscopic features deemed typical of gastric fundic gland polyps. *J Clin Gastroenterol.* 2003;36(5):399–402.
10. Abraham SC, Nobukawa B, Giardiello FM, Hamilton SR, Wu TT. Fundic gland polyps in familial adenomatous polyposis: neoplasms with frequent somatic adenomatous polyposis coli gene alterations. *Am J Pathol.* 2000;157(3):747–754.
11. Odze RD, Marcial MA, Antonioli D. Gastric fundic gland polyps: a morphological study including mucin histochemistry, stereometry, and MIB-1 immunohistochemistry. *Hum Pathol.* 1996;27(9):896–903.

12. Wu TT, Kornacki S, Rashid A, Yardley JH, Hamilton SR. Dysplasia and dysregulation of proliferation in foveolar and surface epithelia of fundic gland polyps from patients with familial adenomatous polyposis. *Am J Surg Pathol*. 1998;22(3):293–298.

13. Bianchi LK, Burke CA, Bennett AE, et al. Fundic gland polyp dysplasia is common in familial adenomatous polyposis. *Clin Gastroenterol Hepatol*. 2008;6(2):180–185.

14. Church JM, McGannon E, Hull-Boiner S, et al. Gastroduodenal polyps in patients with familial adenomatous polyposis. *Dis Colon Rectum*. 1992;35(12):1170–1173.

15. Ranzi T, Castagnone D, Velio P, Bianchi P, Polli EE. Gastric and duodenal polyps in familial polyposis coli. *Gut*. 1981;22(5):363–367.

16. Offerhaus GJ, Giardiello FM, Krush AJ, et al. The risk of upper gastrointestinal cancer in familial adenomatous polyposis. *Gastroenterology*. 1992;102(6):1980–1982.

17. Vasen HF, Bulow S, Myrhoj T, et al. Decision analysis in the management of duodenal adenomatosis in familial adenomatous polyposis. *Gut*. 1997;40(6):716–719.

18. Groves CJ, Saunders BP, Spigelman AD, Phillips RK. Duodenal cancer in patients with familial adenomatous polyposis (FAP): results of a 10 year prospective study. *Gut*. 2002;50(5):636–641.

19. Norton ID, Gostout CJ. Management of periampullary adenoma. *Dig Dis*. 1998;16(5):266–273.

20. Norton ID, Gostout CJ, Baron TH, et al. Safety and outcome of endoscopic snare excision of the major duodenal papilla. *Gastrointest Endosc*. 2002;56(2):239–243.

21. Jenne DE, Reimann H, Nezu J, et al. Peutz-Jeghers syndrome is caused by mutations in a novel serine threonine kinase. *Nat Genet*. 1998;18(1):38–43.

22. Bertario L, Russo A, Sala P, et al. Genotype and phenotype factors as determinants of desmoid tumors in patients with familial adenomatous polyposis. *Int J Cancer*. 2001;95(2):102–107.

23. Bertario L, Russo A, Sala P, et al. Multiple approach to the exploration of genotype-phenotype correlations in familial adenomatous polyposis. *J Clin Oncol*. 2003;21(9):1698–1707.

24. Hodgson SV ME. *Gastrointestinal System*. 2nd ed. New York, NY: Cambridge University Press; 1999.

25. Parc Y, Piquard A, Dozois RR, Parc R, Tiret E. Long-term outcome of familial adenomatous polyposis patients after restorative coloproctectomy. *Ann Surg*. 2004;239(3):378–382.

26. Elayi E, Manilich E, Church J. Polishing the crystal ball: knowing genotype improves ability to predict desmoid disease in patients with familial adenomatous polyposis. *Dis Colon Rectum*. 2009;52(10):1762–1766.

27. Scott RJ, Froggatt NJ, Trembath RC, et al. Familial infiltrative fibromatosis (desmoid tumours) (MIM135290) caused by a recurrent 3′ APC gene mutation. *Hum Mol Genet*. 1996;5(12):1921–1924.

28. Nusliha A, Dalpatadu U, Amarasinghe B, Chandrasinghe PC, Deen KI. Congenital hypertrophy of retinal pigment epithelium (CHRPE) in patients with familial adenomatous polyposis (FAP); a polyposis registry experience. *BMC Res Notes*. 2014;7:734.

29. Chen CS, Phillips KD, Grist S, et al. Congenital hypertrophy of the retinal pigment epithelium (CHRPE) in familial colorectal cancer. *Fam Cancer*. 2006;5(4):397–404.

30. Deibert B, Ferris L, Sanchez N, Weishaar P. The link between colon cancer and congenital hypertrophy of the retinal pigment epithelium (CHRPE). *Am J Ophthalmol Case Rep*. 2019;15:100524.

31. Marchesa P, Fazio VW, Church JM, McGannon E. Adrenal masses in patients with familial adenomatous polyposis. *Dis Colon Rectum*. 1997;40(9):1023–1028.

32. Smith TG, Clark SK, Katz DE, Reznek RH, Phillips RK. Adrenal masses are associated with familial adenomatous polyposis. *Dis Colon Rectum*. 2000;43(12):1739–1742.

33. Boudeau J, Kieloch A, Alessi DR, et al. Functional analysis of LKB1/STK11 mutants and two aberrant isoforms found in Peutz-Jeghers Syndrome patients. *Hum Mutat*. 2003;21(2):172.

34. Aretz S, Koch A, Uhlhaas S, et al. Should children at risk for familial adenomatous polyposis be screened for hepatoblastoma and children with apparently sporadic hepatoblastoma be screened for APC germline mutations? *Pediatr Blood Cancer*. 2006;47(6):811–818.

35. Hirschman BA, Pollock BH, Tomlinson GE. The spectrum of APC mutations in children with hepatoblastoma from familial adenomatous polyposis kindreds. *J Pediatr*. 2005;147(2):263–266.

36. Sanders RP, Furman WL. Familial adenomatous polyposis in two brothers with hepatoblastoma: implications for diagnosis and screening. *Pediatr Blood Cancer*. 2006;47(6):851–854.

37. PDQ Cancer Genetics Editorial Board. *Genetics of Colorectal Cancer (PDQ'): Health Professional Version.* Bethesda, MD: National Cancer Institute; 2002–2020.

38. Spirio L, Olschwang S, Groden J, et al. Alleles of the APC gene: an attenuated form of familial polyposis. *Cell.* 1993;75(5):951–957.

39. Soravia C, Berk T, Madlensky L, et al. Genotype-phenotype correlations in attenuated adenomatous polyposis coli. *Am J Hum Genet.* 1998;62(6):1290–1301.

40. Burt RW. Gastric fundic gland polyps. *Gastroenterology.* 2003;125(5):1462–1469.

41. Brensinger JD, Laken SJ, Luce MC, et al. Variable phenotype of familial adenomatous polyposis in pedigrees with 3' mutation in the APC gene. *Gut.* 1998;43(4):548–552.

42. Giardiello FM, Brensinger JD, Luce MC, et al. Phenotypic expression of disease in families that have mutations in the 5' region of the adenomatous polyposis coli gene. *Ann Intern Med.* 1997;126(7):514–519.

43. Gorlin RJ, Cohen MM Jr., Condon LM, Burke BA. Bannayan-Riley-Ruvalcaba syndrome. *Am J Med Genet.* 1992;44(3):307–314.

44. Lachlan KL, Lucassen AM, Bunyan D, Temple IK. Cowden syndrome and Bannayan Riley Ruvalcaba syndrome represent one condition with variable expression and age-related penetrance: results of a clinical study of PTEN mutation carriers. *J Med Genet.* 2007;44(9):579–585.

45. National Comprehensive Cancer Network. NCCN Clinical Practice Guidelines in Oncology: Genetic/ Familial High-Risk Assessment: Colorectal. https://www.nccn.org/professionals/physician_gls/default. aspx-genetics_colon. Accessed May 6, 2020.

46. Stjepanovic N, Moreira L, Carneiro F, et al. Hereditary gastrointestinal cancers: ESMO Clinical Practice Guidelines for diagnosis, treatment and follow-updagger. *Ann Oncol.* 2019;30(10):1558–1571.

47. Nugent KP, Spigelman AD, Phillips RK. Life expectancy after colectomy and ileorectal anastomosis for familial adenomatous polyposis. *Dis Colon Rectum.* 1993;36(11):1059–1062.

48. Brosens LA, Keller JJ, Offerhaus GJ, Goggins M, Giardiello FM. Prevention and management of duodenal polyps in familial adenomatous polyposis. *Gut.* 2005;54(7):1034–1043.

49. Bulow S, Bjork J, Christensen IJ, et al. Duodenal adenomatosis in familial adenomatous polyposis. *Gut.* 2004;53(3):381–386.

50. Petersen GM. Genetic testing and counseling in familial adenomatous polyposis. *Oncology (Williston Park).* 1996;10(1):89–94; discussion 97–88.

51. Guillem JG, Wood WC, Moley JF, et al. ASCO/SSO review of current role of risk-reducing surgery in common hereditary cancer syndromes. *Ann Surg Oncol.* 2006;13(10):1296–1321.

52. Bertario L, Russo A, Radice P, et al. Genotype and phenotype factors as determinants for rectal stump cancer in patients with familial adenomatous polyposis. Hereditary Colorectal Tumors Registry. *Ann Surg.* 2000;231(4):538–543.

53. Vasen HF, van der Luijt RB, Slors JF, et al. Molecular genetic tests as a guide to surgical management of familial adenomatous polyposis. *Lancet.* 1996;348(9025):433–435.

54. Nieuwenhuis MH, Mathus-Vliegen LM, Slors FJ, et al. Genotype-phenotype correlations as a guide in the management of familial adenomatous polyposis. *Clin Gastroenterol Hepatol.* 2007;5(3):374–378.

55. Ooi BS, Remzi FH, Gramlich T, et al. Anal transitional zone cancer after restorative proctocolectomy and ileoanal anastomosis in familial adenomatous polyposis: report of two cases. *Dis Colon Rectum.* 2003;46(10):1418–1423; discussion 1422–1413.

56. Johnson MD, Mackey R, Brown N, et al. Outcome based on management for duodenal adenomas: sporadic versus familial disease. *J Gastrointest Surg.* 2010;14(2):229–235.

57. Heiskanen I, Kellokumpu I, Jarvinen H. Management of duodenal adenomas in 98 patients with familial adenomatous polyposis. *Endoscopy.* 1999;31(6):412–416.

58. de Vos tot Nederveen Cappel WH, Jarvinen HJ, Bjork J, et al. Worldwide survey among polyposis registries of surgical management of severe duodenal adenomatosis in familial adenomatous polyposis. *Br J Surg.* 2003;90(6):705–710.

59. Penna C, Phillips RK, Tiret E, Spigelman AD. Surgical polypectomy of duodenal adenomas in familial adenomatous polyposis: experience of two European centres. *Br J Surg.* 1993;80(8):1027–1029.

60. Mackey R, Walsh RM, Chung R, et al. Pancreas-sparing duodenectomy is effective management for familial adenomatous polyposis. *J Gastrointest Surg*. 2005;9(8):1088–1093; discussion 1093.

61. Tonelli F, Ficari F, Valanzano R, Brandi ML. Treatment of desmoids and mesenteric fibromatosis in familial adenomatous polyposis with raloxifene. *Tumori*. 2003;89(4):391–396.

62. Hansmann A, Adolph C, Vogel T, Unger A, Moeslein G. High-dose tamoxifen and sulindac as first-line treatment for desmoid tumors. *Cancer*. 2004;100(3):612–620.

63. Lindor NM, Dozois R, Nelson H, et al. Desmoid tumors in familial adenomatous polyposis: a pilot project evaluating efficacy of treatment with pirfenidone. *Am J Gastroenterol*. 2003;98(8):1868–1874.

64. Mace J, Sybil Biermann J, Sondak V, et al. Response of extraabdominal desmoid tumors to therapy with imatinib mesylate. *Cancer*. 2002;95(11):2373–2379.

65. Ishikawa H, Wakabayashi K, Suzuki S, et al. Preventive effects of low-dose aspirin on colorectal adenoma growth in patients with familial adenomatous polyposis: double-blind, randomized clinical trial. *Cancer Med*. 2013;2(1):50–56.

66. Siraj AK, Kumar Parvathareddy S, Pratheeshkumar P, et al. APC truncating mutations in Middle Eastern Population: Tankyrase inhibitor is an effective strategy to sensitize APC mutant CRC To 5-FU chemotherapy. *Biomed Pharmacother*. 2020;121:109572.

67. Cruz-Correa M, Hylind LM, Marrero JH, et al. Efficacy and safety of curcumin in treatment of intestinal adenomas in patients with familial adenomatous polyposis. *Gastroenterology*. 2018;155(3):668–673.

68. Willenbacher E, Khan SZ, Mujica SCA, et al. Curcumin: new insights into an ancient ingredient against cancer. *Int J Mol Sci*. 2019;20(8):E1808.

69. Barnett RM., Borras EN, Samadder J, Vilar E. *Chemoprevention in Hereditary Colorectal Cancer Syndromes*. Cham: Springer; 2018.

70. Nielsen M, Morreau H, Vasen HF, Hes FJ. MUTYH-associated polyposis (MAP). *Crit Rev Oncol Hematol*. 2011;79(1):1–16.

71. Nieuwenhuis MH, Vogt S, Jones N, et al. Evidence for accelerated colorectal adenoma-carcinoma progression in MUTYH-associated polyposis? *Gut*. 2012;61(5):734–738.

72. Win AK, Dowty JG, Cleary SP, et al. Risk of colorectal cancer for carriers of mutations in MUTYH, with and without a family history of cancer. *Gastroenterology*. 2014;146(5):1208–1211, e1201–1205.

73. Nielsen M, Joerink-van de Beld MC, Jones N, et al. Analysis of MUTYH genotypes and colorectal phenotypes in patients with MUTYH-associated polyposis. *Gastroenterology*. 2009;136(2):471–476.

74. Grover S, Kastrinos F, Steyerberg EW, et al. Prevalence and phenotypes of APC and MUTYH mutations in patients with multiple colorectal adenomas. *JAMA*. 2012;308(5):485–492.

75. Sieber OM, Lipton L, Crabtree M, et al. Multiple colorectal adenomas, classic adenomatous polyposis, and germ-line mutations in MYH. *N Engl J Med*. 2003;348(9):791–799.

76. Morak M, Laner A, Bacher U, Keiling C, Holinski-Feder E. MUTYH-associated polyposis-variability of the clinical phenotype in patients with biallelic and monoallelic MUTYH mutations and report on novel mutations. *Clin Genet*. 2010;78(4):353–363.

77. Jones N, Vogt S, Nielsen M, et al. Increased colorectal cancer incidence in obligate carriers of heterozygous mutations in MUTYH. *Gastroenterology*. 2009;137(2):489–494, 494, e481; quiz 725–486.

78. Boparai KS, Dekker E, Van Eeden S, et al. Hyperplastic polyps and sessile serrated adenomas as a phenotypic expression of MYH-associated polyposis. *Gastroenterology*. 2008;135(6):2014–2018.

79. Poulsen ML, Bisgaard ML. MUTYH associated polyposis (MAP). *Curr Genomics*. 2008;9(6):420–435.

80. Goodenberger M, Lindor NM. Lynch syndrome and MYH-associated polyposis: review and testing strategy. *J Clin Gastroenterol*. 2011;45(6):488–500.

81. Win AK, Cleary SP, Dowty JG, et al. Cancer risks for monoallelic MUTYH mutation carriers with a family history of colorectal cancer. *Int J Cancer*. 2011;129(9):2256–2262.

82. Vogt S, Jones N, Christian D, et al. Expanded extracolonic tumor spectrum in MUTYH-associated polyposis. *Gastroenterology*. 2009;137(6):1976–1985, e1971–1910.

83. Wasielewski M, Out AA, Vermeulen J, et al. Increased MUTYH mutation frequency among Dutch families with breast cancer and colorectal cancer. *Breast Cancer Res Treat*. 2010;124(3):635–641.

84. Nascimbeni R, Pucciarelli S, Di Lorenzo D, et al. Rectum-sparing surgery may be appropriate for biallelic MutYH-associated polyposis. *Dis Colon Rectum.* 2010;53(12):1670–1675.

85. Elsayed FA, Kets CM, Ruano D, et al. Germline variants in POLE are associated with early onset mismatch repair deficient colorectal cancer. *Eur J Hum Genet.* 2015;23(8):1080–1084.

86. Weren RD, Ligtenberg MJ, Kets CM, et al. A germline homozygous mutation in the base-excision repair gene NTHL1 causes adenomatous polyposis and colorectal cancer. *Nat Genet.* 2015;47(6):668–671.

87. Quintana I, Mejias-Luque R, Terradas M, et al. Evidence suggests that germline RNF43 mutations are a rare cause of serrated polyposis. *Gut.* 2018;67(12):2230–2232.

88. Taupin D, Lam W, Rangiah D, et al. A deleterious RNF43 germline mutation in a severely affected serrated polyposis kindred. *Hum Genome Var.* 2015;2:15013.

89. Chow E, Lipton L, Lynch E, et al. Hyperplastic polyposis syndrome: phenotypic presentations and the role of MBD4 and MYH. *Gastroenterology.* 2006;131(1):30–39.

90. Herkert JC, Niessen RC, Olderode-Berends MJ, et al. Paediatric intestinal cancer and polyposis due to bi-allelic PMS2 mutations: case series, review and follow-up guidelines. *Eur J Cancer.* 2011;47(7):965–982.

91. Wimmer K, Etzler J. Constitutional mismatch repair-deficiency syndrome: have we so far seen only the tip of an iceberg? *Hum Genet.* 2008;124(2):105–122.

92. Durno CA, Aronson M, Tabori U, Malkin D, Gallinger S, Chan HS. Oncologic surveillance for subjects with biallelic mismatch repair gene mutations: 10 year follow-up of a kindred. *Pediatr Blood Cancer.* 2012;59(4):652–656.

93. Jeghers H, Mc KV, Katz KH. Generalized intestinal polyposis and melanin spots of the oral mucosa, lips and digits; a syndrome of diagnostic significance. *N Engl J Med.* 1949;241(26):1031–1036.

94. Spigelman AD, Williams CB, Talbot IC, Domizio P, Phillips RK. Upper gastrointestinal cancer in patients with familial adenomatous polyposis. *Lancet.* 1989;2(8666):783–785.

95. Aretz S, Stienen D, Uhlhaas S, et al. High proportion of large genomic STK11 deletions in Peutz-Jeghers syndrome. *Hum Mutat.* 2005;26(6):513–519.

96. Lim W, Hearle N, Shah B, et al. Further observations on LKB1/STK11 status and cancer risk in Peutz-Jeghers syndrome. *Br J Cancer.* 2003;89(2):308–313.

97. Giardiello FM, Brensinger JD, Tersmette AC, et al. Very high risk of cancer in familial Peutz-Jeghers syndrome. *Gastroenterology.* 2000;119(6):1447–1453.

98. Srivatsa PJ, Keeney GL, Podratz KC. Disseminated cervical adenoma malignum and bilateral ovarian sex cord tumors with annular tubules associated with Peutz-Jeghers syndrome. *Gynecol Oncol.* 1994;53(2):256–264.

99. Scully RE. Sex cord tumor with annular tubules a distinctive ovarian tumor of the Peutz-Jeghers syndrome. *Cancer.* 1970;25(5):1107–1121.

100. Schreibman IR, Baker M, Amos C, McGarrity TJ. The hamartomatous polyposis syndromes: a clinical and molecular review. *Am J Gastroenterol.* 2005;100(2):476–490.

101. McGarrity TJ, Kulin HE, Zaino RJ. Peutz-Jeghers syndrome. *Am J Gastroenterol.* 2000;95(3):596–604.

102. Amos CI, Keitheri-Cheteri MB, Sabripour M, et al. Genotype-phenotype correlations in Peutz-Jeghers syndrome. *J Med Genet.* 2004;41(5):327–333.

103. van Lier MG, Mathus-Vliegen EM, Wagner A, van Leerdam ME, Kuipers EJ. High cumulative risk of intussusception in patients with Peutz-Jeghers syndrome: time to update surveillance guidelines? *Am J Gastroenterol.* 2011;106(5):940–945.

104. Beggs AD, Latchford AR, Vasen HF, et al. Peutz-Jeghers syndrome: a systematic review and recommendations for management. *Gut.* 2010;59(7):975–986.

105. Latchford A, Cohen S, Auth M, et al. Management of Peutz-Jeghers syndrome in children and adolescents: a position paper from the ESPGHAN Polyposis Working Group. *J Pediatr Gastroenterol Nutr.* 2019;68(3):442–452.

106. Udd L, Katajisto P, Rossi DJ, et al. Suppression of Peutz-Jeghers polyposis by inhibition of cyclooxygenase-2. *Gastroenterology.* 2004;127(4):1030–1037.

107. Latchford AR, Neale K, Phillips RK, Clark SK. Juvenile polyposis syndrome: a study of genotype, phenotype, and long-term outcome. *Dis Colon Rectum.* 2012;55(10):1038–1043.

108. Howe JR, Bair JL, Sayed MG, et al. Germline mutations of the gene encoding bone morphogenetic protein receptor 1A in juvenile polyposis. *Nat Genet.* 2001;28(2):184–187.

109. Zhou XP, Woodford-Richens K, Lehtonen R, et al. Germline mutations in BMPR1A/ALK3 cause a subset of cases of juvenile polyposis syndrome and of Cowden and Bannayan-Riley-Ruvalcaba syndromes. *Am J Hum Genet.* 2001;69(4):704–711.

110. Jass JR, Williams CB, Bussey HJ, Morson BC. Juvenile polyposis – a precancerous condition. *Histopathology.* 1988;13(6):619–630.

111. Chow E, Macrae F. A review of juvenile polyposis syndrome. *J Gastroenterol Hepatol.* 2005;20(11):1634–1640.

112. Boardman LA. Heritable colorectal cancer syndromes: recognition and preventive management. *Gastroenterol Clin North Am.* 2002;31(4):1107–1131.

113. Brosens LA, van Hattem A, Hylind LM, et al. Risk of colorectal cancer in juvenile polyposis. *Gut.* 2007;56(7):965–967.

114. Aretz S, Stienen D, Uhlhaas S, et al. High proportion of large genomic deletions and a genotype phenotype update in 80 unrelated families with juvenile polyposis syndrome. *J Med Genet.* 2007;44(11):702–709.

115. Dahdaleh FS, Carr JC, Calva D, Howe JR. Juvenile polyposis and other intestinal polyposis syndromes with microdeletions of chromosome 10q22-23. *Clin Genet.* 2012;81(2):110–116.

116. Gallione CJ, Repetto GM, Legius E, et al. A combined syndrome of juvenile polyposis and hereditary haemorrhagic telangiectasia associated with mutations in MADH4 (SMAD4). *Lancet.* 2004;363(9412):852–859.

117. Zhou XP, Waite KA, Pilarski R, et al. Germline PTEN promoter mutations and deletions in Cowden/Bannayan-Riley-Ruvalcaba syndrome result in aberrant PTEN protein and dysregulation of the phosphoinositol-3-kinase/Akt pathway. *Am J Hum Genet.* 2003;73(2):404–411.

118. Tan MH, Mester JL, Ngeow J, et al. Lifetime cancer risks in individuals with germline PTEN mutations. *Clin Cancer Res.* 2012;18(2):400–407.

119. Eng C. Will the real Cowden syndrome please stand up: revised diagnostic criteria. *J Med Genet.* 2000;37(11):828–830.

120. Marsh DJ, Kum JB, Lunetta KL, et al. PTEN mutation spectrum and genotype-phenotype correlations in Bannayan-Riley-Ruvalcaba syndrome suggest a single entity with Cowden syndrome. *Hum Mol Genet.* 1999;8(8):1461–1472.

121. National Comprehensive Cancer Network, NCCN Clinical Practice Guidelines in Oncology: Genetic/Familial High-Risk Assessment: Breast, Ovarian, and Pancreatic. Version 1.2020. https://www.nccn.org/professionals/physician_gls/default.aspx-genetics_screening. Accessed May 7, 2020.

122. Hampel H, Bennett RL, Buchanan A, et al. A practice guideline from the American College of Medical Genetics and Genomics and the National Society of Genetic Counselors: referral indications for cancer predisposition assessment. *Genet Med.* 2015;17(1):70–87.

123. Heald B, Mester J, Rybicki L, Orloff MS, Burke CA, Eng C. Frequent gastrointestinal polyps and colorectal adenocarcinomas in a prospective series of PTEN mutation carriers. *Gastroenterology.* 2010;139(6):1927–1933.

124. Stanich PP, Owens VL, Sweetser S, et al. Colonic polyposis and neoplasia in Cowden syndrome. *Mayo Clin Proc.* 2011;86(6):489–492.

125. Riegert-Johnson DL, Gleeson FC, Roberts M, et al. Cancer and Lhermitte-Duclos disease are common in Cowden syndrome patients. *Hered Cancer Clin Pract.* 2010;8(1):6.

126. Robinson S, Cohen AR. Cowden disease and Lhermitte-Duclos disease: an update. Case report and review of the literature. *Neurosurg Focus.* 2006;20(1):E6.

127. Sweetser S, Ahlquist DA, Osborn NK, et al. Clinicopathologic features and treatment outcomes in Cronkhite-Canada syndrome: support for autoimmunity. *Dig Dis Sci.* 2012;57(2):496–502.

128. Seshadri D, Karagiorgos N, Hyser MJ. A case of cronkhite-Canada syndrome and a review of gastrointestinal polyposis syndromes. *Gastroenterol Hepatol (N Y).* 2012;8(3):197–201.

129. Sweetser S, Boardman LA. Cronkhite-Canada syndrome: an acquired condition of gastrointestinal polyposis and dermatologic abnormalities. *Gastroenterol Hepatol (N Y).* 2012;8(3):201–203.

130. Samoha S, Arber N. Cronkhite-Canada syndrome. *Digestion.* 2005;71(4):199–200.

Hereditary Nonpolyposis Colorectal Cancers

Christina Dimopoulos and Xavier Llor

▮ DISEASE-SPECIFIC CANCER EPIDEMIOLOGY

Hereditary colorectal cancers, both polyposis and nonpolyposis, arise from either high-penetrance germline mutations (such as in mismatch repair genes causing Lynch syndrome), moderate-penetrance genes (such as *CHEK2* or the *APC* I1307 variant), and low-penetrance alleles. Nevertheless, in a significant number of cases that are highly suspicious for being hereditary, no pathogenic variants are identified in the known susceptibility genes.

Hereditary nonpolyposis colorectal cancer (HNPCC) accounts for 5% to 10% of all colorectal cancers. HNPCC includes Lynch syndrome, commonly with microsatellite unstable tumors caused by a faulty deoxyribonucleic acid (DNA) mismatch repair system, and the less clear microsatellite stable HNPCC (MSS-HNPCC), also called familial colorectal cancer type X, that does not have DNA mismatch repair deficiency. Also, not well defined is an undetermined percentage of cases that could be related to a number of low-susceptibility alleles, as well as some cases of unclear etiology that result in mismatch repair–deficient tumors but with absence of germline mutations in mismatch repair genes (Lynch-like syndrome).

Lynch Syndrome

Lynch syndrome is an autosomal dominant cancer syndrome due to germline mutations in the MMR genes *MLH1, MSH2, MSH6,* or *PMS2*. *EPCAM* also contributes to the pathogenesis of Lynch syndrome, as deletions at the 3′ end of *EPCAM* cause hypermethylation of the *MSH2* promoter region. This hypermethylation leads to epigenetic silencing of *MSH2* and subsequent loss of MSH2 expression.[1] One in 279 individuals (0.36% of the general population) has Lynch syndrome, making it one of the most common cancer syndromes. The most commonly Lynch syndrome mutated genes in the overall population are *PMS2* (1 in 714 individuals) and *MSH6* (1 in 758). *MLH1* (1 in 1946) and *MSH2* (1 in 2841) are less common.[2] Nevertheless, mutations in *MLH1* and *MSH2* account for over 60% of cancers related to Lynch syndrome, as they have a higher cancer penetrance than *MSH6* and *PMS2*.[3]

About 3% of all colorectal cancers are related to Lynch syndrome. Besides the mentioned differences in terms of cancer risk, there are also important differences related to age at diagnosis among the different MMR genes. Thus, the mean age of colorectal cancer diagnosis in patients with *MLH1* and *MSH2* (including *EPCAM*) mutations is 44 years old, while it is later for *MSH6* (42 to 69 years old), as well as for *PMS2* (61 to 66 years old).[4]

In addition to being implicated in colorectal cancer, Lynch syndrome carries an increased risk of extracolonic cancers. Thus, 2% of all endometrial cancers are related to Lynch syndrome. About 10% to 15% of all inherited ovarian cancers and a not well-defined proportion of inherited gastric cancers are also due to Lynch syndrome. Other Lynch syndrome–related cancers include biliary tract, uroepithelial and kidney, and central nervous system.[5] In terms of location, Lynch syndrome–associated colorectal cancers are more often right-sided, or proximal to the splenic flexure, than sporadic colorectal cancers. There is also a high risk of metachronous colorectal cancer in Lynch syndrome, with 30% of patients developing a second colorectal cancer 10 years after the initial diagnosis.[6] Relatives of patients with mutations who themselves are not carriers do not have an increased risk of cancer, either colorectal or extracolonic.[7]

MSS HNPCC (Familial Colorectal Cancer Type X)

MSS HNPCC are microsatellite stable tumors, and individuals do not have any germline MMR gene mutations. The specific genes that are responsible for MSS HNPCC are not well characterized, but the phenotype is thought to be caused by a combination of single high-penetrance genes, multiple low-penetrance genes, and sporadic colorectal cancer cases. Not having a commonly identified genetic defect, it is difficult to accurately assess its impact in the general group of colorectal cancers. In any case, in a population-based study using Amsterdam criteria[8] as a way to select for families highly enriched with colorectal cancers, this phenotype was as common as Lynch syndrome.[9] It is estimated that about half of the families that meet Amsterdam criteria have MSS HNPCC. While individuals in these families have about a 2-fold increased lifetime risk of colorectal cancers, this risk is lower than in *MLH1*, *MSH2* Lynch syndrome families.[3] Unlike Lynch syndrome, the mean age of colorectal cancer diagnosis is between 50 and 60 years (similar to the mean ages for *MSH6* and *PMS2* Lynch syndrome patients.[10] The location of colorectal cancers in MSS HNPCC tends to be more distal and thus similar to sporadic colorectal cancers, with most tumors found in the rectum and sigmoid colon.[6,9,11] While most studies have not found an increased risk of extracolonic cancers in MSS HNPCC families,[3,9] a recent study based on a national Danish registry found that these patients had an increased risk of gastric, pancreatic, urinary tract, and breast cancers, as well as ocular melanoma. It is unclear, though, the nature of the reported cases, as the group was identified by Amsterdam criteria and MMR-proficient tumors and no genetic data were reported.[12] With regard to histology, MSS HNPCC tumors are more likely to be moderately differentiated without lymphocytic infiltration. This is in contrast to Lynch syndrome, where histology tends to show poor differentiation with lymphocytic infiltrates. Unlike sporadic MSI tumors, both MSS and MSI HNPCC tumors have a low incidence of mucin production.[9]

Moderate-Penetrance Genes and Low-Susceptibility Alleles

Checkpoint kinase 2 (*CHEK2*) is a protein kinase that is involved in cell cycle arrest. *CHEK2* mutations are inherited in an autosomal dominant pattern and have been implicated in colorectal cancer through (1) a truncating mutation that causes a kinase deficiency and (2) a missense polymorphism that leads to an inability to bind and phosphorylate.[13] *CHEK2* is considered a low- to moderate-penetrance allele and accounts for less than 1% of all colorectal cancers. It is estimated that every 1 to 2 in 100 people are *CHEK2* mutation carriers, and this population carries a 5% to 10% lifetime colorectal cancer risk.[14] This risk probably is limited to the two most common founder mutations in populations of European descent: I157T and 1100delC variants.[15,16]

The *APC* gene is responsible for familial adenomatous polyposis (FAP) characterized by the development of hundreds to thousands of colon polyps and invariable cancer development. The *APC* I1307K variant does not cause typical polyposis, but rather it is a low-susceptibility allele for colorectal cancer. This specific pathogenic variant is commonly seen in the Jewish population, particularly, but not exclusively, in the Ashkenazi group, with a reported prevalence in the latter of 6% to 7%.[17] A study of patients with colorectal cancer from Israel found this variant in 11.2% of Ashkenazi Jewish, 2.7% of non-Ashkenazi Jews, and 3.1% of individuals of Arabic descent.[18]

MUTYH is a base excision repair gene that causes *MUTYH*-associated polyposis (MAP). MAP is an autosomal recessive syndrome, and the MAP phenotype only develops when germline mutations are present in both *MUTYH* copies. Biallelic *MUTYH* is considered high penetrance, whereas there are conflicting data regarding the potential increased risk of colorectal cancer with a single germline mutation in one *MUTYH* gene. At most, a heterozygous mutation likely behaves as a moderate-penetrance genetic defect, carrying a 1.5- to 2-fold increased risk of colorectal cancer compared to the general population.[3] An estimated 2.2% of the population is monoallelic for *MUTYH*, and 0.012% is biallelic.[2]

Genome-wide association studies (GWAS) have identified about 100 low-penetrance alleles that are associated with an increased risk of colorectal cancer.[19] Some data suggest that up to 10% of hereditary colorectal cancers can be explained by these loci.[20] Each individual locus carries a small increased risk of colorectal cancer. In order to understand the significance of these alleles, algorithms that approximate the risk of multiple alleles will need to be developed.[21] Compared with individuals that have the median number of these alleles, it has been suggested that those carrying a high number of alleles have three times the risk of developing colorectal cancer.[20]

One study set out to assess individual colorectal cancer risk by using 40,000 individuals to create an algorithm about the combined effects of age, gender, family history, and genotype of 10 known susceptibility loci. The algorithm was shown to not be able to calculate individual colorectal cancer risk; however, when applied to a population, it was able to risk-stratify patients. This could open up the door to risk stratification mechanisms and suggest more rigorous colorectal cancer screening approaches for higher-risk individuals.[22]

It is also worth discussing genes that are historically not associated with colorectal cancer, such as *BRCA1/2* and *p53*. About 0.7% to 1.3% of patients with colorectal cancer are positive for *BRCA1/2*, and a recent meta-analysis showed that there was a 1.22-fold increased risk of colorectal cancer in *BRCA* carriers (1.48 in *BRCA1* but no increased risk in *BRCA2*). The role of *BRCA* genes in colorectal cancer is debated and is thought to be either from the overall prevalence of the mutations or due to pleiotropism (one genetic variant that presents as multiple phenotypes). Studies conducted on the topic so far favor the former explanation. One study found no statistically significant difference in either *BRCA* or *p53* when looking at over 100 hereditary cancer genes in patients with early onset colorectal cancer of unknown etiology versus controls. Another study found no difference in *BRCA* (and other DNA repair genes not classically associated with colorectal cancer) when comparing patients with colorectal cancers of unknown etiology to patients without cancer.[3]

Lynch-Like Syndrome

Lynch-like syndrome is defined by tumors that are MSI but have neither germline MMR mutations (as in Lynch syndrome) nor *MLH1* promoter hypermethylation (as seen in sporadic colorectal cancers).[23] Instead, patients with Lynch-like syndrome often, but not always, have biallelic somatic MMR mutations. Lynch-like syndrome is likely heterogeneous but probably includes some cases that have a genetic basis, as a study showed that patients with Lynch-like syndrome had at least one first-degree relative (FDR) with a solid malignancy and 1.8 FDRs with malignant tumors. These numbers are in comparison to 0.8 FDRs with a solid malignancy in patients with colorectal cancer who were prospectively recruited ($p = 0.014$). In terms of demographics, one study found that the median age for onset of colorectal cancer was 65 in Lynch-like syndrome compared to 76 in patients with sporadic colorectal cancer ($p = 0.04$).[23] Another study showed the onset to be earlier, with age at first cancer diagnosis of 53.7 in Lynch-like syndrome and 48.5 in Lynch syndrome.[24] Given this, some specialists have suggested that patients with Lynch-like syndrome undergo colorectal cancer screening at similar intervals to those with Lynch syndrome.[25] This is not widely accepted among experts, though, at this time. In any case, given the current paucity of data, important consideration should be given to specific personal and family history in order to design surveillance strategies.

Early Onset Colorectal Cancer Early onset colorectal cancer is defined as colorectal cancer that presents prior to age 50. In the last 30 years, the incidence of colorectal cancer in adults ages 20 to 49 has doubled in the United States and some other Western countries, over 12% of new colorectal cancer cases occurring in this age group. It is projected that by 2030, 11% of colon and 23% of rectal cancers will be in adults under age 50. This incidence is in contrast to colorectal cancer in the overall population, which has decreased by over 35% since the 1990s. While it was reported that non-Hispanic black patients make up 16% of the early onset colorectal cancer patients and only 9% of early onset colorectal cancer is seen in non-Hispanic white patients,[14] recent data have shown a substantial narrowing in the differences in incidence of early onset colorectal cancer among the different racial groups in the United States.[26] Compared to older onset colorectal cancer, early onset is more likely to present at a later stage and has a higher incidence of metastatic disease. Younger patients tend to present with tumors in the distal colon and rectum, compared to the proximal colon tumors typically seen in older patients. Histopathology tends to show poorly differentiated tumors with signet ring cell histology and lymphovascular and perineural invasion.

A patient's risk is usually stratified for colorectal cancer by using factors such as age and family history. However, only a minority of patients with early onset colorectal cancer have family history or conditions that would predispose them to colorectal cancer. Rather, about 17% to 35% of younger patients have pathogenic germline variants, a prevalence that is double what is seen in older patients with colorectal cancer. For patients less than 35 years old, about 23% of colorectal cancers are due to germline MMR mutations, 9% due to polyposis genes (including *APC*, *MUTYH*), 2% have other variants (including *BRCA1/2*, *TP53*, *CHEK2*), and 65% have no identifiable germline mutation. For patients less than 50 years old, the breakdown is 10% germline MMR mutations, 3% polyposis genes, 5% other variants, and

80% with no identifiable mutation. Lastly, for patients that are older than 50, the distribution is 3% germline MMR mutation, <1% polyposis genes, 6% other variants, and 90% with no identifiable germline mutations. These statistics demonstrate that the younger a patient is at colorectal cancer diagnosis, the more likely it is due to an inherited cancer syndrome.[14]

In addition to known genes that are implicated in hereditary cancer syndromes, low-susceptibility alleles seem to be significant in early onset colorectal cancer. A recent study developed a polygenic risk score (PRS) based on 95 colorectal cancer–associated single nucleotide polymorphisms that had been identified through a large-scale GWAS.[27] When comparing the highest to the lowest PRS quartile, there was an overall 3.7× higher risk for early onset colorectal cancer versus a 2.9× higher risk for older onset colorectal cancer. This was further subdivided into patients without family history, where the difference between early and older onset was even greater: 4.3× higher risk compared with 2.9×. Patients with Lynch syndrome were removed from the analysis, while genetic mutations related to other, rarer hereditary cancer syndromes were included. This PRS was developed based on people of European ancestry. A PRS will need to be developed and validated in other populations in order for this method to be more broadly generalizable. Combining the PRS with lifestyle and environmental risk factors could more accurately determine which patients would benefit from earlier screening.

▓ DISEASE-SPECIFIC APPROACH TO RISK ASSESSMENT, COUNSELING, AND TESTING

Lynch Syndrome

Clinical Criteria Population-based studies from the United States estimate that 1 in every 279 to 300 individuals has Lynch syndrome. However, the majority of these patients are undiagnosed. Thus, there is a need to develop mechanisms that can reliably identify these patients.[28] Different criteria have been developed over time, based on personal and family history of cancer. Amsterdam criteria[26] and Bethesda guidelines[29] have been used to determine who should be tested for Lynch syndrome. The Amsterdam criteria recommends testing patients for MMR mutations if there are three or more relatives with Lynch syndrome–associated cancers involving at least two generations; one or more of these cancers had to have been diagnosed prior to age 50. The Amsterdam criteria have very low sensitivity, and they are no longer recommended as a tool to select for genetic testing. In fact, 40% of families with known mutations do not fulfill Amsterdam criteria, and 50% of those who meet the criteria do not have a detectable MMR mutation.[1]

The Bethesda and modified Bethesda guidelines were developed as a two-step process, taking advantage of the fact that most Lynch syndrome–related colorectal cancers are MMR deficient. Criteria would be used to select for tumors to undergo screening through either microsatellite instability testing or immunohistochemistry to evaluate mismatch protein expression. Patients with MMR-deficient tumors would be selected for germline testing. These criteria have a much higher sensitivity than Amsterdam criteria but a low specificity of 25%. Nevertheless, even when following these guidelines, up to 28% of patients with MMR mutations will be missed.[1]

Several prediction models have been developed and validated in order to further assist in identifying individuals who should undergo genetic testing for Lynch syndrome.[1] The three current prediction models are MMRpredict, MMRpro, and $PREMM_5$.

- MMRpredict: Estimates the likelihood of having an *MLH1*, *MSH2*, or *MSH6* mutation in patients diagnosed with colorectal cancer prior to age 55. Patients with a score >5% would be advised to undergo genetic testing for Lynch syndrome.[30] The main features of MMRpredict include:
  - Risk assessment is based on age at colorectal cancer diagnosis, gender, proximal versus distal tumor location, and family history of colorectal cancer and/or endometrial cancer
  - Not applicable to extracolonic cancers
  - Unproven usefulness in older patients, as it was validated in a younger population.
- MMRpro: Estimates the probability of having any of the *MLH1*, *MSH2*, or *MSH6* mutations, as well as gene-specific probabilities. Patients with a score >5% would be indicated to undergo genetic testing for Lynch syndrome.[31] The main features of MMRpro include:
  - Takes into account the following for the patient, as well as for first- and second-degree relatives: age at colorectal cancer diagnosis, age at last follow-up, and molecular tumor testing results
  - Not applicable to extracolonic cancers (similar to MMRpredict)
  - Best completed in a cancer clinic with a genetic counselor, given that it requires a complete pedigree (including unaffected family members)[1]
- $PREMM_5$: Predicts the likelihood of a patient having mutations in *MLH1, MSH2, MSH6, PMS2*, and *EPCAM*. The previous model ($PREMM_{1,2,6}$) did not include *PMS2* or *EPCAM* in the risk assessment. Patients with a $PREMM_5$ score >2.5% would be indicated to undergo genetic testing for Lynch syndrome.[4,32] The main features of $PREMM_5$ include:
  - Captures all Lynch syndrome–associated cancers, not just colorectal.
  - Risk assessment is based on age, gender, and personal and family cancer history. Easier to fill out, thus lack of a genetic counselor is not limiting (compared to MMRpro).
  - This model is likely more accurate at estimating the risk of having an *MLH1, MSH2, MSH6*, or *EPCAM* mutation as compared to a *PMS2* mutation (due to the less well-determined penetrance of the latter).[32]

Thus, criteria for MMR germline testing have continued evolving and expanding as genetic testing has become more widely available and reimbursed by payers. These include the recommendation of systematically testing all colorectal and endometrial cancers for MMR deficiency. More recently, some guidelines have expanded the recommendation to include testing for MMR deficiency of all adenocarcinomas of the small bowel, stomach, pancreas, biliary tract, brain, bladder, urothelium, and adrenal glands, regardless of age at diagnosis.[4]

The National Comprehensive Cancer Network (NCCN) guidelines suggest that patients should be evaluated for Lynch syndrome in the following scenarios:

- There is a known Lynch syndrome pathogenic variant in the family
- The patient has a personal history of an MMR-deficient tumor at any age that was detected by immunohistochemistry (IHC), polymerase chain reaction (PCR), or next-generation sequencing (NGS)
- The patient has a personal history of Lynch syndrome–associated cancer, which includes colorectal, endometrial, gastric, ovarian, pancreas, urothelial, glioblastoma, biliary tract, small intestine, sebaceous adenoma and carcinoma, and keratoacanthoma.

- An individual with colorectal or endometrial cancer and any of the following:
  - Diagnosed prior to age 50
  - Diagnosis of another synchronous or metachronous Lynch syndrome–related cancer (including gastric, ovarian, pancreas, urothelial, glioblastoma, biliary tract, small intestine, sebaceous adenoma and carcinoma, and keratoacanthoma)
  - One first- or second-degree relative with a Lynch syndrome–related cancer diagnosed prior to age 50
  - Two or more first- or second-degree relatives with Lynch syndrome–related cancer diagnosed at any age
- Family history of one or more first-degree relatives with colorectal or endometrial cancer diagnosed prior to age 50
- Family history of one or more first-degree relatives with colorectal or endometrial cancer and another synchronous or metachronous Lynch syndrome–related cancer
- Family history of two or more first- or second-degree relatives with Lynch syndrome–related cancers, including at least one diagnosed prior to age 50
- Family history of three or more first- or second-degree relatives with Lynch syndrome–related cancers diagnosed at any age
- An individual with a greater than or equal to 2.5% risk of having an MMR gene pathogenic variant based on the predictive model $PREMM_5$
- An individual with greater than or equal to 5% risk of having an MMR gene pathogenic variant based on the predictive models MMRpro or MMRpredict[4]

If there is a known Lynch syndrome pathogenic variant in the family, then genetic testing for the specific variant can be performed. A patient who turns out to be negative for the familial variant can be treated as an average-risk individual. If there is no known familial Lynch syndrome pathogenic variant, then the patient can undergo germline multigene testing with NGS. For families where there is more than one affected member, the individual with the youngest age at diagnosis, multiple primary malignancies, and colorectal or endometrial cancer can be prioritized for multigene testing.[4]

Tumor Testing to Pre-select for Lynch Syndrome Germline Testing Tumor testing has been an integral part of the Lynch syndrome diagnostic strategy for years. This builds on specific features of Lynch syndrome–associated tumors. The following are important definitions that are relevant to Lynch syndrome tumor testing:

- IHC: A method of staining tumors where antibodies (usually fluorescent) bind to various antigens; in this case, *MLH1, MSH2, MSH6,* or *PMS2* proteins. An abnormal IHC occurs when one of the proteins is not detected in the tumor tissue but it is detected in the nontumor tissue, suggesting that there is a pathogenic variant in the associated gene.
- Microsatellite instability (MSI) analysis: A microsatellite is defined as a region of DNA with repeating nucleotides (either single, such as GGGG, or double, such as CTCTCT). MSI analysis compares the number of microsatellite repeats between healthy and tumor tissue and determines if the same number of repeats are in both tissues. If they are, the tumor is microsatellite stable (MSS); if they differ, the tumor is classified as microsatellite unstable, or MSI. MSI is classified as having 30% or more mutated microsatellite sequences. Microsatellite instability is a surrogate for loss of MMR activity.[1]

- *MLH1* methylation: Hypermethylation of the *MLH1* promoter region silences gene transcription, which produces an MSI tumor phenotype. However, *MLH1* is still intact and has no germline mutation; therefore tumors with epigenetic modification of *MLH1* through methylation are sporadic and not due to Lynch syndrome.
- *BRAF* V600E: BRAF is a serine threonine kinase. It is an activator in the MAPK signaling cascade, which is involved in cellular proliferation. The most common mutation in *BRAF* leads to valine (V) being substituted by glutamic acid (E) at codon 600. This mutation leads to continuous activation of *BRAF*, leading to increased proliferation and tumorigenesis. Mutated *BRAF* is implicated in many cancers, including sporadic colorectal malignancies. If a tumor shows loss of MLH1 and this tumor has the mentioned *BRAF* mutation, the tumor is almost certain to be sporadic and related to methylation of the *MLH1* gene.

The NCCN recommends screening for MMR deficiency of all colorectal and endometrial tumors, as well as all adenocarcinomas of the small bowel, stomach, pancreas, biliary tract, brain, bladder, urothelium, and adrenal glands. If the tumor shows MMR deficiency, germline genetic testing for Lynch syndrome is indicated. Paired tumor somatic and germline testing is also an option that can confirm a somatic origin of the MMR deficiency when no germline mutations are identified.[4] In settings where it is not possible to test the tumors, the Bethesda criteria have traditionally been used to determine which patients should directly undergo genetic testing.[4] In any case, and as mentioned earlier, it seems very likely that only a much more generalized approach to genetic testing can uncover almost all of the individuals with Lynch syndrome. The increasing availability and affordability of genetic tests can eventually allow it.

Two tumor tests can be used, either individually or in combination, to assess tumors for Lynch syndrome: IHC of MMR proteins and MSI. These are effective screening methods, as over 90% of Lynch syndrome tumors lack expression of at least one MMR protein by IHC and are MSI. The sensitivity of MMR IHC when using a colorectal tumor sample is 92% to 94% and the specificity is 88% to 100%. The false-negative rate of MSI testing is about 5% to 15%.[4] When detecting MSI by PCR, mononucleotide markers are more reliable than dinucleotide markers. One study compared two panels of markers in colorectal adenocarcinomas: one comprising two mononucleotide markers and three dinucleotide markers (the National Cancer Institute [NCI] panel) and another made up of five mononucleotide markers (the pentaplex panel). The study found that the sensitivity and positive predictive value (PPV) of the pentaplex panel was 95.8% (95% CI 89% to 103%) and 88.5% (95% CI 79% to 98%), respectively. In comparison, the sensitivity and PPV of the NCI panel was 76.5% (95% CI 61% to 92%) and 65% (95% CI 49% to 81%), respectively. This study also found that using two mononucleotide repeat markers, BAT26 and NR24, had the same PPV as the pentaplex panel. Dinucleotide markers were less reliable to screen for MMR deficiency.[33] MSI can also be detected through NGS, which allows for tens to thousands of microsatellites to be analyzed. Bioinformatics protocols are required for this analysis, and further studies are needed to determine the sensitivity and specificity of MSI by NGS.[4]

With regard to IHC, tumors in Lynch syndrome usually develop after the inactivation of the second allele, as the first one is already inactive due to a pathogenic variant in an MMR gene. This results in lack of expression of the corresponding protein in the tumor tissue, which can be assessed by IHC. MMR proteins work as heterodimers, being MLH1 and MSH2 obligatory components of all types of heterodimers formed. The main heterodimer of MSH2 is formed with MSH6, while the main partner of MLH1 is PMS2. Loss of protein expression most often involves the heterodimer pairs, but loss of only one protein is also seen. If a tumor is found to have a loss of *MSH2, MSH6,* or *PMS2* expression, it is most likely due to a germline mutation causing Lynch syndrome. However, a loss of *MLH1* or both *MLH1/PMS2* in about two-thirds of cases will be an epigenetic event with inactivation of *MLH1* through hypermethylation of the 5′ untranslated region of the gene. This hypermethylation silences gene transcription, which produces an MSI tumor phenotype.

In fact, about 10% of sporadic colorectal cancers[4] and 20% of sporadic endometrial adeno-carcinoma[34] exhibit abnormal IHC and MSI secondary to hypermethylation of the *MLH1* gene promoter region. Therefore, if IHC reveals an absent MLH1 expression, analysis of *MLH1* methylation in the tumor can help identify the overwhelming majority of the sporadic tumors. In this case, genetic testing can be left only for the cases where *MLH1* methylation is not identified. Alternatively, colorectal tumors with loss of *MLH1* expression can be tested for the *BRAF* V600E pathogenic variant. This finding is almost invariably associated with *MLH1* promoter hypermethylation and thus sporadic tumors. This approach is not as sensitive as *MLH1* methylation analysis, but it can be particularly useful in situations where there is limited tumor available for testing. In any case, the absence of a *BRAF* V600E pathogenic variant does not exclude *MLH1* methylation, as only 69% of methylated colorectal cancers contain *BRAF* V600E pathogenic variants. Given this, methylation analysis could also be considered to rule out Lynch syndrome in MSI tumors where no *BRAF* pathogenic variant is found prior to genetic testing or if genetic testing is negative. All three—*MLH1* promoter hypermethylation, *BRAF* V500E pathogenic variant, and abnormal *BRAF* V600E protein expression—correlate with sporadic cancer as opposed to Lynch syndrome. Patients whose tumors have loss of MLH1 protein expression but no *MLH1* promoter methylation and/or wild type *BRAF* (or normal *BRAF* expression) should proceed to germline genetic testing to assess for Lynch syndrome.[4] Unfortunately, *BRAF* V600E mutations are not associated with MMR-deficient endometrial adenocarcinomas; thus, this is not a useful tool in these cases.[35]

IHC has a 5% to 10% false-negative rate. This is largely due to situations where there is a present but inactive or unstable protein to which the antibody can bind. In particular, this is more commonly seen in carriers of *MSH6* and *PMS2* mutations that have a sizable percentage of tumors with normal protein expression on IHC.[36] In these cases, genetic testing can be considered in a patient with normal IHC results if there is clinical suspicion of Lynch syndrome.[1]

Regarding Lynch syndrome–associated colorectal adenomas, about 70% to 79% show loss of MMR protein expression on IHC. This percentage increases with the adenoma size, as well as its degree of dysplasia. However, given this lower sensitivity when compared to testing carried out on samples from adenocarcinomas, a normal MMR protein expression on an adenoma does not rule out Lynch syndrome.

In the specific case of rectal cancers, false-positive IHC has been seen in patients who underwent neoadjuvant chemotherapy and radiation therapy for their malignancy. In these cases, it is not recommended to proceed with IHC; testing should instead be carried out on the pretreatment specimen, and if that is not available, genetic testing is recommended.

As mentioned earlier, the NCCN panel recently extended the recommendation of screening for MMR deficiency to adenocarcinomas of the small bowel, stomach, pancreas, biliary tract, brain, bladder, urothelium, adrenal glands, and sebaceous neoplasms with MSI or IHC, with subsequent genetic testing for Lynch syndrome in the abnormal cases. While there is much less experience regarding the yield of Lynch syndrome diagnosis screening these tumors for MMR deficiency, a large study including more than 50 types of cancers showed MMR deficiency rates as high as 30% for small bowel adenocarcinomas, 6.2% for gastric, and 5.8% for urothelial cancers, with respective Lynch syndrome rates of 12%, 15%, and 37.5% among the MMR-deficient tumors.[36] There is not much information yet regarding rates of *MLH1* promoter methylation or potential presence of *BRAF V600E* mutations in these tumors to use in the overall screening strategy. The authors found a 98.2% concordance between MSI and IHC to ascertain MMR deficiency; therefore either method seems suitable to perform this testing moving forward. This same study showed that 50% of patients with Lynch syndrome who had an MSI tumor had a malignancy that was not colorectal or endometrial. Of these nonclassic tumors (who had Lynch syndrome and MSI), 45% would not have met criteria for genetic testing based on family or personal history. These data make a strong case for this expanded approach of tumor testing in order to dramatically increase Lynch syndrome identification. In fact, this expansion of tumor testing for MMR deficiency is independently supported by the recent approval of immunotherapy agents such as pembrolizumab for all unresponsive solid tumors that demonstrate MMR deficiency.[37]

In the same study, while the majority of patients with Lynch syndrome had MSI tumors, 36% had tumors that were MSS. These MSS tumors were predominantly cancers outside the colon and endometrium, and 78.4% of them had low-penetrance *MSH6* or *PMS2* mutations ($p < 0.001$). Further, 89.2% of these MSS tumors did not have MMR-deficient signatures ($p < 0.001$). In these tumors that were both MSS and MMR deficient, the germline MMR mutations are likely incidental findings rather than the cause of the malignancy.

With regard to sebaceous neoplasms, the sensitivity of IHC was found to be 85% and the specificity 48%, with a false-positive rate of 56%.[38] An established clinical scoring system has been proposed to determine which of these patients with sebaceous neoplasms should be screened for Lynch syndrome, while, as mentioned, the NCCN guidelines propose tumor testing for all these neoplasms.[4] If the primary tumor is not available and there is metastatic disease, IHC and MSI testing can be carried out on the metastatic tissue.[4]

▨ HEREDITARY CANCER SYNDROMES: CLINICAL FEATURES AND CANCER RISKS ACCORDING TO GENETIC DEFECT

Lynch Syndrome

Highly selective criteria, usually only including families with extensive cancer histories, made past estimates of the risk for Lynch syndrome–related cancers prone to significant ascertainment bias. As genetic testing has become more readily available and universal tumor analysis to assess for MMR deficiency is now much more common, a clearer picture on cancer risks and age of onset is emerging. This has resulted in lowering overall risk, as studies have been able to capture the more common but less penetrant genetic defects, particularly mutations in *PMS2*.[39] Thus, the emerging picture of Lynch syndrome is a more heterogenous disease than previously thought, which requires more targeted approaches.

A study with a large number of *MLH1*, *MSH2*, and *MSH6* mutation carriers looking at cancer incidence beyond colorectal and endometrial adenocarcinoma showed that the highest standardized incident ratio (SIR) was for small bowel (SIR 251 for men and 112 for women) and urothelial cancer (SIR 112 for women). The cancers with the earliest mean age at diagnosis were small bowel (46 years old) and ovarian (44 years old). The only noncolon, nonendometrial cancers that had patients diagnosed prior to age 30 were stomach, small bowel, and ovaries. The malignancy with the highest lifetime risk was small bowel in men (12%); the lowest lifetime risk was gastric cancer in women (2.6%).[40]

Tables 7.1 and 7.2 summarize cancer risks and average age at diagnosis for every Lynch syndrome gene. Data was extracted from Cancer Risk tables of the NCCN guidelines: Genetic/Familial High-Risk Assessment: Colorectal (Version 1.2020).[4]

MLH1 *MLH1* has the highest cumulative colorectal cancer risk through age 80, ranging from 46% to 61% as compared to 4.2% in the general population. The average age of presentation is 44. It also carries a high cumulative endometrial cancer risk of 34% to 54%, compared to 3.1% in the general population. Ovarian cancer risk is the third highest, at 4% to 20% as compared to 1.3% in general. Average ages of presentation are 49 and 46 for endometrial and ovarian cancer, respectively.

Along with *MSH2*, *MLH1* mutation carriers have the highest risk of gastric cancer at 5% to 7% versus 0.9% in general (average age 52); small bowel is 0.4% to 11% versus 0.3% (average age 47). Pancreatic cancer is at 6.2% as compared to 1.6% (unclear average age), and biliary tract cancer is from 1.9% to 3.7% versus 0.2% (average age 50). Bladder cancer is at 2% to 7% compared to 2.4% (average age 59), and renal pelvis and/or ureter ranges from 0.2% to 5% (average age 59 to 60). Brain cancer risk is 0.7% to 1.7% versus 0.6% (unclear average age). Incidences for

TABLE 7.1: Cumulative Cancer Risk by Gene

Site	MLH 1 Cumulative Risk for Diagnosis Through Age 80y[b]	MSH 2 Cumulative Risk for Diagnosis Through Age 80y[b]	MSH 6 Cumulative Risk for Diagnosis Through Age 80y[b,e]	PMS 2 Cumulative Risk for Diagnosis Through Age 80y[b,e]	Cumulative Risk for Diagnosis Through Lifetime for General Population[c]
Colorectal	46%–61%	33%–52%	10%–44%	8.7%–20%	4.2%
Endometrial	34%–54%	21%–57%	16%–49%	13%–26%	3.1%
Ovarian	4%–20%	8%–38%	≤1%–13%	3%	1.3%
Renal pelvis and/ or ureter	0.2%–5%	2.2%–28%	0.7%–5.5%	≤1%–3.7%	—[d]
Bladder	2%–7%	4.4%–12.8%	1.0%–8.2%	≤1%–2.4%	2.4%
Gastric	5%–7%	0.2%–9.0%	≤1%–7.9%	Inadequate data	0.9%
Small Bowel	0.4%–11%	1.1%–10%	≤1%–4%	0.1%–0.3%	0.3%
Pancreas	6.20%	0.5%–1.6%	1.4%–1.6%	≤1%–1.6%	1.6%
Biliary tract	1.9%–3.7%	0.02%–1.7%	0.2%–≤1%	0.2%–≤1%	0.2%
Prostate	4.4%–11.6%	3.9%–15.9%	2.5%–11.6%	4.6%–11.6%	11.6%
Breast (female)	10.6%–18.6%	1.5%–12.8%	11.1%–12.8%	8.1%–12.8%	12.8%
Brain	0.7%–1.7%	2.5%–7.7%	0.8%–1.8%	0.6%–≤1%	0.6%

*Data from NCCN guidelines. Genetic/Familial high-risk Assessment: Colorectal v.1 2020

TABLE 7.2: Estimated Average Age at Presentation

Site	MLH 1 Estimated Average Age of Presentation	MSH 2 Estimated Average Age of Presentation	MSH 6 Estimated Average Age of Presentation	PMS 2 Estimated Average Age of Presentation
Colorectal	44 years	44 years	42–69 years	61–66 years
Endometrial	49 years	47–48 years	53–55 years	49–50 years
Ovarian	46 years	43 years	46 years	51–59 years
Renal pelvis and/or ureter	59–60 years	54–61 years	65–69 years	No data
Bladder	59 years	59 years	71 years	71 years
Gastric	52 years	52 years	2 cases reported at age 45 and 81	Inadequate data
Small Bowel	47 years	48 years	54 years	Single case-59 years
Pancreas	No data	No data	No data	No data
Biliary tract	50 years	57 years	No data	No data
Prostate	63 years	59-63 years	63 years	No data
Breast (female)	No data	No data	No data	No data
Brain	No data	No data	43-54 years	40 years

˙Data from NCCN guidelines. Genetic/Familial high-risk Assessment: Colorectal v.1 2020

prostate and breast cancer do not seem to be increased, with reported ranges for the former of 4.4% to 11.6%, which is similar to 11.6% in the general population, and for breast cancer of 10.6% to 18.6% versus 12.8% in the general population.[4] Nevertheless, a study showed that the risk of breast cancer before age 50 in patients with *MLH1* was 6.5% compared to the overall population risk of 2%.[41] This younger age at first diagnosis of breast cancer (as compared to the general population) was corroborated by another study, which showed a mean age of 52.[40]

In terms of gender-based differences, men with *MLH1* have a higher risk of colorectal, gastric, small bowel, biliary, gallbladder, and pancreatic cancer compared to women.[42]

MSH2 and EPCAM *MSH2* and *EPCAM* (through the inactivation of *MSH2* by methylation of its promoter region) have the highest cumulative urinary tract cancer risk through age 80, with bladder cancer risk ranging from 4.4% to 12.8% and renal pelvis and/or ureter between 2.2% and 28%.[4,40] There are gender-based differences in upper urinary tract (renal pelvis and/or ureter) cancers in *MSH2* and *EPCAM* carriers, with 28% risk for men and 12% for women.[43]

With regard to gynecologic cancers, the risk of ovarian cancer is the highest of all MMR genes at 8% to 38% (average age 43); the risk of endometrial cancer is 21% to 57% (average age 47 to 48). *MSH2* also has the second highest cumulative colorectal cancer risk, ranging from 33% to 52% (average age 44). In terms of other gastrointestinal cancers, the risk of gastric cancer is second to *MLH1* at 0.2% to 9% (average age 52). Small bowel is 1.1% to 10% (average age 48), pancreatic is 0.5% to 1.6% (unclear average age), and biliary tract is 0.02% to 1.7% (average age 57). The risk for brain cancer has been estimated at 2.5% to 7.7%. Breast cancer risk ranged from 1.5% to 12.8%, similar to the risk of the general female population.[4] One study that looked at extracolonic cancers in *MLH1, MSH2,* and *MSH6* found that *MSH2* carried the highest risk of prostate cancer, with an SIR of 2.5.[40] Nevertheless, it is far from clear there is an actual association of *MSH2* mutations and prostate cancer, and the reported range in cancer risk is 3.9% to 15.9%.[4]

MSH6 *MSH6* has a 10% to 44% cumulative colorectal cancer risk through age 80, 16% to 49% risk for endometrial cancer, and 1% to 13% for ovarian cancer. Regarding average age of presentation, estimates vary widely for colorectal cancer (42 to 69). For endometrial cancer, it is 53 to 55, and for ovarian cancer, it is 46. For extracolonic gastrointestinal cancers, small bowel is 1% to 4% (average age 54), gastric cancer is 1% to 7.9%, pancreatic is 1.4% to 1.6%, and biliary tract is 0.2% to 1%. There are no data on the average age of presentation in the latter three. For urinary tract cancers, bladder cancer risk ranges from 1% to 8.2% and renal pelvis and/or ureter from 0.7% to 5.5% (average ages 71 and 65 to 69, respectively). Brain cancer cumulative risk is 0.8% to 1.8% (average age 43 to 45). Prostate and breast cancer risk estimates fall within the range of sporadic cases.[4] A study of 841 *MSH6* carriers showed that while colorectal cancer for both males and females is lower (18.2% and 20.3%, respectively, by age 75) than for *MLH1* and *MSH2* mutation carriers, the significant risk of endometrial and ovarian cancer (41.1% and 10.8% through age 75, respectively) results in a very disproportionate burden of cancer for *MSH6* female carriers.[42]

PMS2 While *PMS2* mutations are the most common of all Lynch syndrome–causing genes, *PMS2* has the lowest cumulative cancer risk of any MMR gene, with a colorectal cancer risk of 8.7% to 20%, endometrial cancer risk of 13% to 26%, and ovarian cancer risk of 3%. Average ages at presentation are also later, with estimates of 61 to 66 for colorectal, 49 to 50 for endometrial, and 51 to 59 for ovarian cancer. It is unclear if there is any increased risk for extracolonic gastrointestinal cancers, as well as the other cancers such as bladder, renal pelvis/ureter, and brain. One study of 407 individuals with *PMS2* found that neither men nor women developed colorectal, endometrial, ovarian, or urinary tract cancers prior to age 50. After age 50, the risk of these cancers increased, but the finding was not statistically significant.[42] Prostate and breast cancer risks at 4.6% to 11.6%, and 9.1% to 12.8%, respectively, coincide with general population levels.[4]

▒ POTENTIAL PENETRANCE-MODIFYING GENETIC DEFECTS

Some studies have shown the association of some genetic variants with an altered risk of developing Lynch syndrome–associated cancers. One example of this is a variant in the telomerase gene, *hTERT* rs2075786, which shortens telomeres and has caused Lynch syndrome–associated cancers to present prior to age 45 (RR 2.90; 95% CI 1.02 to 8.26).[44] Two other variants that have been identified include rs16892766 (8q23.3) and rs3802842 (11q23.1). rs16892766 maps to the gene *EIF3H*, a translation factor that can lead to altered cell growth if dysregulated. The role of rs3802842 is unknown, but it is located near a binding site for a microRNA.[45] One study showed that for rs16892766, being homozygous for the C allele (CC) was associated with a 2.16× increased risk of colorectal cancer. For rs3802842, this effect was only seen in female patients: homozygous CC had a hazard ratio (HR) of 3.08, compared to an HR of 1.49 in patients who were heterozygous (AC).[46] A follow-up study found a similar association for rs16892766 (8q23.3) and rs3802842 (11q23.1), but only in patients that were *MLH1* carriers. For rs16892766, patients who were heterozygous (AC) developed colorectal cancer 12 years earlier than those who were homozygous wild type AA ($p = 0.002$). For rs3802842, patients presented with colorectal cancer 10 years earlier if they were homozygous for CC rather than AA; they also had an increased risk with HR 2.67 (95% CI 1.35 to 5.26 and $p = 0.005$). Their study also found that women with *MLH1* who were homozygous for the C allele in rs3802842 had the highest risk of developing colorectal cancer (HR 3.19; 95% CI 1.46 to 7.01 and $p = 0.004$).[45]

Clearly there is a need for more information on the potential effects of genetic variants on cancer risk in Lynch syndrome before this information can be used in defining more personalized approaches to cancer surveillance.

Microsatellite Stable Hereditary Nonpolyposis Colorectal Cancer or Familial Colorectal Cancer Type X

As mentioned earlier, MSS HNPCC is characterized by microsatellite stability, and patients do not have germline MMR gene mutations. Some germline mutations responsible for MSS HNPCC are still being discovered and have been identified through candidate gene analysis, genetic linkage analysis, and genome-wide sequencing. The genes found so far can be placed into four categories: protein glycosylation (*GALNT12*), ribosome biosynthesis (*RPS20* and *BRF1*), DNA repair (*FAN1; WRN* and *ERCC6; POT1, POLE2,* and *MRE11; FAF1;* and *OGG1, MUTYH,* and *NUDT1*), and other (*SEMA4A* and *BMPR1A*). Each of these genes is seen in some families with MSS HNPCC, though so far no "major" susceptibility genes, such as those seen in Lynch syndrome, have been described.[10]

GALNT12 is a gene responsible for protein glycosylation; specifically, it codes for the N-acetylgalactosaminyltransferase enzyme that performs O-linked glycosylation of mucin-type glycans. Glycosylation errors are seen in the majority of colorectal cancers, and germline missense mutations in *GALNT12* have been seen in 2% to 3% of patients with colorectal cancer.[47,48] However, in a study that looked at 103 families that met Amsterdam criteria, none of them had a *GALNT12* mutation.[49] Based on these data, *GALNT12* is felt to be a moderate (rather than high) penetrance susceptibility gene for MSS HNPCC.[10]

RPS20 plays a role in ribosome biosynthesis, as it codes part of the 40S ribosomal subunit. Errors in ribosome biosynthesis are implicated in cancer through p53 activation.[50] Germline missense and truncating mutations in *RPS20* in colorectal cancer have been found in Finnish families, families registered in the UK National Study of Colorectal Cancer Genetics, and a family in Utah. *RPS20* is felt to be a high-penetrance susceptibility gene for MSS HNPCC.[51] Another gene involved in ribosome biosynthesis is *BRF1*. *BRF1* encodes a protein that is part of transcription factor TFIIB, which is part of a complex that initiates transcription by RNA polymerase III. RNA polymerase III then creates RNA for the 5S subunit, a key molecule of the 60S ribosomal subunit.[52] A validation series of 503 families with colorectal cancer found that 10 of them had germline mutations that affected either the expression or function of *BRF1*.[53] *BRF1* is also classified as a high-penetrance susceptibility gene for MSS HNPCC.

FAN1 encodes FANCD2/FANCI-associated nuclease 1, which is responsible for interstrand cross-link repair. A germline nonsense mutation in *FAN1* was found to account for 3% of families with MSS HNPCC in a study conducted in Spain.[54] However, the role of *FAN1* in MSS HNPCC requires further investigation, as a study from the UK National Study of Colorectal Cancer Genetics found no increase in pathogenic *FAN1* variants when comparing cases to controls.[55] Two other genes implicated in DNA repair are *WRN*, a gene involved in double-strand break (DSB) repair, and *ERCC6*, a gene that performs nucleotide excision repair. Heterozygous variants of both *WRN* and *ERCC6* were seen in patients with familial colorectal cancer.[56] Another relevant gene is *FAF1*, which is a tumor suppressor. Missense mutations in *FAF1* have been shown to increase cellular proliferation and make cells resistant to programmed cell death. These identified missense mutations were found to make up 0.4% (2 out of 513) of families with colorectal cancer in an exome sequencing study;[57] therefore, additional data are needed to fully understand the role of *FAF1* in MSS HNPCC.

Three rare but highly penetrant alleles were found through exon sequencing of early onset familial colorectal cancer cases compared to healthy controls. These alleles were *POT1*, which is involved in telomere maintenance; *POLE2*, which is part of the DNA polymerase ε complex; and *MRE11*, which plays a role in DSB repair, homologous recombination, and telomere maintenance. Truncating germline mutations in these three genes were present in case patients more often than in controls.[58]

OGG1, *MUTYH*, and *NUDT1* are involved in base excision repair, which is the main pathway for repairing oxidative DNA damage. *OGG1* repairs 8-oxoguanine DNA glycosylase, which is an enzyme that removes bases that have been mutated by reactive oxygen species (ROS). *MUTYH* uses its adenine glycosylase activity to repair transversion mutations; a transversion is when a purine is substituted for a pyrimidine or vice versa. *NUDT1* hydrolyzes oxidized purines, preventing them from being integrated into DNA. A deficiency in any of these genes leaves transversion mutations unchecked, which leads to carcinogenesis. One study investigated which variants of these genes play a role in MSS HNPCC. They found that *MUTYH*-G382D and *OGG1*-R46Q were associated with increased colorectal cancer risk in these families. They also showed that variant *NUDT1*-D142D had increased risk of colorectal cancer in patients with MSS HNPCC compared to healthy controls (OR = 2.23; 95% CI 1.35 to 3.66 and $p = 0.003$). Patients who were homozygous for this variant presented with colorectal cancer on average 9 years earlier than those who were heterozygous ($p = 0.036$).[59]

SEMA4A is the gene for semaphorine 4A, a membrane protein that plays a role in cell proliferation. Germline missense mutations in *SEMA4A* were found in families with colorectal cancer in Austria, Germany, and the United States.[60] Furthermore, a single nucleotide polymorphism (SNP) of *SEMA4A*: p.Pro682 Ser, was associated with 6% of MSS HNPCC cases vs. 1% of controls ($p = 0.0008$). However, a subsequent study did not find a statistically significant increase in this *SEMA4A* variant in MSS HNPCC families (16%) compared to controls (14%).[61] Therefore, additional studies are needed to further elucidate the role of *SEMA4A* in MSS HNPCC.

The *BMPR1A* gene encodes a type I bone morphogenetic protein receptor, which is part of a serine/threonine kinase family. Both in-frame and truncating splicing mutations were found in genome-wide studies conducted on 18 families from Finland.[62] However, a study was also conducted on 22 families from Newfoundland who had MSS HNPCC and did not detect any *BMPR1A* germline mutations.[63] More studies will be necessary in order to better understand the relationship between *BMPR1A* and MSS HNPCC.

The *TGFBR1* gene plays a role in colorectal cancer through its miRNA binding site. miRNAs bind to a specific target mRNA transcript and are responsible for translational repression and mRNA degradation. *TGFBR1* has a site for let-7 miRNA; when bound tightly, less *TGFBR1* is expressed, which increases the risk of colorectal cancer. SNP rs67687202, which is in linkage disequilibrium with rs868 (a SNP found in the let-7 miRNA binding site of *TGFBR1*), was found to have a significant association with MSS HNPCC in both a discovery set of 27 MSS HNPCC cases and 85 controls ($p = 0.002$), as well as in a replication set of 87 MSS HNPCC cases and 338 controls ($p = 0.041$).[64]

Lynch-Like Syndrome

Lynch-like syndrome comprises tumors that are MSI but do not have germline MMR mutations or *MLH1* promoter hypermethylation. Instead, many patients with Lynch-like syndrome have biallelic somatic mutations. One study sought to characterize which genes were implicated in Lynch-like syndrome and found that the DNA repair genes *WRN, MCPH1, BARD1,* and *REV3L* may play a role. These variants are uncommon in the general population, with an allele frequency of less than 5×10^{-4}, suggesting that these genes are likely involved in pathogenesis.[23] Another study showed that for patients with Lynch-like syndrome, the risk of colorectal cancer by age 70 was 21% (95% CI 9.9 to 41.3) to 40.9% (95% CI 28.3 to 56.4%) for patients with Lynch syndrome.[65] Another study used standardized incidence ratios (SIR) to make this comparison. The SIR is a tool used to determine if the rate of a particular cancer is higher or lower than expected in a given population; an SIR of 1 represents that the incidence of observed cases matches the expected cases. In this case, they found an SIR of 2.12 for colorectal cancer in Lynch-like syndrome versus 6.04 for Lynch syndrome.[24]

It is unclear whether Lynch-like syndrome carries any risk of extracolonic cancers. One study showed that the risk of any cancer by age 70 for Lynch-like syndrome was 27.3% (95% CI 14.5% to 47.8%), compared to 63.7% (95% CI 48.5% to 78.8%) for Lynch syndrome. They also found that compared to the general population, patients with Lynch-like syndrome were shown to have a higher risk of colorectal, gastric, urothelial, and endometrial cancer.[65] However, another study found that there was no statistically significant difference for non-colorectal Lynch syndrome–related cancers for patients with Lynch syndrome compared to those with Lynch-like syndrome.[24]

Constitutional Mismatch Repair Deficiency (CMMRD) Syndrome

This syndrome is due to homozygous pathogenic variants in the MMR genes. In this case, and unlike Lynch syndrome, CMMRD can also be due to biallelic germline variants in the *MSH3*[66] and *MLH3*[67] genes. As opposed to Lynch syndrome, the colon phenotype of these patients ranges from a few polyps to a typical FAP-like phenotype. There is a very limited number of these patients described, and the most commonly involved genes are *PMS2* and *MSH6*, which reflects the higher prevalence of these genetic defects among the MMR genes.[68] Besides the described polyps, the syndrome is characterized by childhood cancers, particularly hematological, as well as brain tumors and colorectal cancers. Patients also commonly present with signs of neurofibromatosis type 1 such as cafe-au-lait spots.[69] As both alleles are mutated at the germline level, the corresponding protein is absent in both tumor and normal tissue. This is in contrast with Lynch syndrome, where expression is retained in normal tissue but lost in tumor tissue, as this is the result of somatic inactivation of the second allele. A consensus panel of the U.S. Multisociety Task Force on Colorectal Cancer put forward a set of suspicion criteria for CMMRD, as well as a suggested surveillance protocol.[70]

▓ CLINICAL MANAGEMENT OF PATIENTS AT INCREASED RISK

Surveillance

Lynch Syndrome: Gene-Specific Approaches The majority of surveillance recommendations for cancer prevention in Lynch syndrome do qualify as category 2A according to the NCCN. Thus, they are based on generally low levels of evidence but uniform consensus on the appropriateness of the particular interventions. On the other hand, as we learn more about the different cancer risks and age of onset of the different cancers by specific gene, there are more widespread attempts to tailor recommendations according to these differences.

The main surveillance strategy for colorectal cancer is high-quality colonoscopy starting at age 20 to 25 for *MLH1* and *MSH2* carriers or 30 to 35 for *MSH6* and *PMS2* carriers. Then repeat screening every 1 to 2 years. In families with *MLH1* and *MSH2* mutations, if an affected family member developed colorectal cancer prior to age 25, screening can be started 2 to 5 years prior to the earliest age of onset. For *MSH6* and *PMS2* families, the cutoff age is before age 30. Patients who could more strongly be advised to have annual (as opposed to biannual) colonoscopy include those with a personal history of adenoma or colorectal cancer, patients with *MLH1* and *MSH2* mutations, those greater than 40 years old, and men.[4]

In addition, the findings on colonoscopy inform management. Patients without pathologic findings or with endoscopically resectable adenomas can continue with the aforementioned 1- to 2-year interval. Patients with colonic adenocarcinomas or adenomas that cannot be endoscopically resected should undergo either segmental or extended colectomy; in those with segmental colectomy, the remaining colonic mucosa is subject to colonoscopy every 1 to 2 years.[4] For patients with *MLH1* and *MSH2* mutations, the cumulative lifetime risk of metachronous colorectal cancer for patients who undergo segmental colectomy is up to 43%. Given these data, patients with *MLH1* or *MSH2* who require surgical resection for colorectal cancer should strongly consider extended colectomy.[4] The risk may be lower for *MSH6* and thus a more conservative approach may be appropriate. There are limited data on *PMS2,* but no marked increase in risk for metachronous colorectal cancers has been seen in the available literature. Therefore, for *PMS2,* consider segmental colectomy.

Prophylactic colectomy is usually not offered as long as the patient understands the need for endoscopic surveillance at a 1- to 2-year interval.[1]

Patients with rectal adenocarcinomas will need proctectomy or total proctocolectomy. The ultimate procedure will depend on the pathogenic variant, location of the adenocarcinoma relative to the anal sphincter, and anticipated need for pelvic radiation.[4]

The protective effect of colonoscopy against colorectal cancer was shown in a prospective Finnish study published in 2000, which looked at families with known Lynch syndrome. The participants were divided into an experimental group, which received a colonoscopy every 3 years, and a control group, which did not receive any colonoscopies. At the end of the 15-year study, those who were undergoing regular colonoscopy surveillance had a 62% reduction in colorectal cancer incidence and a 65% reduction in colorectal cancer mortality compared with the control group.[71] This suggests that colorectal cancer in Lynch syndrome develops through an adenoma-to-carcinoma sequence, which can be intervened upon through performing colonoscopies at regular intervals.[72] However, there are conflicting data as to what the optimal screening interval is and whether screening patients more frequently improves the incidence of colorectal cancer or allows it to be caught at an earlier stage.

One study found that performing colonoscopies every 3 years carried an associated colorectal cancer risk of 10%; decreasing the frequency interval to 1 to 2 years reduced the risk to 6%. Further, with this decreased interval, 90% of the detected interval cancers were localized and early stage.[73] Another study, however, had contradicting results. This study compared the screening intervals of three different countries: Germany, which screens annually; the

Netherlands, which screens every 1 to 2 years; and Finland, which screens every 2 to 3 years. The goal was to see if decreased screening intervals are associated with lower incidence and earlier stage of colorectal cancer. Patients were included if they had a known germline mutation in *MLH1*, *MSH2*, or *MSH6*, as well as patients both with and without a prior colorectal cancer diagnosis. No significant difference was found in the cumulative incidence of first or metachronous colorectal cancer between the three countries, even when taking gender, MMR mutation, age at first colonoscopy, and presence of adenoma at first colonoscopy into account. Further, no significant association was found between the mean colonoscopy intervals and the risk of colorectal cancer (after adjusting for the aforementioned factors). Of the patients followed, 14% were diagnosed with stage III to IV colorectal cancer; there was no significant difference by country or interval since last colonoscopy.[72] The current understanding is that two factors likely play a role in this lack of improved incidence or stage despite decreased colonoscopy intervals. The first is that the MMR mutation inherent to Lynch syndrome pathology causes malignancies to develop at a much faster rate; annual screening may not be frequent enough to catch the adenoma before it progresses to a carcinoma.[74] The second factor is that Lynch syndrome–related colorectal cancer may arise from normal mucosa as opposed to an adenoma precursor, or may arise from submucosal tissue such that it is difficult to detect on surveillance colonoscopy.[72,75]

Endometrial cancer is the most common extracolonic malignancy associated with Lynch syndrome. There are limited data that endometrial biopsy and/or transvaginal ultrasound helps with early detection. In postmenopausal patients, endometrial cancer is often detected based on symptoms; therefore, educating patients about the importance of prompt reporting of abnormal uterine bleeding is key. Patients with abnormal uterine bleeding would then proceed to endometrial biopsy. However, in Lynch syndrome, many patients may develop endometrial cancers when they are premenopausal. In these cases, it is more difficult to rely on symptoms to make the diagnosis. Given this, clinicians can consider endometrial biopsy starting at age 30 to 35 and repeated every 1 to 2 years. With regard to transvaginal ultrasound, it is neither sensitive nor specific enough to aid with screening postmenopausal women for endometrial cancer. Transvaginal ultrasound is not recommended for premenopausal women, given the physiologic variation of endometrial stripe thickness with the menstrual cycle. Hysterectomy reduces the incidence, although not the mortality, of endometrial cancer; it can be considered depending on a number of factors, including the MMR pathogenic variant and a patient's childbearing preferences.[4]

Another gynecologic malignancy with an increased risk in Lynch syndrome is ovarian cancer. There are limited screening tools for ovarian cancer, as neither transvaginal ultrasound nor serum CA-125 have been shown to be sensitive or specific enough in detecting malignancy. Similar to endometrial cancer, one tool is educating patients on the symptoms of ovarian cancer and encouraging them to report these early to a healthcare provider. These symptoms can include bloating, increased abdominal girth, early satiety, constipation, or urinary frequency. In terms of surgical options, bilateral salpingo-oophorectomy (BSO) can reduce the incidence of ovarian cancer. Similar to hysterectomy, the timing of BSO depends on MMR pathogenic variant, childbearing preferences, and whether the patient is premenopausal or postmenopausal.[4] Approaches for gynecological cancer prevention are explained in detail in Chapters 8 and 9.

In addition to gynecologic malignancies, there are various other extracolonic cancers associated with Lynch syndromes; surveillance guidelines for these cancers are outlined in the subsequent paragraphs.

For gastric, duodenal, and distal small bowel cancer surveillance, the data do not support a particular surveillance strategy. However, for patients with risk factors such as male gender, older age, germline *MLH1* or *MSH2* mutations, FDR with these cancers, immigrants from countries with increased incidence of gastric cancer, chronic autoimmune gastritis, gastric intestinal metaplasia, or gastric adenomas, endoscopic surveillance starting at age 40 and repeated every 3 to 5 years (concurrent with colonoscopy) can be considered. Random biopsies should be taken during endoscopy to assess for *Helicobacter pylori* infection status, autoimmune gastritis, and intestinal metaplasia. If detected, *H. pylori* should be treated.[4]

For pancreatic cancer, annual screening with contrast-enhanced magnetic resonance imaging/magnetic resonance cholangiopancreatography (MRI/MRCP) and/or endoscopic ultrasound (EUS) can be initiated at age 50 or 10 years earlier than the youngest family member with an exocrine pancreatic cancer diagnosis. This recommendation applies mainly to patients with *MLH1* mutations who have more than one first- or second-degree relatives (on the side that is presumed to have the Lynch syndrome pathogenic variant) with an exocrine pancreatic cancer. It is unclear if *MSH2, MSH6,* and *PMS2* mutation carriers do have an increased risk of pancreatic cancer. In any case, patients could also consider undergoing screening, particularly if any pancreatic cancers were diagnosed in the family.[4] Approaches for pancreatic cancer prevention are explained in detail in Chapter 10.

While clear evidence showing beneficial effects of urothelial cancer is still lacking, several strategies have been proposed and are commonly used. If done, it is recommended to begin surveillance at age 30 to 35 or 5 years prior to the youngest age at diagnosis if a family member had urothelial cancer before age 40. Educating patients about symptoms of urothelial cancer, such as hematuria, is also key so that patients know to seek prompt medical evaluation. Surveillance strategies for patients with Lynch syndrome may be tailored based on risk groups, which are categorized as follows:

- Low risk: no personal or family history of urothelial cancer OR no *MSH2* mutation
- Intermediate risk: family history of urothelial cancer OR patient has *MSH2* mutation
- High risk: personal history of urothelial cancer

Low-risk patients could undergo surveillance with an annual urine dipstick, cytology, and even NMP22.[43] NMP22, a nuclear matrix protein, has increased sensitivity for detecting urothelial cancer as compared to cytology (55.7% versus 15.8%).[76] Intermediate-risk patients could receive annual urine dipstick, cytology, and NMP22, plus annual renal tract ultrasound. High-risk patients could undergo the same surveillance as low risk, plus annual computed tomography (CT) scan with contrast and a flexible cystoscopy. Cystoscopy is used to detect bladder cancers that may have developed as a result of spread from prior renal pelvis or ureter cancers.[43]

An annual neurologic examination can be considered starting at age 25 to 30 to look for central nervous system malignancies.

As per the prior discussion regarding gene-specific cancer risk, there is controversy surrounding the potential increased risk of breast cancer in Lynch syndrome. The study that found an increased risk in patients with *MLH1* but not *MSH2* recommended that women with *MLH1* start receiving mammograms earlier than women with other MMR mutations. In the UK, annual mammograms begin at age 47 to 50 for women at average risk. For patients with *MLH1*, the recommendation is adjusted for them to begin screening at age 40. In the United States, the age to initiate screening mammograms is undergoing revision. However, for women with *MLH1*, it has been considered to start at age 30 and screen at intervals shorter than a year. Further, ultrasound and/or MRI could be considered as screening modalities, both due to the density of breast tissue in younger patients and to avoid exposing them to radiation.[41] In any case, as it is unclear if there is truly any potential increased risk of breast cancer in Lynch syndrome, most guidelines do not recommend enhanced screening for this cancer, and patients should undergo routine screening for this malignancy as current guidelines indicate. The same applies to prostate cancer.[2]

Gene-Specific Approaches

As mentioned before, each of the four MMR gene mutations confer different risks to colorectal and extracolonic cancers. These differences in risk can be used to tailor the surveillance strategies and screening intervals to each individual.

MLH1 For colorectal, endometrial, ovarian, urothelial, and brain cancer prevention, the guidelines for patients with *MLH1* mutations are the same as described earlier.

For gastric, duodenal, and distal small bowel cancer, patients with *MLH1* can consider having a surveillance esophagogastroduodenoscopy (EGD) every 3 to 5 years starting at age 40. Random biopsies can be obtained to assess for *H. pylori*, autoimmune gastritis, and intestinal metaplasia; *H. pylori* should be treated if detected.[77,78]

For pancreatic cancer, patients with a family history of exocrine pancreatic cancer in more than one first- or second-degree relative (from the side with the presumed pathogenic variant) can start screening at age 50 or 10 years earlier than the youngest family member with an exocrine pancreatic cancer diagnosis. Screening can be performed with an annual contrast-enhanced MRI/MRCP and/or EUS; the interval can be shortened if a concerning finding is seen.[4]

MSH2 *and* EPCAM For colorectal, endometrial, ovarian, and brain cancer prevention, the guidelines for patients with *MSH2* and *EPCAM* mutations are the same as described earlier.

Patients with *MSH2* and *EPCAM* mutations are the ones with the highest risk among all Lynch syndrome patients for urothelial cancer, which includes bladder, ureter, and renal pelvis. These mutation carriers are considered to be at intermediate risk for these malignancies. Thus, it has been suggested to proceed with annual urine dipstick, cytology, and even NMP22 testing, plus annual renal tract ultrasound starting at age 30 to 35 or 5 years prior to the youngest age at diagnosis if a family member had urothelial cancer before age 40.[4,43]

For gastric, duodenal, and distal small bowel cancer, patients with *MSH2* and *EPCAM* mutations can consider having a surveillance EGD every 3 to 5 years starting at age 40. Random biopsies can be obtained to assess for *H. pylori*, autoimmune gastritis, and intestinal metaplasia; *H. pylori* should be treated if detected.[77,78]

For pancreatic cancer, current data do not suggest an increased risk for *MSH2* and *EPCAM* mutation carriers. Nevertheless, the NCCN guidelines suggest pancreatic cancer screening could be done in individuals with a family history of exocrine pancreatic cancer in more than one first- or second-degree relative (from the side with the presumed pathogenic variant). Screening would be considered starting at age 50 or 10 years earlier than the youngest family member with an exocrine pancreatic cancer diagnosis. As with *MLH1* mutation carriers, screening could be performed with an annual contrast-enhanced MRI/MRCP and/or EUS.[4]

MSH6 For endometrial, ovarian, urothelial, gastric, small bowel, and brain cancer prevention, the guidelines for patients with *MSH6* mutations are the same as described earlier.

For colorectal cancer, screening with colonoscopy is recommended every 1 to 2 years starting at age 30 to 35 or 2 to 5 years prior to the youngest age at diagnosis if a family member had colorectal cancer before age 30.[39]

For pancreatic cancer, current data do not suggest an increased risk in *MSH6* mutation carriers. However, the same approach described earlier could be pursued for individuals with a family history of exocrine pancreatic cancer in more than one first- or second-degree relative (from the side with the presumed pathogenic variant), and screening could be considered starting at age 50 or 10 years earlier than the youngest family member with an exocrine pancreatic cancer diagnosis. Screening could also be performed with an annual contrast-enhanced MRI/MRCP and/or EUS.[4]

PMS2 As discussed earlier, increase in cancer risk in these patients is likely limited to colorectum and endometrium and possibly ovarian cancer. There is no evidence to date of higher risk for the other Lynch syndrome–related cancers such as urothelial, gastric, small bowel, pancreas, biliary tract, and brain. Thus, it would be reasonable to limit cancer surveillance to the cancer with increased risk.

For colorectal cancer, the recommendations for screening colonoscopy are the same as for patients with *MSH6*: every 1 to 2 years starting at age 30 to 35 or 2 to 5 years prior to the youngest age at diagnosis if a family member had colorectal cancer before age 30.[39]

For endometrial cancer and ovarian cancer, patients with *PMS2* mutations would be recommended to undergo the same surveillance and appropriately timed BSO as described earlier.

MSS HNPCC (Familial Colorectal Cancer Type X) Given the likely heterogeneous nature of this group and in the absence of a common genetic defect, surveillance recommendations for MSS HNPCC are difficult to formulate. In any case, provided the increased risk of colorectal cancer and younger age at diagnosis than sporadic cases, it is reasonable to enhance colonoscopy screening to at least every 5 years starting at age 40 or 5 to 10 years before the age at which the youngest family member developed colorectal cancer. As most studies have not supported an increased risk of extracolonic cancers, in general no additional cancer surveillance is warranted, but it may be wise to assess case by case according to unique family history features.[11]

Lynch-Like Syndrome There is currently no consensus on how cancer surveillance should be performed in Lynch-like syndrome patients. As this is also likely a heterogeneous group, it seems reasonable at this time to take into account personal and family history in order to design a personalized surveillance approach.

Low Susceptibility Genes: CHEK2, APC I1357K, and Heterozygous MUTYH While there are no strong data that can support specific recommendations, in general it is advised for individuals with pathogenic variants in these three genes to start colorectal cancer screening through colonoscopy at age 40 or 10 years earlier than the age of diagnosis of an FDR with colorectal cancer (if indeed there is such a history) and then repeat no later than every 5 years. The only exception is the heterozygous *MUTYH* carrier with no personal and no family history of colorectal cancer, as data in this case are unclear.[4]

Chemoprevention

Aspirin, ibuprofen, and resistant starch have been studied as forms of chemoprevention in patients with Lynch syndrome. With aspirin, a double-blind randomized control trial showed that patients with an MMR mutation who were taking 600 mg aspirin daily for up to 4 years had a 44% reduced incidence of colorectal cancers at 56 months follow-up. There was a 63% reduction in patients who took aspirin for at least 2 years.[79] In secondary analyses, aspirin also appeared to decrease the risk of extracolonic Lynch syndrome–associated cancers.[1] A randomized double-blind trial (NCT02497820) is currently being conducted to examine the effects of 100, 300, and 600 mg daily of aspirin. If results with the lower doses were comparable, this would make widespread use of aspirin as a chemopreventive agent in Lynch syndrome patients much more acceptable. Meanwhile, based on the cancer protective data with 600 mg daily, some guidelines suggest considering aspirin use at that dose for chemopreventive use in Lynch syndrome.[4,80]

An observational study assessed the effects of aspirin and ibuprofen in patients with MMR mutations. When compared to patients who took aspirin for less than a month, those who took aspirin for a month to 4.9 years had an HR of 0.49; patients who took aspirin for over 5 years had an HR of 0.25. In terms of ibuprofen, patients who took it for a month to 4.9 years had an HR of 0.38 as compared to an HR of 0.26 for those who took it for over 5 years. The study authors translated this to a 60% decrease in colorectal cancer risk in patients who took aspirin for at least a month and a 65% decrease in patients who took ibuprofen for at least a month.[81]

Resistant starch was studied in the same double-blind randomized control trial that looked at chemoprevention with aspirin. Resistant starch is defined as starch that is not digested in the small intestine; it travels to the large intestine and is converted to short-chain fatty acids, where it inhibits tumor proliferation and enhances apoptosis in response to DNA damage.[82] This trial did not show a protective effect of eating 30 g daily of resistant starch, which is meant to mimic a high-fiber diet, against colorectal cancer or other Lynch syndrome–associated cancers.

Role of Behavioral and Environmental Factors on Cancer Risk

A systematic review compiled the findings of 16 studies with regard to how "energy balance" factors, which encompass weight, diet, and physical activity, affect colorectal and endometrial cancer development in patients with Lynch syndrome.[83] With regard to the three studies that looked at endometrial cancer, none of them showed statistical significance between risk of endometrial cancer and body mass index (BMI). However, there was a significant association between taking multivitamin and/or folate supplements and a decreased risk of endometrial cancer.

In terms of colorectal cancer and weight, there was a statistical significance between obesity in early adulthood and development of colorectal cancer, specifically in men, in two out of three studies. The third study, which did not show significance with obesity, observed a 30% increase in risk of developing colorectal cancer with each 5-unit increase in BMI in men. This analysis was further subdivided into MMR gene mutations and showed that patients with *MLH1* and *PMS2* mutations showed a 36% increase in colorectal cancer with each 5-unit increase in BMI in both genders. There was no significance in patients with *MSH2* or *MSH6* mutation carriers. One of the studies looking at obesity in early adulthood also showed that weight gain (between the participants' current weight compared to their weight at age 20) of greater than 21 kg was associated with a 72% increase in colorectal cancer; this was only significant in men.

Regarding colorectal cancer and dietary habits, nine studies were reviewed. One showed that consuming meat and snacks increased the risk of colorectal cancer. The former is consistent with what has been observed in the general population. Two studies focused on supplementation: one of these showed that women had a decreased risk of colorectal cancer if they had ever taken calcium or multivitamins. Regarding fruit consumption, two studies found that high fruit intake reduces colorectal cancer risk. Alcohol use, specifically drinking more than 30 g or about two drinks per day, increased colorectal cancer risk.

Finally, two studies looked at exercise and relation to colorectal cancer. Both showed that exercising confers a protective effect against colorectal cancer, with one showing significance in both men and women who exercised for more than 35 metabolic equivalent of task (MET) hours per week.[83]

In summary, a healthy lifestyle and eating habits likely have a very positive impact on Lynch syndrome patients, and thus these should be strongly encouraged among mutation carriers.

References

1. Kastrinos F, Stoffel EM. History, genetics, and strategies for cancer prevention in Lynch syndrome. *Clin Gastroenterol Hepatol*. 2014;12(5):715–727, quiz e41–43.

2. Win AK, Jenkins MA, Dowty JG, et al. Prevalence and penetrance of major genes and polygenes for colorectal cancer. *Cancer Epidemiol Biomarkers Prev*. 2017;26(3):404–412.

3. Valle L, Vilar E, Tavtigian SV, Stoffel EM. Genetic predisposition to colorectal cancer: syndromes, genes, classification of genetic variants and implications for precision medicine. *J Pathol*. 2019;247(5):574–588.

4. National Comprehensive Cancer Network. Genetic/Familial High-Risk Assessment: Colorectal (Version 1.2020). 2020. Referenced with permission from the NCCN Guidelines' of the National Comprehensive Cancer Network, Inc. 2020. All rights reserved. Accessed October 10, 2020. Available online at www.NCCN. org. NCCN makes no warranties of any kind whatsoever regarding their content, use, or application and disclaims any responsibility for their application or use in any way.

5. Aarnio M, Sankila R, Pukkala E, et al. Cancer risk in mutation carriers of DNA-mismatch-repair genes. *Int J Cancer*. 1999;81(2):214–218.

6. Dominguez-Valentin M, Therkildsen C, Da Silva S, Nilbert M. Familial colorectal cancer type X: genetic profiles and phenotypic features. *Mod Pathol*. 2015;28(1):30–36.

7. Win AK, Young JP, Lindor NM, et al. Colorectal and other cancer risks for carriers and noncarriers from families with a DNA mismatch repair gene mutation: a prospective cohort study. *J Clin Oncol*. 2012;30(9):958–964.

8. Vasen HF, Mecklin JP, Khan, PM, Lynch HT. The International Collaborative Group on Hereditary Non-Polyposis Colorectal Cancer (ICG-HNPCC). *Dis Colon Rectum*. 1991;34(5):424–425.

9. Llor X, Pons E, Xicola RM, et al. Differential features of colorectal cancers fulfilling Amsterdam criteria without involvement of the mutator pathway. *Clin Cancer Res*. 2005;11(20):7304–7310.

10. Peltomäki P, Olkinuora A, Nieminen TT. Updates in the field of hereditary nonpolyposis colorectal cancer. *Expert Rev Gastroenterol Hepatol*. 2020;14(8):707–720.

11. Zetner DB, Bisgaard ML. Familial colorectal cancer type X. *Curr Genomics*, 2017;18(4):341–359.

12. Therkildsen C, Rasmussen M, Smith-Hansen L, et al. Broadening risk profile in familial colorectal cancer type X: increased risk for five cancer types in the national Danish cohort. *BMC Cancer*. 2020;20(1):345.

13. Ma X, Zhang B, Zheng W. Genetic variants associated with colorectal cancer risk: comprehensive research synopsis, meta-analysis, and epidemiological evidence. *Gut*. 2014;63(2):326–336.

14. Stoffel EM, Murphy CC. Epidemiology and mechanisms of the increasing incidence of colon and rectal cancers in young adults. *Gastroenterology*. 2020;158(2):341–353.

15. Liu C, Wang QS, Wang YJ. The CHEK2 I157T variant and colorectal cancer susceptibility: a systematic review and meta-analysis. *Asian Pac J Cancer Prev*. 2012;13(5):2051–2055.

16. Katona BW, Yurgelun MB, Garber J, et al. A counseling framework for moderate-penetrance colorectal cancer susceptibility genes. *Genet Med*. 2018;20(11):1324–1327.

17. Laken SJ, Petersen GM, Gruber SB, et al. Familial colorectal cancer in Ashkenazim due to a hypermutable tract in APC. *Nat Genet*. 1997;14:79–83.

18. Rennert G, Almog R, Tomsho LP, et al. Colorectal polyps in carriers of the APC I1307K polymorphism. *Dis Colon Rectum*. 2005;48(12):2317–2321.

19. Huyghe JR, Bien SA, Harrison TA, et al. Discovery of common and rare genetic risk variants for colorectal cancer. *Nat Genet*. 2019;51(1):76–87.

20. Valle L. Genetic predisposition to colorectal cancer: where we stand and future perspectives. *World J Gastroenterol*. 2014;20(29):9828–9849.

21. Short E, Thomas LE, Hurley J, et al. Inherited predisposition to colorectal cancer: towards a more complete picture. *J Med Genet*. 2015;52(12):791–796.

22. Dunlop MG, Tenesa A, Farrington SM, et al. Cumulative impact of common genetic variants and other risk factors on colorectal cancer risk in 42,103 individuals. *Gut*. 2013;62(6):871–881.

23. Xicola RM, Clark JR, Carroll T, et al. Implication of DNA repair genes in Lynch-like syndrome. *Fam Cancer*. 2019;18(3):331–342.

24. Rodriguez-Soler M, Pérez-Carbonell L, Guarinos C, et al. Risk of cancer in cases of suspected lynch syndrome without germline mutation. *Gastroenterology*. 2013;144(5):926–932 e1; quiz e13–14.

25. Carethers JM. Differentiating Lynch-like from Lynch syndrome. *Gastroenterology*. 2014;146(3):602–604.

26. Wolf AMD, Fontham ETH, Church TR, et al. Colorectal cancer screening for average-risk adults: 2018 guideline update from the American Cancer Society. *CA Cancer J Clin*. 2018;68(4):250–281.

27. Archambault AN, Su Y-R, Jeon J, et al. Cumulative burden of colorectal cancer-associated genetic variants is more strongly associated with early-onset vs late-onset cancer. *Gastroenterology*. 2020;158(5):1274–1286.e12.

28. Hampel H, Frankel WL, Martin E, et al. Screening for the Lynch syndrome (hereditary nonpolyposis colorectal cancer). *N Engl J Med*. 2005;352(18):1851–1860.

29. Umar A, Boland CR, Terdiman P, et al. Revised Bethesda Guidelines for hereditary nonpolyposis colorectal cancer (Lynch syndrome) and microsatellite instability. *J Natl Cancer Inst*. 2004;96(4):261–268.

30. Barnetson RA, Tenesa A, Farrington SM, et al. Identification and survival of carriers of mutations in DNA mismatch-repair genes in colon cancer. *N Engl J Med*. 2006;354(26):2751–2763.

31. Chen S, Wang W, Lee S, et al. Prediction of germline mutations and cancer risk in the Lynch syndrome. *JAMA*. 2006;296(12):1479–1487.

32. Kastrinos F, Uno H, Ukagebu C, et al. Development and validation of the PREMM5 model for comprehensive risk assessment of Lynch syndrome. *J Clin Oncol*. 2017;35(19):2165–2172.

33. Xicola RM, Llor X, Pons E, et al. Performance of different microsatellite marker panels for detection of mismatch repair-deficient colorectal tumors. *J Natl Cancer Inst*. 2007;99(3):244–252.

34. Ryan NAJ, Glaire MA, Blake D, et al. The proportion of endometrial cancers associated with Lynch syndrome: a systematic review of the literature and meta-analysis. *Genet Med*. 2019;21(10):2167–2180.

35. Kawaguchi M, Yanokura M, Banno K, et al. Analysis of a correlation between the BRAF V600E mutation and abnormal DNA mismatch repair in patients with sporadic endometrial cancer. *Int J Oncol*. 2009;34(6):1541–1547.

36. Latham A, Srinivasan P, Kemel Y, et al. microsatellite instability is associated with the presence of Lynch syndrome pan-cancer. *J Clin Oncol*. 2019;37(4):286–295.

37. Marcus L, Lemery SJ, Keegan P, Pazdur R. FDA approval summary: pembrolizumab for the treatment of microsatellite instability-high solid tumors. *Clin Cancer Res*. 2019;25(13):3753–3758.

38. Roberts ME, Riegert-Johnson DL, Thomas BC, et al. A clinical scoring system to identify patients with sebaceous neoplasms at risk for the Muir-Torre variant of Lynch syndrome. *Genet Med.* 2014;16(9):711–716.

39. Suerink M, Rodríguez-Girondo M, van der Klift HM, et al. An alternative approach to establishing unbiased colorectal cancer risk estimation in Lynch syndrome. *Genet Med.* 2019;21(12):2706–2712.

40. Engel C, Loeffler M, Steinke V, et al. Risks of less common cancers in proven mutation carriers with lynch syndrome. *J Clin Oncol.* 2012;30(35):4409–4415.

41. Harkness EF, Barrow E, Newton K, et al. Lynch syndrome caused by MLH1 mutations is associated with an increased risk of breast cancer: a cohort study. *J Med Genet.* 2015;52(8):553–556.

42. Dominguez-Valentin M, Sampson JR, Seppälä TT, et al. Cancer risks by gene, age, and gender in 6350 carriers of pathogenic mismatch repair variants: findings from the Prospective Lynch Syndrome Database. *Genet Med.* 2019;22(1):15–25.

43. Acher P, Kiela G, Thomas K, O'Brien T. Towards a rational strategy for the surveillance of patients with Lynch syndrome (hereditary non-polyposis colon cancer) for upper tract transitional cell carcinoma. *BJU Int.* 2010;106(3):300–302.

44. Bellido F, Guinó E, Jagmohan-Changur S, et al. Genetic variant in the telomerase gene modifies cancer risk in Lynch syndrome. *Eur J Hum Genet.* 2013;21(5):511–516.

45. Talseth-Palmer BA, Brenne IS, Ashton KA, et al. Colorectal cancer susceptibility loci on chromosome 8q23.3 and 11q23.1 as modifiers for disease expression in Lynch syndrome. *J Med Genet.* 2011;48(4):279–284.

46. Wijnen JT, Brohet RM, van Eijk R, et al. Chromosome 8q23.3 and 11q23.1 variants modify colorectal cancer risk in Lynch syndrome. *Gastroenterology.* 2009;136(1):131–137.

47. Clarke E, Green RC, Green JS, et al. Inherited deleterious variants in GALNT12 are associated with CRC susceptibility. *Hum Mutat.* 2012;33(7):1056–1058.

48. Evans DR, Venkitachalam S, Revoredo L, et al. Evidence for GALNT12 as a moderate penetrance gene for colorectal cancer. *Hum Mutat.* 2018;39(8):1092–1101.

49. Segui N, Pineda M, Navarro M, et al. GALNT12 is not a major contributor of familial colorectal cancer type X. *Hum Mutat.* 2014;35(1):50–52.

50. Ajore R, Raiser D, McConkey M, et al. Deletion of ribosomal protein genes is a common vulnerability in human cancer, especially in concert with TP53 mutations. *EMBO Mol Med.* 2017;9(4):498–507.

51. Nieminen TT, O'Donohue MF, Wu Y, et al. Germline mutation of RPS20, encoding a ribosomal protein, causes predisposition to hereditary nonpolyposis colorectal carcinoma without DNA mismatch repair deficiency. *Gastroenterology.* 2014;147(3):595–598.e5.

52. Wang W, Nag S, Zhang X, et al. Ribosomal proteins and human diseases: pathogenesis, molecular mechanisms, and therapeutic implications. *Med Res Rev.* 2015;35(2):225–285.

53. Bellido F, Sowada N, Mur P, et al. Association between germline mutations in BRF1, a subunit of the RNA polymerase III transcription complex, and hereditary colorectal cancer. *Gastroenterology.* 2018;154(1):181–194.e20.

54. Segui N, Mina LB, Lazaro C, et al. Germline mutations in FAN1 cause hereditary colorectal cancer by impairing DNA repair. *Gastroenterology.* 2015;149(3):563–566.

55. Broderick P, Dobbins SE, Chubb D, et al. Validation of recently proposed colorectal cancer susceptibility gene variants in an analysis of families and patients – a systematic review. *Gastroenterology.* 2017;152(1):75–77.e4.

56. Arora S, Yan H, Cho I, et al. Genetic variants that predispose to DNA double-strand breaks in lymphocytes from a subset of patients with familial colorectal carcinomas. *Gastroenterology.* 2015;149(7):1872–1883.e9.

57. Bonjoch L, Franch-Expósito S, Garre P, et al. Germline mutations in FAF1 are associated with hereditary colorectal cancer. *Gastroenterology.* 2020;159(1):227–240.e7.

58. Chubb D, Broderick P, Dobbina SE, et al. Rare disruptive mutations and their contribution to the heritable risk of colorectal cancer. *Nat Commun.* 2016;7:11883.

59. Garre P, Briceño V, Xicola RM, et al. Analysis of the oxidative damage repair genes NUDT1, OGG1, and MUTYH in patients from mismatch repair proficient HNPCC families (MSS-HNPCC). *Clin Cancer Res.* 2011;17(7):1701–1712.

60. Schulz E, Klampfl P, Holzapfel S, et al. Germline variants in the SEMA4A gene predispose to familial colorectal cancer type X. *Nat Commun.* 2014;5:5191.

61. Kinnersley B, Chubb D, Dobbins SE, et al. Correspondence: SEMA4A variation and risk of colorectal cancer. *Nat Commun.* 2016;7:10611.

62. Nieminen TT, Abdel-Rahman WM, Ristimäki A, et al. BMPR1A mutations in hereditary nonpolyposis colorectal cancer without mismatch repair deficiency. *Gastroenterology*. 2011;141(1):e23–e26.

63. Evans DR, Green JS, Woods MO. Screening of BMPR1a for pathogenic mutations in familial colorectal cancer type X families from Newfoundland. *Fam Cancer*. 2018;17(2):205–208.

64. Xicola RM, Bontu N, Doyle BJ, et al. Association of a let-7 miRNA binding region of TGFBR1 with hereditary mismatch repair proficient colorectal cancer (MSS HNPCC). *Carcinogenesis*. 2016;37(8):751–758.

65. Bucksch K, Zachariae S, Aretz S, et al. Cancer risks in Lynch syndrome, Lynch-like syndrome, and familial colorectal cancer type X: a prospective cohort study. *BMC Cancer*. 2020;20(1):460.

66. Adam R, Spier I, Zhao B, et al. Exome sequencing identifies biallelic MSH3 germline mutations as a recessive subtype of colorectal adenomatous polyposis. *Am J Hum Genet*. 2016;99(2):337–351.

67. Olkinuora A, Nieminen TT, Mårtensson E, et al. Biallelic germline nonsense variant of MLH3 underlies polyposis predisposition. *Genet Med*. 2019;21(8):1868–1873.

68. Bodo S, Colas C, Buhard O, et al. Diagnosis of constitutional mismatch repair-deficiency syndrome based on microsatellite instability and lymphocyte tolerance to methylating agents. *Gastroenterology*. 2015;149(4):1017–1029.e3.

69. Bakry D, Aronson M, Durno C, et al. Genetic and clinical determinants of constitutional mismatch repair deficiency syndrome: report from the constitutional mismatch repair deficiency consortium. *Eur J Cancer*. 2014;50(5):987–996.

70. Durno C, Boland CR, Cohen S, et al. Recommendations on surveillance and management of biallelic mismatch repair deficiency (BMMRD) syndrome: a consensus statement by the US Multi-Society Task Force on Colorectal Cancer. *Am J Gastroenterol*. 2017;112(5):682–690.

71. Jarvinen HJ, Aarnio M, Mustonen H, et al. Controlled 15-year trial on screening for colorectal cancer in families with hereditary nonpolyposis colorectal cancer. *Gastroenterology*. 2000;118(5):829–834.

72. Engel C, Vasen HF, Seppälä T, et al. No difference in colorectal cancer incidence or stage at detection by colonoscopy among 3 countries with different Lynch syndrome surveillance policies. *Gastroenterology*. 2018;155(5):1400–1409.e2.

73. Vasen HF, Abdirahman M, Brohet R, et al. One to 2-year surveillance intervals reduce risk of colorectal cancer in families with Lynch syndrome. *Gastroenterology*. 2010;138(7):2300–2306.

74. Sekine S, Mori T, Ogawa R, et al. Mismatch repair deficiency commonly precedes adenoma formation in Lynch syndrome-associated colorectal tumorigenesis. *Mod Pathol*. 2017;30(8):1144–1151.

75. Ahadova A, von Knebel Doeberitz M, Bläker H, Kloor M. CTNNB1-mutant colorectal carcinomas with immediate invasive growth: a model of interval cancers in Lynch syndrome. *Fam Cancer*. 2016;15(4):579–586.

76. Grossman HB, Messing E, Soloway M, et al. Detection of bladder cancer using a point-of-care proteomic assay. *JAMA*. 2005;293(7):810–816.

77. Vasen HF, Blanco I, Aktan-Collan K, et al. Revised guidelines for the clinical management of Lynch syndrome (HNPCC): recommendations by a group of European experts. *Gut*. 2013;62(6):812–823.

78. Kim J, Braun D, Ukaegbu C, et al. Clinical factors associated with gastric cancer in individuals with Lynch syndrome. *Clin Gastroenterol Hepatol*. 2020;18(4):830–837.e1.

79. Burn J, Gerdes AM, Macrae F, et al. Long-term effect of aspirin on cancer risk in carriers of hereditary colorectal cancer: an analysis from the CAPP2 randomised controlled trial. *Lancet*. 2011;378(9809):2081–2087.

80. Rubenstein JH, Enns R, Heidelbaugh J, Barkun A, Clinical Guidelines Committee. American Gastroenterological Association Institute Guideline on the diagnosis and management of Lynch syndrome. *Gastroenterology*. 2015;149(3):777–782; quiz e16–17.

81. Ait Ouakrim D, Dashti SG, Chau R, et al. Aspirin, ibuprofen, and the risk of colorectal cancer in Lynch syndrome. *J Natl Cancer Inst*. 2015;107(9):djv170.

82. Mathers JC, Movahedi M, Macrae F, et al. Long-term effect of resistant starch on cancer risk in carriers of hereditary colorectal cancer: an analysis from the CAPP2 randomised controlled trial. *Lancet Oncol*. 2012;13(12):1242–1249.

83. Coletta AM, Peterson SK, Gatus LA, et al. Energy balance related lifestyle factors and risk of endometrial and colorectal cancer among individuals with Lynch syndrome: a systematic review. *Fam Cancer*. 2019;18(4):399–420.

Risk Assessment and Clinical Management – Uterine Cancer

Burak Zeybek, Whitney Soble, and Elena Ratner

▥ DISEASE SPECIFIC CANCER EPIDEMIOLOGY AND RISK FACTORS

Uterine cancer is the most common gynecologic malignancy in the United States, with an estimated 63,230 new cases and 11,350 deaths from the disease every year.[1] Based on the data from its national cancer database, and Surveillance, Epidemiology and End Results (SEER), the lifetime risk of endometrial cancer is 2.8% and the average age at diagnosis is 62.[2] As opposed to ovarian malignancies, the majority of the cases are diagnosed at an early stage (67% at stage I), as more than 90% of women with uterine cancer have an early presenting symptom (abnormal uterine bleeding).[3] The most common histologic subtype is adenocarcinoma of the endometrium, which is subcategorized into two distinct groups that differ in incidence, response to therapy and prognosis.[4] Type I tumors (80% of endometrial carcinomas), have more favorable outcomes due to grade 1 or 2 endometrioid histology, early stage at diagnosis, retention of hormone receptor status and younger age at onset. On the other hand, type II tumors (20% of endometrial cancers) portend a poorer prognosis, as these represent grade 3 endometrioid tumors and tumors of non-endometrioid histology such as serous, clear cell, mucinous, squamous, transitional cell, mesonephric and undifferentiated. They often lack hormone receptors and there is no clear association with estrogen stimulation.

Hereditary cancer syndromes such as Lynch and Cowden are associated with increased risk of type I malignancies.[4] Lynch accounts for 2 to 5% of all endometrial carcinomas,[5,6] whereas Cowden syndrome is reported to be even rarer.[7]

▥ HEREDITARY CANCER SYNDROMES

Lynch Syndrome

Lynch syndrome (LS) is a highly penetrant autosomal dominant inherited cancer syndrome, which is characterized by germline mutations in DNA mismatch repair genes (MLH1-chromosome 3p.22, MSH2-chromosome 2p21, MSH6-chromosome 2p16.3, PMS2-chromosome 7p22.1) or deletions in the *EPCAM* gene (chromosome 2p21). The mismatch repair system maintains genomic integrity by recognizing base-pair mismatches during DNA replication, which most commonly occur at microsatellites (certain DNA motifs that are typically repeated 5 to 50 times). In the setting of a defective mismatch repair system, the microsatellites become more susceptible to mutations leading to expansion or contraction of these regions. This phenomenon is called microsatellite instability, which is a characteristic feature of tumors related to LS.[8]

The pathogenicity of the disease is described by a two-hit hypothesis, meaning that patients inherit one defective allele, which is followed by inactivation of the second allele via either somatic mutation, loss of heterozygosity or non-inherited methylation of the *MLH1* promoter (epigenetic silencing). Among the four mismatch repair genes, the most common mutation is seen in MSH2 (41%), followed by MLH1 (31%), MSH6 (13%) and PMS2 (9%).[9,10] Pathogenic mutations in PMS2 have a lower penetrance than the mutations in the other three genes. Deletions in *EPCAM* genes lead to silencing of neighboring MSH2 via transcriptional read-through, which is the continuation of transcription beyond a normal stop sign due to failure of RNA polymerase to recognize the signal. The patients with EPCAM deletions demonstrate a mosaic pattern instead of a full spectrum of the disease, as MSH2 is silenced only in the cells where EPCAM is active.[11]

LS is the most common etiology of hereditary endometrial and colon cancers. Based on the available data, the lifetime risk of endometrial cancer is 16 to 61%, and colon cancer is 18 to 61%, which are 2.8% and 4.2%, respectively, in the general population.[12,13] Two to five percent of all endometrial cancers are related to LS.[5,6] The mean age at diagnosis ranges from 46 to 54 years compared with a mean age of 62 in the general population (62 years). Although the majority of the cases are above the age of 45, a significant number of patients (15 to 18%) are diagnosed below the age of 40.[14] The prognosis and survival rates are similar to sporadic cases, as LS-related endometrial cancers are also diagnosed at an early stage.[14,15] The major difference between the two groups is the higher rates of lower uterine segment involvement in LS-related endometrial cancers (25% of cases), which tend to be more invasive than the tumors located in the uterine corpus. Also, synchronous ovarian cancer is reported to represent 21% of the cases.[16]

In addition to colon and endometrial cancers, other types related to LS include ovarian, gastric, small bowel, hepatobiliary, renal pelvis, ureter, certain types of breast and brain, and sebaceous skin tumors.[17,18]

Lynch Syndrome Variants

Muir-Torre Syndrome Muir-Torre syndrome (MTS) is part of the LS family that is characterized by at least one sebaceous skin tumor and one visceral malignancy. It is a rare autosomal dominant disorder caused by germline mutations in mismatch repair genes (MLH1, MSH2, MSH6, PMS2) with a reported frequency of 9.2% in individuals with LS.[19] The most common mutated gene is MSH2, which is found in more than 90% of the patients.[20] Although the majority of the tumors related to MTS (65%) demonstrate microsatellite instability, around one-third of them are microsatellite stable (MSS). This group comprises the second subtype of the syndrome, called MTS II. Different than MTS I, MTS II is caused by germline mutations in a base excision repair *MUTYH* gene on the short arm of chromosome 1 and inherited in an autosomal recessive manner with low to moderate penetrance.[21,22] Table 8.1 shows distinctive features of MTS I and MTS II.

TABLE 8.1: Characteristics of MTS I and MTS II	
MTS I	**MTS II**
2/3 of tumors related to MTS	1/3 of tumors related to MTS
Autosomal dominant	Autosomal recessive
High penetrance	Moderate to low penetrance
Earlier onset tumors	Late onset tumors
MSI	MSS

MTS: Muir-Torre syndrome; MSI: Microsatellite instability; MSS: Microsatellite stable

The most common manifestations of the disease are skin tumors (sebaceous adenomas), which are seen in approximately 68% of the patients. Approximately one-third of sebaceous neoplasms are sebaceous carcinomas. Other skin tumors include keratoacanthoma, basal cell carcinoma with sebaceous differentiation, and cystic sebaceous tumors, which are all rare.[21,23] Although the most common sites for sebaceous tumors are the head and neck in sporadic cases, they are seen on the trunk in patients with MTS. Fordyce spots (ectopic sebaceous glands) on the oral mucosa are also helpful for diagnosis, which are seen in almost all of the MTS patients as opposed to 6.5% of healthy individuals.

Colon cancer is the most common visceral neoplasm that is generally located in the proximal colon (70% of colorectal cancers in LS are located proximal to the splenic flexure as opposed to 30% in sporadic colon cancer) with a median age of onset of 50 years.[20] Endometrial cancer, which is seen in 15% of women with MTS, is the second most common malignancy.

Turcot Syndrome Turcot syndrome (TS) is an historical term used to describe individuals with colorectal cancer or colorectal adenomas in addition to tumors of the central nervous system (CNS). It is divided into two subtypes based on the genetic pathogenesis. The first one is characterized by a pathogenic variant in one of the mismatch repair genes associated with LS, which is inherited as an autosomal recessive trait. The second one is associated with adenomatous polyposis coli gene germline mutation. It is inherited as an autosomal dominant pattern.[24] The most common CNS tumors are gliomas, followed by medulloblastomas, glioblastomas, ependymomas, and astrocytomas. Patients with mismatch repair deficiency have an elevated risk of endometrial cancer similar to patients with LS.

Cowden Syndrome

Cowden syndrome (CS) is an autosomal dominant condition with incomplete penetrance and variable expressivity caused by germline mutations in the phosphatase and tensin (*PTEN*) gene, which plays significant roles in cell cycle, growth, and survival.[25] It includes 9 exons (chromosome 10q23) to encode for a 403 amino acid tumor suppressor protein.[26] PTEN protein specifically down-regulates the phosphatidylinositol 3-kinase (PI3K)/AKT/ mammalian target of rapamycin (mTOR) pathway leading to decreased cellular proliferation and survival.[27] When heterozygosity for the gene is lost by a "second hit" mutation, this break mechanism for mTOR pathway is lost, resulting in development of the disease.

CS is the most common phenotypic presentation of PTEN hamartoma tumor syndrome (PHTS) spectrum, which also includes Bannayan-Riley-Ruvalcaba syndrome (BRRS) and adult

Lhermitte-Duclos disease LDD.[28,29] Segmental overgrowth lipomatosis arteriovenous malformation epidermal nevus (SOLAMEN) syndrome and Autism spectrum disorders with macrocephaly (ASDM) are two other entities that are related to PTEN mutations, but they lack hamartomas.[30,31] There is a female predominance with a rare population prevalence of 1/200,000.[32]

The uterine tumors associated with CS are mostly endometrioid adenocarcinomas, which tend to occur at a younger age (between 30 and 50) when compared to the general population (62 years).[33,34] There are cases in the literature as young as 14 years old.[35] Other histologic types include serous/clear cell (5%), carcinosarcoma (2.7%) and mucinous carcinoma (0.3%).[36] Among women with CS, 12% will present with endometrial cancer as their sentinel malignancy and 10% as their second malignancy.[37]

Affected individuals typically have pathognomonic skin lesions such as trichilemmomas and acral keratosis. Facial papules are the most common findings and are found in up to 86% of the cases.[38] The most frequent extra cutaneous manifestation is thyroid disease, which includes multinodular goiter, Hashimoto's thyroiditis and adenomas, which are seen in more than 50% of the patients.[39] Other benign entities include uterine fibroids, glycogenic acanthosis of esophagus, central nervous system lesions, and gastric, duodenal and colonic polyps. In terms of malignancies, there is increased lifetime risk of thyroid, endometrial, breast, and colon cancers. Among these, breast cancer is the most common malignancy with a lifetime risk of 25 to 50%; however, recent reports indicate a cumulative risk up to 85%.[40] The risk of endometrial cancer is reported to be 13 to 28%, whereas this risk is 3 to 38% and 9 to 18% for non-medullary thyroid cancer and colorectal cancer, respectively.[40,41]

Polymerase Proofreading Associated Polyposis

Polymerase proofreading associated polyposis (PPAP) is an autosomal dominant, highly penetrant cancer syndrome caused by germline mutations in the exonuclease (proofreading) domains of two DNA polymerases (POLE and POLD1).[45] Accurate DNA replication requires polymerases ε (Polε) and δ (Polδ); Polε synthesizes the leading strand, while Polδ serves the same function for the lagging strand.[42] POLE and POLD1 are the main catalytic and proofreading subunits of Polε and Polδ, respectively. Proofreading removes mispaired bases in the daughter strand during replication and the loss of proofreading capability causes multiple mutations in the genome leading to development of malignancies. Initially, two pathogenic mutations (POLE-p.Leu424Val and POLD1-p.Ser478Asn) are related to colorectal adenomas and carcinomas. Subsequently, another mutation (POLD1-p.Pro327Leu) was found in multiple adenoma patients.[43] Among these mutations, POLD1 is also considered to be associated with endometrial cancer.[42,43] A subsequent review of 69 POLE and POLD1 mutation carriers from 29 families revealed that 57.1% of female carriers of POLD1 were diagnosed with endometrial cancer.[44] This should be presented with caution as the high prevalence of uterine cancer in this group might be biased by the inclusion of high-risk families that fulfill the Amsterdam or Bethesda criteria. More data are needed before establishing further recommendations for this group.

POLD1 also participates in mismatch repair and base excision repair; however, as opposed to LS-related tumors, PPAP tumors are MSS.[43] They demonstrate chromosomal instability instead of microsatellite instability (MSI), which leads to development of driver mutations in APC and KRAS genes.[42] This can at least partially explain the increased risk of endometrial cancer in these patients. Besides germline POLD1 mutations, somatic POLE mutations have also been demonstrated to play an important role in approximately 8% of endometrial cancers.[44,46] Similar to the tumors with germline mutations, these tumors are MSS and demonstrate an ultra-mutator phenotype.

The role of a "two-hit" hypothesis has been challenged for POLE- or POLD1-related tumorigenesis. Mice with germline defects in Polε proofreading demonstrate increased mutagenesis and tumor development only in a homozygous state; however, no loss of heterozygosity was found in human endometrial cancers.[44] It still remains possible that "second hits" may occur through mutations elsewhere in the gene. This subject requires further evaluation.

Risk Assessment, Counseling, and Testing

Lynch Syndrome Individuals can be selected for genetic testing to rule out Lynch syndrome, based on three different strategies. These are based on personal and family history of cancer, tumor testing, and prediction models.

A. Family history-based screening: Amsterdam Criteria was initially introduced in 1990 to identify high-risk individuals for LS based on family history. However, it was soon identified to have many limitations and low sensitivity.[47] One of the major limitations was lack of extra-colonic malignancies in the system, which led to revision of the system in 1999.[48] Despite the revision, it still failed to identify more than half of the total and two-thirds of MSH6 mutation carriers.[49-51] Given the limitations of the Amsterdam Criteria, Bethesda guidelines were developed and subsequently revised in 2004, including more useful clinical information to identify individuals at risk.[52,53] Compared to Amsterdam Criteria, these guidelines have shown higher sensitivity (sensitivity: 94%, 95% CI 88–100, specificity: 25%, 95% CI 14–36).[54] However, it did not take into consideration endometrial cancer testing, which greatly decreased the clinical usefulness of these guidelines for referral of high-risk individuals for genetic testing. Therefore, the Society of Gynecologic Oncology (SGO) re-revised these criteria by including endometrial cancer as a sentinel cancer, which currently constitutes a useful approach to identify women at risk (Table 8.2).[55]

TABLE 8.2: Assessment of Lynch
Patients with greater than approximately 5 to 10% chance of having an inherited predisposition to endometrial, colorectal, or related cancers and for whom genetic risk assessment may be recommended
Patients with endometrial or colorectal cancer diagnosed prior to age 50
Patient with endometrial or ovarian cancer with a synchronous or metachronous colorectal or other Lynch-associated tumor* at any age
Patients with endometrial or colorectal cancer and a first-degree relative with a Lynch-associated tumor* diagnosed prior to age 50
Patients with colorectal or endometrial cancer diagnosed at any age with two or more first- or second-degree relatives§ with Lynch-associated tumors,* regardless of age
Patients with a first- or second-degree relative§ who meets the above criteria

* Lynch-related tumors include colorectal, endometrial, stomach, ovarian, pancreas, ureter and renal pelvis, biliary tract, brain (usually glioblastoma as seen in Turcot syndrome) tumors, sebaceous gland adenomas, and keratoacanthomas in Muir-Torre syndrome, and carcinoma of the small bowel.
§ First-degree relatives are parents, siblings, and children. Second-degree relatives are aunts, uncles, nieces, nephews, grandparents, and grandchildren.
Reproduced with permission from Lancaster JM, Powell CB, Kauff ND, et al: Society of Gynecologic Oncologists Education Committee. Society of Gynecologic Oncologists Education Committee statement on risk assessment for inherited gynecologic cancer predispositions, *Gynecol Oncol* 2007 Nov;107(2):159–162.

B. Tumor testing with reflex germline testing: Evaluation of protein products of mismatch repair genes in the tumor through immunohistochemistry is relatively inexpensive and currently available through most pathology laboratories in the United States. It is useful for guidance of germline testing under certain situations. If all four proteins are present after testing, then the presence of LS is ruled out in almost all of the cases. MLH1 loss should be further evaluated for promoter methylation, which is an acquired epigenetic process rather than a germline mutation.[56] Thus, if *MLH1* promoter methylation is confirmed, Lynch syndrome is ruled out. If MLH1 is absent, most of the time will result in absence of PMS2 protein as well, as both proteins exist as a heterodimer in the cell. The only case scenario that does not rule out LS in the setting of all four proteins expressed in the tumor is the presence of a nonsense mutation in any of the genes that leads to full length but non-functional protein product. Therefore, reflex germline testing should still be performed if there is still high clinical suspicion for these individuals.

Another test that is performed on the tumor is MSI testing. Microsatellites are fingerprints of DNA with repetitive sequences of nucleotides that are susceptible to acquiring errors when MMR is defective. These errors cause an inconsistent number of microsatellite nucleotide repeats when compared to normal tissue, which is defined as microsatellite instability. MSI testing is performed via polymerase chain reaction (PCR) to amplify a strand panel of DNA containing nucleotide repeats. The National Cancer Institute (NCI) has designated five microsatellite markers (BAT25, BAT26, D2S123, D5S346, and D17S250) that include two mononucleotide and three dinucleotide repeats. Based on the presence or absence of these markers, MSI testing could be interpreted as one of the following:[53]

- MSI-high: Two or more of the five markers of the core panel show instability. (Currently many labs use a variety of panels as markers. MSI is also considered high when more than 30% of these markers show instability.)
- MSI-low: One of the five markers of the core panel shows instability. (Fewer than 30% of markers show instability if other marker panels are used.)
- MSI-stable: None of the markers show instability.

During the last two decades, considerable evidence has emerged suggesting that dinucleotide markers can be highly polymorphic in the context of LS, leading to decreased specificity of the testing.[57,58] Therefore, most institutions have switched to use of five mononucleotide markers that are more specific and similarly sensitive. In endometrial tumors from unselected patients, MSI testing and IHC have a sensitivity of 80 to 100% and specificity of 60 to 80% for detecting a mutation in an *MMR* gene and they are highly concordant.[59,60]

In individuals with evidence of MSI-H or loss of expression of an MMR protein, further evaluation is warranted with reflex germline testing, which is required for the diagnosis of LS. Knowing the MSI-H status of a solid tumor is also clinically useful, as it may guide treatment planning. Endometrial MSI testing is now further supported by the FDA approval in 2017 of pembrolizumab for unresectable or metastatic defective MMR and MSI-H solid tumors that have progressed following prior treatment and that have no satisfactory alternatives.

In terms of tumor testing, three strategies have been suggested to assess the possibility of LS in a woman,who is affected with colorectal or endometrial cancer.[8]

1. Selective tumor testing after a thorough systematic clinical screen that includes a focused personal and family medical history.

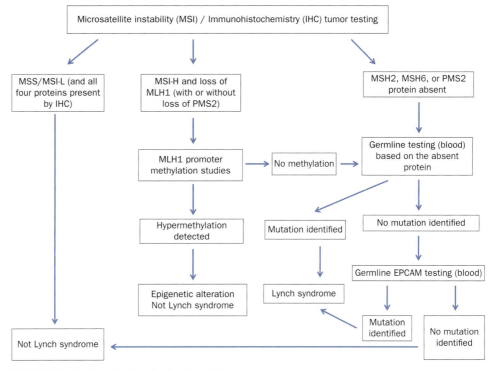

FIGURE 8.1: Testing algorithm for Lynch syndrome.

2. Universal tumor testing (testing of all individuals irrespective of age)

3. Tumor testing on all endometrial or colorectal tumors diagnosed before the age of 60.

NCCN currently recommends universal tumor testing with either MSI or IHC for absence of one of the four DNA MMR proteins.[61] Arguments in favor of this testing approach depends on the fact that approximately 12 to 30% of LS-related endometrial and colorectal cancers will not meet the 2004 Bethesda Guidelines modified to include endometrial cancer as a sentinel tumor.[9,62,63] Cost-effectiveness of this approach has been established and endorsed by various organizations including the Evaluation of Genomic Applications in Practice and Prevention (EGAPP) working group at the Centers for Disease Control and Prevention, the U.S. Multi-Society Task Force on Colorectal Cancer, and the European Society for Medical Oncology.[64–67] SGO also endorses universal molecular screening IHC for the 4 MMR proteins when resources are available in patients with newly diagnosed endometrial cancer.[68] In limited resource settings, a more selective strategy is encouraged that includes patients, who are less than 60, regardless of personal or family history.[68,69] An algorithm for tumor testing is shown in Figure 8.1.

C. Risk prediction models: Three risk prediction models are currently incorporated into NCCN guidelines for risk assessment.[61] The MMRpredict model includes gender, age at diagnosis, tumor location (proximal versus distal), synchronous and/or metachronous tumors, family history of endometrial cancer in any first-degree relative, and age at diagnosis of colorectal cancer in first-degree relatives.[70] Sensitivity and specificity of this model are reported to be 94% and 91%, respectively.[71] The MMRpro model uses age at diagnosis, personal and family history of colorectal and endometrial cancers, MSI status and previous germline testing results to determine the probability of an individual having germline *MLH1*, *MLH2*, or *MSH6* genes.[72] The PREMM5 model includes a personal or family history of colorectal cancer, endometrial cancer, or other Lynch syndrome-associated cancers, types of cancer and ages at diagnosis of first- and second-degree relatives (parents, siblings, children, grandparents, grandchildren, aunts, uncles, nieces, nephews).[73] It assesses the probability of finding a pathogenic mutation in all LS-related genes including MLH1, MSH2, MSH6, PMS2, and EPCAM. Although few studies have compared these models, MMRpro and PREMM models were noted to be superior to MMRpredict in both clinic- and population-based cohorts.[74]

After appropriate assessment, germline testing should be considered in these cases:

- Individuals who meet the criteria in Table 8.2
- Individuals who have a first-, second-, or third-degree relative with a known MMR/EPCAM mutation
- Individuals with a predicted risk for LS > 5% on predictive models (i.e., MMRpro, PREMM5, or MMRpredict). Most recent NCCN guidelines indicate that a lower threshold of $\geq$ 2.5% risk for the PREMM5 model could indicate an MMR gene mutation. Therefore, it might be reasonable to refer individuals for testing based on the $\geq$ 2.5% risk and clinical judgment.[61] However, it is still not clear how this lower threshold applies to the unaffected individuals in general population.

Prior to germline testing, a thorough discussion is crucial. Women should be informed that testing will not identify epigenetic (inactivation of MLH1 by hypermethylation) or somatic (double somatic mutations) alterations. Germline testing will not identify a causative mutation in 10 to 15% of individuals, whose tumor testing showed MLH1 or PMS2 protein loss. For MSH2 or MSH6, this rate is 35–40%.[8] These patients should be managed by cancer genetics professionals based on personal risk factors and family history. The interpretation could be uninformative in the setting of finding variants of uncertain significance (VUS) results. Options for surveillance, chemoprevention, and risk-reducing surgery should also be discussed. Of note, prior to routine tumor testing, counseling is not required, but it is strongly recommended if the screening result is positive.[61]

Cowden Syndrome

The criteria for the diagnosis were first established by the International Cowden Syndrome Consortium in 1996, which was later updated in 2000.[75,76] However, despite the update, the specificity of the criteria still remained low, meaning approximately two-thirds of the individuals with germline PTEN mutations were not identified. Therefore, a multi-center group in the United States updated the criteria in 2013 for the diagnosis, which is also supported by the NCCN guidelines (Table 8.3).[77] According to this model, individuals with no prior family history of PHTS/Cowden syndrome require either three or more major criteria (one of which must be macrocephaly, Lhermitte-Duclos disease, or gastrointestinal hamartomas) or two major plus three minor criteria to be diagnosed with CS. For patients with a family history, the threshold for diagnosis is lower, with the presence of any two major criteria, one major and two minor criteria, or three minor criteria being sufficient. Germline testing criteria is as follows:[78]

- Individual from a family with a known PTEN pathogenic/likely pathogenic mutation
- Individual with Bannayan Ruvalcaba-Riley syndrome (BRRS)
- Individual who meets the clinical diagnostic criteria (Table 8.3)

TABLE 8.3: Revised PTEN Hamartoma Tumor Syndrome Clinical Diagnostic Criteria

Major Criteria

- Breast cancer
- Endometrial cancer (epithelial)
- Thyroid cancer (follicular)
- Gastrointestinal hamartomas (including ganglioneuromas but excluding hyperplastic polyps) ≥ 3
- Lhermitte-Duclos disease (adult)
- Macrocephaly ($\geq$ 97th percentile: 58 cm for females, 60 cm for males)
- Macular pigmentation of the glans penis
- Multiple mucocutaneous lesions (any of the following)
    - Multiple trichilemmomas (≥ 3, at least one biopsy proven)
    - Acral keratosis (≥ 3 palmoplantar keratotic pits and/or acral hyperkeratotic papules)
    - Mucocutaneous neuromas (≥ 3)
    - Oral papillomas (particularly on tongue and gingiva), multiple (≥ 3)
    - *or* biopsy proven *or* dermatologist diagnosed

Minor Criteria

- Autism spectrum disorder
- Colon cancer
- Esophageal glycogenic acanthosis (≥ 3)
- Lipomas (≥ 3)
- Intellectual disability (i.e., IQ ≤ 75)
- Renal cell carcinoma
- Testicular lipomatosis
- Thyroid cancer (papillary or follicular variant of papillary)
- Thyroid structural lesions (e.g., adenoma, multinodular goiter)
- Vascular anomalies (including multiple intracranial developmental venous anomalies)

Operational diagnosis in an individual (either of the following)

1. Three or more major criteria, but one must include macrocephaly, Lhermitte-Duclos disease, or gastrointestinal hamartomas; or
2. Two major and three minor criteria.

Operational diagnosis in a family where one individual meets revised PTEN hamartoma tumor syndrome clinical diagnostic criteria or has a PTEN mutation:

1. Any two major criteria with or without minor criteria;
2. One major and two minor criteria; or
3. Three minor criteria

Reproduced with permission from Pilarski R, Burt R, Kohlman W, et al: Cowden syndrome and the PTEN hamartoma tumor syndrome: systematic review and revised diagnostic criteria, *J Natl Cancer Inst* 2013 Nov 6;105(21):1607–1616.

- Individual who does not meet the clinical diagnostic criteria but has any of the following: adult Lhermitte-Duclos disease (LDD), autism spectrum disorder and macrocephaly, ≥ 2 biopsy proven trichilemmomas, ≥ 2 major criteria (one must be macrocephaly), three major criteria without macrocephaly, one major and ≥ 3 minor criteria, or ≥ 4 minor criteria.
- At-risk individuals (must have any one major or two minor criteria) with a relative with a clinical diagnosis of CS/PHTS or BRRS for whom testing has not been performed.

Testing includes sequencing of the entire coding region, deletion/duplication analysis and the PTEN promoter. Ideally, the proband (affected family member) should be tested first for identification of mutations in the family. This strategy brings up the opportunity to other family members for targeted testing. If there is no established familial PTEN mutation, then the testing should start with the individual, who would most likely have the pathogenic variant based on the clinical presentation. In case of a negative test result, testing for other genes that are related to Cowden-like presentation should be considered. These include AKT1, KLLN, PIK3CA, SDH subunit B, and SDH subunit D.[79,80]

Polymerase Proofreading Associated Polyposis PPAP is a relatively new syndrome (first reported on in 2013) and similar to Lynch, it is related to increased risk of colorectal and endometrial cancers. As there are very few cases in the literature, no testing or management recommendations from any of the national organizations are currently available. Individuals and families who present with LS phenotype but with MSS tumors instead should be tested for germline pathogenic variants in POLD1 and POLE genes. In general, most cancer genetics programs test individuals with multiple polyps with not only APC and MUTYH but panels that also include polymerases.

Clinical Management of Patients at Increased Risk

The management options for individuals at risk for endometrial cancer include surveillance and risk-reducing surgery. Data are limited regarding the role of chemoprevention.

Surveillance The American College of Obstetricians and Gynecologists (ACOG) and NCCN published similar screening guidelines for endometrial cancer in asymptomatic women with LS.[8,61] It suggested an endometrial biopsy from age 30 to 35 every 1 to 2 years. This could be individualized based on family history. Because endometrial cancer is common in patients with LS, the starting age of endometrial sampling could be moved to 5 to 10 years prior to the earliest age of LS-associated cancer of any kind in the family. Patients also should keep a menstrual calendar to evaluate any abnormal bleeding. Studies showed that pelvic ultrasonography (transabdominal or transvaginal) has low sensitivity in detecting endometrial cancer in premenopausal women; therefore, it should not be used alone for screening without endometrial sampling.[81] For postmenopausal women, it might have additional value; however, high-quality data are lacking in this patient cohort. Until more data are available, the standard of care is to perform an endometrial biopsy in both premenopausal and postmenopausal women with LS for endometrial cancer screening.

In women diagnosed with CS, NCCN published similar guidelines in terms of endometrial cancer surveillance as in patients with LS, which included endometrial sampling every one to two years beginning at age 30 to 35.[61] It should be noted that screening with endometrial biopsy does not have a proven benefit in either LS or CS/PTHS. However, given the fact that it is highly sensitive and specific, it is reasonable to screen these patients with this method. Due to the fact that the diagnosis could be made as early as adolescence in CS, patients should track menstrual abnormalities, which requires prompt reporting and further evaluation, irrespective of age. As with LS, the use of transvaginal ultrasound in premenopausal women is not recommended due to the wide variation in normal endometrial lining thicknesses throughout the menstrual cycle. Ultrasound may be ordered in postmenopausal women at the physician's discretion.

PPAP is a relatively new syndrome and high-quality data are lacking for this group. Until more studies are available, frequency of screening strategies (colonoscopy, endometrial biopsy, etc.) and timing of risk-reducing surgery options (colectomy, hysterectomy) should be individualized based on the earliest age of onset of these cancers within the family. In the largest report to date, Palles et al. demonstrated three pedigrees including 23 affected individuals, seven of whom had endometrial cancer.[42] Median age at diagnosis was 45 years (range was 33 to 52). Based on the data, it is reasonable to start screening with endometrial sampling at age 30 (every one to two years).

Risk-Reducing Surgery   Risk-reducing hysterectomy and bilateral salpingo-oophorectomy (RRBSO) is currently the gold standard method for uterine and ovarian cancer risk reduction in individuals with LS.[8,61] The largest study to date is a retrospective study that compared women with germline *MLH1, MLH2,* or *MLH6* mutations, who did or did not undergo hysterectomy with or without BSO.[14] There were no occurrences of endometrial cancer in 61 women who underwent prophylactic hysterectomy. However, 33% of women in the control group were diagnosed with the disease. Similarly, there was no ovarian cancer in RRBSO group, whereas 5% of the control group had the diagnosis. These findings suggest that prophylactic hysterectomy and BSO is effective in preventing these cancers in this patient cohort. Because the risk significantly increases after the age of 40 (endometrial cancer risk is 2 to 4% by the age of 40, and 8 to 17% by the age of 50; these risks are 1 to 2% and 3 to 7%, respectively, for ovarian cancer), the surgery should be discussed with the patients by their early to mid-40s.[8] Preoperative counseling should include reproductive issues, cancer risks at certain ages, degree of protection from ovarian and endometrial cancer, disadvantages of premature menopause (vasomotor symptoms, sexual dysfunction, osteoporosis, cardiovascular effects, cognitive impairment, increased risk of premature death), hormone replacement therapy, and psychosocial and quality of life issues.

In terms of CS and PPAP, risk-reducing hysterectomy should be discussed once childbearing is complete. Oophorectomy is not indicated for CS, as there is no increased risk of ovarian cancer. For PPAP, although no ovarian cancer cases have been reported so far, more data are needed, as it is relatively a new entity.

Some studies demonstrated that uterine serous cancer (USC), which is an aggressive subtype of endometrial cancer, is associated with the BRCA-related cancer spectrum. In a multicenter prospective cohort study, 1083 women, who underwent RRBSO due to a deleterious BRCA1 or BRCA2 mutation, were followed up for a median 5.1 years (interquartile range 3–8.4) after ascertainment, BRCA testing, or RRBSO, whichever occurred last.[82] The uterine cancer incidence in these women was compared with rates expected from the SEER database. A total of 5 serous and/or serous-like carcinomas (4 BRCA1, 1 BRCA2) were diagnosed 7.2 to 12.9 years after RRSO (BRCA1: 0.18 expected, [observed/expected ratio: 22.2, 95% CI: 6.1–56.9; $p < 0.001$], BRCA2: 0.16 expected, [observed/expected ratio: 6.4, 95% CI, 0.2–35.5; $p = 0.15$]). There was no increased risk for endometrioid subtype or sarcoma. Although the relative risk seems to be high, the absolute risk is still low. Therefore, patient preferences should be taken into account for management decisions after appropriate counseling. The literature also did not confirm any association between deleterious BRCA mutations and uterine cancer.[83,84]

Chemoprevention   Data are limited regarding what role chemoprevention may play in reducing the risk of endometrial cancer in women with these syndromes. Based on the available evidence, there is up to 50% risk reduction of endometrial cancer in combined oral contraceptive users in the general population.[85,86] In an observational study that included 1,128 women with a mismatch repair gene mutation, endometrial cancer was diagnosed in 8.7% of women who used hormonal contraceptives for $\geq$ 1 year, compared to 19.2% who used contraceptives for < 1 year.[87] In a prospective multicenter randomized trial that compared combined oral contraceptives (30 micrograms ethynil estradiol, 0.3 mg norgestrel) with Depo-Provera (medroxy-progesterone acetate 150 mg) for prevention of endometrial cancer in patients with LS, both Depo-Provera and combined oral contraceptives induced a dramatic decrease in endometrial epithelial proliferation. The microscopic changes in the endometrium were characteristic of progestin action.[88]

Although more studies are needed to make definitive conclusions, it is reasonable to recommend combined oral contraceptives or progestin therapy, if the patients with these cancer syndromes opt not to undergo risk-reducing surgery.

References

1. Siegel RL, Miller KD, Jemal A. Cancer statistics, 2018. *CA Cancer J Clin.* 2018;68:7–30.
2. http://seer.cancer.gov/statfacts/html/corp.html
3. https://www.cancer.org/cancer/endometrial-cancer/detection-diagnosis-staging/signs-and-symptoms.html
4. Felix AS, Weissfeld JL, Stone RA, et al. Factors associated with Type I and Type II endometrial cancer. *Cancer Causes Control.* 2010;21:1851–1856.
5. Lancaster JM, Powell CB, Chen LM, et al.; SGO Clinical Practice Committee. Society of Gynecologic Oncology statement on risk assessment for inherited gynecologic cancer predispositions. *Gynecol Oncol.* 2015;136:3–7.
6. Kwon JS, Scott JL, Gilks CB, et al. Testing women with endometrial cancer to detect Lynch syndrome. *J Clin Oncol.* 2011 Jun 1;29(16):2247–2252.
7. Tan MH, Mester JL, Ngeow J, et al. Lifetime cancer risks in individuals with germline PTEN mutations. *Clin Cancer Res.* 2012;18:400–407.
8. Committee on Practice Bulletins-Gynecology; Society of Gynecologic Oncology. ACOG Practice Bulletin No. 147: Lynch syndrome. *Obstet Gynecol.* 2014;124:1042–1054.
9. Moreira L, Balaguer F, Lindor N, et al. Identification of Lynch syndrome among patients with colorectal cancer. *JAMA.* 2012;308:1555–1565.
10. Dunlop MG, Farrington SM, Nicholl I, et al. Population carrier frequency of hMSH2 and hMLH1 mutations. *Br J Cancer.* 2000;83:1643–1645.
11. Kempers MJ, Kuiper RP, Ockeloen CW, et al. Risk of colorectal and endometrial cancers in EPCAM deletion-positive Lynch syndrome: a cohort study. *Lancet Oncol.* 2011;12:49–55.
12. Meyer LA, Broaddus RR, Lu KH. Endometrial cancer and Lynch syndrome: clinical and pathologic considerations. *Cancer Control.* 2009;16:14–22. Review.
13. Kwon JS, Scott JL, Gilks CB, et al. Testing women with endometrial cancer to detect Lynch syndrome. *J Clin Oncol.* 2011 1;29:2247–2252.
14. Schmeler KM, Lynch HT, Chen LM, et al. Prophylactic surgery to reduce the risk of gynecologic cancers in the Lynch syndrome. *N Engl J Med.* 2006;354:261–269.
15. Boks DE, Trujillo AP, Voogd AC, et al. Survival analysis of endometrial carcinoma associated with hereditary nonpolyposis colorectal cancer. *Int J Cancer.* 2002;102:198–200.
16. Rossi L, Le Frere-Belda MA, Laurent-Puig P, et al. Clinicopathologic characteristics of endometrial cancer in Lynch syndrome: a French multicenter study. *Int J Gynecol Cancer.* 2017;27:953–960.
17. Watson P, Vasen HF, Mecklin JP, et al. The risk of extra-colonic, extra-endometrial cancer in the Lynch syndrome. *Int J Cancer.* 2008;123:444–449.
18. Win AK, Lindor NM, Young JP, et al. Risks of primary extracolonic cancers following colorectal cancer in Lynch syndrome. *J Natl Cancer Inst.* 2012;104:1363–1372.
19. South CD, Hampel H, Comeras I, et al. The frequency of Muir-Torre syndrome among Lynch syndrome families. *J Natl Cancer Inst.* 2008;100:277–281.

20. Lynch HT, Lynch JF, Attard TA. Diagnosis and management of hereditary colorectal cancer syndromes: Lynch syndrome as a model. *CMAJ*. 2009;181:273–280.

21. John AM, Schwartz RA. Muir-Torre syndrome (MTS): An update and approach to diagnosis and management. *J Am Acad Dermatol*. 2016;74:558–566.

22. Russell AM, Zhang J, Luz J, et al. Prevalence of MYH germline mutations in Swiss APC mutation-negative polyposis patients. *Int J Cancer*. 2006;118:1937–1940.

23. Jones B, Oh C, Mangold E, et al. Muir-Torre syndrome: Diagnostic and screening guidelines. *Australas J Dermatol*. 2006;47:266–269.

24. https://rarediseases.org/rare-diseases/turcot-syndrome

25. Eng C. PTEN: one gene, many syndromes. *Hum Mutat*. 2003;22:183–198.

26. Sansal I, Sellers WR. The biology and clinical relevance of the PTEN tumor suppressor pathway. *J Clin Oncol*. 2004;22:2954–2963.

27. Stambolic V, Suzuki A, de la Pompa JL, et al. Negative regulation of PKB/Akt-dependent cell survival by the tumor suppressor PTEN. *Cell*. 1998;95:29–39.

28. Marsh DJ, Coulon V, Lunetta KL, et al. Mutation spectrum and genotype-phenotype analyses in Cowden disease and Bannayan-Zonana syndrome, two hamartoma syndromes with germline PTEN mutation. *Hum Mol Genet*. 1998;7:507–515.

29. Abel TW, Baker SJ, Fraser MM, et al. Lhermitte-Duclos disease: a report of 31 cases with immunohistochemical analysis of the PTEN/AKT/mTOR pathway. *J Neuropathol Exp Neurol*. 2005;64:341–349.

30. Caux F, Plauchu H, Chibon F, et al. Segmental overgrowth, lipomatosis, arteriovenous malformation and epidermal nevus (SOLAMEN) syndrome is related to mosaic PTEN nullizygosity. *Eur J Hum Genet*. 2007;15:767–773.

31. Butler MG, Dasouki MJ, Zhou XP, et al. Subset of individuals with autism spectrum disorders and extreme macrocephaly associated with germline PTEN tumour suppressor gene mutations. *J Med Genet*. 2005;42:318-321.

32. Nelen MR, Kremer H, Konings IB, et al. Novel PTEN mutations in patients with Cowden disease: absence of clear genotype-phenotype correlations. *Eur J Hum Genet*. 1999;7:267–273.

33. Tan MH, Mester J, Peterson C, et al. A clinical scoring system for selection of patients for PTEN mutation testing is proposed on the basis of a prospective study of 3042 probands. *Am J Hum Genet*. 2011 Jan 7;88:42–56.

34. Starink TM, van der Veen JP, Arwert F, et al. The Cowden syndrome: a clinical and genetic study in 21 patients. *Clin Genet*. 1986;29:222–233.

35. Baker WD, Soisson AP, Dodson MK. Endometrial cancer in a 14-year-old girl with Cowden syndrome: a case report. *J Obstet Gynaecol Res*. 2013;39:876–878.

36. Mahdi H, Mester JL, Nizialek EA, et al. Germline PTEN, SDHB-D, and KLLN alterations in endometrial cancer patients with Cowden and Cowden-like syndromes: an international, multicenter, prospective study. *Cancer*. 2015;121:688–696.

37. Ngeow J, Stanuch K, Mester JL, et al. Second malignant neoplasms in patients with Cowden syndrome with underlying germline PTEN mutations. *J Clin Oncol*. 2014;32:1818–1824.

38. Hanssen AM, Werquin H, Suys E, et al. Cowden syndrome: report of a large family with macrocephaly and increased severity of signs in subsequent generations. *Clin Genet*. 1993;44:281–286.

39. Hall JE, Abdollahian DJ, Sinard RJ. Thyroid disease associated with Cowden syndrome: A meta-analysis. *Head Neck*. 2013;35:1189–1194.

40. Tan MH, Mester JL, Ngeow J, et al. Lifetime cancer risks in individuals with germline PTEN mutations. *Clin Cancer Res*. 2012;18:400–407.

41. Nieuwenhuis MH, Kets CM, Murphy-Ryan M, et al. Cancer risk and genotype-phenotype correlations in PTEN hamartoma tumor syndrome. *Fam Cancer*. 2014;13:57–63.

42. Palles C, Cazier JB, Howarth KM, et al. Germline mutations affecting the proofreading domains of POLE and POLD1 predispose to colorectal adenomas and carcinomas. *Nat Genet*. 2013;45:136–144.

43. Briggs S, Tomlinson I. Germline and somatic polymerase ε and δ mutations define a new class of hypermutated colorectal and endometrial cancers. *J Pathol*. 2013;230:148–153.

44. Church DN, Briggs SE, Palles C, et al. DNA polymerase ε and δ exonuclease domain mutations in endometrial cancer. *Hum Mol Genet*. 2013;22:2820–2828.

45. Bellido F, Pineda M, Aiza G, et al. POLE and POLD1 mutations in 529 kindred with familial colorectal cancer and/or polyposis: review of reported cases and recommendations for genetic testing and surveillance. *Genet Med*. 2016;18:325–332.

46. Cancer Genome Atlas Research Network, Kandoth C, Schultz N, Cherniack AD, et al. Integrated genomic characterization of endometrial carcinoma. *Nature*. 2013;497:67–73.

47. Vasen HF, Mecklin JP, Khan PM, et al. The international collaborative group on hereditary non-polyposis colorectal cancer (ICG-HNPCC). *Dis Colon Rectum*. 1991;34(5):424–425.

48. Vasen HF, Watson P, Mecklin JP, et al. New clinical criteria for hereditary nonpolyposis colorectal cancer (HNPCC, Lynch syndrome) proposed by the International Collaborative group on HNPCC. *Gastroenterology*. 1999;116:1453–1456.

49. Barrow E, Hill J, Evans DG. Cancer risk in Lynch syndrome. *Fam Cancer*. 2013;12:229–240.

50. Barnetson RA, Tenesa A, Farrington SM, et al. Identification and survival of carriers of mutations in DNA mismatch-repair genes in colon cancer. *N Engl J Med*. 2006;354:2751–2763.

51. Plaschke J, Engel C, Krüger S, et al. Lower incidence of colorectal cancer and later age of disease onset in 27 families with pathogenic MSH6 germline mutations compared with families with MLH1 or MSH2 mutations: the German Hereditary Nonpolyposis Colorectal Cancer Consortium. *J Clin Oncol*. 2004;22:4486–4494.

52. Rodriguez-Bigas MA, Boland CR, Hamilton SR, et al. A National Cancer Institute workshop on hereditary nonpolyposis colorectal cancer syndrome: meeting highlights and Bethesda guidelines. *J Natl Cancer Inst*. 1997;89:1758–1762.

53. Umar A, Boland CR, Terdiman JP, et al. Revised Bethesda guidelines for hereditary nonpolyposis colorectal cancer (Lynch syndrome) and microsatellite instability. *J Natl Cancer Inst*. 2004;96:261–268.

54. Syngal S, Fox EA, Eng C, et al. Sensitivity and specificity of clinical criteria for hereditary non-polyposis colorectal cancer associated mutations in MSH2 and MLH1. *J Med Genet*. 2000;37:641–645.

55. Lancaster JM, Powell CB, Kauff ND, et al. Society of Gynecologic Oncologists Education Committee statement on risk assessment for inherited gynecologic cancer predispositions. *Gynecol Oncol*. 2007;107:159–162.

56. Herman JG, Umar A, Polyak K, et al. Incidence and functional consequences of hMLH1 promoter hypermethylation in colorectal carcinoma. *Proc Natl Acad Sci USA*. 1998;95:6870–6875.

57. Xicola RM, Llor X, Pons E, et al; Gastrointestinal Oncology Group of the Spanish Gastroenterological Association. Performance of different microsatellite marker panels for detection of mismatch repair-deficient colorectal tumors. *J Natl Cancer Inst*. 2007;99:244–252.

58. Suraweera N, Duval A, Reperant M, et al. Evaluation of tumor microsatellite instability using five quasimonomorphic mononucleotide repeats and pentaplex PCR. *Gastroenterology*. 2002;123:1804–1811.

59. Stewart A. Genetic testing strategies in newly diagnosed endometrial cancer patients aimed at reducing morbidity or mortality from Lynch syndrome in the index case or her relatives. *PLoS Curr*. 2013 September 16;5. pii: ecurrents.eogt.b59a6e84f27c536e50db4e46aa26309c.

60. Stelloo E, Jansen AML, Osse EM, et al. Practical guidance for mismatch repair-deficiency testing in endometrial cancer. *Ann Oncol*. 2017;28:96–102.

61. National Comprehensive Cancer Network. Genetic/familial high-risk assessment: colorectal. Version 2.2019. NCCN Clinical Practice Guidelines in Oncology. https://www.nccn.org/professionals/physician_gls/pdf/genetics_colon.pdf.

62. Hampel H, Frankel W, Panescu J, et al. Screening for Lynch syndrome (hereditary nonpolyposis colorectal cancer) among endometrial cancer patients. *Cancer Res*. 2006;66:7810–7817.

63. Hampel H, Frankel WL, Martin E, et al. Screening for the Lynch syndrome (hereditary nonpolyposis colorectal cancer). *N Engl J Med*. 2005;352:1851–1860.

64. Evaluation of Genomic Applications in Practice and Prevention (EGAPP) Working Group. Recommendations from the EGAPP Working Group: genetic testing strategies in newly diagnosed individuals with colorectal cancer aimed at reducing morbidity and mortality from Lynch syndrome in relatives. *Genet Med*. 2009;11:35–41.

65. Ladabaum U, Wang G, Terdiman J, et al. Strategies to identify the Lynch syndrome among patients with colorectal cancer: a cost-effectiveness analysis. *Ann Intern Med*. 2011;155:69–79.

66. Palomaki GE, McClain MR, Melillo S, et al. EGAPP supplementary evidence review: DNA testing strategies aimed at reducing morbidity and mortality from Lynch syndrome. *Genet Med*. 2009;11:42–65.

67. Balmaña J, Balaguer F, Cervantes A, et al; ESMO Guidelines Working Group. Familial risk-colorectal cancer: ESMO Clinical Practice Guidelines. *Ann Oncol*. 2013;24(Suppl. 6):vi, 73–80.

68. Society of Gynecologic Oncology. SGO clinical practice statement: screening for Lynch syndrome in endometrial cancer. Chicago (IL): SGO; 2014. https://www.sgo.org/clinical-practice/guidelines/screening-for-lynch-syndrome-in-endometrial-cancer/

69. Buchanan DD, Tan YY, Walsh MD, et al. Tumor mismatch repair immunohistochemistry and DNA MLH1 methylation testing of patients with endometrial cancer diagnosed at age younger than 60 years optimizes triage for population-level germline mismatch repair gene mutation testing. *J Clin Oncol*. 2014;32:90–100.

70. Barnetson RA, Tenesa A, Farrington SM, et al. Identification and survival of carriers of mutations in DNA mismatch-repair genes in colon cancer. *N Engl J Med*. 2006;354:2751–2763.

71. Green RC, Parfrey PS, Woods MO, et al. Prediction of Lynch syndrome in consecutive patients with colorectal cancer. *J Natl Cancer Inst*. 2009;101:331–340.

72. Chen S, Wang W, Lee S, et al. Prediction of germline mutations and cancer risk in the Lynch syndrome. *JAMA*. 2006;296:1479–1487.

73. Kastrinos F, Steyerberg EW, Mercado R, et al. The PREMM(1,2,6) model predicts risk of MLH1, MSH2, and MSH6 germline mutations based on cancer history. *Gastroenterology*. 2011;140:73–81.

74. Kastrinos F, Ojha RP, Leenen C, et al. Comparison of prediction models for Lynch syndrome among individuals with colorectal cancer. *J Natl Cancer Inst*. 2016;108.

75. Eng C. Will the real Cowden syndrome please stand up: revised diagnostic criteria. *J Med Genet*. 2000;37:828–830.

76. Pilarski R, Eng C. Will the real Cowden syndrome please stand up (again)? Expanding mutational and clinical spectra of the PTEN hamartoma tumour syndrome. *J Med Genet*. 2004;41:323–326.

77. Pilarski R, Burt R, Kohlman W, et al. Cowden syndrome and the PTEN hamartoma tumor syndrome: systematic review and revised diagnostic criteria. *J Natl Cancer Inst*. 2013;105:1607–1616.

78. National Comprehensive Cancer Network. Genetic/familial high-risk assessment: breast and ovarian. Version 2.2019. NCCN Clinical Practice Guidelines in Oncology. https://www.nccn.org/professionals/physician_gls/pdf/genetics_screening.pdf

79. Bennett KL, Mester J, Eng C. Germline epigenetic regulation of KILLIN in Cowden and Cowden-like syndrome. *JAMA*. 2010;304:2724–2731.

80. Orloff MS, He X, Peterson C, et al. Germline PIK3CA and AKT1 mutations in Cowden and Cowden-like syndromes. *Am J Hum Genetics*. 2013;92:76–80.

81. Dove-Edwin I, Boks D, Goff S, et al. The outcome of endometrial carcinoma surveillance by ultrasound scan in women at risk of hereditary nonpolyposis colorectal carcinoma and familial colorectal carcinoma. *Cancer*. 2002;94:1708–1712.

82. Shu CA, Pike MC, Jotwani AR, et al. Uterine cancer after risk-reducing salpingo-oophorectomy without hysterectomy in women with BRCA mutations. *JAMA Oncol*. 2016;2:1434–1440.

83. Barak F, Milgrom R, Laitman Y, et al. The rate of the predominant Jewish mutations in the BRCA1, BRCA2, MSH2 and MSH6 genes in unselected Jewish endometrial cancer patients. *Gynecol Oncol*. 2010;119:511–515.

84. Levine DA, Lin O, Barakat RR, et al. Risk of endometrial carcinoma associated with BRCA mutation. *Gynecol Oncol*. 2001;80:395–398.

85. Weiss NS, Sayvetz TA. Incidence of endometrial cancer in relation to the use of oral contraceptives. *N Engl J Med*. 1980;302:551–554.

86. Combination oral contraceptive use and the risk of endometrial cancer. The Cancer and Steroid Hormone Study of the Centers for Disease Control and the National Institute of Child Health and Human Development. *JAMA*. 1987 Feb 13;257(6):796–800.

87. Dashti SG, Chau R, Ouakrim DA, et al. Female hormonal factors and the risk of endometrial cancer in Lynch syndrome. *JAMA*. 2015;314:61–71.

88. Lu KH, Loose DS, Yates MS, et al. Prospective multicenter randomized intermediate biomarker study of oral contraceptive versus Depo-Provera for prevention of endometrial cancer in women with Lynch syndrome. *Cancer Prev Res (Phila)*. 2013;6:774–781.

CHAPTER 9

Risk Assessment and Clinical Management – Ovarian Cancer

Burak Zeybek and Elena Ratner

▓ DISEASE SPECIFIC CANCER EPIDEMIOLOGY AND RISK FACTORS

Ovarian cancer is the second most common gynecologic malignancy and the most common cause of death from gynecologic cancer in the United States with 22,240 new cases and 14,000 deaths annually.[1] It is the fifth leading cause of cancer death in women after cancers of the breast, lung, and endometrium. Based on the National Cancer Database Surveillance, Epidemiology, and End Results (SEER) data from 2011 to 2015, the lifetime risk of developing ovarian cancer is 1.3%, and the median age at diagnosis is 63. The number of new cases and deaths are reported to be 11.6 and 7.2 per 100,000 women per year, respectively.[2]

The high mortality rate of ovarian cancer is due to the fact that most of the patients present with advanced stage disease and screening tests to diagnose early stage disease are still far from ideal. The majority of these neoplasms originate from coelemic epithelium (95%), high-grade serous carcinoma being the most common histologic subtype (75%).[3] Other histologic epithelial subtypes include clear cell, endometrioid, mucinous, Brenner and undifferentiated carcinomas. High-grade serous carcinomas are closely related to fallopian tube and peritoneal carcinomas because of the extreme similarities in histologic features and clinical behaviors. Recent evidence supports that the majority of high-grade serous tumors that have been classified as ovarian (and some peritoneal) cancers actually arise in the fimbrial portion of the fallopian tubes.[4] Due to this close proximity of origin, the primary site of these cancers may not always be determined, possibly leading to underestimation of annual incidence rates of primary fallopian tube (3.3 per 1,000,000)[5] and peritoneal carcinomas (2.7 per 1,000,000).[6]

Certain risk factors are implicated in the etiology of ovarian cancer and based on these factors, women may be categorized into two groups. The high-risk group includes individuals with hereditary cancer syndromes and certain inherited genetic mutations that significantly increase the risk of ovarian cancer. The average-risk group reflects the general population without any of these hereditary cancer syndromes or mutations. At this point, it is important to distinguish a family history of ovarian cancer from familial hereditary ovarian cancer syndrome, as nearly one-third of women with hereditary ovarian carcinoma have no close relatives with cancer.[7] Also the attributed risks are different; one first-degree relative with ovarian cancer increases the lifetime probability of developing it from 1.4 to 5%,[8] whereas this risk is much higher, up to 46%, in a patient with a BRCA1 mutation.[9,10] These well-established risk factors that are used to modify individual risks are summarized in Table 9.1.

Hereditary Cancer Syndromes

Hereditary cancer syndromes are characterized by multiple affected family members, early age of onset, and the presence of multiple or bilateral primary tumors. The syndromes that pose an increased risk of ovarian cancer deserve special attention, as 24% of all ovarian tumors carry germline loss of function mutations in various genes; 75% of them being BRCA1 and BRCA2.[11] For clarification, the term "hereditary breast ovarian cancer syndrome" in this chapter will reflect the syndrome due to mutations in BRCA1 and BRCA2. The moderate-penetrance genes, including BRIP1, RAD51C, and RAD51D, will be reviewed later in this chapter. This topic solely reviews risk assessment and management of ovarian cancer in hereditary cancer syndromes. Breast-related issues in these individuals are discussed elsewhere.

Hereditary Breast Ovarian Cancer Syndrome Hereditary breast and ovarian cancer syndrome (HBOC) is an autosomal dominant inherited cancer syndrome characterized by germline mutations in one or both of the DNA repair genes, BRCA1 and BRCA2.[12] The population incidence of inherited mutations for BRCA1 is approximately 1 out of 974, and for BRCA2 it is about 1 out of 734.[13] In high-risk populations the carrier frequency increases significantly; it is reported to be 1 in 40 in Ashkenazi Jews.[14] The other high-risk populations include women of Swedish, Hungarian, Icelandic, Dutch, or French-Canadian descent.

The two-hit hypothesis, which was first described by Knudson in the setting of retinoblastoma, has also been suggested to explain the pathogenicity of HBOC, meaning that individuals with HBOC inherit one defective allele in BRCA1 or BRCA2 from one of their parents, and the second allele becomes non-functional later in life due to a somatic mutation.[15] The syndrome shows incomplete penetrance, which means that some individuals will not develop cancer even though they carry the deleterious mutation.

Women with HBOC have a 65 to 74% lifetime risk of breast cancer irrespective of the type of BRCA mutation; however, the risk of ovarian cancer differs significantly depending on the mutation status. Women with a BRCA1 mutation have a 39 to 46% lifetime risk of ovarian cancer, whereas it's 12 to 20% in women with a BRCA2 mutation.[10-12] The prevalence of a BRCA1 mutation in women with ovarian cancer is 4.4%, whereas it is 5.6% for BRCA2.[16] Ovarian cancer associated with these mutations is usually high-grade and histologically the type is either serous or endometrioid; however, these patients also show increased sensitivity to platinum-based chemotherapy as well as to PARP inhibitors, and they exhibit favorable survival rates when compared to sporadic cases.[17,18] Mucinous and borderline ovarian tumors are not part of the BRCA-related ovarian tumor spectrum.[19,20]

Individuals with BRCA2 deleterious mutations also face an increased risk of pancreatic cancer, melanoma, prostate cancer and male breast cancer. The risk of pancreatic cancer is three times higher compared to the general population in these individuals with up to a 7% lifetime risk. The risks of male breast cancer and prostate cancer are estimated to be 1 to 10% and 15 to 25%, respectively.[21] In terms of increased risk of melanoma, three large cohort studies found relative risks ranging between 2.5 to 2.7 in these individuals when compared

TABLE 9.1: Risk factors for ovarian cancer	
Risk Factor	**Relative Risk/Odds Ratio**
No risk factor	1.0
Factors that increase risk	
Infertility[122]	2.7 (95% CI, 1.91–3.74)
Endometriosis[123]	
• Clear cell	• 3.05 (95% CI; 2.43–3.84)
• Endometrioid	• 2.04 (95% CI; 1.67–2.48)
• Low grade serous	• 2.11 (95% CI; 1.39–3.20)
PCOS[124]	2.5 (95% CI; 1.08–5.89)
Cigarette smoking*[125]	2.1 (95% CI; 1.7–2.7)
Talc use (all subtypes)[126]	1.31 (95% CI, 1.24–1.39)
• Serous	−1.32 (95% CI, 1.22–1.43)
• Endometrioid	−1.35 (95% CI, 1.14–1.60)
Obesity (per 5 kg/m² over 22)[127]	1.07 (95% CI; 1.02–1.12)
Hormone replacement therapy	
• Combined[128]	1.55 (95% CI, 1.38–1.74)
• Estrogen only[128]	1.58 (95% CI, 1.39–1.80)
• Ant HT use [112]	1.36 (95% CI, 1.28–1.46)
Family history of ovarian cancer (no gene mutation)	
• One first-degree relative[129]	2.96 (95% CI, 2.35–3.72)
• Two first-degree relatives[130]	27
Factors that decrease risk	
Oral contraceptive use[113]	0.58 (95% CI, 0.49–0.68) (ever used)
	0.26 (05% CI, 0.16–0.43) (greater than 10 years of use)
Tubal ligation (overall)[120]	0.70 (95% CI, 0.60–0.75)
Tubal ligation (by histologic subtype)[112]	
• High-grade serous	• 0.92 (95% CI, 0.76–1.11)
• Clear cell	• 0.35 (95% CI, 0.18–0.69)
• Endometrioid	• 0.60 (95% CI, 0.41–0.88)
Breastfeeding[131]	0.79 (less than 6 months) (95% CI, 0.72–0.87)
	0.72 (6–12 months) (95% CI, 0.64–0.81)
	0.67 (≥ 13 months) (95% CI, 0.56–0.79)
Parity[131]	0.72 (para 1) (95% CI, 0.65–0.79)
	0.57 (para 2) (95% CI, 0.41–0.52)
	0.46 (para ≥ 3) (95% CI, 0.41–0.52)
Aspirin use[132]	0.85 (95% CI, 0.83–0.96) 0.85 (95% CI, 0.83–0.96)

*Increases the risk of mucinous carcinoma only and decreases the risk of clear cell carcinoma (RR 0.6, 95% CI 0.3–0.9). Age is the most significant independent risk factor in the general population.
Data include age, early menarche (< 12 years) or late menopause (> 52 years), nulliparity, infertility, polycystic ovarian syndrome, endometriosis, obesity, genetics, cigarette smoking (mucinous type only), long-standing use of estrogen only hormone replacement therapy (> 10 years).

to the general population.[22-24] Evidence also suggests an increased risk of uterine papillary serous carcinoma in women with a BRCA1 mutation.[25,26]

Non BRCA-Associated Hereditary Breast Ovarian Cancer Syndromes (Moderate Penetrance Genes) Approximately 5% of individuals with hereditary ovarian cancer have mutations in genes other than BRCA1 and BRCA2.[27] These genes are also called "moderate penetrance genes," as they are associated with modest elevated risks for ovarian cancer as opposed to BRCA mutations, which are described as "high penetrance genes" due to their high relative risks.

RAD51 Paralogs The RAD51 family of related genes consist of five paralogs: RAD51B, RAD51C, RAD51D, XRCC2, and XRCC3. They encode strand-transfer proteins that play a role in DNA double-strand break repair via homologous recombination.[28] Among these genes, deleterious mutations in RAD51C and RAD51D were shown to be strongly associated with ovarian cancer.[11,28,29] RAD51C mutation is present in approximately 1% of unselected ovarian cancers and the estimated lifetime risk is approximately 9% in these individuals. The cumulative risk before the age of 50 is low, which is approximately 1% by age 49. The average age of ovarian cancer is approximately 60 years.[30] Although the risk for RAD51D is similar to RAD51C until the age of 50 (1%), it escalates to 14% by age 80.[31]

BRIP1 The BRCA1-interacting protein 1 (*BRIP1*) gene protein, also named the Fanconi anemia group J protein, is bound and forms a complex with BRCA1 protein, which plays an important role in double-strand break repair. It is located on the long arm of chromosome 17 at location 23.2 (17q23.2); loss of function mutations in this gene are shown to be associated with moderately increased risk of ovarian cancer. Estimated lifetime risk ranges from 4 to 13%.[32,33]

There are also some moderate penetrance genes that are implicated in an elevated risk of breast cancer but not ovarian cancer. These include CHECK2, NBN, RAD50, FAM175A, and MRE11A.[27] Although some studies confer an elevated risk of ovarian cancer for ATM and PALB2 mutations, current evidence is insufficient for recommending risk-reducing BSO for these individuals.[34]

Low-Risk Loci Single-nucleotide variants are common in the general population and likely account for most of the unexplained hereditary component of ovarian cancer risk. Currently more than 30 low-penetrance single nucleotide polymorphisms have been identified; each confers 1.2 to 1.4 times the risk for epithelial ovarian cancer.[35] In light of current evidence, even in combination, these variants will not increase the risk significantly; women with the highest number of variants are estimated to have a 2.8% absolute lifetime risk of ovarian cancer.[36] This risk might escalate with the identification of new loci in the future; the greater number of polymorphisms in an individual, the greater the attributed risk might be, as these variants may show additive or synergistic effects.

Lynch Syndrome Lynch syndrome (LS) is an autosomal and dominant inherited cancer syndrome, which is characterized by germline mutations in DNA mismatch repair genes (MLH1-chromosome 3p.22, MSH2 chromosome 2p21, MSH6-chromosome 2p16.3, PMS2-chromosome 7p22.1) or deletions in the *EPCAM* gene (chromosome 2p21). The mismatch repair system maintains genomic integrity by recognizing base-pair mismatches during DNA replication. These mismatches most commonly occur at microsatellites, where certain DNA motifs are repeated typically 5 to 50 times. In the setting of defective mismatch repair system, the microsatellites become more susceptible to mutations leading to expansion or contraction of these regions. This phenomenon is called microsatellite instability, which is a characteristic feature of tumors related to LS. Similar to other hereditary cancer syndromes, patients inherit one defective allele, which is followed by inactivation of the second allele via either somatic mutation, loss of heterozygosity or non-inherited methylation of the MLH1 promoter (epigenetic silencing). Among individuals with identifiable germline mutations in the mismatch repair genes based on tumor testing, the most common mutation is seen in MSH2 (41%), followed by MLH1 (31%), MSH6 (13%), and PMS2 (9%).[37] Deletions in the *EPCAM* gene lead to silencing of neighboring MSH2 via transcriptional read-through, which is the continuation of transcription beyond a normal stop sign due to failure of RNA polymerase to recognize the signal. The patients with EPCAM deletions demonstrate a mosaic pattern instead of full spectrum of the disease, as MSH2 is silenced only in the cells where EPCAM is active.[38]

LS is the most common cause of hereditary colon and endometrial cancers and second most common cause of hereditary ovarian cancer. Based on the available data, the lifetime risk of colon cancer is 18 to 61% and endometrial cancer is 16 to 61%, which are 1.7%, and 2.9%, respectively, in the general population.[39,40] The prevalence of the syndrome ranges between 1 in 600 and 1 in 3,000 individuals.[41,42] In addition to colon, endometrial, and ovarian cancers, others types related to LS include gastric, small bowel, hepatobiliary, renal pelvis, ureter, certain types of breast and brain, and sebaceous skin tumors.[43,44] This section will focus on LS-related ovarian cancer. More detailed information regarding other Lynch-related tumors are discussed separately in other chapters.

The lifetime risk of ovarian cancer in LS ranges from 4 to 24%, which approximates a 4 to 14 times higher risk when compared to the general population (Table 9.2).[44-46] Patients with LS-related ovarian cancer typically present at an early age (the median is 45.3 years, and it ranges from 19 to 82) and mostly with high-grade endometrioid histology (53%) when compared to sporadic cases, who are predominantly a high-grade serous type (70%) and their median age at presentation is 63 years.[47] However, the cumulative incidence rate in women < 35 years of age is low, approximately 6%. There is a trend toward MSH2 mutations resulting in higher cumulative risk of ovarian cancer followed by MLH1, MSH6 and PMS2.[40,45,48] This order might reflect the overall mutation frequencies of *MMR* genes in LS; MSH2 and MLH1 account for 90% of the mutations that have been identified in patients, whereas MSH6 accounts for most of the remainder and PMS2

TABLE 9.2: Lifetime ovarian cancer risk based on mutation type in patients with Lynch Syndrome*	
Mutation type	**Lifetime risk of ovarian cancer**
MLH1	11 to 20%
MSH2	15%
MSH6	1%
PMS2	< 1%

*Screening and management of these patients do not differ by genotype. The overall ovarian cancer risk is very low in Lynch syndrome due to EPCAM deletions as compared with MLH1 or MSH2 mutations.

mutations are the rarest.[37] The age at diagnosis does not significantly differ based on the mutation type.[49,50] LS-related ovarian cancer also has more favorable outcomes (the 5-year overall survival rate is 80%) due to the fact that 65% of patients present at stage 1 disease at initial diagnosis as opposed to sporadic cases, 70% of who present with stage 3 (with a 5-year overall survival rate of 28%).[47] High-grade endometrioid tumors are followed by high-grade serous and mixed tumors with rates of 17% and 11%, respectively.[51] The frequency of clear cell carcinoma is similar to mixed tumors (11%). In a systematic review, endometrioid and clear cell tumors were found to be the most common types.[46] Of note, the incidence of synchronous primary endometrial cancers was reported to be 22% in the literature.[52]

Peutz-Jeghers Syndrome (PJS) PJS is an autosomal dominant condition characterized by mutations in serine/threonine kinase 11 (*STK11*) gene. This gene encodes a member of the serine/threonine kinase family, which regulates cell polarity and acts as a tumor suppressor by promoting apoptosis. It is located on the short arm of chromosome 19 at position 13.3 (19p13.3).[53]

The diagnosis of the syndrome is based on clinical findings that is established with any of the following:[54]

- Two or more histologically confirmed PJS-type hamartomatous polyps
- Any number of PJS-type polyps detected in one individual who has a family history of PJS in at least one close relative
- Characteristic mucocutaneous pigmentation in an individual who has a family history of PJS in at least one close relative
- Any number of PJS-type polyps in an individual who also has characteristic mucocutaneous pigmentation.

Molecular genetic testing is used to confirm the diagnosis. The disease shows 100% penetrance, which means that individuals with pathogenic variants in STK11 have definitely shown clinical manifestations. However, the expressivity is variable; some affected individuals may only have one (e.g., polyps or perioral pigmentation) symptom, while some present with a full clinical picture.

In terms of gynecologic malignancies, females with PJS are at risk for ovarian sex cord stromal tumors (OSCSTs) with annular tubules and adenoma malignum of the cervix. OSCSTs with annuler tubules are mostly multifocal small tumors with focal calcification and typically demonstrate a benign course, as opposed to sporadic ones, which are large, unilateral, and associated with a 20% risk of malignancy.[55] The cumulative risk of developing an OSCST is 21% in patients with PJS, in contrast to the risk of 1.6% in the general population. The mean age at diagnosis is typically around 28.

Adenoma malignum is a rare well-differentiated adenocarcinoma with a cumulative risk of <1% in the general population. This risk increases to 10% in patients with PJS. The mean age at diagnosis ranges from 34 to 40.[55]

DICER1 Syndrome DICER1 syndrome is an autosomal dominant disorder that results from germline mutations in the DICER1 gene, which encodes an enzyme (RNase IIIb) required for microRNA (miRNA) synthesis. miRNAs are non-coding small RNAs that are estimated to regulate the expression of over one-third of protein coding genes typically through translational repression or mRNA degradation.[56] These have been implicated in various biological processes including metabolism, cell proliferation, and apoptosis.[57,58] Altered levels have been linked to several human diseases including cancer.[59]

Patients with deleterious DICER1 mutations are susceptible to develop pleiotropic tumors, including pleuropulmonary blastoma (PPB), cystic nephroma, nasal chondromesenchymal hamartomas, and OSCSTs. PPB is the most common primary lung cancer of childhood; over 70% of individuals with PPB have a germline loss of function mutation with a second, tumor-specific missense mutation in the RNase IIIb domain.[60] Most of the germline loss of function mutations are inherited; however, 10–20% may arise *de novo*.

Despite the fact that PPB is the most common tumor, ovarian neoplasms may be the initial manifestation of the syndrome. Sertoli-leydig cell tumors (SLCTs) and gynandroblastoma are the two most common histologic types, which may be associated with androgenic symptoms, such as virilization and abnormal uterine bleeding.[61] Pure SLCTs are rare; they secrete estrogens and renin, which might lead to hypertension and hypokalemia. Abdominal pain and/or increasing abdominal girth are other common symptoms, as these tumors might grow quite large.

The age distribution of risk for SLCTs and gynandroblastoma in DICER1 syndrome varies widely, with a range from 4 to 61 years in the International Ovarian and Testicular Stromal Tumor Registry. The median age at diagnosis is 16.5 years; 95% of individuals are diagnosed by age 40 years.[60] Germline DICER1 mutations are associated with lower risk of recurrence for Sertoli-Leydig cell tumors when compared to those with bi-allelic tumor-specific mutations; however, these individuals are at increased risk for synchronous and metachronous contralateral tumors.

Another gynecologic malignancy that is associated with DICER1 syndrome is the cervical embryonal rhabdomyosarcoma, a very rare tumor that is mostly seen during teen years (mostly < 25 years).[62] It is typically a botyroid variant that most commonly presents with vaginal bleeding, vaginal pressure, or pain.

■ RISK ASSESSMENT, COUNSELING, AND TESTING

Hereditary Breast Ovarian Cancer Syndrome

Current guidelines from multiple organizations, including National Comprehensive Cancer Network (NCCN),[34] Society of Gynecologic Oncology (SGO),[63] American College of Obstetrics and Gynecology (ACOG),[64] National Society of Genetic Counselors,[65] and American College of Medical Genetics and Genomics[65] recommend genetic counseling for individuals who have a family history of breast or ovarian cancer and for all women with epithelial ovarian cancer, irrespective of age and race. The criteria for referral to genetics across different organizations are quite similar and are summarized in Table 9.3. The U.S. Preventive Services Task Force (USPSTF) has also recommended tools such as the Ontario Family History Assessment Tool, Manchester Scoring System, Referral Screening Tool, Pedigree Assessment Tool, and Family History Screen-7, for non-geneticist healthcare providers to guide referrals to genetic counselors.[66] Although these tools were found to be clinically useful (most sensitivity estimates were > 85%), they all have some limitations and there is insufficient evidence to prefer one to another.

TABLE 9.3: Referral Criteria for Hereditary Breast and Ovarian Cancer

Referral Criteria for Further Genetic Evaluation for Hereditary Breast and Ovarian Cancer

Women affected with any of the following:
- Epithelial ovarian, tubal, or peritoneal cancer
- Breast cancer at age 45 or youngers
- Breast cancer with a close relative[a] with breast cancer $\leq$ 50 years or a close relative[a] with epithelial ovarian/tubal/peritoneal cancer at any age
- Breast cancer $\leq$ 50 years with a limited or unknown family history[b]
- Breast cancer with $\geq$ 2 close relatives[a] with breast cancer at any age
- Breast cancer with $\geq$ 2 close relatives[a] with pancreatic cancer or aggressive prostate cancer (Gleason score $\geq$ 7)
- Two breast cancer primaries, with the first diagnosed prior to age of 50
- Triple negative breast cancer $\leq$ 60 years
- Breast cancer and Ashkenazi Jewish ancestry regardless of age
- Pancreatic cancer with $\geq$ 2 close relatives with breast cancer, ovarian/fallopian tube/peritoneal cancer, pancreatic cancer, or aggressive prostate cancer (Gleason score $\geq$ 7)

Women with no cancer history, but with any of the following:
- A first-degree or several close relatives[a] who meet any of the above criteria
- A close relative[a] with a deleterious BRCA1 or BRCA2 mutation
- A close relative[a] with male breast cancer

[a]Close relative is defined as first-degree (parent, sibling, offspring), second-degree (grandparent, grandchild, uncle, aunt, niece, nephew, half-sibling), or third-degree (first cousin, great-grandparent, or great-grandchild).
[b]Limited family history includes fewer than two first- or second-degree female relatives surviving beyond age 45 years.

Initial risk assessment should begin with a detailed personal and family history, which should include at least the following:

- Personal cancer history: type of cancer and age at onset
- Family cancer history that includes at least first- and second-degree relatives from both maternal and paternal sites: type of cancer, age at onset, known hereditary cancer syndrome (any relative), prior genetic testing (any relative), ethnic background
- Ancestry (European Jewish, French Canadian, Icelandic)

Adoption, presence of few female members, and/or removal of ovaries/fallopian tubes in multiple individuals within the family at a young age may mask the hereditary cancer syndrome. Therefore, the threshold to refer these women to genetic counseling should be low.

After risk assessment, if a suspicion for a hereditary cancer syndrome arises, the discussion for genetic testing should be considered as far as the results will aid in diagnosis and/or management options are available for the patient or family members. Before testing is done, a thorough discussion with the individual should be held, which should include the possible outcomes, limitations of testing, effects of testing on family members, financial considerations and laws regarding genetic discrimination. Test results are categorized in four groups; true positive, true negative, uninformative negative, and variant of uncertain clinical significance.[67] True positive indicates detection of a deleterious mutation in the individual. If the test result is positive, the patient should be informed that first-degree relatives (parents, children, sisters, brothers) each have a 50% chance of having the same mutation. True negative indicates that the test result of the individual is negative in the setting of a pathogenic mutation in the family that has previously been identified. The lifetime risk of developing breast/ovarian cancer in these women is the same as the general population and is modified based on the risk factors in Table 9.1. Uninformative negative result is defined as a negative result for deleterious BRCA1 and/or BRCA2 mutations in the individual in the presence of any of the following below:

- The family is not tested.
- The family is tested and there is no known pathogenic mutation in the family. (A pathogenic variant may be present, but available methods cannot detect it.)
- The family carries a pathogenic BRCA variant; however, it could not be detected due to the limitations of the testing method.
- A high-risk pathogenic mutation might be present in a different gene; therefore, a multi-panel testing would be beneficial, if there is high clinical suspicion for a hereditary syndrome.

The interpretation of the BRCA testing results to counsel patients is summarized in Figure 9.1.

Based on the available data, patients without a BRCA mutation and a personal history of breast cancer are not at increased risk of ovarian cancer.[68,69] Women who have a positive family history of ovarian cancer but no deleterious gene mutation should be managed individually based on family history.

Genetic Testing Options for HBOC Genetic testing options for HBOC include BRCA mutation testing and multi-gene panel testing. Ideally, testing should begin with the proband (affected family member) for identification of mutations in the family.[67] This strategy brings up the opportunity to other family members for targeted testing. If the individual belongs to a certain ethnic group (e.g., Ashkenazi Jews, Icelanders, French Canadians), testing for the founder mutations linked to that ancestry could be performed. If the affected family member is not available, it is still reasonable to test the individual after proper counseling, provided that there is high suspicion for a hereditary cancer syndrome. The U.S. Preventive Task Force recommends screening once individuals have reached the age of consent (18 years). Providers should also periodically assess the individuals for changes in family history and update the risk assessment periodically (at least every 5 to 10 years).[70]

BRCA mutation testing BRCA mutation testing includes four options; single-site testing, multi-site panel testing, comprehensive testing, and *BRCA* gene rearrangement testing.[67] Single-site testing targets one specific mutation that has already been identified within the family. This is also called predictive testing. This option is ideal for women with no personal history of breast or ovarian cancer, and there is a known mutation in the family. Multi-site testing includes the testing of the founder mutations in certain ethnic groups or high-risk families. The well-known examples of these mutations are the ones that have already been established in Ashkenazi Jewish population; 185delAG (also known as 187delAG or c.68_69delAG) and 5382insC (also known as 5385insc or c.5266dupC) in BRCA1, 6174delT (c.5946delT) in BRCA2.[71] Approximately 90% of individuals from Ashkenazi Jewish descent

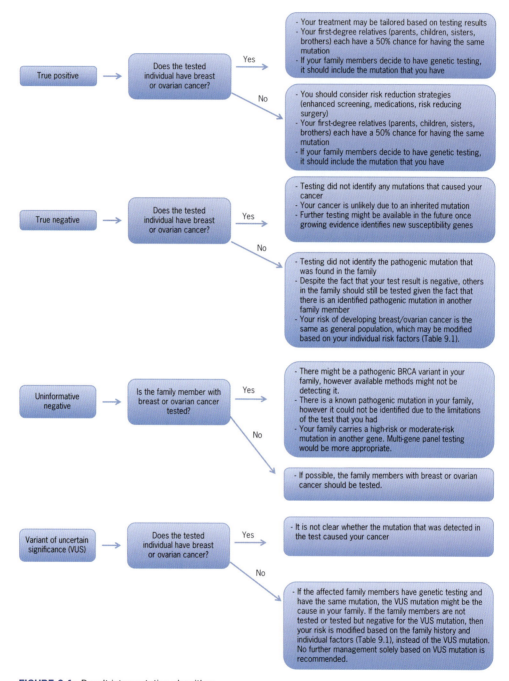

FIGURE 9.1: Result interpretation algorithm.

would have one of these three mutations in the case that they have HBOC.[71,72] There is currently an ongoing debate regarding universal screening versus family history-based selective screening for these high-risk groups. Population-based studies have shown that more than 50% of mutation carriers would have been missed in Ashkenazi Jewish population, if genetic testing is ordered based on family history screening alone.[73] Also, if personal or family history is positive for HBOC-related cancer, 5 to 7% of these individuals have mutations other than BRCA1 and BRCA2.[74,75] Therefore, the risks and benefits of multi-gene panel testing should be discussed with these individuals. Multi-gene testing is also appropriate for women with a limited family history or a family with very few female members.

For individuals with negative multi-site panel testing but still with high suspicion of HBOC, comprehensive testing and rearrangement testing should be considered. In this case scenario, there is always a strong family history; however, the proband is not tested for any reason in the family, so there is no identified mutation that could be used for predictive testing. Comprehensive testing assesses the entire gene sequencing for BRCA1, BRCA2, and the five-site rearrangement panel.[68] The BRCA rearrangement test investigates large-scale rearrangements within the *BRCA* genes that would not have been detected through comprehensive testing. Of note, women, who were tested before 2013 should be considered for re-testing, as there are currently more established pathogenic or likely pathogenic variants for *BRCA* genes.

The other options include next generation whole-exome sequencing (WES), whole-genome sequencing (WGS), and direct-to-consumer BRCA testing. WES identifies protein-coding regions of the genome, which includes approximately 180,000 exons. This constitutes about 1% of the human genome or 30 million base pairs. WGS determines the complete DNA sequence (both coding and non-coding regions) at a single time. Despite the fact that both WES and WGS search the human genome more extensively, they currently do not add more actionable results than multi-gene panel testing.[76] Furthermore, they are expensive and associated with high frequency of Variant of uncertain significance (VUS) results. There are also secondary findings that are unrelated to testing indication.[77] The American College of Medical Genetics and Genomics (ACMG) released a minimum list of genes that should be reported by the clinical laboratory if germline mutations are detected, regardless of the indication of the sequencing test.[78] Therefore WES and WGS are currently not recommended until there is strong evidence of benefit.

Currently the majority of companies in the United States offer panel testing; some only offer well-established high- and moderate-risk gene panel testing, while some do offer panels that assess new, preliminary evidence genes. Panel testing might be the only option in certain laboratories and the costs of these panels might be cheaper than the costs of BRCA-only testing. These tests are especially ideal for individuals with a high suspicion for HBOC and BRCA testing has not identified a pathogenic variant. Women should be counseled regarding increased frequency of VUS results with panel tests. Regarding preliminary evidence gene panels, cancer risk is not well characterized for these genes and there is no guideline from the national organizations for management. Furthermore, the benefits of testing for family members are uncertain for these mutations.

In March 2018, FDA has approved the first direct-to-consumer test to report for BRCA1 and BRCA2 mutations. Direct-to-consumer genetic testing, as a concept, carries many controversies including lack of appropriate pre- and posttest counseling and incomplete assessment of cancer risk due to absence of evaluation for personal and family medical history. Moreover, the test only includes three founder mutations that have been established in Ashkenazi Jewish populations. These mutations are present in approximately 2 to 2.6% of Ashkenazi Jewish women, and approximately 0.1 to 0.2% in other populations.[72,79] It is currently well known that there are more than 1000 known BRCA mutations and many other genes associated with hereditary breast and ovarian cancer; thus, negative tests result will lead to insufficient reassurance in tested individuals. On the other hand, the interpretation of positive test result is also a problem in the setting of incomplete assessment of other risk factors. Based on all these issues, ACOG released a practice advisory that discourages the use of direct-to-consumer testing.

Lynch Syndrome

Identification of high-risk individuals for LS is being assessed in one of two ways:

- Family history-based screening: Amsterdam Criteria was initially introduced in 1990 to identify high-risk individuals for LS based on family history; however, it was soon identified to have many limitations and low sensitivity.[80] One of the major limitations was lack of extra-colonic malignancies in the system, which led to revision of the system in 1999.[81] Despite the revision, it still failed to identify more than half of the total and two-thirds of MSH6 mutation carriers.[40,82,83] Given the limitations of the Amsterdam Criteria, Bethesda guidelines have been developed and subsequently have been revised in 2004 that included more useful clinical information to identify individuals at risk.[84,85] Compared to the Amsterdam Criteria, these guidelines have shown higher sensitivity (sensitivity: 94%, 95% CI 88–100, specificity: 25%, 95% CI 14–36);[86] however, a major problem still persisted; endometrial cancer, which is shown to exceed the risk of colorectal cancer in patients with LS, was still lacking, decreasing the clinical usefulness of these guidelines for referral of high-risk individuals to genetic risk assessment. Therefore, SGO re-revised these criteria by including endometrial cancer as a sentinel cancer, which currently constitutes a useful approach to identify women at risk.[87] Amsterdam II criteria and Bethesda guidelines are shown in Table 9.4.
- Tumor testing with reflex germline testing: Evaluation of protein products of mismatch repair genes in the tumor is relatively inexpensive and currently available through most pathology laboratories in the United States. It is useful for guidance of germline testing under certain situations. If all four proteins are present after testing, then the presence of LS is ruled out in almost all cases. MLH1 loss should be further evaluated for promoter methylation, which is an epigenetic process rather than a germline mutation.[88] If MLH1 is absent, it will result in the absence of PMS2 protein as well, as both proteins exist as a heterodimer in the cell. The only case scenario that does not rule out LS in the setting of all four proteins in existence is the presence of a nonsense mutation in any of the genes that leads to full-length but non-functional protein product. Therefore, reflex germline testing should still be performed, if there is still high clinical suspicion for these individuals.

Another test that is performed on the tumor is microsatellite instability (MSI) testing. Microsatellites are fingerprints of DNA with repetitive sequences of nucleotides that are susceptible to acquiring errors when MMR is defective. These errors cause an inconsistent number of microsatellite nucleotide repeats when compared to normal tissue, which is defined as microsatellite instability. MSI testing is performed via polymerase chain reaction (PCR) to amplify a strand panel of DNA containing nucleotide repeats. The National Cancer Institute (NCI) has designated five microsatellite markers (BAT25, BAT26, D2S123, D5S346, and D17S250) that include two mononucleotide and three dinucleotide repeats. Based on the presence or absence of these markers, MSI testing could be interpreted as one of the following:[85]

TABLE 9.4: Amsterdam II Criteria and Bethesda Guidelines
Amsterdam II Criteria
Three or more relatives with Lynch-related cancer (colorectal, endometrium, small bowel, ureter, renal pelvis) and all of the below
One affected patient should be a first-degree relative of the other two
Two or more successive generations should be affected
Cancer should be diagnosed before the age of 50 at least in one affected relative
Familial adenomatous polyposis should be excluded in colorectal cancer case(s), if any
Tumors should be diagnosed by pathological examination
Bethesda Guidelines (any of the below)
Individuals with endometrial or colorectal cancer diagnosed before age 50
Individuals with endometrial or ovarian cancer with synchronous or metachronous colon or other Lynch-related tumors* at any age
Individuals with colorectal cancer with MSI-H† histology, tumor-infiltrating lymphocytes, peritumoral lymphocytes, Crohn's-like lymphocytic reaction, mucinous-signet ring differentiation, or medullary growth pattern diagnosed before age 60
Individuals with colorectal or endometrial cancer and one or more first-degree relatives§ with Lynch-related tumors; one of the cancers being diagnosed under the age of 50
Individuals with colorectal and endometrial cancer diagnosed at any age with two or more first- or second-degree§ relatives, with Lynch-related tumors, regardless of age

*Lynch-related tumors include colorectal, endometrial, stomach, ovarian, pancreas, ureter and renal pelvis, biliary tract, brain (usually glioblastoma as seen in Turcot syndrome) tumors, sebaceous gland adenomas, and keratoacanthomas in Muir-Torre syndrome, and carcinoma of the small bowel.
†MSI-H: microsatellite instability–high in tumors refers to changes in two or more of the five National Cancer Institute-recommended panels of microsatellite markers.
§First-degree relatives are parents, siblings, and, children. Second-degree relatives are aunts, uncles, nieces, nephews, grandparents, and grandchildren.
Amsterdam II criteria: Modified with permission from Vasen HF, Watson P, Mecklin JP, et al: New clinical criteria for hereditary nonpolyposis colorectal cancer (HNPCC, Lynch syndrome) proposed by the International Collaborative group on HNPCC, Gastroenterology 1999 Jun;116(6):1453-1456.
Bethesda Guidelines: Reproduced with permission from ACOG Practice Bulletin No. 147: *Lynch syndrome, Obstet Gynecol* 2014 Nov;124(5):1042–1054.

- MSI-high: Two or more of the five markers of the core panel show instability. (Currently many labs are using a variety of panels as markers. MSI is also considered high when more than 30% of these markers show instability.)
- MSI-low: One of the five markers of the core panel shows instability (or fewer than 30% of markers show instability if other marker panels are used).
- MSI-stable: None of the markers show instability.

In individuals with evidence of MSI-H or loss of expression of an MMR protein, further evaluation is warranted with reflex germline testing, which is required for the diagnosis of LS.

Knowing the MSI-H status of a solid tumor is clinically useful not only for identification of high-risk individuals for LS, but also for guidance of management, which could incorporate immunotherapy. In 2017, the FDA expanded pembrolizumab approval to include unresectable or metastatic defective MMR and MSI-H solid tumors that have progressed following prior treatment and that have no satisfactory alternatives. Although current NCCN guidelines recommend universal testing of endometrial tumors for defects in a DNA MMR system, there is no recommendation for ovarian tumors at this time. Well-designed clinical trials are needed to assess the impact of immunotherapy on patients with ovarian cancer to make definitive conclusions.

Peutz-Jeghers Syndrome

In large series, 60 to 78% of individuals with PJS had affected relatives and 17 to 40% present as a sporadic case within the family.[89-91] The sporadic cases are caused by *de novo* pathogenic mutations in the *STK11* gene. Referral should be considered for any individual with a personal history of or first-degree relative with;[92]

    (i) $\geq$ 2 histologically confirmed PJ gastrointestinal polyps;

   (ii) $\geq$ 1 PJ gastrointestinal polyp and mucocutanous hyperpigmentation;

  (iii) Ovarian sex cord stromal tumor with annular tubules;

  (iv) Adenoma malignum of the cervix;

   (v) Sertoli cell tumor;

  (vi) Pancreatic cancer and $\geq$ 1 PJ gastrointestinal polyp;

 (vii) Breast cancer and $\geq$ 1 PJ gastrointestinal polyp;

(viii) $\geq$ 1 PJ polyp and a positive family history of PJS.

Although the diagnosis is clinical, identification of a heterozygous pathogenic variant in STK11 by molecular genetic testing also establishes the diagnosis. Molecular testing approaches include single-gene testing, multi-gene testing, and more comprehensive genomic testing.[93] Single-gene testing includes assessment of the entire sequence of STK11 and targeted deletion/duplication analysis. A multi-gene panel includes STK11 and other hereditary cancer syndromes that show overlapping symptoms with PJS. These syndromes and associated genes include juvenile polyposis syndrome (SMAD4, BMPR1A), Cowden syndrome (PTEN), and Carney complex (PRKAR1A), familial adenomatous polyposis (APC), and Lynch syndrome (MLH1, MSH2, MSH6, PMS2). Multi-gene panels could be either laboratory-designed and/or custom phenotype-focused exome analysis that is ordered by the physician. More comprehensive genomic testing (exome or genome sequencing) could be considered when single-gene testing and/or a multi-gene panel fail to confirm a diagnosis. In this case, patients should be informed about increased frequency of VUS results and positive secondary findings that are unrelated to testing indication with the comprehensive test.

If a pathogenic variant in STK11 is identified in an individual, the family members at risk should be tested for that variant and the ones who are positive for the mutation should receive periodic clinical exams and imaging to screen for the manifestations of the disease (e.g., examination of the buccal mucosa and skin of the digits for hyperpigmented macules; upper and lower gastrointestinal endoscopy; mammography; bimanual pelvic examination and pelvic ultrasound). If the pathogenic variant that was detected in the proband cannot be identified in either parent, the two possible scenarios include germline mosaicism in a parent or a *de novo* somatic/germline pathogenic variant in the proband.[94] This is important because the risk to the siblings depends on the genetic status of the parents. Because the disease is inherited in an autosomal dominant way, if a parent is affected, the risk of inheritance to offspring is 50%. In the case of positive germline mosaicism in either parent, the risk is still slightly higher than the general population but subsides significantly when compared to the presence of a STK11 germline pathogenic mutation.[93] The risk to the offspring with a negative family history and no identified STK11 pathogenic variant is unknown. The NCCN recommends surveillance for affected individuals with an annual pelvic exam and pap smear beginning around age 18 to 20. Transvaginal ultrasound may also be considered.[95]

DICER1 Syndrome

Schultz et al. have proposed 15 major and 9 minor indications for DICER1 syndrome testing (Table 9.5). Referral to genetics should be considered for anyone with

- A personal history of at least one major or two minor indications
- One minor indication and a family history of at least one major or one minor indication.[60]

TABLE 9.5: Indications for Genetics Referral/Testing for DICER1[59]
Major Indications
Individuals with
• Pleuropulmonary blastoma (all types)
• Lung cysts during childhood (especially multi-septated, multiple, or bilateral)
• horacic embryonal rhabdomyosarcoma
• Cystic nephroma
• Genito-urinary sarcomas (including undifferentiated sarcomas)
• Ovarian Sertoli-Leydig cell tumors
• Gynandroblastoma
• Cervical or ovarian embryonal rhabdomyosarcoma
• Genito-urinary/gynecologic neuroendocrine tumors
• ultinodular goiter or thyroid cancer in $\geq$ 2 first-degree relatives
• Multinodular goiter or thyroid cancer along with a family history consistent with DICER1 syndrome
• Childhood multinodular goiter or differentiated thyroid cancer
• Pituitary blastoma
• Pineoblastoma
• Ciliary body medulloepithelioma
• Nasal chondromesenchymal hamartoma
Minor Indications
Individuals with
• Lung cyst(s)
• Renal cyst(s)
• Wilms tumor
• Multinodular goiter or differentiated thyroid cancer
• Embryonal rhabdomyosarcoma other than thoracic or gynecologic
• Poorly differentiated neuroendocrine tumor
• Undifferentiated sarcoma
• Macrocephaly
• Consider testing with any childhood cancer in addition to any other minor criteria

Ideally, testing should begin with the proband for identification of mutations in the family. If the proband cannot be tested, it is reasonable to test individuals at risk. Once a pathogenic DICER1 mutation is detected, all first-degree relatives should undergo predictive testing; children less than 7 years of age should be prioritized as they are at greatest risk for PPB. Second- and third-degree relatives should also receive genetic counseling and testing, especially if they have young children.[60]

The preferred method is single-gene testing, which assesses the entire gene sequencing with reflex deletion/duplication analyses. Whenever possible, tumor testing should also be performed concurrently, as the presence of a somatic mutation in the tumor with negative germline testing eliminates the risk of germline inheritance to the offspring. Since there is a 10% of mosaicism rate, testing of the healthy tissue along with the tumor tissue should also be considered, if feasible.

There is currently no surveillance or management guidelines from any of the national organizations for gynecologic manifestations of DICER1 syndrome. Clinicians and family members of the disease should be alert for signs of an abdominal mass, pain or signs of hormone production, such as precocious puberty or virilization that may herald the presence of an ovarian tumor in young girls. Pelvic ultrasounds every 6 to 12 months may be considered starting from childhood and continue at least to age 40, by which time 95% of the Sertoli-Leydig cell tumors and gynandroblastomas are diagnosed.[60]

CLINICAL MANAGEMENT OF PATIENTS AT INCREASED RISK

The management options for individuals at risk for ovarian cancer include screening, chemoprevention, and risk-reducing surgery. The decision regarding when to choose which option, called risk stratification, is extremely important; women with moderate risk would get the most benefit from screening and chemoprevention, while high-risk individuals could be offered preventive surgical strategies at a certain age once benefits of a risk-reducing salpingo-oophorectomy outweigh the risks. To determine the risk category, one of the online risk prediction models, such as BRCAPRO, BODICEA, and QCancer, can be used.[96,97] Traditionally, high risk is defined as a lifetime risk greater than 10%; for moderate- and low-risk methods, these are 3 to 10% and 1 to 2%, respectively. However, it should be noted that all of these online risk prediction models have their own limitations and none of them have been approved by national organizations to guide clinical management decisions in ovarian cancer. Therefore, the thresholds for these risk categories are currently being debated.

Screening

The interest in screening is arising from the fact that survival is related to the stage at diagnosis; it is over 90% in women with stage 1 disease.[98] So far, the two most commonly used screening tools have been the serum Cancer Antigen 125 (CA 125) and pelvic ultrasonography (US). Serum CA 125 values are elevated in approximately 50% of patients with an early stage if ovarian cancer and 80% with an advanced stage.[99] However, its clinical utility is very limited due to the fact that it is also elevated in many benign conditions, such as endometriosis, fibroids, liver disease, inflammatory diseases, and pregnancy. Also, menstrual cycle variations lead to fluctuations of serum levels, which make it less useful in the premenopausal population. In postmenopausal women, its sensitivity is better; however, its positive predictive value is still unacceptably low, which is reported to be around 3%.[100,101]

Pelvic US has also been investigated as a single screening tool in large populations. A prospective cohort study from the University of Kentucky included a total of 46,101 asymptomatic women aged $\geq$ 50 years and women aged $\geq$ 25 years with a documented family history of ovarian cancer.[102] The primary objective was to assess the effects of annual pelvic US on the stage at detection and disease-specific survival of at-risk women. During a median follow-up of 7.9 years (ranging from 9.2 months to 27 years), a total of 71 invasive epithelial ovarian cancers were identified in the screening group; of these 63% (79% type 1 and 58% type 2) were early stage (stage I and II) at diagnosis as opposed to 30% in matched unscreened controls. Also, the disease-specific survival at 5, 10, and 20 years was significantly longer in the screening group (86 $\pm$ 4%, 68 $\pm$ 7%, and 65 $\pm$ 7%, respectively, vs 45 $\pm$ 2%, 31 $\pm$ 2%, and 19 $\pm$ 3%). The sensitivity, specificity, PPV, and NPV of an abnormal screen were 87.2, 98.7, 25, and 99.97%, respectively. Twenty-seven percent of screen-detected malignancies were type I, and 73% were type 2. Although these results are promising, it is difficult to interpret true effects of pelvic US based on this study, as it was not a randomized controlled trial, and the overall incidence rate for ovarian cancer in the screened population was much higher (271 per 100,000) than that of the general population (10.4 per 100,000).[103]

As neither of CA 125 and pelvic US has been noted to be ideal alone, the combination of the two has also been investigated in clinical studies. The largest randomized trial that assessed the utility of CA 125 in combination with transvaginal ultrasound (TVUS) to detect ovarian cancer is the United Kingdom Familial Ovarian Cancer Screening Study (UK-FOCSS), which randomly assigned 202,638 postmenopausal women aged 50 to 74 years to no screening, annual TVUS, or multimodal screening (CA 125 followed by TVUS if CA 125 was abnormal).[104] For the 50,640 women, who were assigned to the multimodal screening arm, an algorithmic guideline (risk of ovarian cancer algorithm or (ROCA) was used. After a median follow-up of 11.1 years, the rates of ovarian cancer were 0.6, 0.7, and 0.7% in no-screening, annual pelvic ultrasound, and multimodal screening groups. Despite the fact that there was a significant stage shift with multi-modal screening (36.1% stage I or II) compared with controls (23.9%), the cumulative ovarian cancer mortality rates were statistically similar during the early years of follow-up (0 to 7 years). However, the survival curves (screening arms vs control arm) began to diverge at around 10 to 12 years from randomization, suggesting a survival benefit beyond 12 years. Therefore, the research committee of this study decided to extend the follow-up period until December 2018 with results of a second mortality analysis expected in the near future.

The stage shift that was seen in UK-FOCSS was also shown in a randomized trial from Japan that included almost 82,467 postmenopausal women, who were assigned into either a screening group (n = 41,688) (annual pelvic US and CA 125 with a cutoff $\geq$ 35 units/mL) or usual care group (n = 40,779).[105] However, there was no decrease in the detection of ovarian cancer at an average follow-up of 9.2 years. Twenty-seven cancers were detected in the 41,688 screened women, whereas 32 were detected in the 40,779 control women. The proportion of stage I ovarian cancer was higher in the screened group (63%) than in the control group (38%), which did not reach statistical significance (P = 0.2285).

The randomized Prostate, Lung, Colorectal, and Ovarian Cancer Screening Trial (PLCO) in the United States evaluated cancer mortality in 68,557 postmenopausal women aged 55 to 74, who were randomly assigned to receive screening with both CA 125 (cutoff $\geq$ 35 units/mL) and TVUS for 4 years followed by CA 125 alone for a further 2 years or usual care from their healthcare provider.[106] During a median follow-up time of 12.4 years, 212 ovarian cancers

(5.7 per 10,000 person-years) were detected in the screening group, whereas there were 176 cases (4.7 per 10,000 person-years) in the usual care group. No difference was found in terms of stage of disease (77% had stage III or IV disease in the screening group vs 78% in the usual care group) and ovarian cancer-related or all-cause mortality. Women in this study were also stratified into average risk (no history of breast or ovarian cancer), moderate risk (one first-degree relative with breast cancer), and high-risk (family history of ovarian cancer, ≥ 2 relatives with breast cancer or personal history of breast cancer) groups; however, screening showed no benefit even in the high-risk group (PPV: 2.8%). Extended follow-up data from this trial up to 19.2 years (median 14.7) also showed there was still no mortality benefit from screening for ovarian cancer with CA-125 and TVUS.[107]

The most important difference of UK-FOCSS from PLCO and Japanese Shizuoka cohort studies was that UK-FOCSS used the ROCA algorithm, while others used a fixed cut-off value of 35 units/mL for CA 125. It was noted that more than half of the screen-detected cancers would have been missed in the multimodal arm of UK-FOCSS, if a predefined cut-off value was used, as CA 125 levels were less than 35 units/mL in these women.

In terms of screening high-risk women, studies focused on shorter screening intervals. A subgroup of high-risk women (n = 4348) in the UK-FOCSS trial underwent multimodal screening sessions every 4 months, including pelvic US and CA 125 interpreted using the ROCA algorithm. Similar to the results in general population, a significant stage shift was observed in the multimodal screening arm (63% stage I-IIIA, compared with 6%) during a median follow-up of 4.8 years.[108] A similar strategy using 3-monthly ROCA was also assessed in high-risk women (n = 3692) in the United States.[109] A total of 19 cancers were detected during the trial; 18 of 19 (prevalent = 4, incident = 6, risk-reducing salpingo-oophorectomy (RRSO) = 9) were detected via screening or risk-reducing salpingo-oophorectomy. Among incident cases, three of six invasive cancers were in the early stage (I/II; 50% vs. 10% historical BRCA1 controls; p = 0.016) and six of nine risk-reducing surgery-related cases were stage I. ROCA caught three of six (50%) incident cases before CA125 exceeded 35 U/mL. Eight of nine patients with stages 0/I/II ovarian cancer were alive at last follow-up (median 6 years).

The distillation of evidence from the aforementioned large cohort studies indicate that there is no proven benefit of ovarian cancer screening in terms of disease related mortality in any of the risk groups. Although there is a potential stage shift, it is still not clear whether this translates into survival benefit. The extended follow-up results of UK-FOCSS are eagerly awaited to clarify this issue. Currently there is no North-American Society that recommends ovarian cancer screening in asymptomatic women, including SGO, USPTFS, NCCN and ACOG. NCCN guidelines indicate that screening with TVUS and CA 125 may be considered at the clinician's discretion starting at age 30 to 35 in women with HBOC who do not elect to undergo a risk-reducing salpingo-oophorectomy.[34] The data also do not support screening for hereditary ovarian cancer syndromes; it again may be considered at the clinician's discretion.

Chemoprevention

It is well known that combined hormonal contraceptives are associated with a decreased risk of ovarian cancer. In a systemic review and meta-analysis that investigated the modifiers of cancer risk in BRCA1 and BRCA2 mutation carriers, risk reduction of ovarian cancer ranged from 33 to 80% in BRCA1 carriers and 58 to 63% in BRCA2 carriers, who used oral contraceptives for more than 1 year.[110] In another meta-analysis, which included a large number of BRCA1 and BRCA2 mutation carriers with (n = 1503) and without (n = 6315) ovarian cancer, the use of oral contraceptives was associated with a 50% reduced risk of ovarian cancer for both BRCA1 (relative risk (RR) 0.51; 95% CI, 0.40–0.65) and BRCA2 (RR 0.52; 95% CI, 0.31–0.87).[111] In an analysis by the Ovarian Cancer Cohort Consortium, which evaluated the effects of hormonal, reproductive, and lifestyle factors on different histologic subtypes of ovarian cancer (3,378 serous, 606 endometrioid, 331 mucinous, 269 clear cell, 1000 other), clear cell (28% risk reduction in users), endometrioid (11% risk reduction), and serous types (18% risk reduction in users) were all shown to have varying degrees of benefit from oral contraceptive use; however, the mucinous type did not have any.[112] The risk reduction was more pronounced with increased duration of use.

A large cohort study from Denmark included all eligible women aged 15 to 49 during 1995 and 2014 to explore the association between hormonal contraceptives (including progestogen types in combined preparations and all progestogen-only products) and ovarian cancer.[113] In this study, women were categorized as never users (no record of being dispensed hormonal contraception), current or recent users (≤1 year after stopping use), or former users (>1 year after stopping use) of different hormonal contraceptives. Compared with never users, current or recent users and former users of any hormonal contraception had decreased risk of ovarian cancer by 42% (RR 0.58; 95% CI, 0.49–0.68) and 23% (RR 0.77, 95% CI, 0.66–0.91), respectively. RRs among current or recent users declined with increasing duration (RR 0.82; 95% CI, 0.59 to 1.12 with ≤ 1 year use, RR 0.26 (0.16 to 0.43) with > 10 years' use). There was little evidence in terms of major differences in risk estimates by tumor type or progestogen content of combined oral contraceptives. Of note, progestogen-only products were not associated with risk reduction.

Based on the available evidence, it is reasonable to recommend combined oral contraceptives for women at high risk for ovarian cancer who wish to avoid pregnancy and opt not to undergo risk-reducing surgery.

Risk-Reducing Surgical Options

Risk-reducing bilateral salpingo-oophorectomy (RRBSO) is currently the gold standard method for ovarian cancer risk reduction in individuals at high risk. RRBSO has been shown to decrease ovarian cancer specific mortality by 80 to 90% and all-cause mortality by 60 to 75% in BRCA mutation carriers.[114,115] Data also suggest that RRBSO combined with a hysterectomy offer overall survival benefits for patients with Lynch syndrome.[116] Current NCCN guidelines recommend women with BRCA1 and BRCA2 mutations undergo RRBSO at age 35 to 40, and 40 to 45, respectively. Women with *BRIP1*, *RAD51C*, and *RAD51D* gene mutations are recommended to undergo surgery at age 45 to 50.[34] The procedure (with hysterectomy) should also be discussed with women with Lynch syndrome who have completed childbearing, usually starting at their early 40s.[34,117]

Preoperative counseling should include reproductive issues, cancer risks at certain ages, degree of protection from ovarian cancer, disadvantages of premature menopause (vasomotor symptoms, sexual dysfunction, osteoporosis, cardiovascular effects, cognitive impairment, increased risk of premature death), hormone replacement therapy, and psychosocial and quality of life issues. Different than BRCA2, BRCA1 mutation carriers are reported to have slightly increased risk of uterine serous cancer, for which risks and benefits of concurrent hysterectomy should also be discussed.[26] The benefits include being able to administer a more simplified hormone replacement therapy, avoidance of systemic progesterone co-administration along with estrogen in patients with breast cancer, and complete removal of cornual fallopian tubes, which eliminates the very small theoretical risk of fallopian tube cancer. The risks of hysterectomy include longer operative time and increased complication rates related to more extensive surgery.

Another issue that should be reviewed is the residual risk of primary peritoneal cancer. In a review from five studies, which included 846 women, the risk has been reported to be 1.7% (ranges from 0.5 to 10.7%).[118] In a large prospective study of 1828 BRCA1/2 carriers, this risk was 4.2% in a 20-year period following the procedure.[119] Currently, no surveillance is recommended for primary peritoneal cancer after RRBSO due to low incidence rates of disease and lack of screening tests with enough sensitivity and positive predictive value.

Due to the evidence indicating that most of the high-grade serous ovarian carcinomas arise from the fallopian tubes, there is increasing interest in bilateral salpingectomy with delayed oophorectomy for women at high-risk of ovarian cancer in order to prevent the consequences of early surgical menopause. Cohort studies so far have been promising in terms of reduced risk of ovarian cancer for average-risk women who had bilateral tubal ligation or bilateral salpingectomy. In a meta-analysis, tubal ligation was associated with a 26 to 30% decrease in ovarian cancer risk in the general population.[120] A nationwide case-control study from Denmark showed that this risk was further decreased by 42% (odds ratio 0.58; 95% CI, 0.36–0.95) if salpingectomy was performed instead of tubal ligation.[121] The results of currently ongoing clinical trials (NCT02321228, NCT01907789) are being awaited in high-risk women to make definitive conclusions. Until that time, salpingectomy alone or with delayed oophorectomy is not the standard of care for risk reduction in these individuals.

References

1. Siegel RL, Miller KD, Jemal A. Cancer statistics, 2017. *CA Cancer J Clin*. 2017;67:7.

2. https://seer.cancer.gov/statfacts/html/ovary.html (accessed on November 19, 2018).

3. Lacey JV, Sherman ME. Ovarian neoplasia. In: Robboy SL, Mutter GL, Prat J, et al. (Eds.), *Robboy's Pathology of the female reproductive tract*, 2nd ed. Oxford: Churchill Livingstone Elsevier; 2009:601.

4. Berek JS, Crum C, Friedlander M. Cancer of the ovary, fallopian tube, and peritoneum. *Int J Gynaecol Obstet*. 2012;119(Suppl. 2):S118.

5. Stewart SL, Wike JM, Foster SL, et al. The incidence of primary fallopian tube cancer in the United States. *Gynecol Oncol*. 2007;107:392.

6. Goodman MT, Shvetsov YB. Rapidly increasing incidence of papillary serous carcinoma of the peritoneum in the United States: fact or artifact? *Int J Cancer*. 2009;124:2231.

7. SGO Clinical Practice Statement: Genetic Testing for Ovarian Cancer. October 2014. https://www.sgo.org/clinical-practice/guidelines/genetic-testing-for-ovarian-cancer.

8. Kerlikowske K, Brown JS, Grady DG. Should women with familial ovarian cancer undergo prophylactic oophorectomy? *Obstet Gynecol*. 1992;80:700.

9. Antoniou A, Pharoah PD, Narod S, et al. Average risks of breast and ovarian cancer associated with BRCA1 or BRCA2 mutations detected in case series unselected for family history: a combined analysis of 22 studies. *Am J Hum Genet*. 2003;72:1117–1130.

10. King MC, Marks JH, Mandell JB. Breast and ovarian cancer risks due to inherited mutations in BRCA1 and BRCA2. New York Breast Cancer Study Group. *Science*. 2003;302:643–646.

11. Walsh T, Casadei S, Lee MK, et al. Mutations in 12 genes for inherited ovarian, fallopian tube, and peritoneal carcinoma identified by massively parallel sequencing. *Proc Natl Acad Sci USA*. 2011;108:18032–18037.

12. Hereditary breast and ovarian cancer syndrome. ACOG Practice Bulletin No. 182. American College of Obstetricians and Gyneoclogists. *Obstet Gynecol*. 2017;130:e110–e126.

13. Antoniou AC, Pharoah PD, McMullan G, et al. A comprehensive model for familial breast cancer incorporating BRCA1, BRCA2 and other genes. *Br J Cancer*. 2002;86:76–83.

14. Whittemore AS, Gong G, Itnyre J. Prevalence and contribution of BRCA1 mutations in breast cancer and ovarian cancer: results from three U.S. population-based case-control studies of ovarian cancer. *Am J Hum Genet*. 1997;60:496–504.

15. Knudson AG Jr. Mutation and cancer: statistical study of retinoblastoma. *Proc Natl Acad Sci USA*. 1971;68:820–823.

16. Nelson HD, Fu R, Goddard K, et al. Risk Assessment, Genetic Counseling, and Genetic Testing for BRCA-Related Cancer: Systematic Review to Update the U.S. Preventive Services Task Force Recommendation. Evidence Synthesis No. 101 (AHRQ Publication No. 12-05164-EF-1). Rockville, MD: Agency for Healthcare Research and Quality; 2013.

17. Norquist B, Wurz KA, Pennil CC, et al. Secondary somatic mutations restoring BRCA1/2 predict chemotherapy resistance in hereditary ovarian carcinomas. *J Clin Oncol*. 2011;29:3008–3015.

18. Moore K, Colombo N, Scambia G, et al. Maintenance olaparib in patients with newly diagnosed sdvanced ovarian cancer. *N Engl J Med*. October 21, 2018.

19. Boyd J, Sonoda Y, Federici MG, et al. Clinicopathologic features of BRCA-linked and sporadic ovarian cancer. *JAMA*. 2000;283:2260–2265.

20. Lakhani SR, Manek S, Penault-Llorca F, et al. Pathology of ovarian cancers in BRCA1 and BRCA2 carriers. *Clin Cancer Res*. 2004;10:2473–2481.

21. Mersch J, Jackson MA, Park M, et al. Cancers associated with BRCA1 and BRCA2 mutations other than breast and ovarian. *Cancer*. 2015;121:269–275.

22. The Breast Cancer Linkage Consortium. Cancer risks in BRCA2 mutation carriers. *J Natl Cancer Inst*. 1999;91:1310–1316.

23. Johannsson O, Loman N, Möller T, et al. Incidence of malignant tumours in relatives of BRCA1 and BRCA2 germline mutation carriers. *Eur J Cancer*. 1999;35:1248–1257.

24. Moran A, O'Hara C, Khan S, et al. Risk of cancer other than breast or ovarian in individuals with BRCA1 and BRCA2 mutations. *Fam Cancer*. 2012;11:235–242.

25. Segev Y, Iqbal J, Lubinski J, et al. The incidence of endometrial cancer in women with BRCA1 and BRCA2 mutations: an international prospective cohort study. *Gynecol Oncol*. 2013;130:127–131.

26. Shu CA, Pike MC, Jotwani AR, et al. Uterine cancer after risk-reducing salpingo-oophorectomy without hysterectomy in women with BRCA mutations. *JAMA Oncol*. 2016;2(11):1434–1440.

27. Norquist BM, Harrell MI, Brady MF, et al. Inherited mutations in women with ovarian carcinoma. *JAMA Oncol*. 2016;2:482–490.

28. Suwaki N, Klare K, Tarsounas M. RAD51 paralogs: roles in DNA damage signalling, recombinational repair and tumorigenesis. *Semin Cell Dev Biol*. 2011;22:898–905.

29. Loveday C, Turnbull C, Ramsay E, et al. Germline mutations in RAD51D confer susceptibility to ovarian cancer. *Nat Genet*. 2011;43:879–882.

30. Sopik V, Akbari MR, Narod SA. Genetic testing for RAD51C mutations: in the clinic and community. *Clin Genet*. 2015;88:303–312.

31. Tung N, Domchek SM, Stadler Z, et al. Counselling framework for moderate-penetrance cancer-susceptibility mutations. *Nat Rev Clin Oncol*. 2016;13:581–588.

32. Rafnar T, Gudbjartsson DF, Sulem P, et al. Mutations in BRIP1 confer high risk of ovarian cancer. *Nat Genet*. 2011;43(11):1104–1107.

33. Ramus SJ, Song H, Dicks E, et al. Germline mutations in the BRIP1, BARD1, PALB2, and NBN genes in women with ovarian cancer. *J Natl Cancer Inst*. 2015 August 27;107(11). pii: djv214.

34. National Comprehensive Cancer Network. Genetic/familial high risk assessment: breast and ovarian. Version 2.2019. NCCN Clinical Practice Guidelines in Oncology. https://www.nccn.org/professionals/physician_gls/pdf/genetics_screening.pdf.

35. Kar SP, Berchuck A, Gayther SA, et al. Common genetic variation and susceptibility to ovarian cancer: current insights and future directions. *Cancer Epidemiol Biomarkers Prev*. 2018;27:395–404.

36. University of Cambridge. Major genetic study identifies 12 new genetic variants for ovarian cancer. https://www.cam.ac.uk/research/news/major-genetic-study-identifies-12-new-genetic-variants-for-ovarian-cancer. Retrieved November 27, 2018.

37. Moreira L, Balaguer F, Lindor N, et al. Identification of Lynch syndrome among patients with colorectal cancer. *JAMA*. 2012;308:1555–1565.

38. Kempers MJ, Kuiper RP, Ockeloen CW, et al. Risk of colorectal and endometrial cancers in EPCAM deletion-positive Lynch syndrome: a cohort study. *Lancet. Oncol*. 2011;12:49–55.

39. Meyer LA, Broaddus RR, Lu KH. Endometrial cancer and Lynch syndrome: clinical and pathologic considerations. *Cancer Control*. 2009;16:14–22. Review.

40. Barrow E, Hill J, Evans DG. Cancer risk in Lynch syndrome. *Fam Cancer*. 2013;12:229–240.

41. Dunlop MG, Farrington SM, Nicholl I, et al. Population carrier frequency of hMSH2 and hMLH1 mutations. *Br J Cancer*. 2000;83:1643–1645.

42. De la Chapelle A. The incidence of Lynch syndrome. *Fam Cancer*. 2005;4:233–237.

43. Watson P, Vasen HF, Mecklin JP, et al. The risk of extra-colonic, extra-endometrial cancer in the Lynch syndrome. *Int J Cancer*. 2008;123:444–449.

44. Win AK, Lindor NM, Young JP. Risks of primary extracolonic cancers following colorectal cancer in Lynch syndrome. *J Natl Cancer Inst*. 2012;104:1363–1372.

45. Bonadona V, Bonaïti B, Olschwang S, et al. Cancer risks associated with germline mutations in MLH1, MSH2, and MSH6 genes in Lynch syndrome. *JAMA*. 2011;305:2304–2310.

46. Aarnio M, Sankila R, Pukkala E, et al. Cancer risk in mutation carriers of DNA-mismatch-repair genes. *Int J Cancer*. 1999;8:214–218.

47. Helder-Woolderink JM, Blok EA, Vasen HF, et al. Ovarian cancer in Lynch syndrome; a systematic review. *Eur J Cancer*. 2016;55:65–73.

48. Vasen HF, Stormorken A, Menko FH, et al. MSH2 mutation carriers are at higher risk of cancer than MLH1 mutation carriers: a study of hereditary nonpolyposis colorectal cancer families. *J Clin Oncol*. 2001;19:4074–4080.

49. Hampel H, Stephans JA, Pukkala E, et al. Cancer risk in hereditary nonpolyposis colorectal cancer syndrome: later age of onset. *Gastroenterology*. 2005;129:415–421.

50. Ketabi Z, Bartuma K, Bernstein I, et al. Ovarian cancer linked to Lynch syndrome typically presents as early-onset, non-serous epithelial tumors. *Gynecol Oncol*. 2011;121:462–465.

51. Ryan NAJ, Evans DG, Green K, et al. Pathological features and clinical behavior of Lynch syndrome-associated ovarian cancer. *Gynecol Oncol*. 2017;144:491–495.

52. Watson P, Butzow R, Lynch HT, et al. The clinical features of ovarian cancer in hereditary nonpolyposis colorectal cancer. International Collaborative Group on HNPCC. *Gynecol Oncol*. 2001;82:223–228.

53. Jenne DE, Reimann H, Nezu J, et al. Peutz-Jeghers syndrome is caused by mutations in a novel serine threonine kinase. *Nat Genet*. 1998;18:38–43.

54. McGarrity TJ, Amos CI, Baker MJ. Peutz-Jeghers syndrome in Gene Reviews' [Internet], Adam MP, Ardinger HH, Pagon RA, et al. eds. Seattle: University of Washington; 1993–2018.

55. Young RH. Sex cord-stromal tumors of the ovary and testis: their similarities and differences with consideration of selected problems. *Mod Pathol*. 2005;Suppl. 2:S81–98. Review.

56. Carthew RW. Gene regulation by microRNAs. *Curr Opin Genet Dev*. 2006;16:203e8.

57. Stadler BM, Ruohola-Baker H. Small RNAs: keeping stem cells in line. *Cell*. 2008;132:563e6.

58. Stefani G, Slack FJ. Small non-coding RNAs in animal development. *Nat Rev Mol Cell Biol*. 2008;9:219e30.

59. Kumar MS, Lu J, Mercer KL, et al. Impaired microRNA processing enhances cellular transformation and tumorigenesis. *Nat Genet*. 2007;39:673e7.

60. Schultz KAP, Williams GM, Kamihara J, et al. DICER1 and associated conditions: identification of at-risk individuals and recommended surveillance strategies. *Clin Cancer Res*. 2018;24:2251–2261.

61. Heravi-Moussavi A, Anglesio MS, Cheng SW, et al. Recurrent somatic DICER1 mutations in nonepithelial ovarian cancers. *N Engl J Med.* 2012;366:234–242.

62. Dehner LP, Jarzembowski JA, Hill DA. Embryonal rhabdomyosarcoma of the uterine cervix: a report of 14 cases and a discussion of its unusual clinicopathological associations. *Mod Pathol.* 2012;25:602–614.

63. Lancaster JM, Powell CB, Chen LM, et al. Society of Gynecologic Oncology statement on risk assessment for inherited gynecologic cancer predispositions. SGO Clinical Practice Committee. *Gynecol Oncol.* 2015;136:3–7.

64. American College of Obstetricians and Gynecologists, Committee on Practice Bulletins–Gynecology, Committee on Genetics, Society of Gynecologic Oncology. Practice Bulletin No 182: Hereditary Breast and Ovarian Cancer Syndrome. *Obstet Gynecol.* 2017;130:e110–e126.

65. Hampel H, Bennett RL, Buchanan A, et al.; Guideline Development Group, American College of Medical Genetics and Genomics Professional Practice and Guidelines Committee and National Society of Genetic Counselors Practice Guidelines Committee. A practice guideline from the American College of Medical Genetics and Genomics and the National Society of Genetic Counselors: referral indications for cancer predisposition assessment. *Genet Med.* 2015;17:70–87.

66. Moyer VA; U.S. Preventive Services Task Force. Risk assessment, genetic counseling, and genetic testing for BRCA-related cancer in women: U.S. Preventive Services Task Force recommendation statement. *Ann Intern Med.* 2014;160:271–281.

67. Nelson HD, Fu R, Goddard K, et al. Risk assessment, genetic counseling, and genetic testing for BRCA-related cancer: systematic review to update the U.S. Preventive Services Task Force recommendation. Evidence Synthesis No. 101. AHRQ Publication No. 12-05164-EF-1. Rockville (MD): Agency for Healthcare Research and Quality; 2013.

68. Kauff ND, Mitra N, Robson ME, et al. Risk of ovarian cancer in BRCA1 and BRCA2 mutation-negative hereditary breast cancer families. *J Natl Cancer Inst.* 2005;97:1382–1384.

69. Ingham SL, Warwick J, Buchan I, et al. Ovarian cancer among 8,005 women from a breast cancer family history clinic: no increased risk of invasive ovarian cancer in families testing negative for BRCA1 and BRCA2. *J Med Genet.* 2013;50:368–372.

70. US Preventive Services Task Force, Owens DK, Davidson KW, Krist AH, et al. Risk Assessment, Genetic Counseling, and Genetic Testing for BRCA-Related Cancer: US Preventive Services Task Force Recommendation Statement. *JAMA.* 2019;322(7):652–665.

71. Frank TS, Deffenbaugh AM, Reid JE, et al. Clinical characteristics of individuals with germline mutations in BRCA1 and BRCA2: analysis of 10,000 individuals. *J Clin Oncol.* 2002;20:1480–1490.

72. Roa BB, Boyd AA, Volcik K, et al. Ashkenazi Jewish population frequencies for common mutations in BRCA1 and BRCA2. *Nat Genet.* 1996;14:185–187.

73. Gabai-Kapara E, Lahad A, Kaufman B, et al. Population-based screening for breast and ovarian cancer risk due to BRCA1 and BRCA2. *Proc Natl Acad Sci USA.* 2014;111:14205–14210.

74. Rosenthal E, Moyes K, Arnell C, et al. Incidence of BRCA1 and BRCA2 non-founder mutations in patients of Ashkenazi Jewish ancestry. *Breast Cancer Res Treat.* 2015;149:223–227.

75. Kauff ND, Perez-Segura P, Robson ME, et al. Incidence of non-founder BRCA1 and BRCA2 mutations in high risk Ashkenazi breast and ovarian cancer families. *J Med Genet.* 2002;39:611–614.

76. Foley SB, Rios JJ, Mgbemena VE, et al. Use of whole genome sequencing for diagnosis and discovery in the cancer genetics clinic. *EBioMedicine.* 2015;2:74–81.

77. Facio FM, Lee K, O'Daniel JM. A genetic counselor's guide to using next-generation sequencing in clinical practice. *J Genet Couns.* 2014;23:455–462.

78. Green RC, Berg JS, Grody WW, et al. ACMG recommendations for reporting of incidental findings in clinical exome and genome sequencing. *Genet Med.* 2013;15:565–574.

79. Ferla R, Calò V, Cascio S, et al. Founder mutations in BRCA1 and BRCA2 genes. *Ann Oncol.* 2007;18(Suppl. 6): vi93–98.

80. Vasen HF, Mecklin JP, Khan PM, et al. The International Collaborative Group on Hereditary Non-Polyposis Colorectal Cancer (ICG-HNPCC). *Dis Colon Rectum.* 1991;34(5):424–425.

81. Vasen HF, Watson P, Mecklin JP, et al. New clinical criteria for hereditary nonpolyposis colorectal cancer (HNPCC, Lynch syndrome) proposed by the International Collaborative Group on HNPCC. *Gastroenterology.* 1999;116:1453–1456.

82. Barnetson RA, Tenesa A, Farrington SM, et al. Identification and survival of carriers of mutations in DNA mismatch-repair genes in colon cancer. *N Engl J Med.* 2006;354:2751–2763.

83. Plaschke J, Engel C, Krüger S, et al. Lower incidence of colorectal cancer and later age of disease onset in 27 families with pathogenic MSH6 germline mutations compared with families with MLH1 or MSH2 mutations: the German Hereditary Nonpolyposis Colorectal Cancer Consortium. *J Clin Oncol.* 2004;22:4486–4494.

84. Rodriguez-Bigas MA, Boland CR, Hamilton SR, et al. A National Cancer Institute Workshop on Hereditary Nonpolyposis Colorectal Cancer Syndrome: meeting highlights and Bethesda guidelines. *J Natl Cancer Inst.* 1997;89:1758–1762.

85. Umar A, Boland CR, Terdiman JP, et al. Revised Bethesda Guidelines for hereditary nonpolyposis colorectal cancer (Lynch syndrome) and microsatellite instability. *J Natl Cancer Inst.* 2004;96:261–268.

86. Syngal S, Fox EA, Eng C, et al. Sensitivity and specificity of clinical criteria for hereditary non-polyposis colorectal cancer associated mutations in MSH2 and MLH1. *J Med Genet.* 2000;37:641–645.

87. Lancaster JM, Powell CB, Kauff ND, et al. Society of Gynecologic Oncologists Education Committee statement on risk assessment for inherited gynecologic cancer predispositions. *Gynecol Oncol.* 2007;107:159–162.

88. Herman JG, Umar A, Polyak K, et al. Incidence and functional consequences of hMLH1 promoter hypermethylation in colorectal carcinoma. *Proc Natl Acad Sci USA.* 1998;95:6870–6875.

89. Lim W, Olschwang S, Keller JJ, et al. Relative frequency and morphology of cancers in STK11 mutation carriers. *Gastroenterology.* 2004;126:1788–1794.

90. van Lier MG, Wagner A, Mathus-Vliegen EMH, et al. High cancer risk in Peutz-Jeghers syndrome: A systematic review and surveillance recommendations. *Am J Gastroenterol.* 2010;105:1258–1264.

91. Resta N, Pierannunzio D, Lenato GM, et al. Cancer risk associated with STK11/LKB1 germline mutations in Peutz-Jeghers syndrome patients: results of an Italian multicenter study. *Dig Liver Dis.* 2013;45:606–611.

92. Hampel H, Bennett RL, Buchanan A, et al.; Guideline Development Group, American College of Medical Genetics and Genomics Professional Practice and Guidelines Committee and National Society of Genetic Counselors Practice Guidelines Committee. A practice guideline from the American College of Medical Genetics and Genomics and the National Society of Genetic Counselors: referral indications for cancer predisposition assessment. *Genet Med.* 2015;17:70–87.

93. McGarrity TJ, Amos CI, Baker MJ. Peutz-Jeghers syndrome. In Adam MP, Ardinger HH, Pagon RA, Wallace SE, Bean LJH, Stephens K, Amemiya A (eds.). GeneReviews® [Internet]. Seattle: University of Washington, 1993–2018.

94. Hernan I, Roig I, Martin B, et al. De novo germline mutation in the serine-threonine kinase STK11/LKB1 gene associated with Peutz-Jeghers syndrome. *Clin Genet.* 2004;66:58–62.

95. National Comprehensive Cancer Network. Genetic/familial high risk assessment: colorectal. Version 1.2018. NCCN Clinical Practice Guidelines in Oncology. https://www.nccn.org/professionals/physician_gls/pdf/genetics_colon.pdf.

96. Chiang PP, Glance D, Walker J, et al. Implementing a QCancer risk tool into general practice consultations: an exploratory study using simulated consultations with Australian general practitioners. *Br J Cancer.* 2015;112(Suppl. 1):S77–83.

97. Parmigiani G, Chen S, Iversen ES Jr., et al. Validity of models for predicting BRCA1 and BRCA2 mutations. *Ann Intern Med.* 2007;147:441–450.

98. Barnholtz-Sloan JS, Schwartz AG, Qureshi F, et al. Ovarian cancer: changes in patterns at diagnosis and relative survival over the last three decades. *Am J Obstet Gynecol.* 2003;189:1120–1127.

99. Carlson KJ, Skates SJ, Singer DE. Screening for ovarian cancer. *Ann Intern Med.* 1994;121:124–132.

100. Einhorn N, Sjövall K, Knapp RC, et al. Prospective evaluation of serum CA 125 levels for early detection of ovarian cancer. *Obstet Gynecol.* 1992;80:14–18.

101. Jacobs I, Davies AP, Bridges J, et al. Prevalence screening for ovarian cancer in postmenopausal women by CA 125 measurement and ultrasonography. *BMJ.* 1993;306:1030–1034.

102. van Nagell JR Jr., Burgess BT, Miller RW, et al. Survival of women with type I and II epithelial ovarian cancer detected by ultrasound screening. *Obstet Gynecol.* October 5, 2018. [Epub ahead of print]

103. State cancer profiles, quick profiles: Kentucky. Available at: https://statecancerprofiles.cancer.gov/quickprofiles/indexphp?statename=Kentucky.

104. Jacobs IJ, Menon U, Ryan A, et al. Ovarian cancer screening and mortality in the UK Collaborative Trial of Ovarian Cancer Screening (UKCTOCS): a randomised controlled trial. *Lancet.* 2016;387:945–956.

105. Kobayashi H, Yamada Y, Sado T, et al. A randomized study of screening for ovarian cancer: a multicenter study in Japan. *Int J Gynecol Cancer.* 2008;18:414–420.

106. Buys SS, Partridge E, Black A, et al. Effect of screening on ovarian cancer mortality: the Prostate, Lung, Colorectal and Ovarian (PLCO) Cancer Screening Randomized Controlled Trial. *JAMA.* 2011;305:2295–2303.

107. Pinsky PF, Yu K, Kramer BS, et al. Extended mortality results for ovarian cancer screening in the PLCO trial with median 15 years follow-up. *Gynecol Oncol.* 2016;143:270–275.

108. Rosenthal AN, Fraser LSM, Philpott S, et al. Evidence of stage shift in women diagnosed with ovarian cancer during phase II of the United Kingdom Familial Ovarian Cancer Screening Study. *J Clin Oncol.* 2017;35:1411–1420.

109. Skates SJ, Greene MH, Buys SS, et al. Early detection of ovarian cancer using the risk of ovarian cancer algorithm with frequent CA125 testing in women at increased familial risk: combined results from two screening trials. *Clin Cancer Res.* 2017;23:3628–3637.

110. Friebel TM, Domchek SM, Rebbeck TR. Modifiers of cancer risk in BRCA1 and BRCA2 mutation carriers: systematic review and meta-analysis. *J Natl Cancer Inst.* 2014 June;106(6):dju091.

111. Iodice S, Barile M, Rotmensz N, et al. Oral contraceptive use and breast or ovarian cancer risk in BRCA1/2 carriers: a meta-analysis. *Eur J Cancer.* 2010;46:2275–2284.

112. Wentzensen N, Poole EM, Trabert B, et al. Ovarian cancer risk factors by histologic subtype: an analysis from the Ovarian Cancer Cohort Consortium. *J Clin Oncol.* 2016;34:2888–2898.

113. Iversen L, Fielding S, Lidegaard Ø, et al. Association between contemporary hormonal contraception and ovarian cancer in women of reproductive age in Denmark: prospective, nationwide cohort study. *BMJ.* 2018 Sept. 26;362:k3609.

114. Domchek SM, Friebel TM, Singer CF, et al. Association of risk-reducing surgery in BRCA1 or BRCA2 mutation carriers with cancer risk and mortality. *JAMA.* 2010;304:967–975.

115. Finch AP, Lubinski J, Møller P, et al. Impact of oophorectomy on cancer incidence and mortality in women with a BRCA1 or BRCA2 mutation. *J Clin Oncol.* 2014;32:1547–1553.

116. Schmeler KM, Lynch HT, Chen LM, et al. Prophylactic surgery to reduce the risk of gynecologic cancers in the Lynch syndrome. *N Engl J Med.* 2006;354:261–269.

117. Committee on Practice Bulletins-Gynecology; Society of Gynecologic Oncology. ACOG Practice Bulletin No. 147: Lynch syndrome. *Obstet Gynecol.* 2014;124:1042–1054.

118. Dowdy SC, Stefanek M, Hartmann LC. Surgical risk reduction: prophylactic salpingo-oophorectomy and prophylactic mastectomy. *Am J Obstet Gynecol.* 2004;191:1113–1123.

119. Finch A, Beiner M, Lubinski J, et al. Salpingo-oophorectomy and the risk of ovarian, fallopian tube, and peritoneal cancers in women with a BRCA1 or BRCA2 Mutation. *JAMA.* 2006;296:185–192.

120. Rice MS, Murphy MA, Tworoger SS. Tubal ligation, hysterectomy and ovarian cancer: a meta-analysis. *J Ovarian Res.* 2012;5:13.

121. Madsen C, Baandrup L, Dehlendorff C, et al. Tubal ligation and salpingectomy and the risk of epithelial ovarian cancer and borderline ovarian tumors: a nationwide case-control study. *Acta Obstet Gynecol Scand.* 2015;94:86–94.

122. Ness RB, Cramer DW, Goodman MT, et al. Infertility, fertility drugs, and ovarian cancer: a pooled analysis of case-control studies. *Am J Epidemiol.* 2002;155:217–224.

123. Pearce CL, Templeman C, Rossing MA, et al. Association between endometriosis and risk of histological subtypes of ovarian cancer: a pooled analysis of case-control studies. *Lancet Oncol.* 2012;13:385–394.

124. Chittenden BG, Fullerton G, Maheshwari A, et al. Polycystic ovary syndrome and the risk of gynaecological cancer: a systematic review. *Reprod Biomed Online.* 2009 Sept.;19(3):398–405.

125. Jordan SJ, Whiteman DC, Purdie DM, et al. Does smoking increase risk of ovarian cancer? A systematic review. *Gynecol Oncol.* 2006;103:1122–1129.

126. Penninkilampi R, Eslick GD. Perineal talc use and ovarian cancer: a systematic review and meta-analysis. *Epidemiology.* 2018;29:41–49.

127. Bhaskaran K, Douglas I, Forbes H, et al. Body-mass index and risk of 22 specific cancers: a population-based cohort study of 5.24 million UK adults. *Lancet.* 2014;384:755–765.

128. Collaborative Group on Epidemiological Studies of Ovarian Cancer, Beral V, Gaitskell K, Hermon C, et al. Menopausal hormone use and ovarian cancer risk: individual participant meta-analysis of 52 epidemiological studies. *Lancet.* 2015;385:1835–1842.

129. Jervis S, Song H, Lee A, et al. Ovarian cancer familial relative risks by tumour subtypes and by known ovarian cancer genetic susceptibility variants. *J Med Genet.* 2014;51:108–113.

130. Foulkes WD, Narod SA. Ovarian cancer risk and family history. *Lancet.* 1997;349:878.

131. Sung HK, Ma SH, Choi JY, et al. The effect of breastfeeding duration and parity on the risk of epithelial ovarian cancer: a systematic review and meta-analysis. *J Prev Med Public Health.* 2016;49:349–366.

132. Burn J, Gerdes AM, Macrae F, et al. Long-term effect of aspirin on cancer risk in carriers of hereditary colorectal cancer: an analysis from the CAPP2 randomised controlled trial. *Lancet.* 2011;378:2081–2087.

CHAPTER 10

Pancreatic Cancer Genetics

Ankit Chhoda, Stephanie Sun, and James J. Farrell

▓ INTRODUCTION

Pancreatic cancer (PC) is a relatively uncommon cancer with a disproportionately high mortality rate. The majority of PC cases involve exocrine pancreatic tissue (93%), while the others involve hormone-producing cells (7%).[1]

In this chapter the discussion of PC will refer to pancreatic ductal adenocarcinoma (PDAC), which is the predominant exocrine pancreatic neoplasm, with particular emphasis on inherited pancreatic cancers. Most PCs are sporadic and account for 90% of the cases.[2] The remainder of cases have inherited risk factors, including known genetic susceptibility or familial risk factors.[3] We outline the PC epidemiology, their molecular and pathological characteristics, associated risk factors, and management strategies for individuals at risk including screening them for target pathology and treatment based on malignant risk. The implications of PC genetics in the therapy of PC will also be reviewed in this chapter.

Pancreatic Cancer Epidemiology

Recent cancer statistics estimate that in 2019 there were 56,770 new cases of PC in the United States, which accounts for only 3.2% of all incident cancers (1,762,450) recorded.[4]

This is in comparison to 145,600 incident cases of colorectal cancer (8.2% of all incident cancers) or 271,270 new cases of breast cancer (15.4% of all incident cancers). PC is the third leading cause of cancer-related deaths in 2019 and is projected to be the cause of 45,750 deaths in 2019 (10.9 deaths per 100,000 people), which represents 7.54% of all cancer-related deaths projected for 2019 in the United States (606,880).[4]

Survival Relative survival statistics are utilized to calculate the survival of an individual with PC as compared to an individual in the general population of the same age, race, and sex. The 5-year relative survival rate of PC is among the lowest of all cancers at just 9%.[4] In contrast, the 5-year relative survival for all stages of prostate cancer combined is 99%; it is 92% for skin melanoma and 90% for female breast cancer. The survival rate of PC is much lower even when compared to other high-mortality cancers, such as lung (18% for the 5-year relative survival rate). Like most cancers, PC has a variable prognosis based on its stage at diagnosis. It has a relative 5-year survival rate of 34% among lesions localized to the primary site, as compared to the stages of nodal spread (11%) and distant metastasis (2.7%). Almost one-third (29%) of patients diagnosed with PC have regional spread at time of diagnosis, and 52% of patients diagnosed already have distant metastases. The survival rate is diminished given that the majority of cases are diagnosed in advanced stages.[5] The survival rate of any cancer is determined by early diagnosis of precancerous and less advanced stages, as well as the efficacy of curative interventions (including either surgical resection and/or chemotherapy, including targeted therapy). While survival rates have generally improved for most cancers since the mid-1970s due to improved treatment and earlier detection, they have not increased in PC patients. As will be discussed later in this chapter, the lack of significant improvement in PC survival rates is related to challenges of earlier detection and limited effective treatments. While interest is growing in modalities to enable screening and earlier detection, early diagnosis without effective treatment is unlikely to truly improve survival and may reflect lead time bias. Hence, reported survival rates of PC, though often an outcome parameter in clinical trials for various treatment modalities, may not truly represent the PC burden.[6] From a clinicopathologic standpoint, no significant difference in histological subtype, patient age, tumor size, tumor location, peripheral invasion, angiolymphatic invasion, lymph node metastasis, or pathological stage is observed when comparing sporadic (n = 651) and familial pancreatic cancer (n = 519).[7] The survival among individuals with familial or genetic risk factors who develop pancreatic cancer while undergoing surveillance is discussed later in the chapter.

Pancreatic Cancer Incidence and Future Trends

The burden of PC can be accurately represented through trends of cancer incidence and mortality. According to SEER statistics, the median age of incidence is 70 (ranges from 65 to 74).[8] Changes in the demographics of the U.S. population, treatment advances, and improved screening and diagnosis will alter trends in cancer incidence and mortality. The cancer incidence rate is defined as the number of new cases per 100,000 people. The incidence of PC is expected to rise in tandem with a growing population of individuals aged 60 and upward. Rahib et al. describe a delay-adjusted average annual percentage change (AAPC) in pancreatic (0.5), thyroid (0.5), and liver (1.9) cancers, in contrast to colorectal, breast, prostate, and lung cancer.[9] The mortality rate of PCs has remained relatively stable since the 1970s. The AAPC of PC from 2006 to 2015 was 0.3 (p < 0.5) for men and 0 for women. In contrast, the AAPC for all cancers overall from 2006 to 2015 was–1.5, representing a general trend of decreasing cancer mortality. PC is progressing to be the second leading cause of cancer-related death by 2030 and warrants significant attention. The Recalcitrant Cancer Research Act signed by President Obama in 2013 further reinforces "scientific frameworks" within the National Cancer Institute (NCI) for pancreas, lung, and other "recalcitrant cancers," which are defined as cancers with survival rates of less than 50%.[10] These scientific frameworks strategize basic, translational, and clinical methods for early diagnosis and treatment for PC.

▓ HISTOPATHOLOGY AND MOLECULAR PROGRESSION

Advances in the molecular basis of pancreatic neoplasms have resulted in a new classification that incorporates molecular characteristics of tumors with their pathological findings. This classification not only enables familial aggregation but also has implications for early detection and personalized therapies for patients.

Ductal Adenocarcinoma

Pancreatic ductal adenocarcinoma (PDAC) is the most common pancreatic neoplasm and results in the highest fatality among solid malignancies. On gross appearance, they form poorly demarcated, firm whitish-yellow masses with associated atrophy.[11] They generally lack well-defined margins, may have central degeneration or cystic change, and are associated with fibrosis of non-neoplastic pancreas. The cancer cells tend to invade the ductal system, and when they occur in the head region, result in the obstruction of the pancreatic duct and biliary, resulting in classical radiologic "double duct" sign. Alternatively, cancer in the tail region leads only to involvement of the pancreatic duct while the bile duct remains unaffected. Significant extrinsic obstructive changes to the pancreatic ductal system may mimic intrapapillary mucinous neoplasms or ductal ectasias. Microscopically, their appearance ranges from a well-differentiated duct to poorly differentiated carcinomas with epithelial differentiation demonstrable only through immunolabeling. A well-differentiated architecture may prevent its differentiation cytologically from chronic pancreatitis. However, certain characteristics including heterogeneous nuclei, histologic disarray, invasion into connective tissue, and perineural and vascular space enables differentiation of PDAC from CP with certainty.[12,13] The neoplastic proliferation within the PDACs is associated with characteristic stromal reaction or desmoplasia, comprising a mixture of dense collagen, fibroblasts, delicate vessels, and inflammatory cells.[13,14] This desmoplastic response results in extensive fibrosis within the pancreatic tissue and can even outnumber the neoplastic pancreatic gland. The desmoplasia of PDAC results in resistance to chemotherapeutic agents and has been the subject of ongoing research with implications for both early diagnosis and treatment. For example, SPARC (secreted protein acidic and rich in cysteine) or osteonectin, is overexpressed and has been targeted by the albuminized form of taxol, nab-pacilitaxel (Figures 10.1 and 10.2).[15]

Precursor Lesions Precursor or precancerous lesions undergo malignant transformation into ductal adenocarcinomas. They have been defined by an NCI-sponsored consensus conference and the definition criteria are listed as following:

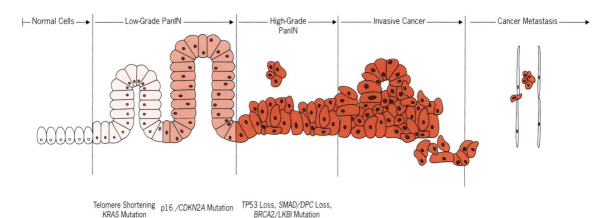

FIGURE 10.1: PDAC progression model (Reproduced with permission from Chhoda A, Lu L, Clerkin BM, et al: Current Approaches to Pancreatic Cancer Screening, Am J Pathol 2019 Jan;189(1):22-35).

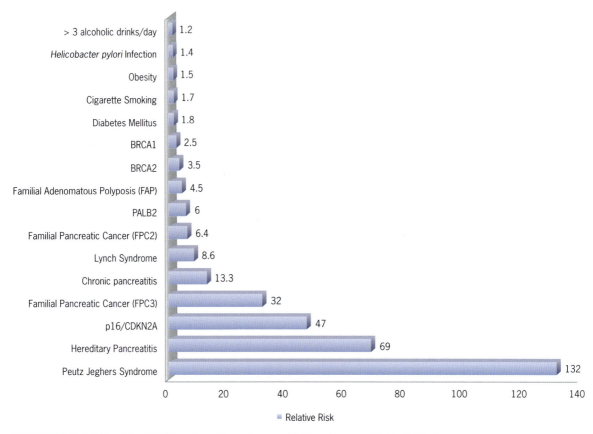

FIGURE 10.2: Relative risk of PDAC conferred by various modifiable and non-modifiable risk factors.

(1) Evidence exists on the association of precancer with an increased risk of cancer.

(2) When a precancer undergoes malignant progression, cancer originates from the cells within the precancerous cells.

(3) A precancer differs from the normal tissue of origin.

(4) A precancer differs from the resultant cancer; it shares some but not all the molecular and phenotypic characteristics of the cancer.

(5) There is an availability of diagnostic method(s) for the precancer.

While among the general population screening for pancreatic cancer is not recommended, screening and surveillance strategies to detect it in high-risk individuals (HRIs) are targeted to identify precursor lesions and PC at early and potentially resectable stages. The following three types of lesions meet these rigorous criteria:

Pancreatic Intraepithelial Neoplasms (PanINs) PanINs are microscopic (generally < 0.5 cm) flat or papillary lesions that originate from the pancreatic duct. They are graded as PanIN 1, 2, or 3 based on the variable mucin content and cellular or architectural atypia. (Figure 10.3[A–C])[16] Pancreatic tumorigenesis has been delineated to occur in stepladder fashion, and early precursor lesions have different immunohistochemical and genetic profiles as compared to advanced lesions (NCI criteria 4).[17] They are smaller than IPMNs, have more

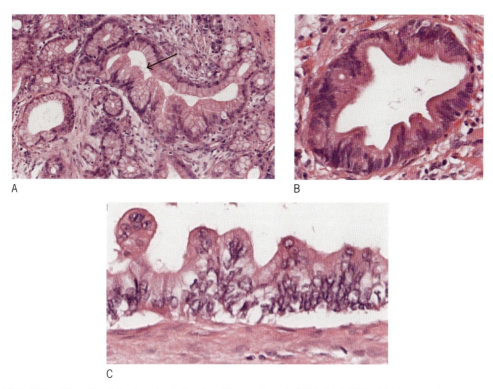

A

B

C

FIGURE 10.3: [A] PanIN1: with minimal cytological and architectural atypia (H&E, 20x) [B] PanIN 2 lesion with moderate cytological atypia, retained nuclear polarity, and partially papillary architecture (H&E, 20x); [C] PanIN-3 lesion with severe atypia, lost
nuclear polarity, and papillary architecture (H&E, 40x) (Reproduced with permission from Distler M, Aust D, Weitz J, Pilarsky C,
Grutzmann R. Precursor lesions for sporadic pancreatic cancer: PanIN, IPMN, and MCN. Biomed Res Int. 2014;2014:474905).

stubby papillae, and lack mucin production, especially in contrast to the intestinal type of
IPMN. PanINs are commonly associated with focal lobular centric atrophy of the pancreatic
parenchyma from surrounding fibrosis around mucinous metaplastic acinar cells. Although
they are potential targets of screening, progress is limited in accurate detection of PanINs in
asymptomatic subjects through cross-sectional imaging and endoscopic ultrasound (EUS).

Intrapapillary Mucinous Neoplasms (IPMNs) IPMNs are mucin-producing epithelial
neoplasms that originate from the pancreatic ductal cells. They are generally > 1 cm in
size, may be single or multicentric, and may arise from the main duct (MD-IPMN), its
contributing branch ducts (BD-IPMN), or have mixed origins (MT-IPMN). The neoplastic
lesions comprise columnar epithelium with delicate papillary projections with luminal
mucin. Microscopically, cells have papillary projections or may be flat and lack ovarian-like
stroma, unlike mucinous cystic neoplasms (MCNs). IPMNs can differentiate along any one
of the four directions: intestinal, gastric, pancreatobiliary, or oncocytic differentiation.[18,19]
There characteristics are summarized as follows:

Gastric type IPMN (low-grade dysplasia) They are characterized by MUC5AC expression.
Histologically, they resemble gastric foveolar epithelium and associated with BD-IPMN
(Figure 10.4[A&B]). [16]

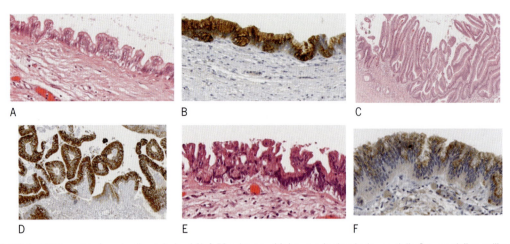

FIGURE 10.4: IPMN gastric foveolar (branch duct) [A & B] subtype with low-grade dysplasia, partially flat, partially papillary architecture, and basally oriented nuclei ([A]; H&E 20x, [B]; MUC5AC 20x); IPMN intestinal subtype [C& D] with low/intermediate dysplasia, long, finger-like papillae, and elongated nuclei ([C]; H&E 4x, [D]; MUC2 10x); IPMN pancreatobiliary subtype [E&F] with high-grade dysplasia, lost nuclear orientation, and complex papillae formation ([E]; H&E 20x, [F]; MUC1 20x) (Reproduced with permission from Distler M, Aust D, Weitz J, Pilarsky C, Grutzmann R. Precursor lesions for sporadic pancreatic cancer: PanIN, IPMN, and MCN. Biomed Res Int. 2014;2014:474905).

1. Intestinal-type IPMN (low- to high-grade dysplasia): They are associated with intestinal programming pathway mucin markers like MUC2 and CDX2. The intestinal type IPMN is characterized by the presence of goblet cells, which are similar to colonic villous adenoma (Figure 10.4[C&D]).

2. Pancreatobiliary-type IPMN (low- to high-grade dysplasia): They are associated with pyloro-pancreatic pathway mucin markers like MUC1 and sometimes MUC6. Pancreatobiliary-type IPMN are characterized by minimal mucin, cuboidal neoplastic cells with enlarged nucleoli and architectural atypia (Figure 10.4[E&F]).

3. Oncocytic-type IPMN/Intraductal oncocytic papillary neoplasm (high-grade dysplasia): They are associated with MUC6 and Heppar 1, and sometimes MUC 1 mucin markers. Their histological characteristics include eosinophilic tumor cells, architectural abnormalities including branching papillae, solid nests, nest-like growth pattern and intraepithelial lumina, and have high mitochondrial concentration. They have variable degrees of dysplasia based on cytologic and architecture features. Though considered precancerous, they have a relatively low rate of overall incidence of malignant progression and are associated with PDAC of colloid or tubular subtypes.[20] A longitudinal study demonstrated significantly higher ($P < 0.001$) 5-year actuarial risk of progression to high-grade dysplasia among MD-IPMNs (63%) than among BD-IPMNs (15%). IPMN lesions are further stratified on the basis of high-risk stigmata (HRS) or worrisome features radiologically.[21,22]

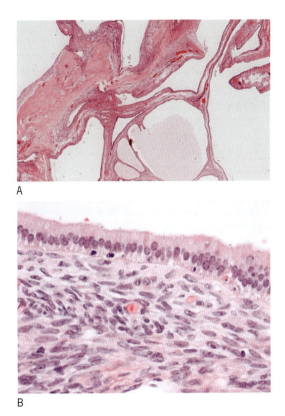

A

B

FIGURE 10.5: MCN [A] with cuboidal to columnar epithelial lining, mild dysplasia, and underlying ovarian type stroma (H&E 2x), and [B] High power view of MCN (H&E 40x) (Reproduced with permission from Distler M, Aust D, Weitz J, Pilarsky C, Grutzmann R. Precursor lesions for sporadic pancreatic cancer: PanIN, IPMN, and MCN. Biomed Res Int. 2014;2014:474905).

Mucinous Cystic Neoplasms (MCNs) These mucin-producing cystic neoplasms arise outside the ductal system within the pancreas. These lesions are almost exclusively found in women and diagnosed at an average age of 50. They are uncommon, with a prevalence of 23% reported among individuals undergoing resection of pancreatic tumors.[23] MCNs are solitary lesions and lack communication with pancreatic ducts. Microscopically, they have tall columnar epithelial cells, characteristic ovarian-like stroma, and mucin-producing epithelium (Figure 10.5[A&B]). The grade of dysplasia is based upon cellular atypia and architectural distortion. Management of MCNs is predominantly surgical due to suitable surgical candidacy in the setting of a generally young age at diagnosis. Their 5-year survival rate in the absence of invasive cancer amounts to 100% and recurrence is unlikely postresection.[24]

Genetics of Pancreatic Ductal Adenocarcinoma Progression

PanIN-PDAC Progression The malignant progression in PC occurs stepwise with accumulation of mutations as shown in Figure 10.1.[25] The understanding of molecular drivers of pancreatic carcinogenesis has substantially increased through the sequencing of genomes and exomes of ductal adenocarcinomas.[26,27] Mutations that target core genes and pathways include *KRAS, p16/CDKN2A, TP53,* and the transforming growth factor-beta (TGF-β) signaling pathway.

KRAS pathway The *KRAS* oncogene (located at the short arm of chromosome 12-12p) encodes for the Kirsten Rat Sarcoma Viral Oncogene Homolog (KRAS) protein. *KRAS* mutation is present among 90% of all PDACs. Its occurrence in low-grade precursor lesions (PanIN-1) supports its early occurrence during PDAC carcinogenesis. Upon stimulation by growth signals, RAS protein results in activation of downstream effectors governing cell division and survival, which include RAF-mitogen and phosphatidyl 3-kinase pathways.[28] RAS protein is activated by transitory GTP binding and has intrinsic GTPase activity, which self-limits its function. However, missense mutations in the *KRAS* oncogene at codon 12, followed by 13 and 61, disable the hydrolysis of GTP, which results in constitutional activation of RAS through GTP binding and cellular proliferation independent of growth signal. The mutation in codon 61 imparts better survival than among codon 12 or 13, implicating prognostic significance to genetic diversity among *KRAS* mutations.[29]

Telomere shortening Telomeres are repetitive nuclear protein complexes found at end chromosomes, which maintain genetic stability. They are non-coding regions of the chromosome and are protective against degradation and end fusion. Early precursor lesions such as PanIN and IPMNs harbor chromosomal abnormalities due to telomere shortening. The inactivation of tumor suppressor genes enables accumulation of resultant genomic instability.

p16/CDKN2A pathway A normal dividing cell transitions from G1 to S phase of the cell cycle and is inhibited by the Rb protein, which is inactivated upon phosphorylation through a complex of cyclin D1 (cycD1) and Cyclin D mediated Kinase 4 (Cdk4).[30] The p16 protein further acts as a competitive inhibitor of cycD1 and Cdk4 and subsequently limits cellular division. Thus, tumorigenesis results from inactivation of the *p16* or *RB* gene, or disinhibition of the *p16* binding domain of Ckd-4, or overexpression of cycD1 and Cdk4. The cell cycle checkpoint protein p16INK4A is encoded by the cyclin-dependent kinase inhibitor 2A gene (*CDKN2A*), which is the most commonly mutated tumor suppressor in PC (95% of the cases). The mutations include epigenetic silencing as a result of methylation of 5′-CpG island within the promoter site, codon missense mutations, or genomic deletion.[31]

TP53 pathway A *TP53* mutation code for p53 protein, which arrests cell cycle upon detection of DNA damage and in response, induces DNA repair or apoptosis. *TP53* mutations occur later in the multistage progression of PDAC and are found in up to 70% of pancreatic neoplasms.[32]

SMAD4 mutation Transforming growth factor-beta (TGF-β) signaling pathway Loss of function of *SMAD4*, a tumor suppressor gene (*DPC4*, SMAD family member 4 gene), is a late event in carcinogenesis (PanIN3-carcinogenesis). It encodes for the Smad4 protein and undergoes homozygous inactivation in 50% of PDACs.[33] Loss of the *SMAD4* gene leads to disinhibition from anti-apoptosis and the growth controlling effect of TGF-β, and results in the selection of more aggressively growing tumors and acquisition of oncogenic mutations. The uncontrolled tumor cells, with the remnant of the TGF-β signaling pathway, undergo epithelial mesenchymal transition, resulting in increased aggressiveness. Tumor-derived TGF-β also induces immunosuppression from suppressed T-cell function and angiogenic spread.[34] Loss of *SMAD4/DPC4* results in aggressive and metastatic disease with poor prognosis, and can be utilized to stratify patients at risk of dissemination and tailor systemic therapeutic regimens.[35,36]

IPMN-PDAC Progression IPMNs have a distinct carcinogenesis pathway with whole genome sequencing that reveals mutations of *KRAS*, *GNAS*, and *RNF3* genes.

KRAS pathway *KRAS* mutations are a predominant molecular driver of IPMN progression due to their incidence in incipient IPMN and an overall incidence of 47 to 81%. However, it has a lower incidence among each grade of IPMN as compared to nearly 100% among PanIN, suggesting alternate signals that result in the activation of the MEK-ERK-MAP kinase pathway.[37]

GNAS pathway *GNAS* mutation occurs at codon 201 and involves the alpha subunit of G protein. This results in constitutional activation of adenylyl cyclase (AC) and downstream cellular proliferation. *GNAS* mutation occurs in incipient IPMNs (lesions of size 0.5 to 1 cm) with a prevalence of 33%, supporting its early occurrence in IPMN progression.[38] GNAS mutations have also been detected in pancreatic juice prior to their radiologic diagnosis.[39] It has been reported in 66% of incident low-grade IPMNs alone, and in the majority of these lesions in combination with *KRAS* mutation (96%).[40] *GNAS* mutation is absent in MCNs and other non-malignant lesions. It has a reported incidence of 66% (96% in combination with *KRAS* among low grade IPMNs, respectively).

RNF43 mutation The *RNF43* gene is a tumor suppressor gene that encodes transmembrane E3 ubiquitin ligase and regulates the WNT signaling pathway. Whole-exome sequencing revealed loss of heterozygosity at the *RNF43* locus (chromosome 17q) in 75% of IPMNs, which was also detected among MCNs.

MCN-PDAC Progression Among MCNs, *KRAS* mutation has been found in some low-grade and the majority of high-grade lesions in a genetic sequencing study.[41] Additionally, a study by Wu et al. established *KRAS* mutation as an initial driver of tumorigenesis, wherein the mutation was found in all grades of MCNs. *GNAS* mutation has not been reported in MCNs to date, a key finding that distinguishes them from IPMNs through mutational analysis of the cystic fluid. *P53* gene mutation has been postulated to impart aggressiveness among MCNs due to its exclusive expression among carcinomas.[42] Genetic alteration in the PI3K pathway involving *PIK3CA* gene mutations also contributes to malignant progression of mucinous tumors.[43] The ovarian-like stroma has been observed to overexpress genes like *STAR* and *ESR*. These genes are related to estrogen metabolism and the canonical WNT signaling pathway, which have been implicated in production of the stromal component of MCNs.[44,45]

▦ PANCREATIC CANCER RISK ASSESSMENT, COUNSELING, AND TESTING

Lifetime risk for the acquisition of PC is 1.6% for both men and women. Among the general population, the U.S. Preventive Services Task Force (USPSTF) designates PC screening among asymptomatic individuals as Grade D, recommending against this service and stating there is moderate or high certainty that screening for PC among asymptomatic individuals is of no net benefit or that harm outweighs any benefit.[46] The unfavorable recommendation is based on its low incidence, lack of sensitive screening modalities, and many of the risk factors remaining unknown. However, there is increasing data to support the role of pancreatic cancer screening in individuals at increased risk. Risk factors are divided into modifiable, non-modifiable, and inherited risk factors. Individuals at increased risk of developing PC, and so eligible for pancreatic cancer screening, include those with certain pancreatic cystic neoplasms, defined familial history of PC often in association with known inherited germ-line mutations, and possibly newonset diabetes.

Non-Modifiable Risk Factors

ABO Blood Group Although the exact mechanism is unknown, the association between PC and the ABO blood group has been known since the 1960s. In western countries, including the United States, the non-O ABO blood group is associated with approximately a 40% increased PC risk (95% CI 26 to 57%).[47] Because A, B, and AB blood groups in total comprise approximately 56% of the population in the United States, the fraction of PC associated with non-O blood groups is nearly 20%, which is comparable to the amount of PC attributable to cigarette smoking and double the amount of PC attributable to high-risk genetic mutations.[47] Additionally, an association between CagA-negative *H. pylori* seropositivity and risk of PC was suggested among individuals with non-O blood type (OR = 2.78[95% CI 1.49–5.20], P = 0.0014). However, this association was lacking among those with O blood type (OR = 1.28, [95% CI 0.62–2.64], P = 0.51).[48]

Mucinous Pancreatic Cysts With the advent of cross-sectional imaging, various pancreatic cystic lesions are diagnosed incidentally among the general population.[49] Among them, mucinous pancreatic cysts histologically include IPMNs and MCNs, and they are considered precancerous. IPMNs originate from the pancreatic ductal system, either from the main duct or its branches, and their management is based on risk stratification based on its size and other radiological characteristics, including high-risk stigmata (which typically proceed to surgical evaluation) and worrisome features (which necessitate further investigation):

- High-risk stigmata (HRS) includes cysts accompanying obstructive jaundice, those with enhancing mural nodules > 5 mm, or main pancreatic duct size > 10 mm in the longest dimension.[50]
- Worrisome features include cysts > 3 cm, enhancing mural nodules < 5 mm, thickened/enhancing cyst walls, main duct size 5 to 9 mm, abrupt change in caliber of pancreatic duct with distal pancreatic atrophy, lymphadenopathy, increased serum level of CA19-9, or cyst growth rate > 5 mm / 2 years or > 10 mm during follow-up.[51,52]

Inherited Risk Factors

Familial Pancreatic Cancer (FPC) The term applies to families with two or more first-degree relatives (FDR) with PC, and the family does not fulfill criteria for known genetic syndromes associated with pancreatic cancer.[53] FPC risk stratification is based on the number of individuals with PC and their relationships to the proband.[54] An elevated risk ratio of 32-fold was found in individuals with three first-degree relatives (lifetime risk, 40%), and 6.4-fold among individuals with two FDRs (lifetime risk, 8 to 12%).[55] A higher risk of PC has also been observed among FPC kindreds with an earlier onset of PC (age < 50 years, standardized incidence ratio = 9.3%).[56] PancPRO is a Mendelian model for PC risk prediction in individuals with FPC. It has been a validated as a tool with an observed-to-predicted PC ratio of 0.83 (95% CI, 0.52 to 1.20) and high discriminatory ability [area under the receiver operating characteristic curve (AUC) of 0.75 (95% CI, 0.68 to 0.81).[57] Some familial aggregation of PC can be attributed to chance or shared environmental factors, such as cigarette smoking and *H. pylori* infection.[58]

Genetic Syndromes Although many genetic defects remain unknown, a number of genetic syndromes associated with PC have been discovered. Because genetic syndromes can produce a variety of cancer types, individuals with genetic susceptibility may not have a specific family history of PC. Inherited cancer syndromes such as hereditary breast ovarian cancer syndrome (HBOC), hereditary pancreatitis (HP), Peutz-Jeghers syndrome (PJS), familial atypical multiple mole melanoma (FAMMM), Lynch syndrome, ataxia-telangiectasia syndrome, and Li-Fraumeni syndrome are associated with an increased risk of developing PC. However, due to their rarity, they account for only a small fraction of PC in total.

The prevalence of various PC susceptibility genes varies depending on the clinical settings. Among PC kindreds enrolled in the National Familial Pancreatic Tumor Registry (NFPTR), a total of 10 *BRCA2* mutation carriers (~6%) from 180 included families were identified.[59] On the other, an Italian study enrolled 225 PC patients, among whom 16 patients had significant family history. *CDKN2A* mutations were found in five of 16 FPC patients (31%). None of the patients had *PALLD*, *PALB2* or *BRCA2* mutation and only one patient harbored a *BRCA1* mutation.[60] Recently, next generation sequencing for 25 cancer susceptibility genes was performed in the lymphocyte DNA from 185 FPC patients. Among the 25 carriers identified, the deleterious mutations included *BRCA2* (11, 5.9%), *ATM* (8, 4.3%), *CDKN2A* (4, 2.16%), *BRCA1* (2, 1.08%), and BARD1(0.54%) each in *BARD1, MSH2, NBN, PALB2,* and *PMS2.* [61]

Hereditary Breast-ovarian Cancer Syndrome (HBOC) This syndrome is characterized by an elevated risk of ovarian and breast cancers due to germline mutations in the *BRCA1, BRCA2, PALB2,* and *ATM* genes involved in DNA repair mechanisms; it carries a high risk of PC.[11] HBOC mutations are also associated with Fanconi anemia, including *FANCC* and *FANCG* genes (Table 10.1).[62–65] Germline mutations in *BRCA1/2* not only impart PC risk but also result in an earlier age of onset (63 for each) as compared to general age of incidence (70 per SEER database).[66] *BRCA2* mutation has been the most commonly identified mutation, with an incidence as high as 17% among FPC.[16] This germline mutation confers a relative risk of 3.5 to 10 for PC.[67,68] *BRCA2* mutation is more common in individuals of Ashkenazi Jewish ancestry, who carry a single mutation, 6174delT, at a frequency of 1.3%.[68] While *BRCA2* codes for Fanconi anemia (FANC) proteins, *BRCA1* directly interacts with them to enable DNA repair prior to the S phase of the cell cycle.[69] *BRCA1* mutation confers 2.5 to 3 times the risk of PC, though its association with PC is not clearly defined and is rarely seen among individuals without a strong family history of breast cancer.[64,65] Among *BRCA* negative individuals, the partner and localizer of the *BRCA2-PALB2* gene is another DNA defect repair gene, which stabilizes *BRCA2* protein during DNA repair.[70] There also appears to be a mechanistic link between ATM mediated kinase and phosphorylation of PALB2 in response to ionizing radiation mediated DNA damage repair.[71,72] A 6-fold higher risk of PC has been demonstrated among individuals with *PALB2* mutations, though robust evidence through population studies is lacking.[73]

Familial Atypical Multiple Mole Melanoma (FAMMM) FAMMM is associated with multiple atypical nevi and malignant melanoma among individuals with one or more affected first-degree or second-degree relatives (SDR). They have an autosomal dominant inheritance pattern and rare germline mutations in the tumor suppressor gene *P16INK4A* (also called *CDKN2A* or multiple tumor suppressor gene). This pattern has been observed in 38% of the individuals with this syndrome.[74,75] PC risk has been associated with this germline mutation, which affects the synthesis of P16 protein involved in cell cycle regulation.[76] Along with the risk of melanoma and non-melanoma skin cancers, a relative risk of 46.6 (CI 24.7 to 76.4) for PC has been observed among *p16* mutation carriers.[77]

Lynch Syndrome Lynch syndrome is generally associated with an increased risk of colon cancer; it is caused by defects in DNA mismatch-repair genes, including *MSH2, MLH1,*

TABLE 10.1: Current Indications for Genetic Testing Among High-Risk Individuals

Hereditary Breast Ovarian Cancer Syndrome (BRCA1/2)[131]

- An individual with known or likely pathogenic *BRCA1/2* gene within family (research based or tumor profiling), or planned for targeted therapy.
- At any age had PC, ovarian cancer, or high grade or metastatic prostate cancer
- Ashkenazi Jewish ancestry with breast cancer
- Individual with breast cancer diagnosed at
- $\leq$ 45 years,
- 46–50 years: 2 primary breast cancers, breast cancer at any age $\geq$1 blood relatives with breast cancer or high-grade prostate cancer, $\geq$1 close blood relative with breast cancer, unknown family history,
- $\leq$ 60 years: triple negative breast cancer, or
- any age: $\geq$1 blood relatives with breast cancer at $\leq$ 50 years, or metastatic prostate cancer or invasive ovarian cancer, or male breast cancer or PC or $\geq$2 blood relatives with breast cancer

Peutz-Jegher Syndrome (STK11/LKB1) (Chromosome 19p)

Presence of 2 or more of these factors:

- $\geq$2 histologically verified PJS hamartomatous polyps or small bowel polyposis,
- Mucocutaneous hyperpigmentation,
- A family history of PJS.

Familial Atypical Multiple Mole Melanoma (p16/CDKN2A)

- $\geq$ 3 invasive melanomas
- Mix of melanoma, PC and/or astrocytoma diagnosis in the individual or family

Hereditary Pancreatitis *PRSS1*(7q), *SPINK1*(5q), *CTRC, CFTR*

- 2 attacks of acute pancreatitis of unknown etiology,
- Idiopathic chronic pancreatitis with disease onset occuring <25 years of age, one FDR or SDR with pancreatitis, unexplained documented episode of childhood pancreatitis that required hospitalization and where there is concern that HP should be excluded.

MSH1, MSH2, PMS2, and *EPCAM*.[78] Patients with Lynch syndrome also have an 8.6-fold increased risk of PC. The pancreatic tumors associated with Lynch syndrome have a classical medullary appearance characterized by microsatellite instability and lymphocytic infiltrates.[79] A recent multicenter study included 3119 patients with Lynch syndrome aged 24 to 75 and investigated their pancreatic cancer risk and survival.[80] The study found a relative cumulative PC incidence of 7.8 (3.3 to 12.3) in *MLH1*, 1.8 (0 to 5.2) in *MSH6*, 0.6 (0-1.9) in *MSH2*, and 0 among *PMS2* gene carriers. The PC risk tailored to each individual's age, sex, and gene variant has also been updated at this website: http://lscarisk.org (last accessed on March 31, 2020).

Peutz-Jeghers Syndrome (PJS) PJS results from rare germline mutations in the *STK11/LKB1* tumor suppressor gene, which encodes for serine/threonine kinase.[81] It has autosomal dominant inheritance and is characterized by mucocutaneous pigmentations in the lips, buccal mucosa, and periorbital area. Individuals with PJS are predisposed to gastric, pancreatic, and small intestinal cancers and non-gastrointestinal malignancies involving the breast, ovary, endometrium, cervix, and testis.[82,83] The relative risk of PC in patients with PJS is 132-fold (95% CI 44 to 261) compared to the general population, and conveys a cumulative lifetime risk as high as 36% from age 15 to 64.[84]

Familial Adenomatous Polyposis (FAP) FAP is characterized by early development of colorectal adenomatous polyps with inevitable malignant progression and colorectal cancer by age 40 due to germline mutations in the *APC* gene,[85] whichis a tumor-suppressor gene that codes for scaffolding proteins that degrade β-catenin and control cell-cycle progression and microtubule stabilization.[86] Along with risk of colon cancers, FAP is associated with a 4.5- to 6-fold risk of PC.[87]

Ataxia-Telangiectasia (AT) Ataxia telangiectasia is an autosomal recessive disorder that occurs from homozygous mutation in the *ATM* gene, which encodes for serine/threonine kinase involved in DNA repair.[88] It is characterized by progressive neurologic abnormalities, telangiectasia of blood vessels of exposed skin and eyes, and immune dysfunction and predisposition to lymphoma and leukemia resulting from hypersensitivity to ionizing radiation.[89] Monoallelic mutations in the *ATM* gene result in an increased risk of breast cancer and doubled risk of PC in comparison with the general population.[90]

Hereditary Pancreatitis (HP) HP is characterized by recurrent pancreatitis starting in childhood, resulting in pancreatic injury and chronic inflammation. This rare syndrome results from germline mutations in *PRSS1, SPINK1, CTRC,* and *CFTR* genes with autosomal dominant inheritance and incomplete penetrance.[91] It causes premature trypsin activation (*PRSS1* mutation) or abnormal inhibitors, including chymotrypsin C-*CTRC* mutation or serine peptidase inhibitor-*SPINK* mutation. Pancreatic carcinogenesis arises from chronic inflammation due to the following proposed mechanisms.[92,93]

- Inflammatory cytokines, including IL-6 and IL-11, which stimulate cellular proliferation through induction of multiple transcription factors, including STAT3 and NF-kB.
- Suppression of immunosurveillance and inhibition of oncogene-induced senescence, which would allow the lesion to develop unchecked.
- Activation of pancreatic stellate cells leading to fibrosis.

These mutations predispose the body to chronic pancreatitis and PC with a standardized incidence ratio of 53.[94] *CFTR* mutation has also been associated with an early age of onset and 5.3-fold increased risk of PC.[95]

Modifiable Risk Factors

Tobacco Exposure Tobacco exposure is a major modifiable risk factor associated with PC that contributes to 20 to 35% of incident cases.[96,97] Tobacco-related carcinogens, including nitrosamines and polycyclic aromatic hydrocarbons and their metabolites, have been postulated to directly contribute to pancreatic inflammation and mutations in proto-oncogenes (*KRAS*) and tumor-suppressor genes (*p53*).[98] A meta-analysis demonstrated relative risk of 1.74 among current cigarette smokers and 1.47 among cigar users. Risk for PC increases with higher intensity and cumulative smoking dose.[97,98] Furthermore, smoking appears to interact with genetic and familial predispositions, causing incremental risk of PC including HP and FPC. These factors decrease the age of onset of PC by 20 years and 10 years, respectively, and increase the risk of their occurrence.[99,100]

Alcohol Intake PC has been attributed to alcohol consumption, though current evidence indicates that it is associated only with heavy alcohol consumption. High alcohol usage has been associated with an increased risk of PC (risk ratio [RR], 1.15; 95% CI 1.06 to 1.25) in a recent meta-analysis.[101] In this study, alcohol consumption has been defined as light (0–12 g per day), moderate ($\geq$12–24 g per day), or heavy alcohol ($\geq$24 g per day). It has been postulated that alcohol and its metabolites (acetaldehyde or ethyl esters) are direct carcinogens and they induce pancreatic inflammation, which in turn contributes to pancreatic carcinogenesis.[98,102]

Diabetes Mellitus (DM) The bidirectional DM-PDAC relationship is an important emerging focus for research and has ushered in endeavors to better understand the relationship between PC, chronic pancreatitis, and diabetes.[103] PC has been demonstrated to be preceded by DM by a few years, and its resection frequently results in resolution of DM among many patients.[104] Conversely, type-2 DM confers a 1.5-fold increased risk of PC over the long term due to endogenous hyperinsulinemia-mediated growth stimulation.[105] Similarly, a Relative risk (RR) of 2.89 for PC was found in a case control study among a DM population, which was further increased to 6.49 through treatment with exogenous insulin and decreased to 2.12 with treatment with oral hypoglycemics. Metformin, in particular, has been shown to reduce PC cancer risks, and improves survival among patients with pre-existing DM and PC.[106] Metformin reduces the levels of circulating insulin and IGF-1 levels and also modulates the mTOR signal pathway.[107] T3cDM or DM secondary to acute or chronic pancreatitis has been associated with PC due to common predisposing risk factors, which lead to exocrine insufficiency.[108] DM among PC patients has been postulated to arise through a paraneoplastic field mechanism attributed to induced insulin resistance from pancreatic polypeptide deficiency,[109] or to adrenomedullin secreted in exosomes.[110] It is currently the basis of several prospective observational studies studying risk of pancreatic ductal adenocarcinoma in new onset diabetics.

Chronic Pancreatitis (CP) This has been associated with PC and been established as a risk factor for PC.[111] A meta-analysis has demonstrated that CP confers an estimated relative risk of 13.3 and can progress to PC over one to two decades.[112] CP is believed to promote carcinogenesis through higher malignant cell survival, autocrine stimulation of a pro-tumorigenic environment, and desmoplasia. Although only 5% of CP patients developed PC over two decades, the risk appeared to be much higher among patients with hereditary predisposition. A recent cohort study reported an older age of onset and a substantial smoking history (> 60 pack/years) in a high proportion of patients with CP.[111,113]

H. Pylori Infection A meta-analysis of six studies (involving 2335 individuals) supports significant association between *H. pylori* seropositivity and development of PC (AOR 1.38, 95% CI 1.08–1.75; P=0.009.[114] In a study by Nilsson et al., 16s ribosomal subunit DNA was found in 75% of exocrine PC specimens.[115] While the exact mechanism is unknown, *H. pylori* infection has been demonstrated to promote a pro-inflammatory state leading to cell turnover and accumulation of DNA damage. The infection also induces transcription factors like nuclear factor-KB, serum response element (SRE), activator protein-1, pro-inflammatory cytokines like IL-8, and angiogenic factors including VEGF.[116]

Interaction of Genetic and Environmental Risk Factors About four to five million alterations in a single DNA building block or single nucleotide polymorphism (SNP) occur among every individual's genome. These SNPs have been utilized to identify predilection gene risk, (G), which may interact with environmental risk factors, (E). The risk factors for PC, being a rare disease, can be analyzed via case-control studies. The gene-to-environment interaction (G x E) has been studied through logistic regression and their modifications, among case-control and cohort studies.

Smoking and Genes Interaction between smoking and genetic risk factors, especially those with a role in carcinogen metabolism, DNA repair, inflammation, hormone metabolism, and chromatin-remodeling, have been investigated. Variants of *CYP1A2* and *NAT1* genes, which are involved in metabolism of aromatic amines, have been demonstrated to cause gender-specific PC susceptibility to tobacco carcinogen and dietary mutagens.[117] *CAPN10*, a diabetes susceptibility gene, may also be associated with elevated risk of PC among a high-risk cohort of smokers.[118,119] The *CTLA-4* gene is associated with negative regulation of T-cell mediated antitumor immunosurveillance.[120] Smoking has also been demonstrated to interact with PC risk associated with *CTLA-4 49G>A* gene variant (with at least one A allele) ($p=0.037$).[121]

Alcohol and Genes Alcohol and its major metabolite, acetaldehyde, have a role in pancreatic tumorigenesis and progression. The pancreas has the ability to metabolize alcohol through oxidative as well as non-oxidative pathways.[122] Alcohol intake has an interaction with PC risk associated with *CTLA-4 49G>A* gene variant (with at least one A allele) ($p=0.042$).[121] Alcohol consumption also interacts with SNPs within the IGF axis genes including *IGF2R* ($p=0.03$) and *IRS1* genotypes ($p=0.019$).

Anthropometric Factors and Genes PC risks from elevated BMI have been demonstrated to interact with genetic variations associated with feeding/fasting status and energy expenditure. A study investigated modification of PC risk from obesity- and diabetes-related genetic polymorphisms of *FTO, PPARγ, NR5A2, AMPK* and *ADIPOQ* genes.[123] It demonstrated significant interaction of BMI with two *FTO* gene variants (*FTO* IVS1-27777C>A and IVS1-23525A>T). The study also revealed a weak association of BMI with *ADIPOQ* Ex3+117 CT/CC variant ($p=0.03$). Elevated BMI, either current or in the past, has also been demonstrated to interact with *IGF-1* polymorphism.[124] Previously, Haplotype analysis of *IGF1* gene has also revealed synergistic interaction of *IGF1* Ex4-177 G>CC allele with diabetes in risk of PC.[125]

Dietary Factors and Genes Dietary intake has been hypothesized to interact with genes associated with metabolism, antioxidant defense, and DNA repair. Superoxide dismutase 2 (*SOD2*) catalyzes the dismutation of superoxides resulting in hydrogen peroxide, which is reduced by catalase or forms reactive hydroxyl radicals that initiate lipid peroxidation chain reactions and are broken by Vitamin E. Superoxide dismutase 2 (*SOD2*) has been demonstrated to slow PC growth.[126] AA genotype of *SOD2 1221G>A* causes elevated PC risk with low Vitamin E intake and vice versa ($p=0.002$).[127] A case-control study has revealed significantly higher PC risk due to the absence of minor *CAT rs12807961* polymorphisms and higher total grain intake (OR:2.48[1.5-4.09], $p=0.0007$) and the presence of *GAA* polymorphism rs3816257(OR:1.9[1.28-2.83], p $p=0.0005$).[128]

■ GENETIC COUNSELING AND TESTING

Genetic testing and counseling is crucial in PC screening endeavors.[53] Both activities are intertwined as testing must be accompanied with pre- and posttest counseling. This not only enables the implementation of recommendations and acts as the first screening filter but also enables communication of risk of PC to patients and relatives. Moreover, it enables patient-centered care through clarification of risks and benefits in order to allay fears among the population undergoing testing even in the setting of unknown genetic predisposition.[129]

Counseling for patients has also been beneficial when PC susceptibility genes were unknown. Based on the American Society of Clinical Oncology policy statement update on genetic testing for cancer susceptibility, genetic counseling and testing must be performed in the following circumstances:

1. *Testing should be performed when individuals meet characteristic features for a genetic cancer susceptibility condition.* Acquisition of complete personal and family history for features indicating genetic cancer susceptibility is a prerequisite for counseling patients about known mutations that predispose to PC: *BRCA1/2, STK11/LB1, PRSS1* and *p16/CDKN2A, ATM.* The characteristics indicating genetic testing for PC-associated genetic syndromes have been summarized in Table 10.1. Direct to consumer testing are microarray-based single nucleotide polymorphism SNP testing, which is commonly used to test individuals for ancestry. As compared to confirmatory testing they have lower accuracy, limited clinical utility, and inadequate consenting and have not been validated for clinical use.

2. *The test can be adequately interpreted.* Each genetic test has its false positive and false negative rates and may have ambiguous results. In the setting of a false positive, the individual will experience undue distress and be subjected to closer surveillance, while a false negative may risk a missed diagnosis. Being cognizant of both these scenarios and being able to interpret, apply, and educate the patient and family about the same is vital during testing for hereditary cancers.

3. *Testing results aid in diagnosis or influence the medical or surgical management of the patient or family members at hereditary risk of cancer.* In case of PC the individuals with positive genetic diagnosis are identified as high-risk individuals. They undergo frequent surveillance and undergo curative resection in case of radiological and histological evidence of progression.

4. *Per NCCN guidelines germline testing are indicated for any individual diagnosed with PC.*[130] This includes a panel of multiple genes, which would enable diagnosis of genetic syndromes that can be missed by reliance on history of the patient.

5. *Additionally, pathogenic variants are provided through tumor profiling that warrant germline testing for mutations like BRCA1/2 , which rarely have somatic mutations.*[131] However, somatic pathogenic /likely pathogenic variants for genes such as *STK11, p53* are common and these mutations are rarely indicative of germline mutations.

▦ CLINICAL MANAGEMENT OF PATIENTS AT INCREASED RISK

While most PCs are considered sporadic, in some individuals they can be attributed to familial aggregation (7%), chronic diseases with genetic predisposition, and high-risk genetic syndromes (3%).[132] Based on the current evidence on the relative risk for PC imparted by various environmental and genetic risk factors, they can be stratified into low (<5), moderate (5 to 10), and high (>10) risk (Figure 10.2). These individuals are classified as high-risk individuals (HRI) and have an elevated lifetime PC risk (RR at least 5-fold) due to familial or genetic predisposition. In 2011, recommendations for PC screening, surveillance of HRI, and their subsequent management were formulated by an international consortium of 49 multidisciplinary international experts, the Consortium for Pancreas Screening (CAPS).[133]

Target Population

The screening recommendations within the research protocol have been implemented at various centers as a prospective clinical trial (CAPS5 study); their target groups/cohorts are summarized in Table 10.2.

Age of Initiation and Termination of Screening The average age of diagnosis of PC among individuals with familial PC is 68.18 years, but genetic anticipation may result in earlier age of onset in successive affected generations.[56] To date, the CAPS recommendation for the age of screening initiation for PC is 50 years.[133] This age is determined on the basis of natural history of the cancer's progression and also by RR imparted by particular genetic or familial syndromes. On the basis of evidence gathered from natural history studies, *PRSS1* mutation carriers with hereditary pancreatitis undergo initial screening at age 40 years, or

TABLE 10.2: Current Indications for Pancreatic Cancer Screening in High-Risk Individuals	
SCREENING GROUPS	**DESCRIPTION**
Familial pancreatic cancer relatives	1. 55 years old or 10 years younger than the age of youngest relative with pancreatic cancer, and 2. Come from a family with two or more members with a history of pancreatic cancer (two of whom have a first-degree relationship consistent with familial pancreatic cancer), and 3. Have a first-degree relationship with at least one of the relatives with pancreatic cancer. If there are two or more affected blood relatives, at least one must be a first-degree relative of the individual being screened.
Germline mutation carrier (risk ~10% or higher)	Group 1 germline mutation carriers with an estimated lifetime risk of pancreatic cancer of ~10% or higher 1. 50 years old or 10 years younger than the age of the youngest relative with pancreatic cancer, and 2. The patient is a carrier of a confirmed *FAMMM (p16/CDKN2A), BRCA2, or PALB2* mutation, and there is one or more pancreatic cancer diagnoses in the family, one of whom is a first- or second-degree relative of the subject to be screened.
Germline mutation carrier (risk ~5%)	Group 2 germline mutation carriers with an estimated lifetime risk pancreatic cancer of ~5% 1. 55 years old or 10 years younger than the age of the youngest relative with pancreatic cancer, and 2. The patient is a carrier of a confirmed BRCA1, ATM or HNPCC (hereditary non-polyposis colorectal cancer or Lynch syndrome, hMLH1, hMSH2, PMS1, hMSH6, EpCAM) gene mutation, and there is > 1 pancreatic cancer in the family, one of whom is a first- or second-degree relative of the subject to be screened.
Hereditary pancreatitis	1. Hereditary pancreatitis with confirmed gene mutations that predispose to chronic pancreatitis, such as PRSS1, PRSS2, CTRC) and age 50 or older (these patients have an estimated lifetime risk for pancreatic cancer of 40%), or 20 years since their first attack of pancreatitis, whichever age is younger.
Peutz-Jeghers syndrome	1. At least 30 years old, and 2. At least two of three criteria diagnostic of Peutz-Jeghers syndrome (characteristic intestinal hamartomatous polyps, mucocutaneous melanin deposition, or family history of PJS, or 3. Known STK11 gene mutation carrier.

10 years before the youngest age of presentation within the pancreatic cancer kindred.[134] Among patients with PJS, screening begins at age of 30 given the younger age of onset. The age to begin screening is a crucial parameter for timely detection of precancerous lesions but also affects the health costs and psychological stress among HRIs.

Imaging Modalities for Screening

MRI/MRCP MRI has been accepted as a standard modality for detection of small asymptomatic pancreatic lesions. It is not associated with radiation exposure, is non-invasive, and enables better characterization of pancreatic cysts as compared to EUS in a comparative study.[135] In conjunction with MR cholangiography, MRI achieves fairly high diagnostic accuracy (84% sensitivity and 97% specificity) for PC detection.[136] Many of the early PC lesions without discrete solid masses and associated ductal or cystic changes can be reliably detected by MRI/MRCP. Diffusion weighted imaging (DWI) represents another advancement in MRI that can be used to detect the Brownian movements of water molecules. This modality has higher sensitivity in diagnosis of cell density, edema, fibrosis, and altered functionality of cellular membranes.[137] The pooled diagnostic sensitivity and specificity of DWI is 0.91 (95% CI 0.84 to 0.95) and 0.86 (95% CI 0.76 to 0.93), respectively.[133,138]

Endoscopic Ultrasound EUS is another screening modality for PC used for the diagnosis of cystic lesions, chronic pancreatitis-like changes, and discrete solid lesions. On the basis of a blinded multicenter comparative trial, a 55% agreement rate between MRI and EUS was found for the diagnosis of clinically relevant lesions.[135] The modalities involved detection of cystic lesions by EUS and solid lesions by MRI, but had good agreement for lesion site (100%) and size (Spearman coefficient, 0.83). The diagnostic modality was not associated with radiation exposure but has demerits of high interobserver variation, the invasive nature of the test, and the risks associated with patient sedation.[139]

Endoscopic Retrograde Cholangiopancreatography ERCP has been used as an imaging modality for PC screening. It enables diagnosis of pancreatic ductal abnormalities (graded by Cambridge classification)[140] and can also be used to acquire pancreatic juice and biliary samples for diagnostic cytology. However, the procedure is associated with post-procedural pancreatitis, which has been demonstrated to occur at a rate of 4 to 7% in a clinical setting.[141,142] Despite it usage in earlier studies, ERCP has been replaced by EUS as an imaging modality.[143–145]

CT Scan Pancreatic cancer lesions can be detected through various imaging modalities. CT scans as a surveillance tool have low accuracy and are associated with risks of radiation exposure. However, as a staging modality, CT accurately determines resectability of the cancer and visualization of the upper abdomen.[146]

Biomarker Screening

The evidence for biomarker screening is mostly based on the general population and currently the evidence can only be extrapolated to HRIs. Due to low population incidence and required accuracy, biomarkers remain elusive for the moment and screening for precursor and PC lesions is based on radiologic modalities.

Pancreatic Juice and Pancreatic Cyst Biomarkers Molecular analysis of duodenal aspirate for pancreatic juice or cystic fluid can also be utilized for diagnosis of precancerous or early stage PC, especially those undetectable on imaging. Its biologic mechanism is based on enrichment from protein secreted or DNA released from upstream pancreatic ductal system.[147] The specimen procured from duodenal aspirate and biopsy is analyzed for genetic alterations, including *KRAS* mutations, *GNAS* for cystic precursors, and loss of heterozygosity (LOH) at *CDKN2A, RNF43, SMAD4, TP53,* and *VHL*. The evidence on the accuracy of these tests for identification of precursor lesions is scarce, including among HRIs.

A study by Kanda et al. demonstrated *GNAS* mutations in the pancreatic juice of 64.1% of IPMN specimen.[39] Moreover, *TP53* mutations were detected in the pancreatic juice from 29 of 43 patients with PC, and four of eight patients with advanced precursor lesions (PanIN-3 and IPMNs with high-grade dysplasia).[71] Another study utilized a next generation sequencing assay for mutational analysis of pancreatic juice for 12 genes and included 31 HRIs. Among these HRIs, abnormal TP53/SMAD4 concentration was found among three individuals, two of whom had the most abnormalities on pancreatic imaging.[148] The study demonstrated that mutant TP53/SMAD4 concentrations had sensitivity of 61.1% and specificity of 95.7% (AUC 0.819) in distinguishing resection specimens containing PC or high-grade dysplasia from other subjects. These studies support a vital complementary role for mutational analysis of pancreatic juice along with pancreatic imaging.

Treatment of Patients at Risk

Screening for PC is recommended among HRIs through cross-sectional or endoscopic imaging. Pancreatic lesions detected through surveillance may either undergo curative-intent resection or observation. Screening and subsequent management are both recommended at high-volume centers with multidisciplinary teams, per guidelines and based on recent evidence.

Solid Lesions Surgical resection is recommended for solid lesions ≥1 cm or those detected on multimodalities, which warrant prior confirmatory histologic diagnosis through biopsy. The evidence on management of indeterminate solid lesions, however, is not clear. Total prophylactic pancreatectomy is not recommended for asymptomatic lesions among HRIs.[133] If selected, surgical resection must be performed at high-volume centers with lower operative mortality and morbidity.[149]

Cystic Lesions MCN and IPMN are precursor cystic lesions, which are classified and managed, based on consensus guidelines. Symptomatic cysts (associated with pain, pancreatitis, or jaundice) and those with high-risk stigmata (HRS) should be considered for surgery.[50] Cysts with worrisome features warrant surveillance through EUS and require histologic analysis through FNA. Among cysts with worrisome features, surgical resection should be considered if cysts have main duct involvement, high-grade dysplasia, or a mural nodule > 5 mm. A recent systematic review, which included low risk and non-low risk (worrisome features and HRS) patients, found the 10-year progression risk of low- and high-risk IPMNs to be 8% and 25%, respectively.[150] Moreover, radiologic classification of cystic lesions had 70% histologic correlation among sporadic cystic lesions.[151] These studies were based on sporadic cystic lesions incidentally detected among general populations; data to guide a threshold for resection among HRIs are lacking. The choice of surgery for lesions in HRI is not completely clear. Total pancreatectomy (TP) enables complete excision of field defect and results in brittle diabetes and exocrine insufficiency. Surgical resection targets gross as well as microscopically negative margins since survival is significantly decreased by residual invasive cancer.[152] Intraoperative frozen section is utilized during pancreatic resection, though it is accompanied with challenges of grading PanINs.

During surveillance of HRIs and subsequent management of detected lesions, the risk of leaving behind premalignant lesions competes with surgical complications and inaccurate preoperative diagnosis. A systematic review reported a pooled proportion of overall surgery of 6% (95% CI 4.1 to 7.9, p<0.001, I2=60.91%) and proportion of unnecessary surgery of 68.1% (95% CI 59.5 to 76.7, p<0.001, I2=4.05%).[153]

Chronic Pancreatitis-Like Changes CP-like changes within the pancreatic parenchyma and ductal system have been postulated to be associated with PanINs. They have been associated with advanced grades of PanIN and malignant progression among sporadic patients with IPMNs.[154,155] They undergo diagnosis and grading through endoscopic modalities, followed by procurement of a tissue sample and a subsequent pathology review. These findings thereby have been linked as potential targets for screening to the associated PC risks. Many PC surveillance studies have found CP-like lesions, which were thereby diagnosed with precursor, or early cancerous, lesions.

Follow-up HRIs with no imaging abnormalities are generally observed and undergo surveillance. The appropriate time interval for re-imaging remains unclear. Although a 12-month follow-up period was favored, such a consensus position was not evidence-based. A study by Bartsch et al. included individuals at risk of FPC and found 24 months to be an optimal follow-up interval for individuals with unremarkable baseline imaging.[156]

Appraisal of Screening Programs

"Successful screening" is defined as detection and treatment of high-grade lesions, including PanIN-3, IPMNs, MCNs with high-grade dysplasia, and early resectable T1N0M0 margin-negative PC. Patient information, screening modalities, and outcome measures of various screening studies have been summarized in Table 10.3.[107,143–145,156–176]

Survival Benefit PC screening targets detection of high-grade precursor lesions and early cancers but delineation of survival benefit from lead-time bias is imperative. A systematic review showed higher rates of curative resection (60% vs 25%, $P = 0.011$) and prolonged survival (14.5 months vs. 4 months, $P < 0.001$) among HRIs undergoing PC screening.[177] Two large cohort studies have displayed higher survival among HRIs undergoing surveillance as compared to symptomatic sporadic PDACs.[171,176]

Economic Burden Studies investigating cost-effectiveness of PC surveillance have been performed but are inconsistent in terms of diagnostic modality utilized and target groups screened. An incremental cost-effectiveness ratio of $16,885/life-year saved was demonstrated through one-time screening by EUS and ERCP. This conclusion was based on prerequisites of ≥16% prevalence of dysplasia and EUS sensitivity of ≥84%.[178] For patients with *CDKN2A (p16)*-Leiden mutation, surveillance through MRI/MRCP was estimated at $4,545.[179] This was in contrast to the life saved cost of over $350,000 for PC surveillance of PJS patients based on American Gastroenterology Association guidelines.[180] Besides the heterogeneity in study methods, the studies did not account for intangible components of screening such as psychological stress and quality of life.

TABLE 10.3: Description of Screening Programs

Authors, Year, Country	Individuals' HRI distribution	Age[a]	Follow-up time[b]	Interventions screening tests [confirmation]	Diagnostic yield	Surgery	Pathology diagnosed
Bretnall et al. 1999, USA[157]	n=14 FPC kindreds	41 [28–65]	Surgical: 12–30 Non surgical: 15 [8–17]	EUS [CT, ERCP]	EUS: 10/14, ERCP: 7/13 CT: 3/8	7	Dysplasia-7
Rulayak et al. 2001, USA[158]	n=35 FPC kindreds		[1–48]	EUS, ERCP	EUS: 22/34 ERCP:11/22	12	Dysplasia-12 PDAC-0
Kimmey et al. 2002, USA[143]	n=46, FPC kindreds	NA	up to 60	EUS [ERCP]	EUS: 24/46 ERCP: 13/28	12	Dysplasia-12
Canto et al. 2004, USA[144]	n=38 FPC PJS	56	22.4 [11.3–50.5]	EUS [FNA, ERCP, MDCT]	EUS: 29/38 ERCP: 23/23 FNA: 1, 2/17	7 (4WP, 3DP)	T2N1-1 PanIN3/IPMN borderline-2 SCA/PanIN1-2-4
Canto et al. 2006, USA[145]	n=78 FPC-72 PJS-6 control-149	52 [32–77]	[3-12]	EUS [FNA, ERCP, MDCT]	EUS :17/78 ERCP: 14/65	7, 1 outside institution	PanIN3-1 IPMN-HGD-1 benign (low PanIN, IPMN, CP) -4 M1PDAC -1
Poley et al. 2009, Netherlands[159]	n=44 FPC-12 p16-13 PJS2 HBOC:5 p53-1	50 [32–75]	NA	EUS [MRI, CT]	EUS-10/44 (mass (n=3), cystic (n=7))	3	PDAC-3
Langer et al. 2009[160]	n=76 FPC-32, p16-44	60 [35–85]	44 [5–93]	EUS, MRI [EUS-FNA]	EUS-25/44 MRI-18/44	7	PanIN1-2/IPMN -4 SCA -2, None-1

(Continued)

TABLE 10.3: Description of Screening Programs (Continued)

Authors, Year, Country	Individuals' HRI distribution	Age[a]	Follow-up time[b]	Interventions screening tests [confirmation]	Diagnostic yield	Surgery	Pathology diagnosed
Verna et al. 2010, USA[161]	n=51 FPC, HBOC, p16, LS	52 [29–77]	initial screening	EUS, MRI [FNA, ERCP]	EUS-20/31 MRI-11/33 ERCP-3/7	5	PDAC-2 BD-IPMN-MGD + PanIN2-3
Ludwig et al. 2011, USA[162]	n=109 FPC	54 [33–86]	initial screening	MRI, CT [EUS, FNA]	MRI-16/98 EUS-9/15	6	PanIN3-1 PanIN2-1 PDAC-1 SCA-1 IPMN-2
Schneider et al. 2011, Germany[163]	n=72 FPC HBOC p16	63c [31–91]	44c	MRI/EUS	MRI/EUS-26/72	10	PDAC-1, SCA-3, PanIN3-1, IPMN- 2, PanIN1/2-2 No pathology-1
Vasen et al. 2011, Netherlands[164]	n=79 p16	56c [39–72]	48c [0–120]	MRI/MRCP	MRI/MRCP: 7 PDAC, 9 Precursor	5	PDAC-5
Al-Sukhni et al. 2012, Canada[165]	n=262 FPC-159 HBOC-73 p16-11 PJS-7 HP-2	54 [22–89]	50 [0–96]	MRI/MRCP [EUS, MRI, CT, ERCP]	MRI/MRCP, 4	6	PDAC-3 PNET-1 BD-IPMN/PanIN-2
Canto et al. 2012, USA[166]	n=216: FPC-195 HBOC-19 PJS-2	56.1 [28–79]	28.8 [14–47.2]	EUS, MRI, CT [EUS-FNA]	EUS, MRI, CT, EUS-FNA-92	5	PNET-1 MD-IPMN-1 BD-IPMN-HGD/ PanIN3-2 PanIN1-2, BD-IPMN-LGD, MGD-2

TABLE 10.3: Description of Screening Programs

Authors, Year, Country	Individuals' HRI distribution	Age[a]	Follow-up time[b]	Interventions screening tests [confirmation]	Diagnostic yield	Surgery	Pathology diagnosed
Potjer et al. 2013, Netherlands[167]	n=241 FPC-116, p16-116, HBOC-9	FPC:54 [38–72] p16:54 [38–72]	FPC: 36 [0–110] p16: 34 [0–127]	MRI, EUS	PDAC: FPC 1 p16: 8 cystic lesion: FPC : 52 p16: 18	FPC: 12 P16: 7	FPC : PDAC -1 IPMN/PanIN: LGD-6 HGD-3 SCA-3 p16: PC-6 PanIN/IPMN: LGD-1
Sud et al. 2014, USA[168]	n=30	51.28 [20–75]	[0–36]	EUS [FNA]	EUS:16/30	3	PDAC-2 IPMN-LGD-1
Del Chiaro et al. 2015, USA[169]	n=40 FPC-32 p16-4 HBOC-4	49.9 [23–76]	12.9 [0–36]	MRI [EUS]	MRI:16/40 [EUS]	5	PDAC-3 BD-IPMN- 1 MT-IPMN-1
Mocci 2015, Spain[170]	n=41 FPC-24, HBOC-12 family PDAC-4	68.9 [45–93]	24	EUS, CT [MRI, FNA]	EUS-16/38 MRI-4/12	1	PNET-1, benign -1, HGD -1
Vasen et al. 2016, Netherlands[171]	n=411 p16:178 FPC:214 HBOC:19	46-56 [25–81]	[16–53]	MRI ± EUS [EUS], CT [EUS-FNA]	MRI: p16: PDAC:13/178 cyst: 26/178 FPC: PDAC:3/224 cyst: 112/224 HBOC: PDAC:1 cyst: 2	30 p16:11 FPC:16 HBOC:3	p16: PDAC-9 IPMN/PanIN-2 FPC: PDAC-1, PNET-1 PanIN-3/IPMN with HGD-4 PanIN1-2/IPMN with LGD- 6 SCA-4

(Continued)

TABLE 10.3: Description of Screening Programs (Continued)

Authors, Year, Country	Individuals' HRI distribution	Age[a]	Follow-up time[b]	Interventions screening tests [confirmation]	Diagnostic yield	Surgery	Pathology diagnosed
Hanrick et al. 2016, Netherlands[107]	n=139 FPC-68 p16-38 HBOC-23 PJS-7 p53-3	51 [20–73]	12	MRI+/EUS	MRI+/EUS:9	2	PDAC-1 PanIN2-1
Bartsch 2016, Germany[156]	n=253 non p16 HRI FPC, HBOC	48 [25–81]	28 [1–152]	MRI+EUS	MRI+/EUS: 134/253	21	PDAC-2 PNET-1 PanIN 1--5 BD-IPMN- LGD/ MGD-6BD-IPMN-HGD-1 panIN-3-3 SCA-3
Konnings et al. 2017, Netherlands[172]	n=186 FPC-98 p16-53 HBOC-30 PJS-11 p534	52 [19–75]	44 [0–120]	MRI+/EUS	MRI+/EUS: 100/186	3	PDAC-2 PanIN-2-1MT-IPMN+MGD-1
Devee et al.[173]	n=86 p16-53 Lynch: 3 HBOC-64 FAP:1 ATM: 1 PJS-5 p53-12	48.5 [40–58]	29.8 [21.7–43.5]	EUS+/MRI/MRCP, CT	EUS: 22/64 EUS-FNA: 4 MRI: 6/35 CT:8/44	-	no PDACs or high-grade PRL

TABLE 10.3: Description of Screening Programs

Authors, Year, Country	Individuals' HRI distribution	Age[a]	Follow-up time[b]	Interventions screening tests [confirmation]	Diagnostic yield	Surgery	Pathology diagnosed
Barnes et al.[174]	n=186 FPC-98 p16-53 HBOC-30 PJS-11 p53-4	56 [42–70]	2 [1–3]c	MRI, EUS, EUS-FNA	MRI: 28 cysts	0	0
Gangi 2018 et al.[175]	n=58 FPC-39 1FDR: 9 HBOC-9 PJS-1	60 ± 11yr	5	EUS+/FNA, stable lesions MRI/MRCP	EUS: 3 cysts 21 subcentimetric lesions FNA: 2 atypical cells	1	IPMN –LGD:1 Benign etiology:1
Canto 2018[176]	n=354 FPC-297 p16-4 HBOC-41 PJS-10 PRSS-1 Lynch syndrme-1	56.4 (29–81)	5.4	EUS+/RI/MRCP, CT	EUS+/ MRI/MRCP, CT: 10 PRL, 14 PDAC	20	PDAC: 14 High-grade PRL: 10: IPMN-HGD: 6 PanIN3: 5

[a]Expressed in years as mean [range].
[b]Expressed in months as mean [range].
[c]Central tendency is median.
FPC- (familial pancreatic cancer), p16- p16/CDKN2A mutation, HBOC (hereditary breast ovarian cancer), PJS (Peutz-Jeghers syndrome), p53 (individuals with p53 mutation), LGD, MGD, HGD (low-, moderate-, and high-grade dysplasia), PNET (pancreatic neuroendocrine tumor), PDAC (pancreatic adenocarcinoma), MD-IPMN (main duct intrapapillary mucinous neoplasm), BD-IPMN (branch duct intrapapillary mucinous neoplasm), MT-IPMN (mixed duct intrapapillary mucinous neoplasm), PanIN (pancreatic intraepithelial neoplasia), SCA (serous cyst adenoma), MRI/MRCP (magnetic resonance imaging/ cholangiopancreatography), EUS (endoscopic ultrasound), FNA (fine needle aspiration), WP (Whipple's procedure), and DP (distal pancreatectomy).

Psychological Stress Any individual undergoing screening or prior genetic testing has multiple psychological stressors. They include perceived mortality risk, procedure discomfort, cancer-related anxiety, and general emotional distress. A higher perceived risk was reported among FPC family members as compared to *BRCA2* mutation carriers.[181] Interestingly, the study demonstrated a decline in perceived risk, cancer-related worries, intrusive thoughts, and anxiety toward the next procedure over time. Individuals with higher baseline levels of risk perception and distress may benefit from comprehensive risk assessment and psychological support. Another study investigated the psychological aspect of screening endeavors and found clinical depression or anxiety in 9% of patients. Procedure-related discomfort was found in 14% and 15% of those undergoing EUS and MRI, respectively. No correlation was observed between cancer-related worries and surveillance outcomes (pancreatectomy or shortening of surveillance intervals), and a favorable surveillance benefit-to-risk ratio (88%).[182] Levels of anxiety and depression are not well defined for individuals who tested false positive for PC.

IMPACT OF GENETIC RISK FACTORS ON PANCREATIC CANCER THERAPIES

Recent evidence supports germline testing and determination of somatic mutation in newly diagnosed PC. The actionable somatic mutations include fusions (*ALK, NRG1, NTRK, ROS1*), mutations (*BRAF, BRCA1/2, HER2, KRAS, PALB2*), and mismatch repair (MMR) deficiency.[130]

Platinum-Based Therapies

Loss-of-function mutations in *BRCA1* and/or *BRCA2* genes predispose cells to DNA double-strand breaks due to the absence of homologous recombinant repair (HRR) and subsequent genomic instability.[183] The PC cells deficient in DNA repair mechanisms have been hypothesized to be prone to platinum-based chemotherapy, which acts via DNA crosslinking.[184] Among *BRCA1/2* mutated cases, the latest NCCN guidelines support the use of gemcitabine plus cisplatin as some of the first-line chemotherapeutic agents.[130] A study by Golan and colleagues, which included patients with stage III/IV PC, supported significantly longer overall survival (OS) among patients receiving a platinum-based regimen (median OS: 22 months) as compared to a non-platinum regimen (median OS: 9 months).[185]

Another retrospective cohort study sequenced 36 patients with metastatic PC and found superior improved response among patients with somatic or germline mutation in DNA damage repair genes: *BRCA1, BRCA2, PALB2, MSH2,* and *FANCF.*[186] Kaplan–Meier analysis demonstrated a higher median OS among patients with somatic or germline *BRCA1/2* mutations in comparison to those without these mutations (15 vs. 5 months), though the association lacked statistical significance (HR=0.64[95% CI, 0.32–1.29], p=0.17). The multivariate Cox regression model, however, revealed a significant improvement in OS upon presence of *BRCA1/2* mutations (adjusted HR=0.32[95% CI, 0.11–0.94], p=0.04).

Poly Adenosine Diphosphate–Ribose Polymerase (PARP) inhibitor

BRCA 1/2 mutation carriers, due to lack of HRR, are sensitive to poly (adenosine diphosphate–ribose) polymerase (PARP) inhibition due to the trapping of PARP on DNA at sites of single-strand breaks. These processes cause accumulation of double-strand breaks in replicating cells and subsequent tumor-cell death.[188] Recently, a randomized control trial investigated the efficacy of olaparib, a PARP inhibitor, among patients with *BRCA1/2* germline mutation and metastatic PC with stable response to gemcitabine. Patients who received maintenance olaparib (n=92) had significantly longer median progression-free survival than patients receiving a placebo (n=52) (7.4 months vs. 3.8 months; HR for disease progression or death: 0.53; 95% confidence interval [CI], 0.35 to 0.82; P=0.004).[189]

Immune Checkpoint Inhibitor

T-cell mediated immunity is responsible for immunosurveillance of abnormal surface markers and helps in fighting infections and cancers.[190] A blockade of interaction between the checkpoint ligands and their cognate receptors results in a potent antitumor response.[191] A subset of cells deficient in mismatch repair (MMR), due to somatic or germline mutations, have a high burden of mutant neoantigens that predisposes them to an immune checkpoint blockade with antibodies to programmed death receptor–1 (PD-1). The clinical efficacy of pembrolizumab, an anti-PD-L1 antibody, was evaluated among eight PC patients with MMR deficient malignancies. In the proof-of-concept study, an overall response rate of 62.5% and complete response rate of 25% was observed.[192] It was granted accelerated FDA approval for patients with unresectable or metastatic MMR-deficient solid tumors with progression or unsatisfactory response to alternate treatment options. Most of the clinical studies on immune checkpoint inhibitors for PC are underway and these agents exacerbate autoimmune mediated adverse effects.[193] Per the recommendations of the NCCN panel, off-label utilization of these agents outside of a clinical trial is strongly discouraged.[187]

Anaplastic Lymphoma Kinase (ALK) Protein Inhibitor

Among patients with PC onset <50 years, the rare occurrence of an anaplastic lymphoma kinase (*ALK*) gene in a genomic profiling study has been reported.[194] Among five PC patients diagnosed <50 years (attributing for 1.3% incidence), three of four patients treated with ALK protein inhibitor demonstrated clinical stability, resolution of CA19-9, and radiographic response.

▦ FUTURE DIRECTIONS

Current imaging modalities are sensitive for the early detection of cystic lesions. However, smaller lesions such as small PanIN require better characterization for early diagnosis and are not easily visualized through regular imaging. Early diagnosis of PC requires better biomarkers or panels of biomarkers and more robust imaging protocols. These improvements are vital in order to balance preventing overdiagnosis of clinically non-significant lesions and a "missed diagnosis" of high-grade precursors and early PC. We describe herein novel biomarkers and imaging modalities, which have been used in the general population and need to be investigated for earlier and more accurate diagnosis of PC among HRIs.

Novel Biomarkers

Circulating Free DNA (cfDNA) cfDNA are fragments of DNA released from cells as a part of metabolism, further increased by rapid cellular turnover. The DNA originates from lysis of CTCs or micrometastasis, from necrosis and apoptosis, or active cellular secretion.[195] CfDNA panels are based on the detection of *KRAS* mutation or alteration of the methylation pattern of CpG islands within the KRAS promoter site. They have been demonstrated to differentiate PC from chronic pancreatitis.[196,197] A recent CANCERSEEK test, to detect cfDNA and proteins, had a diagnostic sensitivity of up to 95% and specificity of > 99% for non-metastatic cancers and enabled anatomic localization in 81% of PC cases.[198]

Circulating MicroRNA MicroRNA are 17 to 25 evolutionarily conserved nucleotide-noncoding RNAs that regulate translation of mRNA in the posttranscriptional stage or facilitate its degradation.[199,200] Early PC has been consistently associated with four miRNAs, miR-21, miR-155, miR-196a, and miR-210, which are good candidates as biomarkers for early PC and have been observed in precancerous lesions such as IPMN and PanIN.[201,202] Among them, miR-196a has prognostic significance and has been associated with advanced unresectable stages of PC (p=0.001) and poor median survival (p=0.007).[203]

Exosomal Biomarkers

Exosomal biomarkers are another class of diagnostic molecular markers that comprise cell-secreted circulating extracellular microvesicles enclosed in bilayer membranes and contain enriched biomaterials of protein, lipid, DNA, and RNA. Exosomal miRNA, the RNAase stable biomarkers, have been demonstrated to be significantly elevated among patients with PC and IPMN (p<0.05 and had 5 to 20% higher AUC as compared to circulating biomarkers.[204]

Novel Imaging Modalities

In addition to the conventional imaging, novel imaging techniques used to diagnose very small early pancreatic adenocarcinomas or even PanIN lesions have evolved.

Contrast Enhanced Endoscopic Ultrasound Contrast enhanced EUS utilizes inert gas microbubbles in order to visualize the microvasculature and larger blood vessels. Focal lesions among pancreatic parenchyma have different vascular enhancements based on etiology: pancreatic adenocarcinoma is hypo-enhancing while neuroendocrine tumors are hyper-enhancing. Among the general population, pooled sensitivity of CE-EUS in differential diagnosis of PDAC was demonstrated to be 94% (95% CI, 0.91–0.95), and the specificity was 89% (95% CI, 0.85–0.92).[205] Currently, the FDA has not approved its use in the United States and its use is restricted to Europe and Asia.

Confocal Laser Endomicroscopy (CFLE) CFLE is an imaging modality that provides real-time visualization of mucosal gland tissue structure. The technique involves passage of a needle-based miniprobe through a 19G FNA needle. Among cystic lesions including IPMNs "finger-like structures" ($P = 0.004$) were observed to be a significant finding with a sensitivity of 59%, specificity of 100%, positive predictive value (PPV) of 100%, and negative predictive value (NPV) of 50%.[206] This technique has limited adoptability due to high interobserver variability, poor sensitivity, and high heterogeneity within the cystic lesion.

Endoscopic Ultrasound Elastography EUS elastography is a novel imaging modality that enables visualization of tissue elasticity distribution during the EUS procedure through changes in the EUS image of tissues with vascular pulsations and respiratory movements. A meta-analysis revealed cumulative sensitivity and specificity of qualitative EUS for the diagnosis of malignant pancreatic masses to be 0.98 (95% confidence interval [CI] 0.93–1.00) and 0.69 (95% CI 0.52–0.82), respectively, and for quantitative EUS elastography to be 0.96 (95% CI 0.86–0.99) and 0.76 (95% CI 0.58–0.87), respectively.[207] Though EUS elastography is limited by interobserver and intraobserver variability, it can be used as a supplemental method to EUS-FNA or during surveillance of a post-negative histologic review.

Molecular Probe-based Omaging Due to alteration of cellular composition among PCs, certain molecular markers can be tagged through antibody-based probes and have been considered as pertinent targets for probe-based imaging techniques.[208] These molecular targets arise from the neo-vasculature and tumor microenvironment.[209] The evidence accumulated in this area has arisen mostly from preliminary studies and their safety and efficacy needs more exploration through clinical studies. Moreover, in order to stand as a viable diagnostic modality, these imaging techniques must meet the prerequisite of sensitivity and specificity >90%.

CONCLUSION

Validated among individuals with familial or genetic risk factors, PC screening seems to be feasible based on various studies conducted over the past two decades. However, the surveillance programs to date have been limited to research settings and high-risk groups, and their more general applicability is presently uncertain. The preferred screening modality and interval of follow-up among the initially screened population also remain mostly empirical as a result of the paucity of evidence on optimal follow-up strategy. HRIs comprise only about 10% of PDAC patients, and early detection of sporadic PCs among individuals with no apparent predispositions have only been recently addressed.[210]

Due to ethical and economic considerations, randomized studies with control subjects are not feasible. In order to address various challenges for PC screening, prospective studies with larger samples and longer lengths of follow-up are imperative. These cohort studies require systematic reporting of imaging modalities and outcome measures, and for both to be coupled with access to stored biosamples taken throughout the duration of follow-up.

References

1. Gold EB, Goldin SB. Epidemiology of and risk factors for pancreatic cancer. *Surg Oncol Clin N Am.* 1998;7(1):67–91.
2. Carrera S, Sancho A, Azkona E, et al. Hereditary pancreatic cancer: related syndromes and clinical perspective. *Hered Cancer Clin Pract.* 2017;15:9.
3. Matsubayashi H, Takaori K, Morizane C, et al. Familial pancreatic cancer: Concept, management and issues. *World J Gastroenterol.* 2017;23(6):935–948.
4. Siegel RL, Miller KD, Jemal A. Cancer statistics, 2019. *CA: A Cancer Journal for Clinicians.* 2019;69(1):7–34.
5. Noone AM, Krapcho M, Miller D, et al. (eds). SEER Cancer Statistics Review, 1975–2015, National Cancer Institute. Bethesda, MD (based on November 2017 SEER data submission, last accessed on January 26, 2018). https://seer.cancer.gov/csr/1975_2015/. Published April 2018.
6. Welch HG, Schwartz LM, Woloshin S. Are increasing 5-year survival rates evidence of success against cancer? *JAMA.* 2000;283(22):2975–2978.
7. Singhi AD, Ishida H, Ali SZ, et al. A histomorphologic comparison of familial and sporadic pancreatic cancers. *Pancreatology.* 2015;15(4):387–391.
8. https://seer.cancer.gov/statfacts/html/pancreas.html (SEER database for statistics on Pancreatic Cancer), last accessed on March 7, 2019.
9. Rahib L, Smith BD, Aizenberg R, et al. Projecting cancer incidence and deaths to 2030: the unexpected burden of thyroid, liver, and pancreas cancers in the United States. *Cancer Res.* 2014;74(11):2913–2921.

10. https://www.congress.gov/bill/112th-congress/senate-bill/3566?q=%7B%22search%22%3A%5B%22recal-citrant+cancer%22%5D%7D&s=2&r=1 (Congress bill introduced in September 2012), last accessed on March 7, 2019.

11. Hruban RH, Klimstra DS. *Tumors of the pancreas: atlas of tumor pathology*. Washington, DC: American Registry of Pathology and Armed Forces Institute of Pathology; 2006.

12. Hong SM, Goggins M, Wolfgang CL, et al. Vascular invasion in infiltrating ductal adenocarcinoma of the pancreas can mimic pancreatic intraepithelial neoplasia: a histopathologic study of 209 cases. *Am J Surg Pathol*. 2012;36(2):235–241.

13. Hirai I, Kimura W, Ozawa K, et al. Perineural invasion in pancreatic cancer. *Pancreas*. 2002;24(1):15–25.

14. Infante JR, Matsubayashi H, Sato N, et al. Peritumoral fibroblast SPARC expression and patient outcome with resectable pancreatic adenocarcinoma. *J Clin Oncol*. 2007;25(3):319–325.

15. Von Hoff DD, Ervin T, Arena FP, et al. Increased survival in pancreatic cancer with nab-paclitaxel plus gemcitabine. *N Engl J Med*. 2013;369(18):1691–1703.

16. Distler M, Aust D, Weitz J, et al. Precursor lesions for sporadic pancreatic cancer: PanIN, IPMN, and MCN. *Biomed Res Int*. 2014;474905.

17. Wilentz RE, Iacobuzio-Donahue CA, Argani P, et al. Loss of expression of Dpc4 in pancreatic intraepithelial neoplasia: evidence that DPC4 inactivation occurs late in neoplastic progression. *Cancer Res*. 2000;60(7):2002–2006.

18. Furukawa T, Kloppel G, Volkan Adsay N, et al. Classification of types of intraductal papillary-mucinous neoplasm of the pancreas: a consensus study. *Virchows Arch*. 2005;447(5):794–799.

19. Yamada S, Fujii T, Shimoyama Y, et al. Clinical implication of morphological subtypes in management of intraductal papillary mucinous neoplasm. *Ann Surg Oncol*. 2014;21(7):2444–2452.

20. Strauss A, Birdsey M, Fritz S, et al. Intraductal papillary mucinous neoplasms of the pancreas: radiological predictors of malignant transformation and the introduction of bile duct dilation to current guidelines. *Br J Radiol*. 2016;89(1061):20150853.

21. Schnelldorfer T, Sarr MG, Nagorney DM, et al. Experience with 208 resections for intraductal papillary mucinous neoplasm of the pancreas. *Arch Surg*. 2008;143(7):639–646.

22. Tanaka M, Fernández-Del Castillo C, Kamisawa T, et al. Revisions of international consensus Fukuoka guidelines for the management of IPMN of the pancreas. *Pancreatology*. 2017;17(5):738–753.

23. Valsangkar NP, Morales-Oyarvide V, Thayer SP, et al. 851 resected cystic tumors of the pancreas: a 33-year experience at the Massachusetts General Hospital. *Surgery*. 2012;152(3 Suppl. 1):S4–12.

24. Yamao K, Yanagisawa A, Takahashi K, et al. Clinicopathological features and prognosis of mucinous cystic neoplasm with ovarian-type stroma: a multi-institutional study of the Japan pancreas society. *Pancreas*. 2011;40(1):67–71.

25. Chhoda A, Lu L, Clerkin BM, et al. Current approaches to pancreatic cancer screening. *Am J Pathol*. 2019;189(1):22–35.

26. Jones S, Zhang X, Parsons DW, et al. Core signaling pathways in human pancreatic cancers revealed by global genomic analyses. *Science*. 2008;321(5897):1801–1806.

27. Biankin AV, Waddell N, Kassahn KS, et al. Pancreatic cancer genomes reveal aberrations in axon guidance pathway genes. *Nature*. 2012;491(7424):399–405.

28. Jancik S, Drabek J, Radzioch D, et al. Clinical relevance of KRAS in human cancers. *J Biomed Biotechnol*. 2010;150960.

29. Witkiewicz AK, McMillan EA, Balaji U, et al. Whole-exome sequencing of pancreatic cancer defines genetic diversity and therapeutic targets. *Nat Commun*. 2015;6:6744.

30. Sherr CJ. Cancer cell cycles. *Science*. 1996;274(5293):1672–1677.

31. Schutte M, Hruban RH, Geradts J, et al. Abrogation of the Rb/p16 tumor-suppressive pathway in virtually all pancreatic carcinomas. *Cancer Res*. 1997;57(15):3126–3130.

32. Scarpa A, Capelli P, Mukai K, et al. Pancreatic adenocarcinomas frequently show p53 gene mutations. *Am J Pathol*. 1993;142(5):1534–1543.

33. Hahn SA, Schutte M, Hoque AT, et al. DPC4, a candidate tumor suppressor gene at human chromosome 18q21.1. *Science*. 1996;271(5247):350–353.

34. Siegel PM, Massague J. Cytostatic and apoptotic actions of TGF-beta in homeostasis and cancer. *Nat Rev Cancer*. 2003;3(11):807–821.

35. Iacobuzio-Donahue CA, Fu B, Yachida S, et al. DPC4 gene status of the primary carcinoma correlates with patterns of failure in patients with pancreatic cancer. *J Clin Oncol*. 2009;27(11):1806–1813.

36. Crane CH, Varadhachary GR, Yordy JS, et al. Phase II trial of cetuximab, gemcitabine, and oxaliplatin followed by chemoradiation with cetuximab for locally advanced (T4) pancreatic adenocarcinoma: correlation of Smad4(Dpc4) immunostaining with pattern of disease progression. *J Clin Oncol*. 2011;29(22):3037–3043.

37. Schonleben F, Qiu W, Bruckman KC, et al. BRAF and KRAS gene mutations in intraductal papillary mucinous neoplasm/carcinoma (IPMN/IPMC) of the pancreas. *Cancer Lett*. 2007;249(2):242–248.

38. Matthaei H, Wu J, Dal Molin M, et al. GNAS sequencing identifies IPMN-specific mutations in a subgroup of diminutive pancreatic cysts referred to as "incipient IPMNs." *Am J Surg Pathol*. 2014;38(3):360–363.

39. Kanda M, Knight S, Topazian M, et al. Mutant GNAS detected in duodenal collections of secretin-stimulated pancreatic juice indicates the presence or emergence of pancreatic cysts. *Gut*. 2013;62(7):1024–1033.

40. Wu J, Matthaei H, Maitra A, et al. Recurrent GNAS mutations define an unexpected pathway for pancreatic cyst development. *Sci Transl Med*. 2011;3(92):92ra66.

41. Conner JR, Marino-Enriquez A, Mino-Kenudson M, et al. Genomic characterization of low- and high-grade pancreatic mucinous cystic neoplasms teveals recurrent KRAS alterations in "high-risk" lesions. *Pancreas*. 2017;46(5):665–671.

42. Jimenez RE, Warshaw AL, Z'Graggen K, et al. Sequential accumulation of K-ras mutations and p53 overexpression in the progression of pancreatic mucinous cystic neoplasms to malignancy. *Ann Surg*. 1999;230(4):501–509; discussion 509–511.

43. Garcia-Carracedo D, Chen ZM, Qiu W, et al. PIK3CA mutations in mucinous cystic neoplasms of the pancreas. *Pancreas*. 2014;43(2):245–249.

44. Sano M, Driscoll DR, De Jesus-Monge WE, et al. Activated Wnt signaling in stroma contributes to development of pancreatic mucinous cystic neoplasms. *Gastroenterology*. 2014;146(1):257–267.

45. Fukushima N, Sato N, Prasad N, et al. Characterization of gene expression in mucinous cystic neoplasms of the pancreas using oligonucleotide microarrays. *Oncogene*. 2004;23(56):9042–9051.

46. Final Update Summary: Pancreatic Cancer: Screening - US Preventive Services Task Force (https://www.uspreventiveservicestaskforce.org/uspstf/recommendation/pancreatic-cancer-screening, last accessed on March 31, 2020).

47. Risch HA, Lu L, Wang J, et al. ABO blood group and risk of pancreatic cancer: a study in Shanghai and meta-analysis. *Am J Epidemiol*. 2013;177(12):1326–1337.

48. Risch HA, Yu H, Lu L, et al. ABO blood group, Helicobacter pylori seropositivity, and risk of pancreatic cancer: a case-control study. *J Natl Cancer Inst*. 2010;102(7):502–505.

49. Scheiman JM, Hwang JH, Moayyedi P. American gastroenterological association technical review on the diagnosis and management of asymptomatic neoplastic pancreatic cysts. *Gastroenterology*. 2015;148(4):824–848, e822.

50. Kim TH, Song TJ, Hwang J-H, et al. Predictors of malignancy in pure branch duct type intraductal papillary mucinous neoplasm of the pancreas: a nationwide multicenter study. *Pancreatology*. 2015;15(4):405–410.

51. Kang MJ, Jang J-Y, Kim SJ, et al. Cyst growth rate predicts malignancy in patients with branch duct intraductal papillary mucinous neoplasms. *Clin Gastroenterol Hepatol*. 2011;9(1):87–93.

52. Kwong WT, Lawson RD, Hunt G, et al. Rapid growth rates of suspected pancreatic cyst branch duct intraductal papillary mucinous neoplasms predict malignancy. *Dig Dis Sci*. 2015;60(9):2800–2806.

53. Brand RE, Lerch MM, Rubinstein WS, et al. Advances in counselling and surveillance of patients at risk for pancreatic cancer. *Gut*. 2007;56(10):1460–1469.

54. Klein AP, Brune KA, Petersen GM, et al. Prospective risk of pancreatic cancer in familial pancreatic cancer kindreds. *Cancer Res*. 2004;64(7):2634–2638.

55. Grover S, Syngal S. Hereditary pancreatic cancer. *Gastroenterology*. 2010;139(4):1076–1080, e1072.

56. Brune KA, Lau B, Palmisano E, et al. Importance of age of onset in pancreatic cancer kindreds. *J Natl Cancer Inst*. 2010;102(2):119–126.

57. Wang W, Chen S, Brune KA, et al. PancPRO: risk assessment for individuals with a family history of pancreatic cancer. *J Clin Oncol.* 2007;25(11):1417–1422.

58. Maisonneuve P, Lowenfels AB. Epidemiology of pancreatic cancer: an update. *Dig Dis.* 2010;28(4-5):645–656.

59. Couch FJ, Johnson MR, Rabe KG, et al. The prevalence of BRCA2 mutations in familial pancreatic cancer. *Cancer Epidemiol Biomarkers Prev.* 2007;16(2):342–346.

60. Ghiorzo P, Fornarini G, Sciallero S, et al. CDKN2A is the main susceptibility gene in Italian pancreatic cancer families. *J Med Genet.* 2012;49(3):164–170.

61. Chaffee KG, Oberg AL, McWilliams RR, et al. Prevalence of germ-line mutations in cancer genes among pancreatic cancer patients with a positive family history. *Genet Med.* 2018;20(1):119–127.

62. The Breast Cancer Linkage C. Cancer Risks in *BRCA2* Mutation Carriers. *JNCI: Journal of the National Cancer Institute.* 1999;91(15):1310–1316.

63. van Asperen CJ, Brohet RM, Meijers-Heijboer EJ, et al. Cancer risks in BRCA2 families: estimates for sites other than breast and ovary. *J Med Genet.* 2005;42(9):711–719.

64. Brose MS. Cancer risk estimates for *BRCA1* mutation carriers identified in a risk evaluation program. *CancerSpectrum Knowledge Environment.* 2002;94(18):1365–1372.

65. Thompson D, Easton DF. The Breast Cancer Linkage C. Cancer Incidence in BRCA1 Mutation Carriers. *JNCI: Journal of the National Cancer Institute.* 2002;94(18):1358–1365.

66. Kim DH, Crawford B, Ziegler J, et al. Prevalence and characteristics of pancreatic cancer in families with BRCA1 and BRCA2 mutations. *Fam Cancer.* 2009;8(2):153–158.

67. Murphy KM, Brune KA, Griffin C, et al. Evaluation of candidate genes MAP2K4, MADH4, ACVR1B, and BRCA2 in familial pancreatic cancer: deleterious BRCA2 mutations in 17%. *Cancer Res.* 2002;62(13):3789–3793.

68. Risch HA, McLaughlin JR, Cole DEC, et al. Population BRCA1 and BRCA2 mutation frequencies and cancer penetrances: a kin–cohort study in Ontario, Canada. JNCI: *Journal of the National Cancer Institute.* 2006;98(23):1694–1706.

69. Folias A, Matkovic M, Bruun D, et al. BRCA1 interacts directly with the Fanconi anemia protein FANCA. *Hum Mol Genet.* 2002;11(21):2591–2597.

70. Jones S, Hruban RH, Kamiyama M, et al. Exomic sequencing identifies PALB2 as a pancreatic cancer susceptibility gene. *Science.* 2009;324(5924):217.

71. Kanda M, Sadakari Y, Borges M, et al. Mutant TP53 in duodenal samples of pancreatic juice from patients with pancreatic cancer or high-grade dysplasia. *Clin Gastroenterol Hepatol.* 2013;11(6):719–730.

72. Guo Y, Feng W, Sy SM, et al. ATM-dependent phosphorylation of the Fanconi anemia protein PALB2 promotes the DNA damage response. *J Biol Chem.* 2015;290(46):27545–27556.

73. Casadei S, Norquist BM, Walsh T, et al. Contribution of inherited mutations in the *BRCA2*-interacting protein PALB2 to familial breast cancer. (1538-7445 (Electronic)).

74. Goldstein AM, Chan M, Harland M, et al. Features associated with germline CDKN2A mutations: a GenoMEL study of melanoma-prone families from three continents. *J Med Genet.* 2007;44(2):99–106.

75. Goldstein AM, Chan M, Harland M, et al. High-risk melanoma susceptibility genes and pancreatic cancer, neural system tumors, and uveal melanoma across GenoMEL. *Cancer Res.* 2006;66(20):9818–9828.

76. Goldstein AM, Fraser MC, Struewing JP, et al. Increased risk of pancreatic cancer in melanoma-prone kindreds with p16INK4 mutations. *N Engl J Med.* 1995;333(15):970–974.

77. de Snoo FA, Bishop DT, Bergman W, et al. Increased risk of cancer other than melanoma in CDKN2A founder mutation (p16-Leiden)-positive melanoma families. *Clin Cancer Res.* 2008;14(21):7151–7157.

78. Kastrinos F, Stoffel EM. History, genetics, and strategies for cancer prevention in Lynch syndrome. *Clin Gastroenterol Hepatol.* 2014;12(5):715–727.

79. Kastrinos F, Mukherjee B, Tayob N, et al. Risk of pancreatic cancer in families with Lynch syndrome. *JAMA.* 2009;302(16):1790–1795.

80. Moller P, Seppala TT, Bernstein I, et al. Cancer risk and survival in path_MMR carriers by gene and gender up to 75 years of age: a report from the Prospective Lynch Syndrome Database. *Gut.* 2018;67(7):1306–1316.

81. Jenne DE, Reimann H, Nezu J, et al. Peutz-Jeghers syndrome is caused by mutations in a novel serine threonine kinase. *Nat Genet.* 1998;18(1):38–43.

82. Grover S, Syngal S. Hereditary pancreatic cancer. *Gastroenterology*. 2010;139(4):1076–1080.

83. Tomlinson IP, Houlston RS. Peutz-Jeghers syndrome. *J Med Genet*. 1997;34(12):1007–1011.

84. Giardiello FM, Brensinger JD, Tersmette AC, et al. Very high risk of cancer in familial Peutz–Jeghers syndrome. *Gastroenterology*. 2000;119(6):1447–1453.

85. Kastrinos F, Syngal S. Inherited colorectal cancer syndromes. *Cancer J*. 2011;17(6):405–415.

86. Galiatsatos P, Foulkes WD. Familial adenomatous polyposis. *Am J Gastroenterol*. 2006;101(2):385–398.

87. Giardiello FM, Offerhaus GJ, Lee DH, et al. Increased risk of thyroid and pancreatic carcinoma in familial adenomatous polyposis. *Gut*. 1993;34(10):1394–1396.

88. Roberts NJ, Jiao Y, Yu J, et al. *ATM* mutations in patients with hereditary pancreatic cancer. *Cancer Discov*. 2012;2(1):41–46.

89. Roberts NJ, Jiao Y, Yu J, et al. *ATM* mutations in patients with hereditary pancreatic cancer. *Cancer Discov*. 2011;2(1):41–46.

90. Swift M, Chase CL, Morrell D. Cancer predisposition of ataxia-telangiectasia heterozygotes. *Cancer Genet Cytogenet*. 1990;46(1):21–27.

91. Howes N, Lerch MM, Greenhalf W, et al. Clinical and genetic characteristics of hereditary pancreatitis in Europe. *Clin Gastroenterol Hepatol*. 2004;2(3):252–261.

92. Gukovsky I, Li N, Todoric J, et al. Inflammation, autophagy, and obesity: common features in the pathogenesis of pancreatitis and pancreatic cancer. *Gastroenterology*. 2013;144(6):1199–1209.

93. Masamune A, Watanabe T, Kikuta K, et al. Roles of pancreatic stellate cells in pancreatic inflammation and fibrosis. *Clin Gastroenterol Hepatol*. 2009;7(11 Suppl.):S48–54.

94. Lowenfels AB, Maisonneuve P, DiMagno EP, et al. Hereditary pancreatitis and the risk of pancreatic cancer. International Hereditary Pancreatitis Study Group. *J Natl Cancer Inst*. 1997;89(6):442–446.

95. Maisonneuve P, Marshall BC, Lowenfels AB. Risk of pancreatic cancer in patients with cystic fibrosis. *Gut*. 2007;56(9):1327–1328.

96. Lowenfels AB, Maisonneuve P. Epidemiology and prevention of pancreatic cancer. *Jpn J Clin Oncol*. 2004;34(5):238–244.

97. Iodice S, Gandini S, Maisonneuve P, et al. Tobacco and the risk of pancreatic cancer: a review and meta-analysis. *Langenbecks Arch Surg*. 2008;393(4):535–545.

98. Duell EJ. Epidemiology and potential mechanisms of tobacco smoking and heavy alcohol consumption in pancreatic cancer. *Mol Carcinog*. 2012;51(1):40–52.

99. Rulyak SJ, Lowenfels AB, Maisonneuve P, et al. Risk factors for the development of pancreatic cancer in familial pancreatic cancer kindreds. *Gastroenterology*. 2003;124(5):1292–1299.

100. Lowenfels AB, Maisonneuve P, Whitcomb DC, et al. Cigarette smoking as a risk factor for pancreatic cancer in patients with hereditary pancreatitis. *JAMA*. 2001;286(2):169–170.

101. Wang Y-T, Gou Y-W, Jin W-W, et al. Association between alcohol intake and the risk of pancreatic cancer: a dose-response meta-analysis of cohort studies. *BMC Cancer*. 2016;16:212.

102. Yeo TP, Lowenfels AB. Demographics and epidemiology of pancreatic cancer. *Cancer J*. 2012;18(6):477–484.

103. Andersen DK, Andren-Sandberg Å, Duell EJ, et al. Pancreatitis - Diabetes - Pancreatic Cancer: Summary of an NIDDK-NCI Workshop. *Pancreas*. 2013;42(8). doi:10.1097/MPA.1090b1013e3182a1099ad1099d.

104. Permert J, Ihse I, Jorfeldt L, et al. Improved glucose metabolism after subtotal pancreatectomy for pancreatic cancer. *Br J Surg*. 1993;80(8):1047–1050.

105. Ding XZ, Fehsenfeld DM, Murphy LO, et al. Physiological concentrations of insulin augment pancreatic cancer cell proliferation and glucose utilization by activating MAP kinase, PI3 kinase and enhancing GLUT-1 expression. *Pancreas*. 2000;21(3):310–320.

106. Amin S, Mhango G, Lin J, et al. Metformin improves survival in patients with pancreatic ductal adenocarcinoma and pre-existing diabetes: a propensity score analysis. *Am J Gastroenterol*. 2016;111(9):1350–1357.

107. Yue W, Yang CS, DiPaola RS, et al. Repurposing of metformin and aspirin by targeting AMPK-mTOR and inflammation for pancreatic cancer prevention and treatment. *Cancer Prev Res (Phila)*. 2014;7(4):388–397.

108. Andersen DK, Korc M, Petersen GM, et al. Diabetes, pancreatogenic diabetes, and pancreatic cancer. *Diabetes*. 2017;66(5):1103–1110.

109. Hart PA, Baichoo E, Bi Y, et al. Pancreatic polypeptide response to a mixed meal is blunted in pancreatic head cancer associated with diabetes mellitus. *Pancreatology*. 2015;15(2):162–166.

110. Sah RP, Nagpal SJS, Mukhopadhyay D, et al. New insights into pancreatic cancer-induced paraneoplastic diabetes. *Nat Rev Gastroenterol Hepatol*. 2013;10(7):423–433.

111. Lowenfels AB, Maisonneuve P, Cavallini G, et al. Pancreatitis and the risk of pancreatic cancer. International Pancreatitis Study Group. *N Engl J Med*. 1993;328(20):1433–1437.

112. Raimondi S, Lowenfels AB, Morselli-Labate AM, et al. Pancreatic cancer in chronic pancreatitis; aetiology, incidence, and early detection. *Best Pract Res Clin Gastroenterol*. 2010;24(3):349–358.

113. Hao L, Zeng X-P, Xin L, et al. Incidence of and risk factors for pancreatic cancer in chronic pancreatitis: A cohort of 1656 patients. *Dig Liver Dis*. 2017;49(11):1249–1256.

114. Trikudanathan G, Philip A, Dasanu CA, et al. Association between Helicobacter pylori infection and pancreatic cancer. A cumulative meta-analysis. *JOP*. 2011;12(1):26–31.

115. Nilsson HO, Stenram U, Ihse I, et al. Helicobacter species ribosomal DNA in the pancreas, stomach and duodenum of pancreatic cancer patients. *World J Gastroenterol*. 2006;12(19):3038–3043.

116. Takayama S, Takahashi H, Matsuo Y, et al. Effects of Helicobacter pylori infection on human pancreatic cancer cell line. *Hepatogastroenterology*. 2007;54(80):2387–2391.

117. Suzuki H, Morris JS, Li Y, et al. Interaction of the cytochrome P4501A2, SULT1A1 and NAT gene polymorphisms with smoking and dietary mutagen intake in modification of the risk of pancreatic cancer. *Carcinogenesis*. 2008;29(6):1184–1191.

118. Fong PY, Fesinmeyer MD, White E, et al. Association of diabetes susceptibility gene *calpain-10* with pancreatic cancer among smokers. *J Gastrointest Cancer*. 2010;41(3):203–208.

119. Fesinmeyer MD, Stanford JL, Brentnall TA, et al. Association between the peroxisome proliferator-activated receptor gamma Pro12Ala variant and haplotype and pancreatic cancer in a high-risk cohort of smokers: a pilot study. *Pancreas*. 2009;38(6):631–637.

120. Appleman LJ, Berezovskaya A, Grass I, et al. CD28 costimulation mediates T cell expansion via IL-2-independent and IL-2-dependent regulation of cell cycle progression. *J Immunol*. 2000;164(1):144–151.

121. Yang M, Sun T, Zhou Y, et al. The functional cytotoxic T lymphocyte-associated Protein 4 49G-to-A genetic variant and risk of pancreatic cancer. *Cancer*. 2012;118(19):4681–4686.

122. Herreros-Villanueva M, Hijona E, Banales JM, et al. Alcohol consumption on pancreatic diseases. *World J Gastroenterol*. 2013;19(5):638–647.

123. Tang H, Dong X, Hassan M, et al. Body mass index and obesity- and diabetes-associated genotypes and risk for pancreatic cancer. *Cancer Epidemiol Biomarkers Prev*. 2011;20(5):779–792.

124. Nakao M, Hosono S, Ito H, et al. Interaction between IGF-1 polymorphisms and overweight for the risk of pancreatic cancer in Japanese. *Int J Mol Epidemiol Genet*. 2011;2(4):354–366.

125. Suzuki H, Li Y, Dong X, et al. Effect of insulin-like growth factor gene polymorphisms alone or in interaction with diabetes on the risk of pancreatic cancer. *Cancer Epidemiol Biomarkers Prev*. 2008;17(12):3467–3473.

126. Cullen JJ, Weydert C, Hinkhouse MM, et al. The role of manganese superoxide dismutase in the growth of pancreatic adenocarcinoma. *Cancer Res*. 2003;63(6):1297–1303.

127. Tang H, Dong X, Day RS, et al. Antioxidant genes, diabetes and dietary antioxidants in association with risk of pancreatic cancer. *Carcinogenesis*. 2010;31(4):607–613.

128. Jansen RJ, Robinson DP, Stolzenberg-Solomon RZ, et al. Polymorphisms in metabolism/antioxidant genes may mediate the effect of dietary intake on pancreatic cancer risk. *Pancreas*. 2013;42(7):1043–1053.

129. Axilbund JE, Brune KA, Canto MI, et al. Patient perspective on the value of genetic counselling for familial pancreas cancer. *Hered Cancer Clin Pract*. 2005;3(3):115–122.

130. https://www.nccn.org/professionals/physician_gls/pdf/pancreatic.pdf (NCCN guidelines for *BRCA1/2* testing). Last accessed on March 7, 2019.

131. https://www.nccn.org/professionals/physician_gls/pdf/genetics_screening.pdf (NCCN guidelines for *BRCA1/2* testing). Last accessed on March 7, 2019.

132. Bartsch DK, Gress TM, Langer P. Familial pancreatic cancer: current knowledge. *Nat Rev Gastroenterol Hepatol*. 2012;9(8):445–453.

133. Canto MI, Harinck F, Hruban RH, et al. International Cancer of the Pancreas Screening (CAPS) Consortium summit on the management of patients with increased risk for familial pancreatic cancer. *Gut.* 2013;62(3):339–347.

134. Ulrich CD, Consensus Committees of the European Registry of Hereditary Pancreatic Diseases MM-CPSGIAoP. Pancreatic cancer in hereditary pancreatitis: consensus guidelines for prevention, screening and treatment. *Pancreatology.* 2001;1(5):416–422.

135. Harinck F, Konings I, Kluijt I, et al. A multicentre comparative prospective blinded analysis of EUS and MRI for screening of pancreatic cancer in high-risk individuals. *Gut.* 2016;65(9):1505–1513.

136. Adamek HE, Albert J, Breer H, et al. Pancreatic cancer detection with magnetic resonance cholangiopancreatography and endoscopic retrograde cholangiopancreatography: a prospective controlled study. *Lancet.* 2000;356(9225):190–193.

137. Robertis RD, De Robertis R. Diffusion-weighted imaging of pancreatic cancer. *World J Radiol.* 2015;7(10):319.

138. Niu X-K, Bhetuwal A, Das S, et al. Meta-analysis of quantitative diffusion-weighted MR imaging in differentiating benign and malignant pancreatic masses. *J Huazhong Univ Sci Technolog Med Sci.* 2014;34(6):950–956.

139. Topazian M, Enders F, Kimmey M, et al. Interobserver agreement for EUS findings in familial pancreatic-cancer kindreds. *Gastrointest Endosc.* 2007;66(1):62–67.

140. Axon AT. Endoscopic retrograde cholangiopancreatography in chronic pancreatitis. Cambridge classification. *Radiol Clin North Am.* 1989;27(1):39–50.

141. Cheng CL, Sherman S, Watkins JL, et al. Risk factors for post-ERCP pancreatitis: a prospective multicenter study. *Am J Gastroenterol.* 2006;101(1):139–147.

142. Williams EJ, Taylor S, Fairclough P, et al. Risk factors for complication following ERCP; results of a large-scale, prospective multicenter study. *Endoscopy.* 2007;39(9):793–801.

143. Kimmey MB, Bronner MP, Byrd DR, et al. Screening and surveillance for hereditary pancreatic cancer. *Gastrointest Endosc.* 2002;56(4 Suppl):S82–86.

144. Canto MI, Goggins M, Yeo CJ, et al. Screening for pancreatic neoplasia in high-risk individuals: an EUS-based approach. *Clin Gastroenterol Hepatol.* 2004;2(7):606–621.

145. Canto MI, Goggins M, Hruban RH, et al. Screening for early pancreatic neoplasia in high-risk individuals: a prospective controlled study. *Clin Gastroenterol Hepatol.* 2006;4(6):766–781; quiz 665.

146. Kaneko OF, Lee DM, Wong J, et al. Performance of multidetector computed tomographic angiography in determining surgical resectability of pancreatic head adenocarcinoma. *J Comput Assist Tomogr.* 2010;34(5):732–738.

147. Chen R, Pan S, Yi EC, et al. Quantitative proteomic profiling of pancreatic cancer juice. *Proteomics.* 2006;6(13):3871–3879.

148. Suenaga M, Yu J, Shindo K, et al. Pancreatic juice mutation concentrations can help predict the grade of dysplasia in patients undergoing pancreatic surveillance. *Clin Cancer Res.* 2018;24(12):2963–2974.

149. Finks JF, Osborne NH, Birkmeyer JD. Trends in hospital volume and operative mortality for high-risk surgery. *N Engl J Med.* 2011;364(22):2128–2137.

150. Choi SH, Park SH, Kim KW, et al. Progression of unresected intraductal papillary mucinous neoplasms of the pancreas to cancer: a systematic review and meta-analysis. *Clin Gastroenterol Hepatol.* 2017;15(10):1509–1520.

151. Baiocchi GL, Portolani N, Missale G, et al. Intraductal papillary mucinous neoplasm of the pancreas (IPMN): clinico-pathological correlations and surgical indications. *World J Surg Oncol.* 2010;8:25.

152. Matthaei H, Hong S-M, Mayo SC, et al. Presence of pancreatic intraepithelial neoplasia in the pancreatic transection margin does not influence outcome in patients with R0 resected pancreatic cancer. *Ann Surg Oncol.* 2011;18(12):3493–3499.

153. Paiella S, Salvia R, De Pastena M, et al. Screening/surveillance programs for pancreatic cancer in familial high-risk individuals: a systematic review and proportion meta-analysis of screening results. *Pancreatology.* 2018;18(4):420–428.

154. LeBlanc JK, Chen JH, Al-Haddad M, et al. Endoscopic ultrasound and histology in chronic pancreatitis: how are they associated? *Pancreas.* 2014;43(3):440–444.

155. Takenaka M, Masuda A, Shiomi H, et al. Chronic pancreatitis finding by endoscopic ultrasonography in the pancreatic parenchyma of intraductal papillary mucinous neoplasms is associated with invasive intraductal papillary mucinous carcinoma. *Oncology.* 2017;93(Suppl. 1):61–68.

156. Bartsch DK, Slater EP, Carrato A, et al. Refinement of screening for familial pancreatic cancer. *Gut.* 2016;65(8):1314–1321.

157. Brentnall TA, Bronner MP, Byrd DR, et al. Early diagnosis and treatment of pancreatic dysplasia in patients with a family history of pancreatic cancer. *Annals of Internal Medicine.* 1999;131(4):247–255.

158. Rulyak SJ, Brentnall TA. Inherited pancreatic cancer: surveillance and treatment strategies for affected families. *Pancreatology.* 2001;1(5):477–485.

159. Poley JW, Kluijt I, Gouma DJ, et al. The yield of first-time endoscopic ultrasonography in screening individuals at a high risk of developing pancreatic cancer. *Am J Gastroenterol.* 2009;104(9):2175–2181.

160. Langer P, Kann PH, Fendrich V, et al. Five years of prospective screening of high-risk individuals from families with familial pancreatic cancer. *Gut.* 2009;58(10):1410–1418.

161. Verna EC, Hwang C, Stevens PD, et al. Pancreatic cancer screening in a prospective cohort of high-risk patients: a comprehensive strategy of imaging and genetics. *Clin Cancer Res.* 2010;16(20):5028–5037.

162. Ludwig E, Olson SH, Bayuga S, et al. Feasibility and yield of screening in relatives from familial pancreatic cancer families. *Am J Gastroenterol.* 2011;106(5):946–954.

163. Schneider R, Slater EP, Sina M, et al. German national case collection for familial pancreatic cancer (FaPaCa): ten years experience. *Fam Cancer.* 2011;10(2):323–330.

164. Vasen HFA, Wasser M, van Mil A, et al. Magnetic resonance imaging surveillance detects early-stage pancreatic cancer in carriers of a p16-Leiden mutation. *Gastroenterology.* 2011;140(3):850–856.

165. Al-Sukhni W, Borgida A, Rothenmund H, et al. Screening for pancreatic cancer in a high-risk cohort: an eight-year experience. *J Gastrointest Surg.* 2012;16(4):771–783.

166. Canto MI, Hruban RH, Fishman EK, et al. Frequent detection of pancreatic lesions in asymptomatic high-risk individuals. *Gastroenterology.* 2012;142(4):796–804.

167. Potjer TP, Schot I, Langer P, et al. Variation in precursor lesions of pancreatic cancer among high-risk groups. *Clin Cancer Res.* 2013;19(2):442–449.

168. Sud A, Wham D, Catalano M, et al. Promising outcomes of screening for pancreatic cancer by genetic testing and endoscopic ultrasound. *Pancreas.* 2014;43(3):458–461.

169. Del Chiaro M, Verbeke CS, Kartalis N, et al. Short-term results of a magnetic resonance imaging-based Swedish screening program for individuals at risk for pancreatic cancer. *JAMA Surg.* 2015;150(6):512–518.

170. Mocci E, Guillen-Ponce C, Earl J, et al. PanGen-Fam: Spanish registry of hereditary pancreatic cancer. *Eur J Cancer.* 2015;51(14):1911–1917.

171. Vasen H, Ibrahim I, Ponce CG, et al. Benefit of surveillance for pancreatic cancer in high-risk individuals: outcome of long-term prospective follow-up studies from three European expert centers. *J Clin Oncol.* 2016;34(17):2010–2019.

172. Konings IC, Harinck F, Poley JW, et al. Prevalence and progression of pancreatic cystic precursor lesions differ between groups at high risk of developing pancreatic cancer. *Pancreas.* 2017;46(1):28–34.

173. DaVee T, Coronel E, Papafragkakis C, et al. Pancreatic cancer screening in high-risk individuals with germline genetic mutations. *Gastrointest Endosc.* 2018;87(6):1443–1450.

174. Barnes CA, Krzywda E, Lahiff S, et al. Development of a high risk pancreatic screening clinic using 3.0 T MRI. *Fam Cancer.* 2018;17(1):101–111.

175. Gangi A, Malafa M, Klapman J. Endoscopic ultrasound-based pancreatic cancer screening of high-risk individuals: a prospective observational trial. *Pancreas.* 2018;47(5):586–591.

176. Canto MI, Almario JA, Schulick RD, et al. Risk of neoplastic progression in individuals at high risk for pancreatic cancer undergoing long-term surveillance. *Gastroenterology.* 2018;155(3):740–751.

177. Lu C. Screening for pancreatic cancer in familial high-risk individuals: A systematic review. *World J Gastroenterol.* 2015;21(28):8678.

178. Rulyak SJ, Kimmey MB, Veenstra DL, Brentnall TA. Cost-effectiveness of pancreatic cancer screening in familial pancreatic cancer kindreds. *Gastrointest Endosc.* 2003;57(1):23–29.

179. Bruenderman E, Martin RC. A cost analysis of a pancreatic cancer screening protocol in high-risk populations. *Am J Surg*. 2015;210(3):409–416.

180. Latchford A, Greenhalf W, Vitone LJ, et al. Peutz-Jeghers syndrome and screening for pancreatic cancer. *The British Journal of Surgery*. 2006;93(12):1446–1455.

181. Maheu C, Vodermaier A, Rothenmund H, et al. Pancreatic cancer risk counselling and screening: impact on perceived risk and psychological functioning. *Fam Cancer*. 2010;9(4):617–624.

182. Harinck F, Nagtegaal T, Kluijt I, et al. Feasibility of a pancreatic cancer surveillance program from a psychological point of view. *Genet Med*. 2011;13(12):1015–1024.

183. Tutt A, Ashworth A. The relationship between the roles of BRCA genes in DNA repair and cancer predisposition. *Trends Mol Med*. 2002;8(12):571–576.

184. Lowery MA, Kelsen DP, Stadler ZK, et al. An emerging entity: pancreatic adenocarcinoma associated with a known BRCA mutation: clinical descriptors, treatment implications, and future directions. *Oncologist*. 2011;16(10):1397–1402.

185. Golan T, Kanji ZS, Epelbaum R, et al. Overall survival and clinical characteristics of pancreatic cancer in BRCA mutation carriers. *Br J Cancer*. 2014;111(6):1132–1138.

186. Sehdev A, Gbolahan O, Hancock BA, et al. Germline and somatic DNA damage repair gene mutations and overall survival in metastatic pancreatic adenocarcinoma patients treated with FOLFIRINOX. *Clin Cancer Res*. 2018;24(24):6204–6211.

187. NCCN Guidelines for Pancreatic Adenocarcinoma (Version 3.2019 J, 2019). Last accessed on March 29, 2020.

188. Bryant HE, Schultz N, Thomas HD, et al. Specific killing of BRCA2-deficient tumours with inhibitors of poly(ADP-ribose) polymerase. *Nature*. 2005;434(7035):913–917.

189. Golan T, Hammel P, Reni M, et al. Maintenance olaparib for germline BRCA-mutated metastatic pancreatic cancer. *N Engl J Med*. 2019;381(4):317–327.

190. Dunn GP, Bruce AT, Ikeda H, et al. Cancer immunoediting: from immunosurveillance to tumor escape. *Nat Immunol*. 2002;3(11):991–998.

191. Topalian SL, Drake CG, Pardoll DM. Immune checkpoint blockade: a common denominator approach to cancer therapy. *Cancer Cell*. 2015;27(4):450–461.

192. Le DT, Durham JN, Smith KN, et al. Mismatch repair deficiency predicts response of solid tumors to PD-1 blockade. *Science*. 2017;357(6349):409–413.

193. Johansson H, Andersson R, Bauden M, et al. Immune checkpoint therapy for pancreatic cancer. *World J Gastroenterol*. 2016;22(43):9457–9476.

194. Singhi AD, Ali SM, Lacy J, et al. Identification of targetable ALK rearrangements in pancreatic ductal adenocarcinoma. *J Natl Compr Canc Netw*. 2017;15(5):555–562.

195. Stroun M, Maurice P, Vasioukhin V, et al. The origin and mechanism of circulating DNA. *Ann N Y Acad Sci*. 2000;906:161–168.

196. Liggett T, Melnikov A, Yi QL, et al. Differential methylation of cell-free circulating DNA among patients with pancreatic cancer versus chronic pancreatitis. *Cancer*. 2010;116(7):1674–1680.

197. Gall TMH, Belete S, Khanderia E, et al. Circulating tumor cells and cell-free DNA in pancreatic ductal adenocarcinoma. *Am J Pathol*. 2019;189(1):71–81.

198. Cohen JD, Li L, Wang Y, et al. Detection and localization of surgically resectable cancers with a multi-analyte blood test. *Science*. 2018;359(6378):926–930.

199. Croce CM, Calin GA. miRNAs, cancer, and stem cell division. *Cell*. 2005;122(1):6–7.

200. Bloomston M, Frankel WL, Petrocca F, et al. MicroRNA expression patterns to differentiate pancreatic adenocarcinoma from normal pancreas and chronic pancreatitis. *JAMA*. 2007;297(17):1901.

201. Ho AS, Huang X, Cao H, et al. Circulating miR-210 as a novel hypoxia marker in pancreatic cancer. *Transl Oncol*. 2010;3(2):109–113.

202. Wang J, Chen J, Chang P, et al. MicroRNAs in plasma of pancreatic ductal adenocarcinoma patients as novel blood-based biomarkers of disease. *Cancer Prev Res (Phila)*. 2009;2(9):807–813.

203. Kong X, Du Y, Wang G, et al. Detection of differentially expressed microRNAs in serum of pancreatic ductal adenocarcinoma patients: miR-196a could be a potential marker for poor prognosis. *Dig Dis Sci.* 2011;56(2):602–609.

204. Goto T, Fujiya M, Konishi H, et al. An elevated expression of serum exosomal microRNA-191, - 21, -451a of pancreatic neoplasm is considered to be efficient diagnostic marker. *BMC Cancer.* 2018;18(1):116.

205. Gong TT, Hu DM, Zhu Q. Contrast-enhanced EUS for differential diagnosis of pancreatic mass lesions: a meta-analysis. *Gastrointest Endosc.* 2012;76(2):301–309.

206. Li F, Malli A, Cruz-Monserrate Z, et al. Confocal endomicroscopy and cyst fluid molecular analysis: Comprehensive evaluation of pancreatic cysts. *World J Gastrointest Endosc.* 2018;10(1):1–9.

207. Ying L, Lin X, Xie ZL, et al. Clinical utility of endoscopic ultrasound elastography for identification of malignant pancreatic masses: a meta-analysis. *J Gastroenterol Hepatol.* 2013;28(9):1434–1443.

208. Dimastromatteo J, Brentnall T, Kelly KA. Imaging in pancreatic disease. *Nat Rev Gastroenterol Hepatol.* 2017;14(2):97–109.

209. Foygel K, Wang H, Machtaler S, et al. Detection of pancreatic ductal adenocarcinoma in mice by ultrasound imaging of thymocyte differentiation antigen 1. *Gastroenterology.* 2013;145(4):885–8943.

210. Chari ST, Kelly K, Hollingsworth MA, et al. Early detection of sporadic pancreatic cancer: summative review. *Pancreas.* 2015;44(5):693–712.

Risk Assessment and Clinical Management – Genito-Urinary Tract Cancer

Soum D. Lokeshwar, Jamil S. Syed, and Preston C. Sprenkle

▦ INTRODUCTION

The genito-urinary system involves organs responsible for the production and storage of urine as well as those related to male sexual function. Cancer within this system presents a unique challenge to providers as patients often present with non-specific symptoms. However, cancer in many of these organs have genetic components that may aide in the early diagnosis and individualized treatment of patients. This chapter discusses the background and genetics of kidney, bladder, prostate, and testicular cancer. Table 11.1 provides a brief summary of the hereditary cancer syndromes.

▦ KIDNEY CANCER

A hereditary component exists in a small but non-negligible proportion of patients with kidney cancer. There are a number of well-described hereditary kidney cancer syndromes with a variety of renal and extrarenal manifestations. A clinical suspicion based on young age of diagnosis, presentation with bilateral or multifocal tumors, or strong family history of kidney cancer should prompt consideration for genetic testing. Surgical intervention is guided by the principle of nephron sparing when feasible and thresholds for intervention are dependent on the hereditary syndrome and size of the tumors. In this section we describe various hereditary kidney cancer syndromes along with indications for genetic testing and general principles regarding when to intervene surgically (Table 11.2).

Epidemiology and Genetic Risk

The median age of diagnosis for kidney cancer is 64 years.[1] For the year 2021 it is estimated that there will be more than 76,000 new cases of kidney cancer with more than 14,000 associated deaths in the United States.[1] Solid neoplastic lesions of the kidney include both benign and malignant pathology. In a patient with a renal mass, the likelihood of malignancy and risk of synchronous metastasis is related to the size of the mass based on imaging. Masses

TABLE 11.1: Hereditary GU Cancer Syndromes

Cancer	Hereditary Condition	Genes	Associated Symptoms	GU Specific
Kidney	VHL	VHL Chromosome 13	Retinal angiomas, endolymphatic sac tumors, benign CNS hemangioblastomas, pancreatic cysts, islet tumors, epididymal cystadenomas, pheochromocytomas	Clear cell RCC
	HPRC	MET Chromosome 7	GU specific	Bilateral multifocal type 1 papillary RCC
	HLRCC	FH Chromosome 1	Multiple cutaneous piloleiomyomas, multiple early-onset uterine leiomyomas	Papillary type II RCC
	BHD	BHD Chromosome 17	Pulmonary cysts, fibrofolliculomas, thyroid nodules	Chromophobe RCC, oncocytomas, hybrid renal tumors
	SDRCC	SDH Chromosome 10	Paragangliomas of the head and neck, classical pheochromocytomas, GI stromal tumors	RCC, papillary, sarcomatoid kidney cancers
Bladder	Lynch	MLH1, MSH2, MSH6, PMS2 Chromosome 2,3,5 or 7	Colorectal cancer, cancer of the endometrium, ovary, stomach, small bowel, pancreato-biliary system, skin pathologies, brain	Prostate and bladder tumors
	RB	RB Chromosome 13	Retinoblastomas, osteosarcoma, soft tissue sarcomas, skin melanomas, lung cancer, breast cancer, head and neck cancer, uterine cancer, brain tumors	Bladder cancer
	Costello	HRAS Chromosome 11	Intellectual disability, facial abnormalities, excess skin, flexible joints, hypertrophic cardiomyopathy, short stature, renal anomalies	Bladder papillomata and bladder transitional cell carcinoma
	Apert	FGFR2 Chromosome 10	Craniofacial abnormalities, hand and foot malformations, developmental delay, hearing loss, overriding aorta and other cardiac abnormalities, pyloric stenosis, other organ malignancies	Bladder cancer Undescended testicles
Prostate	HBOC	BRCA1 & 2 Other tumor suppressor genes Chromosome 13 &17	Ovarian and breast cancer	Prostate cancer
	HOBX13	HOXB13 Chromosome 22	GU specific	Prostate cancer
Testicular	Peutz-Jeghers	STK11/LKB1 Chromosome 19	Gastrointestinal hamartomatous polyps, mucocutaneous pigmentation, breast, ovarian, uterine, and lung cancer	Sertoli cell tumors
	Carney Complex	PRKAR1A Chromosome 17	Multiple endocrine gland tumors, cardiac myxomas, abnormal skin pigmentation, melanotic schwannomas, breast myxomatosis	Sertoli cell tumors often bilateral

TABLE 11.2: Familial Kidney Cancer Subtypes

Syndrome	Predisposing Gene (Chromosome)	Renal Tumor Histology and Other Major Clinical Manifestations	Recommended Management for Renal Tumors	Kidney Cancer Screening
von Hippel-Lindau disease (VHL)	VHL (3p25)	Clear cell RCC, often multifocal Retinal angiomas Central nervous system hemangioblastomas Pheochromocytoma Other tumors	Active surveillance <3 cm Surgical excision ≥3 cm, preference for nephron-sparing approaches	Annual renal ultrasound, abdominal MRI every other year
Hereditary papillary renal carcinoma (HPRC)	MET (7q31)	Multiple, bilateral type 1 papillary RCC	Active surveillance <3 cm Surgical excision ≥3 cm, preference for nephron-sparing approaches	Annual renal ultrasound, abdominal MRI every other year
Hereditary leiomyomatosis and renal cell carcinoma (HLRCC)	Fumarate hydratase (FH) (1q42-43)	Type 2 papillary RCC most common Collecting duct carcinoma Leiomyomas of skin or uterus Uterine leiomyosarcomas Low-grade variants of RCC also seen in children	Surgical excision, preference for PN, but only when wide margins can be achieved	Abdominal MRI yearly
Succinate dehydrogenase-deficient RCC (SDH-RCC)	SDHA SDHB (1p36.13), SDHC (1q23.3), SDHD (11q23.1), SHDAF2	SDH-associated RCC (chromophobe, clear cell, type 2 papillary RCC; or oncocytoma), variable aggressiveness Paragangliomas (benign and malignant) Papillary thyroid carcinoma	Surgical excision, preference for PN, but only when wide margins can be achieved	Abdominal MRI every other year
Birt-Hogg-Dube syndrome (BHD)	Folliculin (17p11.2)	Multiple chromophobe RCC, hybrid oncocytic tumors, oncocytomas Clear cell RCC (occasionally) Papillary RCC (occasionally) Facial fibrofolliculomas Lung cysts Spontaneous pneumothorax	Active surveillance <3 cm Surgical excision ≥3 cm, preference for nephron-sparing approaches	Abdominal MRI every other year
PTEN hamartoma tumor syndrome (Cowden syndrome)	PTEN (10q23)	Papillary RCC or other histology Breast tumors (malignant and benign) Epithelial thyroid carcinoma	Active surveillance <3 cm Surgical excision ≥3 cm, preference for nephron-sparing approaches	Renal Ultrasound or abdominal MRI every year
BAP1 tumor predisposition syndrome	BAP1 (3p21.2)	Clear cell RCC, can be high grade	Surgical excision, preference for nephron-sparing approaches	Abdominal MRI every other year

Adapted with permission from Schmidt LS, Linehan WM. Genetic predisposition to kidney cancer, Semin Oncol 2016 Oct;43(5):566-574.

that are 3 to 4 cm in diameter have an estimated 80 to 85% chance of harboring malignancy with a 2% risk of metastasis while those above 7 cm have a 95% chance of being malignant with a 15 to 20% chance of having synchronous metastasis.[2] Most kidney cancers are thought to occur secondary to *de novo* events. Established risk factors associated with kidney cancer development include smoking, hypertension, and obesity.[3] Several case-control studies suggest an association of renal cell cancer (RCC) with agricultural work and with herbicide and insecticide exposure.[4]

It has been increasingly recognized that a significant proportion of patients may harbor a genetic predisposition to developing kidney cancer. About 5 to 8% of kidney cancers are thought to be associated with a hereditary influence.[5] Management strategies for kidney cancer in patients with a familial predisposition can be challenging as most clinicians do not routinely work within these patient populations. From surveillance to surgical treatment, decision-making is complex, especially in a patient who may present with bilateral or multiple tumors. Furthermore, the clinician should be aware of extrarenal manifestations associated with certain syndromes and the possibility of secondary *de novo* tumors.[6]

Clinical Presentation

The presentation of kidney cancer can vary. With the widespread use of cross-sectional imaging, the "incidentaloma" has become a frequently used term. Historically, a triad of flank pain, mass. and hematuria was the hallmark of kidney cancer but in the era of modern imaging, it has become a rare presentation. A migration toward diagnosing patients with lower-stage kidney cancer has been seen and these patients may not have symptoms related to local tumor growth. In a contemporary series, less than 5% of patients present with symptoms and greater than 50% of renal masses are diagnosed incidentally with imaging obtained for unrelated issues.[7] Of all patients diagnosed with kidney cancer, regardless of whether or not they have associated symptoms, about 30% will have synchronous metastasis. In patients who do present with clinical symptoms it is likely due to metastatic disease, local tumor growth with possible hemorrhage or a paraneoplastic process. Paraneoplastic syndromes can be found in 10 to 20% of patients with kidney cancer.[8] Described paraneoplastic syndromes associated with kidney cancer include the following:

1. Stauffer's syndrome: Reversible hepatitis not associated with liver metastases.
2. Anemia or polycythemia.
3. Elevated erythrocyte sedimentation rate, C-reactive protein, alkaline phosphatase, and calcium.

Physical Examination/Labwork/Imaging

Physical exams can be an important part of the diagnostic workup for a patient with a renal mass though most patients with localized disease will have a normal exam. Findings of a large mass, or adenopathy, may be indicative of advanced disease. Varicoceles most notably of the right testicle can be indicative of tumor thrombus within the vena cava or vena cava compression. Skin assessment is also crucial in the physical exam for someone with a renal mass as patients with familial syndromes often have dermatologic findings.

There are no urinary or serum biomarkers used to diagnose kidney cancer at the present time. Labwork that is routinely obtained at our institution for patients with a newly diagnosed, presumed malignant mass includes a complete blood count with differential, comprehensive metabolic panel, LDH, and urinalysis.

Gold standard imaging for the evaluation of renal masses includes multi-phase contrast-enhanced MRI or CT scan. If a patient has a renal mass detected on ultrasound, it should be confirmed with contrast-enhanced cross-sectional imaging. Patients with chronic kidney disease (CKD) may be at risk from iodinated and gadolinium-based contrast agents. It has been shown, however, that patients with stage III-IV cancer can receive a contrast-enhanced CT without an increased risk of acute kidney injury (AKI), emergent dialysis, and short-term mortality when compared to those with normal kidney function.[9] In addition to abdominal imaging, a chest X-ray should be obtained in all patients with a newly diagnosed renal mass and consideration for a CT scan should be made in those patients with respiratory symptoms, concern for metastasis, or abnormal X-ray findings. Bone scans and brain imaging are not routinely performed unless there is clinical suspicion for involvement of the respective organs.

Management

The management of renal masses involves complex decision-making. Management strategies for localized disease are dependent on a number of factors that include but are not limited to patient preference, co-morbidities, renal function, tumor size and location, and clinical stage. For localized tumors, the mainstay treatment options include active surveillance, nephron sparing procedures for amenable masses (ablation, cryotherapy, or partial nephrectomy), and radical nephrectomy. For the remainder of this section, we will focus on the hereditary kidney cancer syndromes and their management.

Hereditary Cancer Syndromes

There are several well-described kidney cancer syndromes. The vast majority are inherited in an autosomal dominant fashion with a younger age (~46 years) of diagnosis being a risk factor for a familial syndrome. The syndromes that will be discussed in this chapter include Von Hippel-Lindau (VHL), hereditary papillary renal cell carcinoma (HPRC), hereditary leiomyomatosis and renal cell carcinoma (HLRCC), Birt-Hogg-Dube (BHD), tuberous sclerosis complex (TSC), BRCA-1 associated protein 1 (BAP1), Cowden syndrome (PTEN), microphthalmia associated transcription factor (MITF), hereditary hyperparathyroidism jaw tumour syndrome (*CDC73*), and succinate dehydrogenase renal cell carcinoma (SDHRCC).

VHL A germline VHL mutation occurs in 1 out of every 35,000 people.[10] VHL is a tumor suppressor gene on the short arm of chromosome 3 and when mutated is unable to form the E3 ubiquitin ligase complex that regulates the degradation of regulatory proteins, including the hypoxia inducible cactor (HIF-1, HIF-2). The resultant over-accumulation of intracellular HIF results in upregulation of vascular endothelial growth factor and other regulatory proteins impacting cellular growth and development.[11] Patients with VHL can develop retinal angiomas, endolymphatic sac tumors, benign CNS hemangioblastomas, pancreatic cysts and islet tumors, epididymal cystadenomas, and pheochromocytomas. Clear cell RCC develops with early (third to fifth decade in age) and is often bilateral and multifocal with an estimated penetrance of 50%. It should be noted that in patients with VHL, cysts can harbor malignancy and as such are not scored using the Bosniak criteria, which is based on CT imaging criteria to define cysts of the kidney into categories that are distinct from one another in terms of the likelihood of malignancy.

HPRC HPRC is a highly penetrant yet rare disorder. The gene responsible for HPRC is MET and is localized to the long arm of chromosome 7. This disorder is inherited in an autosomal dominant fashion, however, and represents a mutation in a proto-oncogene. MET mutations lead to activation of tyrosine kinase, which allows cell proliferation.[12] The disorder is characterized by bilateral and multifocal Type I papillary RCC. Of the classically described kidney cancer syndromes, it is the least common, and there are no extrarenal findings. Early age of onset, bilateral/multifocal papillary tumors, and family history of papillary RCC could be used for considering genetic testing. However, because this syndrome is extremely rare (30 known families), genetic testing even among patients with bilateral and multifocal RCC often leads to negative results.[13,14]

HLRCC HLRCC is an autosomal dominant disorder characterized by papillary type II RCC with a 20% penetrance or as HLRCC-associated RCC with an aggressive clinical behavior necessitating early surgical intervention with wide resection. Metastatic progression is not uncommon. Patients may present with clinical manifestations that include painful cutaneous leiomyomas (Figure 11.1) that are flesh colored or uterine leiomyomas in women. The HLRCC locus has been mapped to the long arm of chromosome 1, the site of the fumarate hydratase (FH) tumor suppressor gene.[15]

BHD BHD is an autosomal dominant disorder that is characterized by bilateral, multifocal, chromophobe RCC, oncocytomas, or hybrid renal tumors with a 20 to 40% penetrance. The disorder is rare with an incidence of approximately 1 in 200,000 individuals.[16] Patients with BHD may present with clinical manifestations that include fibrofolliculomas (Figure 11.2) of the head and neck, pulmonary cysts, and spontaneous pneumothorax. The BHD gene has been mapped to the short arm of chromosome 17, which encodes the tumor suppressor gene product folliculin (FLCN).[17] Fortunately, kidney cancer in BHD tends to be of lower grade with a hybrid of chromophobe and oncocytic characteristics and portends a better prognosis when compared to kidney cancer seen in other hereditary syndromes.

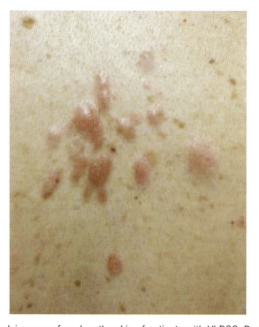

FIGURE 11.1: Cutaneous leiomyoma found on the skin of patients with HLRCC. Reproduced with permission from Nguyen KA, Syed JS, Shuch B. Hereditary Kidney Cancer Syndromes and Surgical Management of the Small Renal Mass, Urol Clin North Am 2017 May;44(2):155-167.

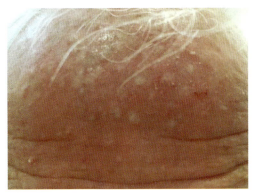

FIGURE 11.2: Cutaneous fibrofolliculomas commonly found on the skin of the head or neck of patients with BHD. Reproduced with permission from Nguyen KA, Syed JS, Shuch B. Hereditary Kidney Cancer Syndromes and Surgical Management of the Small Renal Mass, Urol Clin North Am 2017 May;44(2):155-167.

TSC TSC is inherited in an autosomal dominant fashion with an incidence of approximately 1 in 10,000. Most cases are secondary to alterations in TSC1 or TSC2 genes, which are located on chromosomes 9 and 16, respectively.[14] TSC1/2 act as tumor suppressors and mutations can lead to upregulation of HIF.[18] More than half of all patients with TSC have been reported to develop renal manifestations including angiomyolipomas and renal cysts. Kidney cancer can develop in 5% of patients with a wide range of histology.[19] In the central nervous system hamartomas and giant cell astrocytomas can develop. Dermatologic manifestations include facial angiofibromas, shagreen patches, ash leaf spots, and periungual fibromas.

BAP1 BAP1 tumor predisposition has been associated with the BAP1 gene located on chromosome 3p2 and has been estimated to be represented in 15% of all clear cell kidney cancers though other histologies have been reported.[20] Other cancers involved with BAP1 alterations include uveal and cutaneous melanomas and mesotheliomas. BAP1 alterations in kidney cancer are associated with higher-grade disease and surgical excision is recommended with a preference for nephron sparing if feasible.

PTEN Cowden syndrome results from germline mutations of the phosphatase and tensin homolog tumor suppressor gene localized to 10q22, which together are termed PTEN hamartoma syndrome. The incidence of Cowden syndrome is 1 in 200,000 people.[21] Patients with Cowden syndrome carry a 34% chance of developing kidney cancer. Other cancers associated with Cowden syndrome include female breast cancer and thyroid cancer. Hair follicle lesions called trichilemmomas have been associated with Cowden syndrome in addition to neurologic signs and symptoms including macrocephaly, ataxia, and tremors. Given the lifetime risk of developing RCC in patients with Cowden syndrome, routine surveillance with a yearly CT or MRI has been suggested for surveillance.

MITF MITF has been proposed as an oncogene implicated in melanoma and RCC.[22] MITF regulates HIF-1α and is normally suppressed; the mutated version activates HIF-1α, potentially contributing to the development of RCC. Renal tumor histology and other major clinical manifestations have yet to be clearly defined and a definitive diagnosis is reached by genetic testing.

CDC73 Hereditary hyperparathyroidism jaw tumor syndrome is an inherited autosomal dominant disorder caused by mutations in *CDC73* and characterized by susceptibility to parathyroid adenomas, ossifying jaw fibromas, and renal abnormalities, most commonly renal cysts, but also clear cell kidney cancer.[23,24]

SDRCC Patients with SDRCC develop extra-adrenal pheochromocytomas or otherwise termed paragangliomas of the head and neck or classical pheochromocytomas.[25] Gastrointestinal stromal tumors are also associated with this syndrome. This syndrome involves loss of the succinate dehydrogenase complex, which is a mitochondrial enzyme that functions in the electron transport chain. Individuals with germline mutation of one of the multiple genes encoding the complex, including *SDHA, SDHB, SDHC, SDHD,* and *SHDAF2,* are at increased risk for RCC. Kidney cancer can develop in 5 to 15% of patients with succinate dehydrogenase associated paraganglioma syndromes and 25% may present with bilateral tumors.[26] Clear cell, papillary, and sarcomatoid characteristics have all been seen in those with SDRCC.[27]

Genetic Testing Genetic testing can be used to identify germline mutations in patients. For patients with a genetic predisposition to kidney cancer, knowing the type of disorder can help with decision-making regarding screening, when to proceed with surgery, how to conduct surveillance, and how to direct family members with regards to screening for renal and extrarenal malignancy. The treating clinician is responsible for recognizing patients who may benefit from genetic counseling and testing. Patients who have a family history and present at an early age with kidney cancer are at risk of having a genetic predisposition, so consideration for genetic testing can be made. A commonly used age as a cutoff for genetic testing is tumors diagnosed in patients is ≤ 46 years old.[28] Patients with bilateral tumors or multifocal tumors may be referred for genetic counseling as well. In addition, those with at least one first- or second-degree family member with kidney cancer can be considered for genetic counseling. The American College of Medical Genetics and Genomics guidelines recommends that patients meet with a genetic counselor for assessing suitability prior to genetic testing.[29] Individual genes can then be tested based on clinical suspicion. From the results, sequence variations are then classified as pathogenic or likely pathogenic.[29] The identification of a patient with a mutation should lead to the notification of family members who may be at risk. In this scenario, at-risk individuals could be screened for early identification of a renal tumor to help prevent metastasis. Furthermore, a clinician can take necessary steps to initiate appropriate referrals for multidisciplinary care for patients and their family members. It should be mentioned that next-generation sequencing has revolutionized molecular diagnostics to allow for panel testing. Compared with sequential single-gene testing, panel testing offers an expedited evaluation of multiple genes and can result in a higher identification rate of germline alterations.[30] Furthermore, panel testing allows an evaluation of hereditary syndromes that may not be discernable by clinical diagnosis.[31]

Imaging in Patients with Hereditary Predisposition to Kidney Cancer In patients with a diagnosed hereditary risk of kidney cancer, lifelong surveillance is crucial as the risk of developing kidney cancer is much higher compared to the general population. Yearly imaging is usually obtained for patients with hereditary kidney cancer. For patients with VHL at our institution, yearly abdominal imaging with CT or MRI is performed. There is risk of secondary malignancy with radiation exposure from yearly CT scanning. As such, alternating with abdominal ultrasound can be considered. In patients with BHD, annual abdominal imaging is performed with CT or MRI. For patients with HPRC, ultrasound is not recommended for detection or follow-up of renal lesions as they can be difficult to see due to their isoechoic appearance and surveillance with CT or MRI is preferred.[32] Annual screening/surveillance with CT or MRI is performed at our institution for patients with SDRCC or HLRCC.

Surgical Intervention Historically, radical nephrectomy was the gold standard for renal masses. In patients with bilateral renal masses as frequently seen in patients with hereditary syndromes, the outcome was bilateral nephrectomy and placement of dialysis. It has been subsequently shown that nephron sparing techniques with enucleation of individual tumors to spare nephrons has equivalent cancer control and can obviate the need for dialysis.[33] The decision of when to intervene with surgery for patients with hereditary kidney cancer that is localized is determined by the pathologic aggressiveness associated with the disorder. The "3 cm" rule has been used as a trigger for intervention in patients with certain hereditary kidney cancer syndromes. For patients with BHD, VHL, and HPRC, surveillance is performed until the largest tumor of the respective kidney measures 3 cm. This size represents the threshold for surgery of the mass and any other lesions of the respective kidney.[34] The risk of metastatic spread in these syndromes with tumors less than 3 cm is very rare; however, for patients with HLRCC or SDRCC the 3 cm rule does not apply. In these instances, tumors are more aggressive and represent a metastatic risk even if < 3 cm. Hence, early removal of the mass is recommended. For patients with kidney tumors associated with the less well-characterized hereditary conditions, the role of active surveillance remains unclear. For these patients, prompt removal of renal masses should be recommended to avoid the risk of metastasis.[35]

Bladder Cancer

Bladder cancer is a neoplasm with a high morbidity and mortality for patients.[36] A diagnosis of advanced bladder cancer is often life changing as it generally involves invasive surgery and/or chemoradiation. Therefore, the early detection and risk stratification of bladder cancer is at the forefront of bladder cancer research. Although environmental factors are by far the prevailing cause of bladder cancer, there exist a few genetic predispositions. This includes well-described hereditary bladder cancer syndromes that result in a constellation of symptoms. With the aid of imaging, genetic tests, and clinical suspicion based on familial history, it may be possible to accurately screen and diagnose patients prior to the development of metastatic or advanced disease. In this section we discuss the background of bladder cancer, the genetic risk and hereditary cancer syndromes associated with bladder cancer, and how to diagnose and counsel these patients.

Epidemiology and Genetic Risk Bladder cancer is one of the most common cancers in the United States.[1] In 2020 it is estimated that there were more than 81,400 new cases of bladder cancer with 17,980 estimated deaths. In men, bladder cancer is the fourth most common cancer, and it comprises 7% of all cancer cases. Approximately 62,100 new cases of bladder cancer patients are in males and 19,300 in females, with more men than women dying of the disease as well (13,050 and 4,930, respectively).[1]

Bladder cancer is an umbrella term used to describe any neoplasm affecting the bladder and/or the urinary tract. Bladder tumors can include malignant and benign tumors. Bladder tumors include a myriad of types. By far the most common type is urothelial cell carcinoma (UCC) or transitional cell carcinoma comprising more than 90% of all cases.[37] These tumors arise from the transitional epithelium that lines the bladder. As transitional cells line much of the urinary collecting system, these tumors may arise in the bladder, urethra, ureters, and the kidney. Next most common is squamous cell cancer of the bladder with 2 to 5% of presenting cases in the United States.[38] Squamous cell cancer, although uncommon in the United States, is common in countries where schistosomiasis is endemic, such as Egypt.[39] The other less common cases of bladder cancer are adenocarcinoma, small cell carcinoma, and sarcoma.

The primary risk factors for bladder cancer are generally thought to be environmental exposure. As the bladder is responsible for urine storage, the urothelium can be exposed to toxins and carcinogens concentrated in the urine. Tobacco smoking is the most recognized risk factor for bladder cancer, but other risk factors include industrial chemical exposure, obesity, radiation exposure, and schistosomiasis infection.[40] Although not well understood, there exists a genetic risk of bladder cancer. It may cause some patients to be at a higher risk for developing bladder cancer and possibly with a higher malignant potential.

There is a reported almost 2-fold increase in bladder cancer risk among first-degree relatives of patients with UCC.[41] In a population-based study of twins, the estimated genetic heritability of bladder cancer was 31%.[42] Inherited genetic factors have also been investigated. N-acetyltransferase 2 (NAT2) variants and glutathione S-transferase mu 1 (GSTM1)-null genotypes increase a carrier's risk of developing bladder cancer.[43] A NAT2 mutation may also confer additional susceptibility to bladder cancer in smokers as it is involved in detoxification and bioactivation of carcinogens.[44] Eight common sequence variants are associated with bladder cancer, which are located at 4p16.3, 5p15.33, 2q37.1, 3q28, 8q24.21, 8q24.3, 19q12, and 22q13.1.[45-47] Although variants in these locations have been identified and associated with bladder cancer, the majority increase risk by <20%.[48]

Clinical Presentation The median age of presentation for bladder cancer is 73, with 90% of patients with this disease diagnosed over the age of 55.[1] Approximately 70% of patients presenting with bladder tumors will have superficial, non-life threatening but often recurrent, disease. Approximately 30% of patients present with muscle invasive disease, which has the potential for distant metastasis to other organs and organ systems.[37]

The most common presentation for bladder cancer is painless hematuria,[49] which may present on routine urinalysis as microscopic hematuria or be visible gross hematuria. About 20% of patients who present with painless gross hematuria have bladder cancer.[50] Microscopic hematuria related bladder cancer has an incidence of 2 to 5%.[51] According to the American Urological Association (AUA), asymptomatic microhematuria is defined as three or more red blood cells per high-powered field on urinalysis. Bladder-cancer-associated hematuria should be of higher suspicion in older patients who have a history of smoking. Other clinical presentations include pain in the pubic region or during micturition, trouble voiding, and constitutional symptoms such as fatigue. As there is no routine screening for bladder cancer, patients may not present until they have a large tumor burden.

Physical Examination/Labwork/Imaging Examining for a suspicion of bladder cancer may be challenging. For the clinical presentation of voiding symptoms or hematuria, the history is crucial to rule out more benign causes. Hematuria may be caused by a plethora of benign conditions including kidney stones, urinary tract infection, vigorous exercise or microtrauma, recent urological procedure, or idiopathic microhematuria. History should include the standard record of symptoms but should also include a detailed family history of cancer. The social history of a patient including smoking history and environmental exposures should also be elucidated. Bladder cancer may also present with disease processes that may be hereditary in nature.

Physical examination for bladder cancer should include a full comprehensive exam including a focused genito-urinary exam including a digital rectal exam. In advanced cases of bladder cancer, a solid pelvic mass may be felt. The lymph nodes of the genitals and pelvis should be examined for lymphadenopathy. The digital rectal exam may aid in ruling out benign prostatic hyperplasia or BPH. Percussion and palpation of the flanks should also be performed. Positive signs of pain may indicate upper urinary tract lesions, renal stones, or ureteral obstruction.

For patients presenting with microhematuria, the AUA[52] recommends evaluation of microscopic hematuria by examination of urinary sediment through formal urinalysis. For patients older than 35 years of age, cystoscopy should be performed in the workup of asymptomatic microhematuria or gross hematuria. In patients younger than 35 this can be performed at the physician's discretion but tobacco smokers or those with environmental exposure should undergo cystoscopy evaluation.

According to the AUA,[52] radiologic evaluation should also be performed in patients with asymptomatic microhematuria or suspicion of bladder cancer. The use of a multiphasic CT (with and without IV contrast) including sufficient phases to view the renal parenchyma, to aid in the rule out of renal malignancy, should be performed. In patients who cannot undergo a CT scan, an MRU with and without IV contrast is acceptable. Although urine cytology and urine markers are used in some practices, this is not recommended as part of a routine evaluation.

Hereditary Cancer Syndromes The early identification and recognition of hereditary cancer syndromes may aid in the early diagnosis of bladder cancer or other related disease within a syndrome. This identification may aid in screening of the patient as well as familial screening. Syndromes associated with bladder cancer include Lynch syndrome, hereditary RB, Costello syndrome, and Apert syndrome.

Lynch Syndrome Lynch syndrome, also referred to as hereditary nonpolyposis colorectal cancer, is a hereditary cancer syndrome caused by mutations in the DNA mismatch-repair genes: MLH1, MSH2, MSH6, EPCAM and PMS2. Patients who carry these genetic mutations have a higher likelihood of developing many types of tumors, most commonly colorectal cancer. Extracolonic manifestations include cancer of the endometrium, ovaries, stomach, small bowel, pancreatobiliary system, skin pathologies, brain, and the genito-urinary system including the bladder.[53] In Western countries, Lynch syndrome has a prevalence of 1:370 to 1:2000.[54] In a Dutch study performed on 95 families with germline mutations in MLH1, MSH2 and MSH6, the relative risk for developing bladder cancer before the age of 70, in mutation carriers and first-degree relatives, was 4.2 (95% CI 2.2 to 7.2) for men and 2.2 (95% CI 0.3 to 8.0) for women when compared to the general population. This relative risk was most pronounced in those with the MSH2 mutation.[55]

Hereditary RB Hereditary retinoblastoma (RB) is a rare childhood tumor that arises in the retina either unilaterally or bilaterally and is caused by an inactivating mutation in the RB1 gene (q14 on chromosome 13).[56] Survivors of retinoblastoma during childhood have a higher risk of developing other cancers later in life. These include osteosarcoma, soft tissue sarcomas, skin melanomas, lymphoma, lung cancer, breast cancer, cancer of the head and neck region, uterine cancer, brain tumors, and bladder cancer. In a study of 144 survivors of hereditary RB the standardized morality ratio (SMR) for bladder cancer was 26.31 (95% CI 8.54 to 61.41).[57] Retinoblastoma confers cancer risk on survivors not only by gene mutation but also due to radiation treatment exposure early in life.

Costello Syndrome Costello syndrome is an autosomal dominant disorder that is also called faciocutaneoskeletal syndrome.[58] It is caused by an activating mutation in HRAS. This is a germline mutation in regulators and components of the RAS/MAPK pathway. Costello syndrome occurs in about 1 in 300,000 births.[59] It is characterized by intellectual disability, distinct facial features, excess skin, flexible joints, hypertrophic cardiomyopathy, short stature, and a susceptibility to certain tumors.[60] Renal anomalies are present in over 80% of fetuses with Costello syndrome.[61] These patients also may have a number of other genito-urinary findings but also have a higher likelihood of bladder papillomata and bladder cancer. Bladder transitional cell carcinomas have been reported in adolescent children.[62] In total, about 1% of Costello syndrome children develop transitional cell carcinoma of the bladder.

Apert Syndrome Apert syndrome is an autosomal dominant craniosynostosis syndrome caused by mutations of the FGFR2 gene.[63] It presents as craniofacial abnormalities, hand and foot malformations, developmental delays, hearing loss, overriding aorta and other cardiac abnormalities, pyloric stenosis, undescended testicles, and a higher risk for some malignancies. Apert syndrome affects about 1 in every 65,000 to 200,000 births.[64] Although early-onset low-grade papillary carcinoma of the bladder has been reported in very young patients with Apert and FGFR2 mutation,[65] the risk associated with developing bladder cancer is not well studied.

Genetic Testing and Counseling

Genetic testing in bladder cancer may play a key role in the early identification and risk stratification of patients with a susceptibility for bladder cancer. Additionally, the characterization of genetic mutations in patients with bladder cancer can aid urologists in tailoring treatment for the individual patient. For hereditary syndromes, genetic testing may play a role in screening methods. For patients who present with a first-degree relative with bladder cancer, genetic testing and counseling should be offered. Identifiable hereditary genetic syndromes present the opportunity for early genetic counseling and screening.

Hereditary Syndrome	Risk of Bladder Tumor	Recommendations
Lynch	RR: 4.2 (95% CI 2.2 to 7.2) men 2.2 (95% CI 0.3 to 8.0) women	Smoking cessation Risk counseling Urinalysis with urine cytology (25 to 35 years old);[66] however, this screening remains controversial[67] and should include shared decision-making.
RB	SMR: 26.31 (95% CI 8.54 to 61.41)	Smoking cessation Counseling on increased risk of many cancers later in life No established guidelines regarding bladder screening
Costello	1% risk	Risk counseling Shared decision-making on screening urinalysis for hematuria >10 years. However, there are no established guidelines regarding bladder screening. Refer to urologist
Apert	Reported cases in childhood	Counseling on increased risk starting in childhood; no established guidelines regarding bladder screening

Management The management of bladder cancer is multifaceted and requires complex decision-making involving the provider and the patient. Management begins at the primary care level with the identification of risk factors and alarm signs indicating the potential for bladder cancer. The use of a urinalysis is an inexpensive and risk-free test for patients presenting with hematuria. The management of hereditary syndrome related bladder cancer differs in the age of screening and risk counseling in patients. This risk counseling primarily takes place prior to patients seeking specialized care. Non-muscle invasive bladder cancer of low malignant potential can be treated with repeat cystoscopies and bladder tumor cauterization. More advanced disease may require chemotherapy, radiation, surgery, or some combination of all three. Surgery for muscle-invasive bladder cancer can be a partial or more often, radical, cystectomy with intestinal diversion. The duty of the urologist is to find the ideal individualized therapy for the patient.

Prostate Cancer

The prostate is a walnut-shaped organ that secretes alkaline fluid, which makes up about 70% of the ejaculate. Prostate cancer has a well-studied genetic component and can present with more aggressive disease in patients of certain race and familial history. Clinical suspicion of hereditary prostate cancer should warrant genetic testing and counseling for family members. Early diagnosis, surveillance, and treatment of prostate cancer results in a lower mortality rate. In this section we will give a background on prostate cancer, genetic testing, and hereditary considerations for screening and counseling.

Epidemiology and Genetic Risk Prostate cancer is the most common cancer in men. It is also the second most common cause of cancer death in men. The estimated number of new cases of prostate cancer in the United States for 2020 is 191,930. The estimated number of deaths from prostate cancer in 2020 in the United States is 33,330.[1]

Although both prostate cancer and benign prostatic hyperplasia (BPH) are associated with age, there is no defined connection between the two diseases.[68] Prostate cancer and BPH also occur in different zones of the prostate. BPH growth occurs around the urethra in a zone called the transition zone. Prostate cancer usually occurs in the peripheral zone of the prostate.

The most well-defined risk factor for prostate cancer is age; older patients have a higher risk of developing the disease.[69] Approximately 64% of new prostate cancer cases in the United states were diagnosed in men over the age of 65.[70] Prostate cancer is also more common among African American men. They also have a much higher prostate cancer mortality rate when compared to Caucasian American men (RR: 1.84 CI 95%: 1.22 to 2.79).[71] The cause for this increased mortality has been speculated to be a combination of genetic factors and socioeconomic factors. However, in a multiple-cohort study of 306,100 patients, African American men with nonmetastatic prostate cancer had comparable prostate cancer specific mortality as that of Caucasian men when they had similar access to care and standardized treatment protocols.[72]

Prostate cancer has a well-studied genetic component. In a large study of twins (44,788 pairs) in Northern Europe, cancer heritable factors were studied. Prostate cancer had a statistically significant effect from heritable factors, or the proportion of susceptibility to cancer that was accounted for by genetics (42%, 95% CI 29 to 50%). More specifically, the absolute risk of prostate cancer in the twin of an affected person up to the age of 75 was 0.18 for monozygotic twins and 0.03 for dizygotic twins.[42] Similarly, patients in the Massachusetts Male Aging Study cohort who had a family history of prostate cancer had a 3.8-fold relative risk of prostate cancer compared to those men with no family history.[73] Prostate cancer also has associated genes that can afford greater susceptibility to the development of prostate cancers and some genetic mutation. These will be discussed in detail in the later sections.

Physical Exam/Labwork/Imaging   Prostate cancer presents a unique challenge for physicians as it does not always present with symptoms in patients. Occasionally patients with prostate cancer will present with lower urinary tract symptoms (LUTs). However, LUT are highly associated with BPH due to the anatomical location of both diseases. As BPH often occurs in the transitional zone of the prostate, benign growth of the prostate results in narrowing of the prostatic urethra causing voiding and storage symptoms. However, prostate cancer generally occurs in the peripheral zone, which is not directly in contact with the urinary tract. Prostate cancer therefore may not cause symptoms until a much more advanced stage, when it metastasizes to the bone and causes pain.[74]

The prostate specific antigen (PSA) blood test is used to screen patients for prostate cancer. The American Urological Association (AUA) has clear guidelines on prostate cancer screening.[75]

1. The AUA does not recommend PSA screening in men under 40
2. The AUA does not recommend routine screening in men aged 40–54 at average risk
3. The AUA strongly recommends shared decision-making for men aged 55 to 69 in considering PSA screening
4. The AUA allows for routine screening every two years or more in those men who have participated in shared decision-making
5. The AUA does not recommend routine PSA screening in men over 70 or in men who do not have a life expectancy greater than 10 to 15 years

Routine screening for men younger than 55 may be indicated for those with a family history of metastatic or lethal adenocarcinomas spanning multiple generations, affected first-degree relatives, and disease that developed at younger ages. Earlier screening may also be beneficial to African American men.

Although there are age related changes to PSA values, the general practice is to use a PSA value of 3 or 4 as a suspicion for prostate cancer. A PSA value greater than 4 has a positive predictive value of about 30%, in that about one in three men with a PSA value over 4 will have prostate cancer detectable on biopsy.[76] For patients with an elevated PSA a urologist will engage in shared decision-making about additional testing and whether surveillance PSAs can be continued or if prostate biopsy may be indicated. Magnetic resonance imaging of the prostate as well as more specific urine and serum markers have been introduced to help improve decision-making about whether to perform a prostate biopsy. MRI-targeted prostate biopsy is considered the most accurate way to diagnose prostate cancer in men with concerning biomarker findings but has technical considerations and is not yet ubiquitously available.[77]

Hereditary Cancer Syndromes and Hereditary Prostate Cancer   Prostate cancer has been linked to certain genetic mutations and cancer syndromes. Hereditary prostate cancer, for example, has an overall relative risk in the development of prostate cancer in a man with a pedigree of prostate cancer of 2.3 (95% CI 2.21 to 2.39), as well as for aggressive prostate cancer at 2.31 (95% CI 2.16 to 2.46).[78] This risk increases with the number of first-degree relatives with prostate cancer. In patients with two or more affected first-degree family members the relative risk of developing prostate cancer was 4.39 (95% CI 2.61 to 7.39) compared to those with no familial history of prostate cancer.[79] In the following section we discuss some other genetic mutations and syndromes that may lead to a higher chance of developing prostate cancer. Prostate cancer related syndromes include hereditary breast and ovarian cancer syndrome, hereditary prostate cancer, Lynch syndrome, and gene mutations including *HOXB13* and others.

HBOC, BRCA, and Prostate Cancer Hereditary breast and ovarian cancer syndrome (HBOC) is a genetic cancer syndrome considered when multiple first-degree relatives are diagnosed with cases of breast and ovarian cancer. HBOC may be caused by genetic mutations TP53, PTEN, CDH1, ATM, BRCA and other tumor suppressor genes. Men with a pedigree of HBOC have a relative risk of developing prostate cancer of 1.46 (95% CI 1.43 to 1.5) and a relative risk of early onset of 2.05 (95% CI 1.86 to 2.26).[78]

BRCA1 and 2 genetic mutations have been well studied for their role in breast cancer. BRCA1 and 2 genetic mutations also play a role in prostate cancer. In a study of Ashkenazi Israelis with BRCA founder mutations, the incidence of prostate cancer among male first-degree relatives with a founder mutation was almost 30% by the age of 80.[80] A similar study found that a rare mutation in BRCA2 increased the relative risk of early-onset prostate cancer (<55 years old) to 7.8 (95% CI 1.8 to 9.4).[81] BRCA2 mutation carriers have been shown to have a lower mean age at diagnosis and may have more aggressive tumors, with shorter median survival time.[82] Due to the nature of BRCA associated prostate cancer, patients with a known BRCA mutation or with first-degree relatives with BRCA mutations should be screened carefully and at a younger age. As BRCA2 may confer a higher likelihood of more aggressive disease, shared decision making should include discussion of earlier treatment and active surveillance.

HOXB13 and Other Genetics HOXB13 is a gene that encodes transcription factor homeobox B13 on chromosome 17q21-22. Genetic mutations in *HOXB13* have been investigated for their role in susceptibility to prostate cancer. In men who inherited a rare mutation of *HOXB13*, their risk of prostate cancer increased 10–20-fold (1.4% compared to 0.1% $p = 8.5 \times 10^{-7}$).[83]

Patients with Lynch syndrome also have a higher relative risk of developing prostate cancer (RR 1.15 95% CI 1.12 to 1.19).[78] Other candidate genes that have been identified including HPC1, PCAP, HPCX, CAPB, ELAC2/HPC2, HPC20, KLF6, AMACR, MSR1, NBS1, and CHEK2.[84]

Genetic Testing and Counseling Patients with a strong familial history of prostate, breast, or ovarian cancer should have a higher suspicion for prostate cancer, especially in those with an elevated PSA. The American College of Medical Genetics' guidelines on prostate cancer state the following warrant consideration for genetic testing:

1. Three or more first-degree relatives with prostate cancer; or
2. Two or more first-degree relatives diagnosed with prostate cancer at age ≤55, or
3. Gleason grade >7 prostate cancer and a family history of ≥2 individuals with breast, ovarian, or pancreatic cancer.[85]

Currently there are no uniform guidelines for genetic testing of prostate cancer; however, in men with a known genetic risk factor for prostate cancer the NCCN guidelines for early detection of prostate cancer suggest shared decision-making and consideration of earlier screening for prostate cancer beginning as early as age 40.[86]

Management The management of prostate cancer depends on the staging and grading of the disease. For patients with clinically localized low-risk prostate cancer, active surveillance may be the safest option. For nonmetastatic, or localized, prostate cancer, surgical removal of the prostate, radiation, and ablation therapies are all options. For men with metastatic disease, hormone ablation therapy with or without radiation or chemotherapy, are management options. Ultimately prostate cancer is a disease where shared decision-making is an essential part of diagnosis and management, with careful surveillance and early detection playing large roles in reducing morbidity and mortality.

Specifically, to patients at high risk for prostate cancer such as those with familial prostate cancer or genetic syndromes, management begins with risk counseling and early screening. For patients with the BRCA1 or 2 mutations, screening using PSA testing should begin at 40 after shared decision-making. For men with familial history of prostate cancer, annual PSA testing should be discussed starting at the age of 40 to 45. Currently there is no established genetic therapy to specifically target familial prostate cancer.

Testicular Cancer

The testicles play a vital role in sexual reproduction in men. The testes are responsible for the production of sperm and contain Leydig cells, which produce testosterone. During development, the testicles descend from the abdomen through the inguinal canal and into the scrotum. With a strong genetic component, men with a familial history of testicular cancer may benefit from earlier screening as the treatment of advanced testicular cancer may cause sexual and reproductive side effects as well as negatively impact survival. In the following section we discuss the genetic risks associated with testicular cancer as well as workup and management.

Epidemiology and Genetic Risk Testicular cancer has an estimated 9,610 new cases in 2020 in the United States, with 440 men succumbing to the disease.[1] Testicular cancer is an uncommon cancer with a lifetime risk of 1 in 250 for men. Unlike the other GU malignancies, testicular cancer has a younger average age of diagnosis of 33 years. However, the disease may present in men over the age of 55 (8%) and in children and teens (6%). The incidence of testicular cancer has been increasing in the past two decades.

Testicular cancer is an umbrella term used to describe various types of malignancies that affect the testes. According to the World Health Organization classification of testicular tumors, the majority of testicular tumors can be broadly divided into sex cord stromal tumors and germ cell tumors. Germ cell tumors, which make up about 95% of the cases,[87] include both germ cell tumors derived from germ cell neoplasia in situ and those that are not derived from germ cell neoplasia in situ. The former includes seminomas, and non-seminomatous germ cell tumors including embryonal carcinoma, yolk sac tumors, teratomas, and trophoblastic tumors. Sex cord stromal tumors (5%) include those of Leydig, Sertoli, and granulosa cell tumors. There are also less common tumors defined by the WHO in 2016.

The risk factors for testicular cancer include genetic and environmental factors. One of the most common risk factors for testicular cancer is cryptorchidism, also known as an undescended testicle.[88] Cryptorchidism increases the likelihood of testicular cancer by almost 5-fold.[89] Environmental factors such as diet and post-natal exposures have also been discussed as potential risk factors, but they remain controversial.[90]

Greater than 40% of testicular cancer is attributed to genetic effects. This makes testicular cancer the cancer with the third-highest rate of cause linked to genetic effects after thyroid and endocrine tumors.[91,92] In a large twin study of 203,691 individuals in the Nordic countries, a monozygotic twin had a 13.8% (5.7 to 29.6%) chance of developing testicular cancer if their twin had testicular cancer.[92] In a study of 49,492 cancer patients compiled by the U.S. National Cancer Institute, first-degree relatives of a patient with testicular cancer had a relative risk of 7.07 (5.34 to 9.37) of developing testicular cancer. The parent-to-child relative risk was 4.31 (2.05 to 7.95).[93] With a known genetic risk of testicular cancer, genetic counseling and testing may be imperative in screening patients at higher risk.

Physical Exam/Labwork/Imaging Testicular cancer may commonly present as a painless scrotal mass, scrotal pain, or on routine imaging.[94] The workup for a patient suspected to have testicular cancer begins with a comprehensive history. A detailed background on the presenting symptom should be elicited, such as if it was brought on by trauma. Familial history including first-degree relatives with other cancers is helpful in diagnosis. Furthermore, any history of cryptorchidism, infertility, or genetic syndrome may raise suspicion. A history should be followed by a comprehensive physical exam with a focus on the scrotum and genitalia. Both testicles should be carefully identified within the scrotum and palpated. As inguinal hernias may present with similar symptoms (pain in the scrotum with a painless mass), the inguinal canals should be palpated. The scrotum should be examined for signs of infection or trauma. Pelvic and genital lymph nodes should be palpated for signs of lymphadenopathy.

For patients with a suspicion of testicular cancer, the AUA has certain guidelines. Patients with a solid mass in the testes identified on imaging or physical exam should be managed as malignant neoplasm until proven otherwise. A scrotal ultrasound with Doppler should be obtained. For patient with a solid mass suspicious for malignant neoplasm, serum tumor markers such as AFP, hCG, and LDH should be measured prior to surgical removal of the testicle by radical orchiectomy. Patients with normal tumor markers and indeterminate findings on imaging and physical exam should undergo repeat imaging in six to eight weeks. MRI should not be used as the initial evaluation imaging;[95] however, for staging purposes an MRI or CT scan of the abdomen in a man with testicular cancer is indicated to evaluate for metastasis.

Hereditary Testicular Cancer Syndromes and Genetics Testicular cancer has been linked to a few hereditary testicular cancer syndromes. In the following section we discuss hereditary cancer syndromes including Peutz-Jeghers syndrome and Carney complex, with a link to testicular cancer as well as some of the genetics behind testicular cancer.

Peutz-Jeghers Syndrome

Peutz-Jeghers syndrome (PJS) is an autosomal dominant genetic disorder characterized by the development of gastrointestinal hamartomatous polyps and mucocutaneous pigmentation.[96] This syndrome is most often caused by germline mutations in the *STK11/LKB1* gene on chromosome 19p13.3.[97] PJS is associated with an increased risk for cancers in other sites, including the breast, ovary, uterus, cervix, lung, and testes. PJS has a prevalence between 1 in 29,000 and 1 in 200,000.[84] Sertoli cell tumors of the testes have been linked to PJS. In a case series of eight children with PJS with a mean age of 6.5 years, Sertoli cell tumors were reported.[98] Furthermore, testicular tumors in boys with PJS often present with similar features as females with PJS who have ovarian sex cord annular tubules. These boys present with sexual precocity and gynecomastia.[99]

Carney Complex

Carney complex is a rare, autosomal dominant genetic disorder associated with one of the multiple endocrine neoplasia syndromes. Most commonly it affects multiple endocrine glands such as the thyroid, pituitary, and adrenal glands. It is also associated with cardiac myxomas, abnormal pigmentation of the skin, melanotic schwannomas, breast myxomatosis, and testicular tumors.[100] Bilateral sex cord stromal testicular tumors present in patients with Carney complex. In a cohort of 26 patients with the complex with testicular tumors, 61% presented with bilateral testicular tumors.[101] The typical presenting tumor is a large, calcifying Sertoli cell tumor. As these tumors often present bilaterally, it may present a challenge in management and future fertility.

Genetic Testing and Counseling Testicular cancer as it presents earlier in life may present difficulty in early counseling and fertility. Some genes associated with testicular cancer include KITLG, SPRY4, PRKAR1A, and STK11(LKB1). Currently, routine screening for testicular cancer in asymptomatic men is not recommended. Genetic testing for testicular cancer is still undergoing development although a susceptible gene on chromosome xq27 is currently undergoing investigation.[102] Although genetic testing for high-risk families is still not available, interest for testing among family members is high. In a study of 229 participants from 47 multiple-case familial testicular cancer families, 66% expressed interest in genetic testing.[103]

Patients with PJS or Carney complex and their caregivers should be informed of the increased risk of testicular cancer. These patients do not necessarily need routine screening; however, there should be a lower threshold of suspicion when patients present with a painless scrotal mass or scrotal discomfort. In families with a history of testicular cancer, especially if multiple members have had testicular cancer, counseling should include having a lower threshold of suspicion for intra-scrotal pain or masses and serial monthly testicular self-examination. In those patients with cryptorchidism, counseling should include the increased risk of testicular cancer. Men with testicular cancer should also be counseled of the increased risk of tumor in the contralateral testicle as their risk for cancer in the other testicle is about 2% over 15 years.[104]

Management For proven cases of testicular cancer, patients should be counseled on the increased risk of infertility and given the option for sperm banking. Sperm banking should be offered to patients as young as 13; patients as young as 14 to 17 have been shown to be good candidates.[105]

Surgical removal of the tumor is the initial step in management in almost all cases. For patients with localized low-stage testicular cancer, surgical management only with orchiectomy or testis-sparing surgery may be sufficient. For patients with more advanced disease including distal metastasis on CT or MRI staging imaging, platinum-based chemotherapy, radiation, and/or surgery may be indicated. Ultimately, testicular cancer may have many psychological and physiological long-term effects and patients should be extensively counseled prior to treatment.

References

1. Siegel RL, Miller KD, Jemal A. Cancer statistics, 2020. *CA: A Cancer Journal for Clinicians.* 2020;70:7–30.
2. Frank I, Blute ML, Cheville JC, et al. Solid renal tumors: An analysis of pathological features related to tumor size. *Journal of Urology.* 2003;170:2217–2220.

3. Tsivian M, Moreira DM, Caso JR, et al. Cigarette smoking is associated with advanced renal cell carcinoma. *J Clin Oncol*. 2011;15:2027–2031.

4. Andreotti G, Beane Freeman LE, Shearer JJ, et al. Occupational pesticide use and risk of renal cell carcinoma in the agricultural health study. *Environ Health Perspect*. 2020;128:67011.

5. Gudbjartsson T, Jónasdóttir TJ, Thoroddsen Á, et al. A population-based familial aggregation analysis indicates genetic contribution in a majority of renal cell carcinomas. *Int J Cancer*. 2002;100:476–479.

6. Bratslavsky G, Linehan WM. Long-term management of bilateral, multifocal, recurrent renal carcinoma. *Nat Rev Urol*. 2010;7:267–275.

7. Jayson M, Sanders H. Increased incidence of serendipitously discovered renal cell carcinoma. *Urology*. 1998;51:203–205.

8. Gold PJ, Fefer AF, Thompson JA. Paraneoplastic manifestations of renal cell carcinoma. *Semin Urol Oncol*. 1996 Nov.;14(4):216–222.

9. McDonald JS, McDonald RJ, Lieske JC, et al. Risk of acute kidney injury, dialysis, and mortality in patients with chronic kidney disease after intravenous contrast material exposure. *Mayo Clin Proc*. 2015;90:1046–1053.

10. Maher ER, Iselius L, Yates JR, et al. Von Hippel-Lindau disease: a genetic study. *J Med Genet*. 1991;28:443–447.

11. Maranchie JK, Vasselli JR, Riss J, et al. The contribution of VHL substrate binding and HIF1-α to the phenotype of VHL loss in renal cell carcinoma. *Cancer Cell*. 2002;1:247–255.

12. Schmidt LS, Nickerson ML, Angeloni D, et al. Early onset hereditary papillary renal carcinoma: germline missense mutations in the tyrosine kinase domain of the MET proto-oncogene. *The J of Urology*. 2004;172:1256–1261.

13. Lindor NM, Dechet CB, Greene MH, et al. Papillary renal cell carcinoma: analysis of germline mutations in the MET proto-oncogene in a clinic-based population. *Genet Test*. 2001;5:101–106.

14. Nguyen KA, Syed JS, Shuch B. Hereditary kidney cancer syndromes and surgical management of the small renal mass. *Urol Clin North Am*. 2017;44:155–167.

15. Toro JR, Nickerson ML, Wei M-H, et al. Mutations in the fumarate hydratase gene cause hereditary leiomyomatosis and renal cell cancer in families in North America. *Am J Hum Genet*. 2003;73:95–106.

16. Birt AR, Hogg GR, Dubé WJ. Hereditary multiple fibrofolliculomas with trichodiscomas and acrochordons. *Arch Dermatol*. 1977;113:1674–1677.

17. Toro JR, Wei MH, Glenn GM, et al. BHD mutations, clinical and molecular genetic investigations of Birt-Hogg-Dubé syndrome: a new series of 50 families and a review of published reports. *J Med Genet*. 2008;45:321–331.

18. Liu MY, Poellinger L, Walker CL. Up-regulation of hypoxia-inducible factor 2α in renal cell carcinoma associated with loss of Tsc-2 tumor suppressor gene. *Cancer Res*. 2003;63:2675–2680.

19. Bjornsson J, Short MP, Kwiatkowski DJ, et al. Tuberous sclerosis-associated renal cell carcinoma: clinical, pathological, and genetic features. *Am J Pathol*. 1996;149:1201–1208.

20. Peña-Llopis S, Vega-Rubín-De-Celis S, Liao A, et al. BAP1 loss defines a new class of renal cell carcinoma. *Nat Genet*. 2012;44:751–759.

21. Nelen MR, Padberg GW, Peeters EAJ, et al. Localization of the gene for Cowden disease to chromosome 10q22-23. *Nat Genet*. 1996;13:114–116.

22. Garraway LA, Widlund HR, Rubin MA, et al. Integrative genomic analyses identify MITF as a lineage survival oncogene amplified in malignant melanoma. *Nature*. 2005;436:117–122.

23. van der Tuin K, Tops CMJ, Adank MA, et al. CDC73-related disorders: clinical manifestations and case detection in primary hyperparathyroidism. *J Clin Endocrinol Metab*. 2017;102(12):4534–4540.

24. Carlo MI, Hakimi AA, Stewart GD, et al. Familial kidney cancer: implications of new syndromes and molecular insights. *Eur Urol*. 2019;76:754–764.

25. Neumann HPH, Pawlu C, Pęczkowska M, et al. Distinct clinical features of paraganglioma syndromes associated with SDHB and SDHD gene mutations. *JAMA*. 2004;292:943–951.

26. Williamson SR, Eble JN, Amin MB, et al. Succinate dehydrogenase-deficient renal cell carcinoma: detailed characterization of 11 tumors defining a unique subtype of renal cell carcinoma. *Mod Pathol*. 2015;28:80–94.

27. Gill AJ, Pachter NS, Chou A, et al. Renal tumors associated with germline SDHB mutation show distinctive morphology. *Am J Surg Pathol*. 2011;35(10):1578–85.

28. Shuch B, Vourganti S, Ricketts CJ, et al. Defining early-onset kidney cancer: implications for germline and somatic mutation testing and clinical management. *J Clin Oncol.* 2014;32:431–437.

29. Hampel H, Bennett RL, Buchanan A, et al. A practice guideline from the American College of Medical Genetics and Genomics and the National Society of Genetic Counselors: referral indications for cancer predisposition assessment. *Genet Med.* 2015;17:70–87.

30. Kurian AW, Hare EE, Mills MA, et al. Clinical evaluation of a multiple-gene sequencing panel for hereditary cancer risk assessment. *J Clin Oncol.* 2014;32:2001–2009.

31. Nguyen KA, Syed JS, Espenschied CR, et al. Advances in the diagnosis of hereditary kidney cancer: initial results of a multigene panel test. *Cancer.* 2017;123:4363–4371.

32. Gaur S, Turkbey B, Choyke P. Hereditary renal tumor syndromes: update on diagnosis and management. *Semin Ultrasound CT MR.* 2017;38:59–71.

33. Walther MM, Thompson N, Linehan W. Enucleation procedures in patients with multiple hereditary renal tumors. *World J Urol.* 1995;13:248–250.

34. M WM, Choyke Peter L, Glenn G, et al. Renal cancer in families with hereditary renal cancer: prospective analysis of a tumor size threshold for renal parenchymal sparing surgery. *J Urol.* 1999;161:1475–1479.

35. Blackwell RH, Li B, Kozel Z, et al. Functional implications of renal tumor enucleation relative to standard partial nephrectomy. *Urology.* 2017;99:162–168.

36. Saginala K, Barsouk A, Aluru JS, et al. Epidemiology of bladder cancer. *Med Sci.* 2020;8:15.

37. Kaufman DS, Shipley WU, Feldman AS. Bladder cancer. *Lancet.* 2009;374:239–249.

38. Martin JW, Carballido EM, Ahmed A, et al. Squamous cell carcinoma of the urinary bladder: Systematic review of clinical characteristics and therapeutic approaches. *Arab J Urol.* 2016;14:183–191.

39. Shokeir AA. Squamous cell carcinoma of the bladder: pathology, diagnosis and treatment. *BJU international.* 2004;93:216–220.

40. Lokeshwar S, Klaassen Z, Terris M. A contemporary review of risk factors for bladder. *Clinics in Oncology.* 2016;1:1–3.

41. Aben KK, Witjes JA, Schoenberg MP. Familial aggregation of urothelial cell carcinoma. *Int J Cancer.* 2002;98:274–278.

42. Lichtenstein P, Holm NV, Verkasalo PK, et al. Environmental and heritable factors in the causation of cancer: analyses of cohorts of twins from Sweden, Denmark, and Finland. *New Engl J Med.* 2000;343:78–85.

43. Burger M, Catto JW, Dalbagni G, et al. Epidemiology and risk factors of urothelial bladder cancer. *Eur Urol.* 2013;63:234–241.

44. Gu J, Liang D, Wang Y, et al. Effects of N-acetyl transferase 1 and 2 polymorphisms on bladder cancer risk in Caucasians. *Mutat Res.* 2005;581:97–104.

45. Rothman N, Garcia-Closas M, Chatterjee N, et al. A multi-stage genome-wide association study of bladder cancer identifies multiple susceptibility loci. *Nat Genet.* 2010;42:978–984.

46. Kiemeney LA, Thorlacius S, Sulem P, et al. Sequence variant on 8q24 confers susceptibility to urinary bladder cancer. *Nat Genet.* 2008;40:1307–1312.

47. Kiemeney LA, Sulem P, Besenbacher S, et al. A sequence variant at 4p16.3 confers susceptibility to urinary bladder cancer. *Nat Genet.* 2010;42:415–419.

48. Gu J, Wu X. Genetic susceptibility to bladder cancer risk and outcome. *Per Med.* 2011;8:365–374.

49. Pashos CL, Botteman MF, Laskin BL, et al. Bladder cancer: epidemiology, diagnosis, and management. *Cancer Pract.* 2002;10:311–322.

50. Cha EK, Tirsar L-A, Schwentner C, et al. Accurate risk assessment of patients with asymptomatic hematuria for the presence of bladder cancer. *World J Urol.* 2012;30:847–852.

51. Grossfeld GD, Litwin MS, Wolf JS, et al. Evaluation of asymptomatic microscopic hematuria in adults: the American Urological Association best practice policy—part I: definition, detection, prevalence, and etiology. *Urology.* 2001;57:599–603.

52. Davis R, Jones JS, Barocas DA, et al. Diagnosis, evaluation and follow-up of asymptomatic microhematuria (AMH) in adults: AUA guideline. *The J Urol.* 2012;188:2473–2481.

53. Lynch HT, Boland CR, Gong G, et al. Phenotypic and genotypic heterogeneity in the Lynch syndrome: diagnostic, surveillance and management implications. *Eur J Hum Genet.* 2006;14:390–402.

54. Haraldsdottir S, Rafnar T, Frankel WL, et al. Comprehensive population-wide analysis of Lynch syndrome in Iceland reveals founder mutations in MSH6 and PMS2. *Nat Commun*. 2017;8:14755.

55. van der Post RS, Kiemeney LA, Ligtenberg MJ, et al. Risk of urothelial bladder cancer in Lynch syndrome is increased, in particular among MSH2 mutation carriers. *J Med Genet*. 2010;47:464–470.

56. Friend SH, Bernards R, Rogelj S, et al. A human DNA segment with properties of the gene that predisposes to retinoblastoma and osteosarcoma. *Nature*. 1986;323:643–646.

57. Fletcher O, Easton D, Anderson K, Gilham C, Jay M, Peto J. Lifetime risks of common cancers among retino-blastoma survivors. *J Natl Cancer Inst*. 2004;96:357–363.

58. Costello J. A new syndrome: mental subnormality and nasal papillomata. *Aust Paediatr J*. Jun;13(2):114-8.

59. Abe Y, Aoki Y, Kuriyama S, et al. Prevalence and clinical features of Costello syndrome and cardio-facio-cutaneous syndrome in Japan: Findings from a nationwide epidemiological survey. *Am J Med Genet A*. 2012;158:1083–1094.

60. Gripp KW, Morse LA, Axelrad M, et al. Costello syndrome: clinical phenotype, genotype, and management guidelines. *Am J Med Genet A*. 2019;179:1725–1744.

61. Myers A, Bernstein JA, Brennan ML, et al. Perinatal features of the RASopathies: Noonan syndrome, cardio-faciocutaneous syndrome and Costello syndrome. *Am J Med Genet A*. 2014;164:2814–2821.

62. Gripp KW. Tumor predisposition in Costello syndrome. *American Journal of Medical Genetics, Part C: Seminars in Medical Genetics*. 2005;137C:72–77.

63. Tan AP, Mankad K. Apert syndrome: magnetic resonance imaging (MRI) of associated intracranial anomalies. *Childs Nerv Syst*. 2018;34:205–216.

64. Fearon JA. Treatment of the hands and feet in Apert syndrome: an evolution in management. *Plast Reconstr Surg*. 2003;112:1–12; discussion 3–9.

65. Andreou A, Lamy A, Layet V, et al. Early-onset low-grade papillary carcinoma of the bladder associated with Apert syndrome and a germline FGFR2 mutation (Pro253Arg). *Am J Med Genet A*. 2006;140A:2245–2247.

66. Lindor NM, Petersen GM, Hadley DW, et al. Recommendations for the care of individuals with an inherited predisposition to Lynch syndrome: a systematic review. *JAMA*. 2006;296:1507–1517.

67. Bernstein IT, Myrhøj T. Surveillance for urinary tract cancer in Lynch syndrome. *Fam Cancer*. 2013;12:279–284.

68. Miah S, Catto J. BPH and prostate cancer risk. *Indian J Urol*. 2014;30:214–218.

69. Gann PH. Risk factors for prostate cancer. *Rev Urol*. 2002;4(Suppl. 5):S3–S10.

70. Bechis SK, Carroll PR, Cooperberg MR. Impact of age at diagnosis on prostate cancer treatment and survival. *J Clin Oncol*. 2011;29:235–241.

71. Freeman VL, Durazo-Arvizu R, Keys LC, et al. Racial differences in survival among men with prostate cancer and comorbidity at time of diagnosis. *Am J Public Health*. 2004;94:803–808.

72. Dess RT, Hartman HE, Mahal BA, et al. Association of black race with prostate cancer-specific and other-cause mortality. *JAMA Oncol*. 2019;5:975–983.

73. Kalish LA, McDougal WS, McKinlay JB. Family history and the risk of prostate cancer. *Urology*. 2000;56:803–806.

74. Muralidharan A, Smith MT. Pathobiology and management of prostate cancer-induced bone pain: recent insights and future treatments. *Inflammopharmacology*. 2013;21:339–363.

75. Carter HB, Albertsen PC, Barry MJ, et al. Early detection of prostate cancer: AUA Guideline. *J Urol*. 2013;190:419–426.

76. Adhyam M, Gupta AK. A review on the clinical utility of PSA in cancer prostate. *Indian J Surg Oncol*. 2012;3:120–129.

77. Ahdoot M, Wilbur AR, Reese SE, et al. MRI-targeted, systematic, and combined biopsy for prostate cancer diagnosis. *New Engl J Med*. 2020;382:917–928.

78. Beebe-Dimmer JL, Kapron A, Fraser AM, et al. Relative risks of prostate cancer associated with different family cancer histories. *J Clin Oncol*. 2019;37:1505.

79. Kiciński M, Vangronsveld J, Nawrot TS. An epidemiological reappraisal of the familial aggregation of prostate cancer: a meta-analysis. *PloS One*. 2011;6:e27130.

80. Giusti RM, Rutter JL, Duray PH, et al. A twofold increase in BRCA mutation related prostate cancer among Ashkenazi Israelis is not associated with distinctive histopathology. *J Med Genet*. 2003;40:787–792.

81. Agalliu I, Karlins E, Kwon E, et al. Rare germline mutations in the BRCA2 gene are associated with early-onset prostate cancer. *Br J Cancer*. 2007;97:826–831.

82. Tryggvadóttir L, Vidarsdóttir L, Thorgeirsson T, et al. Prostate cancer progression and survival in BRCA2 mutation carriers. *J Natl Cancer Inst*. 2007;99:929–935.

83. Ewing CM, Ray AM, Lange EM, et al. Germline mutations in HOXB13 and prostate-cancer risk. *N Engl J med*. 2012;366:141–149.

84. Gallagher DJ, Feifer A, Coleman JA. Genitourinary cancer predisposition syndromes. *Hematol Oncol Clin North Am*. 2010;24:861–883.

85. Zhen JT, Syed J, Nguyen KA, et al. Genetic testing for hereditary prostate cancer: current status and limitations. *Cancer*. 2018;124:3105–3117.

86. Network NCC. NCCN guidelines, version 2. 2019, prostate cancer. 2019.

87. Chung P, Warde P. Testicular cancer: germ cell tumours. *BMJ Clin Evid*. 2016;2016:1807.

88. Cheng L, Albers P, Berney DM, et al. Testicular cancer. *Nat Rev Dis Primers*. 2018;4:29.

89. Purdue MP, Devesa SS, Sigurdson AJ, McGlynn KA. International patterns and trends in testis cancer incidence. *Int J Cancer*. 2005;115:822–827.

90. Gurney J, Stanley J, Shaw C, Sarfati D. Ethnic patterns of hypospadias in New Zealand do not resemble those observed for cryptorchidism and testicular cancer: evidence of differential aetiology? *Andrology*. 2016;4:82–86.

91. Litchfield K, Levy M, Orlando G, et al. Identification of 19 new risk loci and potential regulatory mechanisms influencing susceptibility to testicular germ cell tumor. *Nat Genet*. 2017;49:1133.

92. Mucci LA, Hjelmborg JB, Harris JR, et al. Familial risk and heritability of cancer among twins in Nordic countries. *JAMA*. 2016;315:68–76.

93. Sampson JN, Wheeler WA, Yeager M, et al. Analysis of heritability and shared heritability based on genome-wide association studies for thirteen cancer types. *J Natl Cancer Inst*. 2015;107:djv279.

94. Baird DC, Meyers GJ, Hu JS. Testicular cancer: aiagnosis and treatment. *Am Fam Physician*. 2018;97:261–268.

95. Stephenson A, Eggener SE, Bass EB, et al. Diagnosis and treatment of early stage testicular cancer: AUA guideline. *J Urol*. 2019;202:272–281.

96. Nevozinskaya Z, Korsunskaya I, Sakaniya L, et al. Peutz-Jeghers syndrome in dermatology. *Acta Dermatovenerol Alp Pannonica Adriat*. 2019;28:135–137.

97. Hearle N, Schumacher V, Menko FH, et al. Frequency and spectrum of cancers in the Peutz-Jeghers syndrome. *Clin Cancer Res*. 2006;12:3209–3215.

98. Ulbright TM, Amin MB, Young RH. Intratubular large cell hyalinizing sertoli cell neoplasia of the testis: a report of 8 cases of a distinctive lesion of the Peutz-Jeghers syndrome. *Am J Surg Pathol*. 2007;31:827–835.

99. McGarrity TJ, Kulin HE, Zaino RJ. Peutz-Jeghers syndrome. *Am J Gastroenterol*. 2000;95:596–604.

100. Vindhyal MR, Elshimy G, Elhomsy G. Carney Complex. StatPearls. Treasure Island (FL): StatPearls Publishing. Copyright © 2020, StatPearls Publishing LLC.; 2020.

101. Washecka R, Dresner MI, Honda SA. Testicular tumors in Carney's complex. *J Urol*. 2002;167:1299–1302.

102. Rapley EA, Crockford GP, Teare D, et al. Localization to Xq27 of a susceptibility gene for testicular germ-cell tumours. *Nat Genet*. 2000;24:197–200.

103. Peters JA, Vadaparampil ST, Kramer J, et al. Familial testicular cancer: Interest in genetic testing among high-risk family members. *Genet Med*. 2006;8:760–770.

104. Fosså SD, Chen J, Schonfeld SJ, et al. Risk of contralateral testicular cancer: a population-based study of 29,515 U.S. men. *J Natl Cancer Inst*. 2005;97:1056–1066.

105. Williams DH. Sperm banking and the cancer patient. *Ther Adv Urol*. 2010;2:19–34.

106. Schmidt LS, Linehan WM. Genetic predisposition to kidney cancer. *Semin Oncol*. 2016;43:566–574.

CHAPTER 12

Genetic Predisposition to Gastric Cancer

Tannaz Guivatchian and Elena M. Stoffel

▩ OVERVIEW, EPIDEMIOLOGY, AND SUBTYPES

Gastric cancer is currently the fifth most common cause of cancer and the third-leading cause of cancer death worldwide, accounting for 1.3 million incident cases and 819,000 deaths annually.[1] The incidence of gastric cancer varies geographically, with incidence highest in East Asia and South America and lowest in Western countries. While the incidence of gastric cancer is declining overall (possibly due to treatment of *H. pylori* infection), incidence of cancers arising from the gastric cardia continues to increase in developed countries (including the United States) for unknown reasons.[2] There are gender differences in gastric cancer, with incidence 2- to 3-fold higher in men compared to women.[2]

Gastric cancers can be divided according to histopathologic subtype. The majority (90%) are adenocarcinomas, with the remaining 10% comprised of lymphomas, leiomyosarcomas, gastrointestinal stromal tumors (GISTs), and other tumor subtypes. Gastric lymphomas are most often B-cell lymphomas, with T-cell lymphoma being rare in the stomach.[2,3] MALT-lymphoma is a type of gastric lymphoma most often associated with *H. pylori* infection. This review will focus on gastric adenocarcinomas.

Gastric adenocarcinomas have historically been subdivided based on location (cardia versus non-cardia) and histology (Lauren's classification, intestinal 60% versus diffuse 30%). Intestinal adenocarcinomas of the stomach are the most common, often presenting as gastric masses or ulcers, with histopathology demonstrating cohesive cells forming gland-like tubular structures. The main pathway for development of intestinal gastric cancer, referred to as Correa's cascade, begins with *H. pylori* infection leading to chronic gastritis, followed by atrophic gastritis, intestinal metaplasia, dysplasia, and finally carcinoma.[4] Diffuse gastric cancers (DGC) differ from intestinal gastric cancers in that DGCs often present with *linitis plastica* and/or peritoneal carcinomatosis as neoplastic epithelial cells with signet ring morphology infiltrating the stomach wall, often without an obvious ulcer or mass lesion. Downregulation or mutation of *E-cadherin (CDH1)*, a tumor suppressor trans-membrane glycoprotein involved in cell to cell adhesion, is instrumental to the development of diffuse gastric cancer.[2,3,5]

Interestingly, new data suggest a possible correlation between the molecular characteristics of gastric adenocarcinomas with both epidemiology and disease prognosis. A collaborative effort led by the U.S. National Institutes of Health (NIH) and Cancer Genome Atlas (TCGA) employed genomic profiling (genome/exome/methylome DNA sequencing) to identify four molecular subtypes of gastric adenocarcinoma:[6] the Epstein-Barr virus subtype (EBV), microsatellite instability subtype (MIS), genomically stable subtype (GS), and chromosomal instability subtype (CIN). Investigations into the clinical features suggest that both the EBV associated subtype and GS subtypes tend to occur more often in younger patients. The CIN subtype has a predilection for the proximal stomach, while the MIS subtype is more commonly in the distal stomach. The EBV associated subtype appears to have the best prognosis, while the GS subtype appears to have the worst. Furthermore, the GS subtype appears to have limited response to adjuvant chemotherapy while the CIN subtype has the best response.[7] As we continue to learn more about the heterogeneity of gastric cancers, we have opportunities to gain insights regarding their pathogenesis.

RISK FACTORS FOR GASTRIC CANCER

Both genetic predisposition and environmental exposures increase an individual's risk of developing gastric cancer. Advanced age, male gender, tobacco use, and family history have all been associated with an increased risk for gastric cancer in population based studies.[2] In Western countries, lower socioeconomic status is associated with an increased risk of gastric cancer. Additionally, diets high in salt, high in smoked foods, and lower in fruits and vegetables are also recognized as risk factors. Chronic inflammation likely plays an important role in the development of gastric cancer. Conditions leading to chronic inflammation such as autoimmune gastritis and smoking increase an individual's risk while there is some evidence that statins and nonsteroidal anti-inflammatories (NSAIDs) have an inverse relationship with the risk of gastric cancer, possibly by decreasing inflammation.[2,8] For cancers arising from the gastric cardia, GERD and obesity are known risk factors, which may be one reason why the increase in incidence of gastric cardia cancers in the Western world coincides with the rise in obesity.[2] Non-cardia gastric cancers, which account for the majority of gastric cancers worldwide, have been linked to specific dietary factors and/or *H. pylori* infection.

H. pylori infection has been implicated in anywhere from 65 to 80% of all gastric cancers worldwide,[2] which prompted the World Health Organization to categorize *H. pylori* as a class 1 carcinogen.[9] It was first identified in 1983 in pivotal work published by Marshall and Warren.[10] Individuals with *H. pylori* infection are at risk for the development of peptic ulcer disease, gastric adenocarcinoma, and MALT lymphoma.[8,11] Several virulence factors have been identified in *H. pylori* that are associated with a higher risk of gastric cancer, the most well studied of which is the CagA (cytokine associated gene A) protein, which is now considered a bacterial oncoprotein. Another more recently identified virulence factor is VacA, which additionally creates a pro-inflammatory environment.[8,9] Eradication of *H. pylori* is a standard of care and can lead to remission in up to 80% of cases of early MALT lymphomas.[8,12]

GENETIC PREDISPOSITION TO GASTRIC CANCER

Although 90% of gastric cancers are believed to be sporadic, 10% exhibit familial aggregation and 1 to 3% have been linked to hereditary cancer syndromes.[13–15] Pathogenic germline

TABLE 12.1: Hereditary Gastric Cancer Syndromes

Hereditary Condition	Gene(s)	Other Commonly Associated Cancer Types	Estimated Risk of Gastric Cancer (Lifetime)
Hereditary diffuse gastric cancer	CDH1, CTNNA1	Lobular breast cancer	Up to 70%[15]
Familial intestinal gastric cancer	Unknown	None	Increased
Familial adenomatous polyposis (FAP)	APC	Colon, thyroid, small bowel	1 to 15%, highest in Asian populations[41,54,55]
MUTYH-associated polyposis (MAP)	MUTYH (biallelic)	Colon, thyroid	Increased
Gastric adenocarcinoma and proximal polyposis syndrome (GAPPS)	Exon 1B promoter region APC	None	Increased
Lynch syndrome	MSH2, MLH1, MSH6, PMS2, EPCAM	Colon, uterine, ovarian, pancreas, small intestine, brain, prostate, genito-urinary	5–20%[41,43–46]
Peutz-Jeghers syndrome	STK11	Colon, small intestine, breast, pancreas, ovarian, testicular, lung	5–29%[46,80]
Juvenile polyposis syndrome	SMAD4, BMPR1A	Colon, small intestine, pancreas	5–30%[46,77]
PTEN hamartoma syndrome	PTEN	Breast, thyroid, endometrial	Possibly increased
Li-Fraumeni syndrome	TP53	Sarcomas, breast, brain, adrenal cortex, colon, lung	3–20%[46,85,86]
Hereditary breast and ovarian cancer syndrome	BRCA1, BRCA2	Breast, ovarian, pancreas, prostate	Possibly increased

variants in several genes have been associated with increased risk of gastric cancer including hereditary diffuse gastric cancer (HDGC), Lynch syndrome, familial adenomatous polyposis (FAP), gastric adenocarcinoma and proximal polyposis syndrome (GAPPS), MUTYH-associated polyposis (MAP), Peutz-Jeghers syndrome (PJS), juvenile polyposis syndrome (JPS), PTEN hamartoma syndrome, hereditary breast ovarian cancer, and Li-Fraumeni syndrome (Table 12.1).

When evaluating a patient with gastric cancer, the patient's complete personal medical history, family history of cancer (including all cancer types diagnosed in first- and second-degree relatives and ages at diagnosis), and histopathologic subtype (diffuse versus intestinal) should be considered to determine diagnostic approach and management (Figure 12.1).

HEREDITARY DIFFUSE GASTRIC CANCER

Hereditary diffuse gastric cancer (HDGC) is an autosomal dominant familial syndrome often characterized by early onset, diffuse gastric cancer affecting relatives in multiple generations. Signet ring cells infiltrating the stomach lining are the hallmark histopathologic finding in diffuse gastric cancers (Figure 12.2).[14] In 1998, Guilford et al. documented the association between germline CDH1/E-cadherin mutations and familial diffuse gastric cancer in a large Maori family in New Zealand with 25 members affected with gastric cancer.[16]

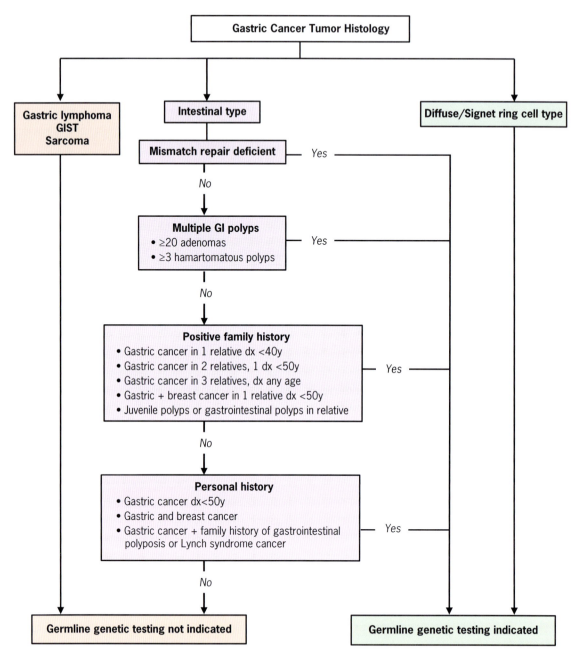

FIGURE 12.1: Approach to genetic testing for gastric cancer.

Pathogenic germline variants in the *CDH1* gene are found in roughly 25 to 50% of families meeting clinical criteria for hereditary diffuse gastric cancer.[14] To date, over 155 different mutations in the *CDH1* gene have been associated with diffuse gastric cancer, and gene mutations in the *CTNNA1* gene have also been reported in three families meeting clinical criteria for HDGC (Table 12.1).[15]

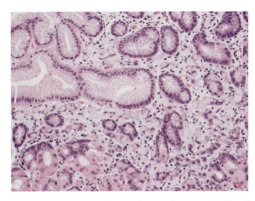

FIGURE 12.2: Signet ring cell gastric adenocarcinoma in gastric mucosal biopsies from a patient with a pathogenic germline variant in *CDH1*.

For carriers of *CDH1* pathogenic germline variants, the lifetime risk of developing gastric cancer is higher than is seen in any other genetic syndrome.[15] While lifetime risks of diffuse gastric cancer approaching 70% for men and 56% for women with *CDH1* mutations have been reported, a recent study found lower penetrance, estimating gastric cancer risks at 37% and 25%, respectively.[17] Additionally, pathogenic variants in *CDH1* are associated with an increase in risk for lobular breast cancer in women, with a cumulative risk of 42% by age 80.[15] There is some evidence suggesting the risk of colon cancer and prostate cancer may also be slightly increased.[14,15,18,19]

Clinical Features

Clinical criteria used to identify families with HDGC were outlined by the International Gastric Cancer Linkage Consortium in 2010, and updated in 2015.[14,15] Genetic testing for germline variants in *CDH1* should be offered to patients with any one of the following:

- 2+ cases of gastric cancer regardless of age in first- or second-degree relatives with at least one confirmed to have diffuse pathology
- one case of DGC diagnosed before the age of 40
- personal or family history of DGC or lobular breast cancer, one of which is diagnosed before the age of 50

Additionally, genetic testing for *CDH1* should be considered in the following cases:

- bilateral lobular breast cancer or a family history of 2+ cases of lobular breast cancer diagnosed before the age of 50
- a personal or family history of cleft lip/palate in a patient with DGC
- in situ signet ring cells and/or pagetoid spread of signet ring cells.

The overall prognosis of diffuse gastric cancer is poor with a 10% 5-year survival rate.[15,20] This poor prognosis is mainly due to the fact that most patients present at advanced stages with *linitis plastica* and/or peritoneal carcinomatosis. Diagnosis is often challenging as symptoms of diffuse gastric cancer are often vague, such as abdominal discomfort or bloating. Furthermore, the gastric mucosa appears endoscopically normal in most cases, as the signet ring cells are submucosally infiltrative and rarely form exophytic masses and/or ulcers. Yet although the stomach may appear normal, careful histopathologic review of gastrectomy specimens from asymptomatic *CDH1* carriers identifies multifocal signet ring cell carcinoma in the vast majority of patients.[13,14,18-24] A review of asymptomatic *CDH1* mutation carriers in a Dutch population who underwent prophylactic gastrectomy identified premalignant or malignant changes in 27 out of 28 patients.[19]

There appears to be significant variability in penetrance in families with germline *CDH1* pathogenic mutations, with lifetime risk for developing diffuse gastric cancer ranging from 40 to 80%. A recent study of endoscopic surveillance in patients with germline *CDH1* mutations identified signet ring cells in 12 of 20 patients, and half of those affected reported no family history of gastric cancer.[25]

Management

Once an individual is known to carry a pathogenic germline mutation in *CDH1*, options for gastric cancer risk reduction include total prophylactic gastrectomy versus endoscopic surveillance. Numerous studies have demonstrated the limited sensitivity of endoscopic biopsies for identifying malignant or pre-malignant lesions in HDGC; therefore, expert clinical opinion currently recommends total prophylactic gastrectomy as the preferred management strategy.[14,15] International consortium guidelines stress the importance of a multidisciplinary approach for patients with HDGC. Patients should have the opportunity to meet with a genetic counselor, gastroenterologist, surgeon, dietician, psychologist, and breast oncologist. Patients at risk for HDGC should undergo genetic testing as early as age 16, depending on family history, as there are rare cases of gastric cancers presenting before age 20.[14,15]

Unfortunately sensitivity of endoscopic surveillance with mapping biopsies is low, and multiple studies have shown that the foci of DGC or signet ring cells are often missed.[13,14,18,20,24-28] In one of the largest studies evaluating post-operative outcomes after prophylactic gastrectomy in HDGC patients, van der Kaaij *et al.* evaluated 26 patients with HDGC. Pre-operative EGD surveillance noted signet ring cell foci in endoscopic biopsies in 16 of 26 patients; however, review of surgical gastrectomy specimens identified signet ring sells in 23 of 26.[28] Additionally, the international consortium pooled all the studies of a comparison between endoscopic surveillance and prophylactic gastrectomy available at the time. In their review, they noted that in the cases in which endoscopic surveillance biopsies were negative, greater than 80% of the cases had early invasive signet ring cell carcinomas on gastrectomy. Additional cases were found to have pre-malignant pathology findings as well.[14] In a recent study of patients with *CDH1* germline mutations undergoing surveillance at the University of Michigan, 40% had SRCC on surveillance biopsies. Furthermore, 40% of those with normal endoscopic biopsies had SRCC identified on gastrectomy specimens.[25]

Studies are underway, seeking to improve diagnostic yield of endoscopic biopsies. At present, endoscopic surveillance with 30 minutes of inspection time combined with at least five biopsies from various parts of the stomach plus targeted biopsies of pale areas (known as the Cambridge protocol) appears to provide the best diagnostic yield of signet ring cells, although overall sensitivity is still low-moderate.[13,22,25] While the use of chromoendoscopy with Congo red or methylene blue had previously been employed to improve the yield of endoscopic surveillance biopsies[23] these agents are no longer recommended due to potential toxicity. At this time there are no data to support that narrow band imaging or endoscopic ultrasound offer any incremental benefit. A phase II study evaluating the use of confocal endoscopic micros-copy compared to standard Cambridge protocol biopsies is currently underway.[29]

For many patients the idea of a prophylactic gastrectomy can be daunting due to the potential for procedural and post-procedural morbidity. Nevertheless, for known carriers of a pathogenic germline *CDH1* mutation, the international consortium recommends consideration of total prophylactic gastrectomy, regardless of endoscopic findings, as the most effective intervention to reduce gastric cancer mortality.[15] There is still insufficient evidence to support an optimal age at which patients should undergo gastrectomy. Guidelines recommend surgery be considered around 20 to 30 years of age and a recent analysis using Markov modeling suggested the optimal age for gastrectomy was 30 for women and 30 to 39 for men, based on age-specific incidence rates.[30] Even so, the variability in cancer phenotypes and penetrance observed among families with *CDH1* mutations continue to fuel debate about the optimal timing and absolute indications for prophylactic gastrectomy.[17] All patients should undergo a baseline upper endoscopy with multiple biopsies (40+ as per Cambridge protocol) and evaluate for gross lesions, Barrett's esophagus, or other potential anatomic features that may impact surgical planning. The surgical approach for prophylactic gastrectomy should include a total gastrectomy with Roux-en-Y reconstruction with the jejuno-jejunal anastomosis at least 50 cm distal to the esophago-jejunal junction to reduce the risk of bile acid reflux.[14,15]

Overall mortality from gastrectomy is 1 to 2%; however, 10 to 20% of individuals report some degree of procedure-related morbidity. Nearly all patients will experience weight loss after surgery and require lifelong vitamin B12 supplementation. Most patients are ultimately able to return to their normal activity level and work within six months and report good quality of life overall.[14,15,26,27,31]

In terms of breast cancer risk reduction, as the lifetime risk for breast cancer is 42% for women with germline *CDH1* mutations, recommendations call for enhanced breast cancer surveillance with an annual breast MRI and mammogram as the sensitivity of mammogram alone is limited for detection of lobular breast cancers. Prophylactic mastectomy can also be considered. There have been reports suggesting a modest increase in the risk for colon cancer, and early colonoscopy can be considered.[14,15]

FAMILIAL INTESTINAL GASTRIC CANCER

Familial intestinal gastric cancer (FIGC) is defined as non-diffuse gastric cancer exhibiting an autosomal dominant pattern of inheritance.[14,32,33] The clinical criteria for diagnosis of FIGC varies depending on the incidence of gastric cancer in the population. In countries with high incidence of gastric cancer, such as Japan, criteria similar to the Amsterdam criteria for colon cancer are used for a clinical diagnosis: gastric cancer diagnosed in at least three relatives, across two consecutive generations, with one diagnosis before the age of 50. In these higher incidence populations utilizing the Amsterdam criteria, only 0.9% of 3632 families with gastric cancer met criteria for FIGC.[33] In the Western countries such as the United States and United Kingdom with a lower incidence of gastric cancer, clinical criteria for familial intestinal gastric cancer specify at least two first- or second-degree relatives with intestinal gastric cancer with at least one diagnosed before the age of 50 or three or more relatives with intestinal gastric cancer at any age.[33,34]

The etiology of FIGC is unknown in most cases and may involve a combination of both genetic and environmental factors. *H. pylori* infection is thought to play a role in its development, as well as smoking, diet, and other environmental factors.[35] To date there is no known genetic alteration associated with FIGC specifically. However; it is possible that some of these familial cases may be attributable to other hereditary conditions associated with high or moderate penetrance genetic alterations. Lynch syndrome was first described by Warthin *et al.* in 1985[36] as familial gastric cancer; however, as incidence of gastric cancer has fallen in the general population, colorectal cancer has replaced it as the most prevalent malignancy in families with germline MMR gene mutations. As gastric cancers can be prominent in other known hereditary cancer syndromes (Table 12.1), multigene panel testing is justified in patients meeting clinical criteria for FIGC.

There are no standardized criteria for endoscopic management in patients meeting clinical criteria for FIGC. However, Corso *et al.* have recommended yearly endoscopic surveillance beginning at age 60.[37]

Lynch Syndrome

Lynch syndrome (previously known as hereditary nonpolyposis colorectal cancer or HNPCC) is among the most common of the hereditary cancer syndromes, with a population prevalence estimated at 1 in 300.[38] Lynch syndrome has been implicated in 3% of colorectal cancers and is also associated with an increased risk for other cancers, predominantly gastrointestinal and gynecologic malignancies.[39,40] Cancers are characterized by phenotypes of defective DNA mismatch repair and often develop at younger ages.[39]

Genetics and Clinical Features Pathogenic germline variants in one of the four DNA mismatch repair (MMR) genes (*MSH2, MLH1, MSH6, PMS2*) as well as the *EPCAM* gene (directly upstream to *MSH2)* have been implicated in the pathogenesis of Lynch syndrome.[41] Germline MMR gene variants predispose to development of rapidly growing neoplasms. Immunhistochemical (IHC) staining of Lynch-associated tumors will often show the absence of one or more of the MMR proteins. Additionally, most Lynch syndrome cancers are microsatellite instable (MSI-H) and/or hypermutated.[39] Both MSI analysis and IHC staining are employed to screen colorectal and endometrial cancers for Lynch syndrome; however, the sensitivity and specificity of DNA mismatch repair phenotypes for identifying Lynch-associated gastric cancers remain to be determined.

In contrast to the lifetime risk for colorectal cancer and endometrial cancer of 75% and 40 to 60%, respectively, in Western countries the risk for gastric cancer in Lynch syndrome patients has been estimated at 5 to 20%.[40–46] While Aarino *et al.* found a 19% cumulative lifetime risk of developing gastric cancer among Finnish Lynch syndrome families,[44] most other studies have found lower risks of gastric cancer across different populations. Watson *et al.* examined 6041 patients across four different countries (Finland, Denmark, Holland, and Omaha, USA) and concluded that the risk of developing gastric cancer by the age of 70 was 5.8%.[43]

Several studies in Asian countries, which have higher rates of gastric cancer in the general population, have also reviewed the risk of developing gastric cancer in Lynch syndrome. In a study of Chinese families meeting Amsterdam criteria, Cai *et al.* noted an overall rate of gastric cancer of 7%, although it accounted for 44.5% of all extra-colonic tumors, which is similar to the rates in Western countries.[47] In contrast, gastric cancer is often the most prominent malignancy in Lynch syndrome families in Japan and Korea.[47,48] Park *et al.*'s analysis of the Korean Hereditary Tumor registry found a 3.2-fold higher risk of gastric cancer in Lynch syndrome mutation carriers compared to the general population. This risk was even more dramatic in younger groups with a relative risk of 11.3 in the 30-year-olds and 5.5 in the 40-year-olds. They noted the mean age of gastric cancer diagnosis was 47.[48]

The risk for gastric cancer may vary based on the underlying MMR gene mutation. Broeke *et al.*, in a study of 284 Lynch syndrome families, found no increase in risk of gastric cancer in *PMS2* mutation carriers, although their overall sample size was small.[49] In a Swedish study by Karimi *et al.*, the risk of gastric cancer was higher among *MLH1* and *MSH2* mutation carriers with a trend toward higher rates in *MSH6* mutation carriers that did not meet statistical significance.[50] In a review of the Prospective Lynch Syndrome Database, Moller *et al.* determined that gastric cancer and upper GI cancers occurred at a higher rate in older adults, with a cumulative risk of gastric cancer of 7% in *MLH1* mutation carriers and 8% in *MSH2* mutation carriers.[45] A recent analysis of 3828 patients diagnosed with Lynch syndrome ascertained through a commercial genetic testing laboratory also identified mutations in *MLH1* and *MSH2*, older age, and male sex as risk factors.[51]

Management Screening and surveillance recommendations for Lynch syndrome focus primarily on colon and endometrial cancers with annual colonoscopies beginning between 20 and 25 years of age. Although the benefit of endometrial surveillance remains unproven, guidelines suggest an annual pelvic exam with annual endometrial biopsy and transvaginal ultrasound begin at age 30 to 35, with consideration of prophylactic total abdominal hysterectomy, and bilateral salpingo-oopherectomy is recommended once childbearing is complete.[52]

Although the need for upper GI surveillance has been a topic of debate, most guidelines recommend a baseline EGD between 30 and 35 with a surveillance exam every 2 to 5 years.[46,52] A family history of a gastric or upper GI tract malignancy should prompt closer monitoring. *H. pylori* should always be eradicated given that it is a class I carcinogen.[41]

Familial Adenomatous Polyposis (FAP)

Genetics and Clinical Features FAP is an autosomal dominant polyposis syndrome characterized by development of hundreds to thousands of adenomatous polyps in the colon, often beginning in adolescence. In attenuated FAP, patients present with fewer colorectal polyps, often at a later age. Germline pathogenic variants in the *APC* tumor suppressor gene are identified in >90% of individuals with classic adenomatous polyposis (again, up to thousands of colorectal adenomas) and there are more than 300 known mutations in the *APC* gene associated with variable clinical phenotypes.[35] The most common extra-colonic malignancies in FAP include duodenal, ampullary, and thyroid cancers.[53,54]

Gastric cancers are relatively rare in FAP, especially in Western countries (<1% cumulative risk), comparable to the rate of gastric cancer in the general population.[41,53,54] However, in Asian countries such as Japan or Korea, the risk of gastric cancer is 7- to 10-fold increased among individuals with FAP compared to the general population.[54] Park *et al.* reported a gastric cancer rate of 2.7% in their Korean FAP population, while others have reported rates approaching 15%.[41,55] It is important to note that while many patients with FAP develop dense gastric polyposis, these are usually fundic gland polyps (FGP), which are histopathologically distinct and appear to have a low malignant potential (0.5 to 1% progress to cancer).[41] FGPs in patients with FAP may exhibit low-grade dysplasia; few (<3%) appear to feature high-grade dysplasia.[56,57] Gastric adenomas are relatively uncommon, found in 6–14% of FAP patients in Western populations,[35,56,58] but incidence appears to be much higher in Asian populations 36–50%.[55,58] Gastric adenomas are often found in the antrum, whereas FGPs cluster in the fundus and cardia, sparing the antrum. However, gastric adenomas can develop in other parts of the stomach where they can be hard to detect, especially in patients with dense polyposis. Larger polyp size is associated with a higher likelihood of an adenoma, justifying endoscopy biopsy and/or removal of polyps that are larger (>1 cm) or stand out from the rest.

In a recent review of FAP patients followed through a large hereditary colon cancer registry from 1979 through 2016, Mankaney et al. reported that 10 of 767 FAP patients (1.3%) developed gastric cancer; however, it is worth noting that most of the gastric cancers were diagnosed in 2012–2016, suggesting a possible rise in incidence.[53] Additionally, they identified several worrisome endoscopic features associated with the development of gastric cancers: fundic gland polyps carpeting the proximal stomach, growth of these polyps during surveillance, and the development of heaped up tissue or mounds within the background of carpeting polyps.[53]

Management   Currently, EGD is recommended every 1 to 3 years for FAP surveillance. While the interval depends mostly on the duodenal polyp burden and Spigelman stage, experts have proposed that gastric polyp burden and size and degree of dysplasia should also be used in determining the surveillance interval. Gastric polyps >1 cm should be resected. Prophylactic gastrectomy is not recommended in the absence of severe dysplasia.[35,53]

Gastric Adenocarcinoma and Proximal Polyposis Syndrome (GAPPS)

Genetics and Clinical Features   Worthley et al. first described GAPPS in three families from the United States, Canada, and Australia.[59] He proposed the following diagnostic criteria:

- gastric polyps restricted to the body and fundus with no evidence of colorectal or duodenal polyposis,
- >100 polyps carpeting the proximal stomach in the index case or >30 polyps in a first-degree relative of another case,
- predominantly FGPs, some having regions of dysplasia (or a family member with either dysplastic FGPs or gastric adenocarcinoma),
- an autosomal dominant pattern of inheritance.

Since then, GAPPS has been reported in various ethnic populations, including Asians.[60–62] It is an autosomal dominant condition with diffuse fundic gland polyposis of the oxyntic mucosa of the stomach in the fundus and body with antral sparing. The fundic gland polyps may have evidence of dysplasia and there is an increased risk of gastric adenocarcinoma. Li et al. identified hotspot point mutations in the promoter 1B region of the *APC* gene as the underlying germline mutation leading to the condition based on germline testing of six families.[60] Interestingly, GAPPS differs significantly from FAP in that there does not appear to be an increased risk of polyposis elsewhere in the GI tract (e.g., no colorectal polyposis).[62]

At this time, the absolute risk for gastric cancer in GAPPS is unknown, although there are reports of individuals developing metastatic adenocarcinoma while under endoscopic surveillance.[62] Affected individuals may develop complications of gastric polyposis including bleeding/anemia, which may require surgical intervention.

Management There are currently no surveillance guidelines specifically for GAPPS; however, affected patients should be followed closely based on their phenotype with endoscopic resection of large polyps and a low threshold for gastrectomy in the setting of dysplasia.[62]

MUTYH-Associated Polyposis (MAP)

Genetics and Clinical Features MUTYH-associated polyposis (MAP) is an autosomal recessive colon polyposis syndrome first identified by Al-Tassan *et al.* in 2002.[63] It is associated with biallelic mutations in the *MUTYH* base excision repair gene.[64] There also appear to be a number of founder mutations in different populations. For instance, in European populations (German and Italian), there appear to be two specific mutations in the *MUTYH* gene that are found in up to 1.14% of healthy individuals.[65] While monoallelic carriers do not appear to have a significant increase in colon cancer risk, biallelic mutations are associated with polyposis and increased risk of colorectal cancer. Patients with MAP may present with either a "classic" polyposis phenotype with >100 adenomas or the "attenuated" multiple adenoma phenotype with 5 to 100 adenomas. Compared to FAP, patients with MAP often have a milder presentation, developing colon cancer at a later age (median age is in the 40s) with an overall lower adenoma burden.[66]

In addition to the increased risk of colon cancer in MAP, there appears to also be an increased risk of extracolonic malignancies in MAP, especially upper GI tract polyps and cancers.[40] In a review of 133 patients with MAP, Poulsen *et al.* found either fundic gland polyps or gastric cancer in 8%.[67] Interestingly, in a Korean population of gastric cancer specimens, Kim *et al.* found 2 of 95 specimens with advanced gastric cancer had somatic *MUTYH* gene mutations, suggesting that germline *MUTYH* mutations might play a role in pathogenesis of gastric cancer.[68] Additional research is needed to better understand gastric cancer risks associated with MAP.

Management At this time, surveillance for MAP focuses mainly on the colorectum. While EGD is recommended for evaluation of duodenal polyps, there are no formal recommendations regarding surveillance for gastric cancer in MAP.

The Hamartomatous Polyposis Syndromes

The hamartomatous polyposis syndromes are a group of rare hereditary disorders in which patients develop hamartomatous polyps within and occasionally outside the GI tract. These include Peutz-Jeghers syndrome, juvenile polyposis syndrome, and Cowden/PTEN hamartoma tumor syndrome. Although most of the morbidity from gastrointestinal hamartomas is due to occult blood loss and small intestinal obstructions, the risks for gastric and other cancers are increased.

Juvenile Polyposis Syndrome

Genetics and Clinical Features Juvenile polyposis syndrome (JPS) is the most common of the autosomal dominant hamartomatous polyp syndromes, affecting about 1 in 100,000 individuals. Clinical criteria for JPS include at least one of the following: five or more juvenile polyps in the colon, juvenile polyps throughout the GI tract, or a family history of JPS and any number of juvenile polyps in the colon.[69,70] It was first described in 1964 by McColl *et al.*[71] and in 1979, Watanabe *et al.* described a gastric form named juvenile polyposis of the stomach, first seen in the Japanese population.[72]

Juvenile polyps have a classic pathologic appearance of mucin filled cystic dilation of epithelial tubules embedded in abundant lamina propria containing macrophages, fibroblasts, and myofibroblasts.[73] JPS patients often present with chronic GI bleeding, anemia, abdominal pain, diarrhea, or prolapsed rectal polyps. Fifteen percent of patients also have congenital defects such as malrotation of the gut and cleft palate.[73]

Germline mutations in two genes, *SMAD4* and *BMPR1A,* have been associated with JPS. Overall sensitivity of genetic testing is 20 to 60%; thus, a significant proportion of patients who meet clinical criteria have no identifiable germline mutation.[69,70,73] Seventy-five percent of cases of JPS are familial and 25% are considered *de novo* mutations.[69] Up to 20% of patients with *SMAD4* mutations have symptoms and signs of hereditary hemorrhagic telangiectasia (HHT).[69,73,74]

It is thought that juvenile polyps can develop adenomatous changes, and this is what leads to the development of adenocarcinoma. A literature review of 271 JPS patients across 12 countries found that 50 of 271 had juvenile polyps exhibiting adenomatous changes and 47 of them developed carcinomas.[75] Larger polyps are also associated with higher rates of dysplasia.[76] The risk of developing gastric cancer appears to be higher in *SMAD4* mutation carriers, ranging from 5 to 30%.[46,77] One study by Ishida *et al.* reviewed 171 Japanese patients with JPS and calculated an overall lifetime risk of any malignancy by age 70 was 86.2%, and the lifetime risk of gastric cancer was 73%.[70]

Peutz-Jeghers Syndrome

Genetics and Clinical Features Peutz-Jeghers syndrome (PJS) is an autosomal dominant condition characterized by mucocutaneous pigmention, hamartomatous GI polyps, and increased risk for gastrointestinal and other cancers.[69,78] Clinical criteria include any one of the following: two or more histologically confirmed Peutz-Jeghers polyps, any number of PJ polyps in an individual with a family history, characteristic mucocutaneous pigmentation in an individual with a family history, and/or any number of PJ polyps in an individual with the characteristic mucocutaneous pigmentation (Table 12.1).[78]

The hamartomatous polyps most often involve the small intestine followed by the colon and stomach. Presenting symptoms often include intussusception, bowel obstruction, and GI bleeding, developing at median age 11.[69] Peutz-Jeghers polyps have a typical appearance on pathology including the classic arborization of smooth muscle into the polyp fronds.[78,79]

The *STK11* gene, which is a tumor suppressor gene, has been found to be mutated in 30 to 70% of patients meeting clinical criteria for PJS.[79] Although it is an autosomal dominant condition, it appears that 25% of cases are *de novo* mutations.[69]

Patients with PJS syndrome have a high risk of various types of malignancies.[69,76] Giardiello *et al.* reported a 93% cumulative risk of developing malignancy and specifically a 29% risk of developing gastric cancer in their meta-analysis of 210 patients;[79,80] however, recent studies have found the overall gastric malignancy risk to be lower, ranging from 5 to 20%.[46]

PTEN Hamartoma Tumor Syndrome PTEN hamartoma tumor syndrome (PHTS) includes Cowden's syndrome, Bannayan-Riley-Ruvalcaba syndrome, and Proteus syndrome. Originally these three were considered distinct entities, but they are now felt to be part

TABLE 12.2: Gastric Cancer Screening Recommendations[51]	
Hereditary Condition	**Gastric Cancer Screening Recommendations**
Hereditary diffuse gastric cancer	Prophylactic gastrectomy strongly considered (otherwise annual EGD with extensive biopsies per Cambridge protocol, although endoscopic surveillance has limited sensitivity)
Familial intestinal gastric cancer	Consider EGD, test for *H. pylori* and treat if positive
FAP	EGD every 1 to 3 years based on gastroduodenal polyp burden, remove gastric polyps >1 cm
MAP	Baseline EGD age 30 to 35; repeat based on polyp burden
GAPPS	Consider EGD every 1 to 2 years, with removal of large polyps; consider gastrectomy if high-grade dysplasia
Lynch syndrome	EGD every 2 to 5 years, at age 30 to 35
Peutz-Jeghers syndrome	Baseline EGD and small bowel imaging at age 8 and surveillance q2–3 years; otherwise resume screening age 18, remove polyps >1 cm
Juvenile polyposis syndrome	EGD every 1 to 3 years starting at age 15; removal of large polyps and consider gastrectomy if high-grade dysplasia or if polyp burden cannot be managed endoscopically
PTEN hamartoma syndrome	Consider EGD q2–3 years
Li-Fraumeni syndrome	EGD every 2 to 5 years starting at age 25
Hereditary breast and ovarian cancer syndrome	No clear recommendations

of the spectrum of the same disorder, associated with a germline mutation in the *PTEN* gene.[81,82]

Cowden's syndrome is a rare autosomal dominant condition with variable penetrance occurring in 1:200,000 people.[82] Individuals with Cowden's syndrome develop multiple hamartomas and neoplasms arising from all three germ layers (ectoderm, mesoderm, and endoderm). Germline mutations in the *PTEN* gene, a tumor suppressor gene, are found in 80% of patients with Cowden's syndrome.[82] There is a vast spectrum of malignancies associated with Cowden's syndrome with the most common being breast, thyroid, and gynecologic malignancies (Table 12.2). Furthermore, multiple studies have noted the presence of polyps throughout the GI tract with hamartomatous polyps and ganglioneuromas being the hallmark polyp type.[46,76,83,84] For a long time, there was no clear evidence of increased risk of gastrointestinal cancers in spite of the hamartomatous polyps in the GI tract. More recently, however, there is some indication of increased risk of both upper and lower tract GI cancers, including gastric cancer, but the magnitude of risk increase remains unknown.[46] Heald *et al.* noted 9% of subjects with germline *PTEN* mutations had colon cancer, but there were no gastric cancers reported in their cohort.[84] A case report by Al-Thihli *et al.* in 2009, documented a case of Cowden's syndrome presenting with gastric carcinoma.[83]

Hamartomatous Polyposis Management Although each of the hamartomatous polyposis syndromes have different screening/surveillance recommendations for various cancer types, overall the recommendations for screening for gastric neoplasia are similar and the goal of upper endoscopy is to remove all large polyps (>1 cm).[35,52,79] Typically gastric polyps can be managed endoscopically; however, in rare cases, surgery may be necessary for management of significant polyp burden that leads to iron deficiency, hypoalbuminemia, or if there is the presence of dysplasia.[69,74]

Different studies advocate different upper GI screening protocols for JPS. The ACG consensus guidelines recommend starting both colon cancer and gastric cancer surveillance with colonoscopy and EGD beginning from age 12 to 15 with repeat endoscopy every 1 to 3 years depending on polyp burden.[52] For patients with *SMAD4* mutation, cardiovascular examination and screening for HHT should also be considered.[52,74] PJS has very similar recommendations, although given the risk of developing complications from the hamartomatous polyps at a young age, small bowel imaging and endoscopic evaluation can begin as early as age eight.[35,52,78]

Since the phenotype of Cowden's syndrome is variable, there is still debate about the ideal time to start endoscopic screening. A colonoscopy should be repeated every 1 to 3 years depending on polyp burden while EGD should be done every 2 to 3, although a shorter interval is recommended if there is duodenal polyposis.[52] Neither Bannayan-Riley-Ruvalcaba nor Proteus syndrome have been shown to be associated with an increased risk of GI malignancy.

Li-Fraumeni Syndrome

Genetics and Clinical Features Li-Fraumeni syndrome (LFS) is a rare autosomal dominant condition in which patients are at risk for developing multiple primary tumors. The most common malignancies associated with LFS are sarcomas, as well as carcinomas of the breast, brain, and adrenal cortex;[35] however, risk for gastrointestinal cancers is also increased. The syndrome was first described by Li and Fraumeni in 1988 and updated clinical diagnostic criteria were proposed by Birch *et al.* in 1994: a proband with any childhood tumor or a sarcoma, brain tumor or adrenal cortical tumor before the age of 45, plus a first- or second-degree relative with a typical LFS tumor at any age, plus an additional first- or second-degree relative in the same lineage with any cancer before the age of 60.[35]

A number of studies have reviewed the risk of gastric cancer in LFS. Nichols *et al.* reviewed clinical cohorts compiled by Dana Farber Cancer Institute and the National Cancer Institute; among the 185 families with *TP53* mutations, there were a total of 738 cancers, of which 23 were gastric cancers. Of note, nine of them were diagnosed in Japanese individuals with the median age of diagnosis 30 years younger than the general population.[85] A follow-up study focused on gastric or gastroesophageal cancers in 21 patients diagnosed at a median age of 36; interestingly, a pathology review of the gastric cancers revealed both intestinal and diffuse type (signet ring cell) tumors.[86]

Management Li-Fraumeni syndrome has extensive management recommendations including intensive surveillance for breast cancer and annual whole-body MRI. An upper endoscopy and colonoscopy are recommended every 2 to 5 years beginning at age 25.

Hereditary Breast and Ovarian Syndrome

Genetics and Clinical Features

As its name implies, hereditary breast and ovarian cancer syndrome is primarily associated with an elevated risk of breast and ovarian cancer. The primary genes responsible for this syndrome are pathogenic germline variants in *BRCA1* and *BRCA2*, genes involved in double-stranded DNA repair. The risk for gastric cancer appears to be increased in *BRCA1* and *BRCA2* mutation carriers, although the magnitude of risk remains unclear.[46,77] Brose *et al.* studied 483 *BRCA1* mutation carriers at two different academic institutions and noted a 4-fold increased risk of gastric cancer in a 10-year follow-up period.[87] Johannsson *et al.* studied both *BRCA1* and *BRCA2* mutation carriers and found risk of gastric cancer to be more pronounced among *BRCA1* mutation carriers where gastric cancers accounted for 3.4% of all tumors with a 6-fold increased risk of gastric cancer in females.[88] Finally, Friedenson *et al.* reviewed observational studies of *BRCA1* and *BRCA2* families and identified increased risk of gastric cancer in six of 17 population studies, with overall relative risk of 1.7.[89]

Management At this time, there are no recommendations for screening or surveillance for gastric cancer for patients with germline mutations in *BRCA1* or *BRCA2*.

GENETIC COUNSELING

Patients with personal or family history suggestive of possible genetic predisposition to gastric cancer should be counseled about the potential benefits and risks of genetic testing and should be informed about the various possible outcomes of a genetic test, including positive result (pathogenic germline variant present), negative result (no pathogenic germline variant present), or variant of uncertain significance (VUS).[14,15] Patients should be aware of the potential implications the testing could have on their medical care and the potential need for heightened surveillance and/or surgery depending on the gene mutation. Individuals identified as carriers of pathogenic germline variants should be educated on the potential risks to their children and other family members and the importance of sharing genetic test results with at-risk family members.[90]

When determining whether or not a patient should undergo genetic evaluation (Figure 12.1), an accurate and complete family history should be obtained, including age of onset of different cancer types in all first- and second-degree relatives.[91] In general, younger age of onset or multiple family members with malignancy should prompt consideration of genetic referral. The criteria for genetic testing continue to evolve and the cost of genetic testing continues to decrease. The ideal candidate for genetic testing in a family would be someone affected with one or more of the characteristic tumors/phenotypes; however, in many cases only cancer-unaffected individuals may be available for germline testing.[91]

GASTRIC CANCER RISK REDUCTION

Identifying individuals with genetic predisposition to gastric cancer (and/or other types) offer opportunities for early detection and prevention. For example, in families with HDGC, prophylactic gastrectomy would be offered given the difficulty identifying early stage lesions with endoscopic surveillance. By offering genetic testing to family members, additional high-risk individuals can be successfully identified and preventive surveillance and screening implemented.

Population-based endoscopic screening for gastric cancer is not currently recommended in Western countries given the overall low incidence of gastric cancer. However, in Asian populations, there are population-based gastric cancer screening protocols in place and the high incidence of gastric cancer associated with specific germline mutations discussed here justifies endoscopic surveillance. For individuals with familial gastric cancer with or without an identified germline mutation, modifying lifestyle and environmental factors is important, especially smoking cessation. *H. pylori* should be actively tested for and eradicated whenever it is found.

CONCLUSION

Overall, 1 to 3% of gastric cancers arise in individuals with an underlying genetic cause. Eliciting a detailed family cancer history and recognizing red flags in patients' clinical presentation and tumor phenotypes are of utmost importance, as early diagnosis of cancer predisposition syndromes can improve outcomes and provide opportunities for cancer early detection/prevention in families at high risk for gastric and other tumors.

References

1. Global Burden of Disease Cancer C, Fitzmaurice C, Allen C, *et al.* Global, regional, and national cancer incidence, mortality, years of life lost, years lived with disability, and disability-adjusted life-years for 32 cancer groups, 1990 to 2015: a systematic analysis for the global burden of disease study. *JAMA Oncol.* 2017;3:524–548.

2. Karimi P, Islami F, Anandasabapathy S, *et al.* Gastric cancer: descriptive epidemiology, risk factors, screening, and prevention. *Cancer Epidemiol Biomarkers Prev.* 2014;23:700–713.

3. Ansari S, Gantuya B, Tuan VP, *et al.* Diffuse gastric cancer: a summary of analogous contributing factors for its molecular pathogenicity. *Int J Mol Sci.* 2018;19.

4. Correa P. Human gastric carcinogenesis: a multistep and multifactorial process—First American Cancer Society Award Lecture on Cancer Epidemiology and Prevention. *Cancer Res.* 1992;52:6735–6740.

5. Lauren P. The two histological main types of gastric carcinoma: diffuse and so-called intestinal-type carcinoma: an attempt at a histo-clinical classification. *Acta Pathol Microbiol Scand.* 1965;64:31–49.

6. Cancer Genome Atlas Research N. Comprehensive molecular characterization of gastric adenocarcinoma. *Nature.* 2014;513:202–209.

7. Sohn BH, Hwang JE, Jang HJ, *et al.* Clinical significance of four molecular subtypes of gastric cancer identified by The Cancer Genome Atlas Project. *Clin Cancer Res.* 2017.

8. Wang F, Meng W, Wang B, *et al.* Helicobacter pylori-induced gastric inflammation and gastric cancer. *Cancer Lett.* 2014;345:196–202.

9. Amieva M, Peek RM Jr. Pathobiology of Helicobacter pylori-induced gastric cancer. *Gastroenterology.* 2016;150:64–78.

10. Marshall BJ, Warren JR. Unidentified curved bacilli in the stomach of patients with gastritis and peptic ulceration. *Lancet.* 1984;1:1311–1315.

11. Noto JM, Peek RM Jr. Helicobacter pylori: an overview. *Methods Mol Biol.* 2012;921:7–10.

12. Zullo A, Hassan C, Cristofari F, *et al.* Effects of Helicobacter pylori eradication on early stage gastric mucosa-associated lymphoid tissue lymphoma. *Clin Gastroenterol Hepatol.* 2010;8:105–110.

13. Chen Y, Kingham K, Ford JM, *et al.* A prospective study of total gastrectomy for CDH1-positive hereditary diffuse gastric cancer. *Ann Surg Oncol.* 2011;18:2594–2598.

14. Fitzgerald RC, Hardwick R, Huntsman D, *et al.* Hereditary diffuse gastric cancer: updated consensus guidelines for clinical management and directions for future research. *J Med Genet.* 2010;47:436–444.

15. van der Post RS, Vogelaar IP, Carneiro F, *et al.* Hereditary diffuse gastric cancer: updated clinical guidelines with an emphasis on germline CDH1 mutation carriers. *J Med Genet.* 2015;52:361–374.

16. Guilford P, Hopkins J, Harraway J, *et al.* E-cadherin germline mutations in familial gastric cancer. *Nature.* 1998;392:402–405.

17. Xicola RM, Li S, Rodriguez N, *et al.* Clinical features and cancer risk in families with pathogenic CDH1 variants irrespective of clinical criteria. *J Med Genet.* 2019;56:838–843.

18. Hansford S, Kaurah P, Li-Chang H, *et al.* Hereditary diffuse gastric cancer syndrome: CDH1 mutations and beyond. *JAMA Oncol.* 2015;1:23–32.

19. Kluijt I, Siemerink EJ, Ausems MG, *et al.* CDH1-related hereditary diffuse gastric cancer syndrome: clinical variations and implications for counseling. *Int J Cancer.* 2012;131:367–376.

20. Chun YS, Lindor NM, Smyrk TC, *et al.* Germline E-cadherin gene mutations: is prophylactic total gastrectomy indicated? *Cancer.* 2001;92:181–187.

21. Barber M, Murrell A, Ito Y, *et al.* Mechanisms and sequelae of E-cadherin silencing in hereditary diffuse gastric cancer. *J Pathol.* 2008;216:295–306.

22. Lim YC, di Pietro M, O'Donovan M, *et al.* Prospective cohort study assessing outcomes of patients from families fulfilling criteria for hereditary diffuse gastric cancer undergoing endoscopic surveillance. *Gastrointest Endosc.* 2014;80:78–87.

23. Shaw D, Blair V, Framp A, *et al.* Chromoendoscopic surveillance in hereditary diffuse gastric cancer: an alternative to prophylactic gastrectomy? *Gut.* 2005;54:461–468.

24. Suriano G, Yew S, Ferreira P, *et al.* Characterization of a recurrent germ line mutation of the E-cadherin gene: implications for genetic testing and clinical management. *Clin Cancer Res.* 2005;11:5401–5409.

25. Jacobs MF, Dust H, Koeppe E, *et al.* Outcomes of endoscopic surveillance in individuals with genetic predisposition to hereditary diffuse gastric cancer. *Gastroenterology.* 2019;157:87–96.

26. Hebbard PC, Macmillan A, Huntsman D, *et al.* Prophylactic total gastrectomy (PTG) for hereditary diffuse gastric cancer (HDGC): the Newfoundland experience with 23 patients. *Ann Surg Oncol.* 2009;16:1890–1895.

27. Seevaratnam R, Coburn N, Cardoso R, *et al.* A systematic review of the indications for genetic testing and prophylactic gastrectomy among patients with hereditary diffuse gastric cancer. *Gastric Cancer.* 2012;15(Suppl. 1): S153–163.

28. van der Kaaij RT, van Kessel JP, van Dieren JM, *et al.* Outcomes after prophylactic gastrectomy for hereditary diffuse gastric cancer. *Br J Surg.* 2018;105:e176–e82.

29. Ruff S, Curtin B, Quezado M, *et al.* Evaluation of confocal endoscopic microscopy for detection of early-stage gastric cancer in hereditary diffuse gastric cancer (HDGC) syndrome. *J Gastrointest Oncol.* 2019;10:407–411.

30. Laszkowska M, Silver E, Schrope B, *et al.* Optimal timing of total gastrectomy to prevent diffuse gastric cancer in individuals with pathogenic variants in CDH1. *Clin Gastroenterol Hepatol/* 2020 Apr;18(4):822–829.

31. Newman EA, Mulholland MW. Prophylactic gastrectomy for hereditary diffuse gastric cancer syndrome. *J Am Coll Surg.* 2006;202:612–617.

32. Oliveira C, Pinheiro H, Figueiredo J, *et al.* Familial gastric cancer: genetic susceptibility, pathology, and implications for management. *Lancet Oncol.* 2015;16:e60–70.

33. Setia N, Clark JW, Duda DG, *et al.* Familial gastric cancers. *Oncologist.* 2015;20:1365–1377.

34. Caldas C, Carneiro F, Lynch HT, *et al.* Familial gastric cancer: overview and guidelines for management. *J Med Genet.* 1999;36:873–880.

35. Sereno M, Aguayo C, Guillen Ponce C, *et al.* Gastric tumours in hereditary cancer syndromes: clinical features, molecular biology and strategies for prevention. *Clin Transl Oncol.* 2011;13:599–610.

36. Classics in oncology. Heredity with reference to carcinoma as shown by the study of the cases examined in the pathological laboratory of the University of Michigan, 1895–1913. By Aldred Scott Warthin. 1913. *CA Cancer J Clin.* 1985;35:348–359.

37. Corso G, Roncalli F, Marrelli D, *et al.* History, pathogenesis, and management of familial gastric cancer: original study of John XXIII's family. *Biomed Res Int.* 2013;2013:385132.

38. Hampel H, Frankel WL, Martin E, *et al.* Screening for the Lynch syndrome (hereditary nonpolyposis colorectal cancer). *N Engl J Med.* 2005;352:1851–1860.

39. Rodriguez-Bigas MA, Boland CR, Hamilton SR, *et al.* A National Cancer Institute Workshop on Hereditary Nonpolyposis Colorectal Cancer Syndrome: meeting highlights and Bethesda guidelines. *J Natl Cancer Inst.* 1997;89:1758–1762.

40. Goodenberger M, Lindor NM. Lynch syndrome and MYH-associated polyposis: review and testing strategy. *J Clin Gastroenterol.* 2011;45:488–500.

41. Fornasarig M, Magris R, De Re V, *et al.* Molecular and pathological features of gastric cancer in Lynch syndrome and familial adenomatous polyposis. *Int J Mol Sci.* 2018;19.

42. Wang Y, Wang Y, Li J, *et al.* Lynch syndrome related endometrial cancer: clinical significance beyond the endometrium. *J Hematol Oncol.* 2013;6:22.

43. Watson P, Vasen HFA, Mecklin JP, *et al.* The risk of extra-colonic, extra-endometrial cancer in the Lynch syndrome. *Int J Cancer.* 2008;123:444–449.

44. Aarnio M, Mecklin JP, Aaltonen LA, *et al.* Life-time risk of different cancers in hereditary non-polyposis colorectal cancer (HNPCC) syndrome. *Int J Cancer.* 1995;64:430–433.

45. Moller P, Seppala TT, Bernstein I, *et al.* Cancer risk and survival in path_MMR carriers by gene and gender up to 75 years of age: a report from the Prospective Lynch Syndrome Database. *Gut.* 2018;67:1306–1316.

46. Stoffel EM. Heritable gastrointestinal cancer syndromes. *Gastroenterol Clin North Am.* 2016;45:509–527.

47. Cai SJ, Xu Y, Cai GX, *et al.* Clinical characteristics and diagnosis of patients with hereditary nonpolyposis colorectal cancer. *World J Gastroenterol.* 2003;9:284–287.

48. Park YJ, Shin KH, Park JG. Risk of gastric cancer in hereditary nonpolyposis colorectal cancer in Korea. *Clin Cancer Res.* 2000;6:2994–2998.

49. Ten Broeke SW, van der Klift HM, Tops CMJ, *et al.* Cancer risks for PMS2-associated Lynch syndrome. *J Clin Oncol.* 2018;36:2961–2968.

50. Karimi M, von Salome J, Aravidis C, *et al.* A retrospective study of extracolonic, non-endometrial cancer in Swedish Lynch syndrome families. *Hered Cancer Clin Pract.* 2018;16:16.

51. Kim J, Braun D, Ukaegbu C, *et al.* Clinical factors associated with gastric cancer in individuals with Lynch syndrome. *Clin Gastroenterol Hepatol.* 2019.

52. Syngal S, Brand RE, Church JM, *et al.* ACG clinical guideline: genetic testing and management of hereditary gastrointestinal cancer syndromes. *Am J Gastroenterol.* 2015;110:223–262; quiz 63.

53. Mankaney G, Leone P, Cruise M, *et al.* Gastric cancer in FAP: a concerning rise in incidence. *Fam Cancer.* 2017;16:371–376.

54. Walton SJ, Frayling IM, Clark SK, *et al.* Gastric tumours in FAP. *Fam Cancer.* 2017;16:363–369.

55. Park SY, Ryu JK, Park JH, *et al.* Prevalence of gastric and duodenal polyps and risk factors for duodenal neoplasm in korean patients with familial adenomatous polyposis. *Gut Liver.* 2011;5:46–51.

56. Bianchi LK, Burke CA, Bennett AE, *et al.* Fundic gland polyp dysplasia is common in familial adenomatous polyposis. *Clin Gastroenterol Hepatol.* 2008;6:180–185.

57. Bertoni G, Sassatelli R, Nigrisoli E, *et al.* Dysplastic changes in gastric fundic gland polyps of patients with familial adenomatous polyposis. *Ital J Gastroenterol Hepatol.* 1999;31:192–197.

58. Ngamruengphong S, Boardman LA, Heigh RI, *et al.* Gastric adenomas in familial adenomatous polyposis are common, but subtle, and have a benign course. *Hered Cancer Clin Pract.* 2014;12:4.

59. Worthley DL, Phillips KD, Wayte N, *et al.* Gastric adenocarcinoma and proximal polyposis of the stomach (GAPPS): a new autosomal dominant syndrome. *Gut.* 2012;61:774–779.

60. Li J, Woods SL, Healey S, *et al.* Point mutations in exon 1B of APC reveal gastric adenocarcinoma and proximal polyposis of the stomach as a familial adenomatous polyposis variant. *Am J Hum Genet.* 2016;98:830–842.

61. Mitsui Y, Yokoyama R, Fujimoto S, *et al.* First report of an Asian family with gastric adenocarcinoma and proximal polyposis of the stomach (GAPPS) revealed with the germline mutation of the APC exon 1B promoter region. *Gastric Cancer.* 2018;21:1058–1063.

62. Rudloff U. Gastric adenocarcinoma and proximal polyposis of the stomach: diagnosis and clinical perspectives. *Clin Exp Gastroenterol.* 2018;11:447–459.

63. Al-Tassan N, Chmiel NH, Maynard J, *et al.* Inherited variants of MYH associated with somatic G:C-->T:A mutations in colorectal tumors. *Nat Genet.* 2002;30:227–232.

64. Win AK, Reece JC, Dowty JG, *et al.* Risk of extracolonic cancers for people with biallelic and monoallelic mutations in MUTYH. *Int J Cancer.* 2016;139:1557–1563.

65. Aretz S, Tricarico R, Papi L, *et al.* MUTYH-associated polyposis (MAP): evidence for the origin of the common European mutations p.Tyr179Cys and p.Gly396Asp by founder events. *Eur J Hum Genet.* 2014;22:923–929.

66. Lipton L, Tomlinson I. The multiple colorectal adenoma phenotype and MYH, a base excision repair gene. *Clin Gastroenterol Hepatol.* 2004;2:633–688.

67. Poulsen ML, Bisgaard ML. MUTYH associated polyposis (MAP). *Curr Genomics.* 2008;9:420–435.

68. Kim CJ, Cho YG, Park CH, *et al.* Genetic alterations of the MYH gene in gastric cancer. *Oncogene.* 2004;23:6820–6822.

69. Schreibman IR, Baker M, Amos C, *et al.* The hamartomatous polyposis syndromes: a clinical and molecular review. *Am J Gastroenterol.* 2005;100:476–490.

70. Ishida H, Ishibashi K, Iwama T. Malignant tumors associated with juvenile polyposis syndrome in Japan. *Surg Today.* 2018;48:253–263.

71. McColl I, Busxey HJ, Veale AM, *et al.* Juvenile Polyposis Coli. *Proc R Soc Med.* 1964;57:896–897.

72. Watanabe A, Nagashima H, Motoi M, *et al.* Familial juvenile polyposis of the stomach. *Gastroenterology.* 1979;77:148–151.

73. Chow E, Macrae F. A review of juvenile polyposis syndrome. *J Gastroenterol Hepatol.* 2005;20:1634–1640.

74. Brosens LA, Langeveld D, van Hattem WA, *et al.* Juvenile polyposis syndrome. *World J Gastroenterol.* 2011;17:4839–4844.

75. Agnifili A, Verzaro R, Gola P, *et al.* Juvenile polyposis: case report and assessment of the neoplastic risk in 271 patients reported in the literature. *Dig Surg.* 1999;16:161–166.

76. Wirtzfeld DA, Petrelli NJ, Rodriguez-Bigas MA. Hamartomatous polyposis syndromes: molecular genetics, neoplastic risk, and surveillance recommendations. *Ann Surg Oncol.* 2001;8:319–27.

77. van der Post RS, Carneiro F. Emerging concepts in gastric neoplasia: heritable gastric cancers and polyposis disorders. *Surg Pathol Clin.* 2017;10:931–945.

78. Beggs AD, Latchford AR, Vasen HF, *et al.* Peutz-Jeghers syndrome: a systematic review and recommendations for management. *Gut.* 2010;59:975–986.

79. Giardiello FM, Trimbath JD. Peutz-Jeghers syndrome and management recommendations. *Clin Gastroenterol Hepatol.* 2006;4:408–415.

80. Giardiello FM, Brensinger JD, Tersmette AC, *et al.* Very high risk of cancer in familial Peutz-Jeghers syndrome. *Gastroenterology.* 2000;119:1447–53.

81. Marsh DJ, Kum JB, Lunetta KL, *et al.* PTEN mutation spectrum and genotype-phenotype correlations in Bannayan-Riley-Ruvalcaba syndrome suggest a single entity with Cowden syndrome. *Hum Mol Genet.* 1999;8:1461–1472.

82. Pilarski R, Eng C. Will the real Cowden syndrome please stand up (again)? Expanding mutational and clinical spectra of the PTEN hamartoma tumour syndrome. *J Med Genet.* 2004;41:323–326.

83. Al-Thihli K, Palma L, Marcus V, *et al.* A case of Cowden's syndrome presenting with gastric carcinomas and gastrointestinal polyposis. *Nat Clin Pract Gastroenterol Hepatol.* 2009;6:184–189.

84. Heald B, Mester J, Rybicki L, *et al.* Frequent gastrointestinal polyps and colorectal adenocarcinomas in a prospective series of PTEN mutation carriers. *Gastroenterology.* 2010;139:1927–1933.

85. Nichols KE, Malkin D, Garber JE, *et al.* Germ-line p53 mutations predispose to a wide spectrum of early-onset cancers. *Cancer Epidemiol Biomarkers Prev.* 2001;10:83–87.

86. Masciari S, Dewanwala A, Stoffel EM, *et al.* Gastric cancer in individuals with Li-Fraumeni syndrome. *Genet Med.* 2011;13:651–657.

87. Brose MS, Rebbeck TR, Calzone KA, *et al.* Cancer risk estimates for BRCA1 mutation carriers identified in a risk evaluation program. *J Natl Cancer Inst.* 2002;94:1365–1372.

88. Johannsson O, Loman N, Moller T, *et al.* Incidence of malignant tumours in relatives of BRCA1 and BRCA2 germline mutation carriers. *Eur J Cancer.* 1999;35:1248–1257.

89. Friedenson B. BRCA1 and BRCA2 pathways and the risk of cancers other than breast or ovarian. *MedGenMed.* 2005;7:60.

90. Robson ME, Bradbury AR, Arun B, *et al.* American Society of Clinical Oncology Policy Statement Update: Genetic and Genomic Testing for Cancer Susceptibility. *J Clin Oncol.* 2015;33:3660–3667.

91. Corso G, Figueiredo J, La Vecchia C, *et al.* Hereditary lobular breast cancer with an emphasis on E-cadherin genetic defect. *J Med Genet.* 2018;55:431–441.

CHAPTER 13

Endocrine Cancers

Jianliang Man, Norman G. Nicolson, and Tobias Carling

▥ INTRODUCTION

The term *endocrine cancers* most commonly refers to cancers of the thyroid, parathyroid, adrenal glands, and endocrine tumors arising in the pancreas and intestinal tract. Most lesions in these glands are benign, but both benign and malignant endocrine tumors can be associated with multiple neoplasia syndromes. This chapter will discuss benign and malignant endocrine neoplasms and the genetic underpinnings of each.

▥ NON-MEDULLARY THYROID CANCER

Risk Assessment and Management

Most thyroid cancers present as new thyroid nodules that are discovered by patients or clinicians by physical exam or incidentally on imaging. It is important to note that most thyroid nodules discovered in the general population are benign—only 5 to 10% are malignant. Risk factors for any form of thyroid malignancy include radiation exposure (especially in childhood), extreme age ranges (children or elderly), female sex, and family history.[1-3]

While most non-medullary thyroid cancers (NMTC) are sporadic, 3 to 9% of cases present in familial clusters with at least two first-degree relatives also with this cancer.[4] Individuals with one or more first-degree relatives with NMTC will have a 4- to 10-fold increase in their own risk for the disease.[5] Therefore, it is essential to obtain detailed personal and family histories upon discovery of a new thyroid nodule. A history of rapid increase in size, dyspnea, dysphagia, hoarseness. and new onset of Horner's syndrome all suggest the possibility of cancer. A focused physical exam should evaluate the entirety of the neck and note the size, firmness, and mobility of the nodule, and features such as lymphadenopathy or adherence to neighboring structures increase the suspicion for malignancy.[1-3]

The next step in workup is to perform thyroid function testing and focused thyroid ultrasound. Thyroid ultrasound is a sensitive and specific imaging modality for thyroid nodules and can provide helpful clues as to the nature of the lesion, such as size, internal calcifications, solid versus cystic components, associated lymphadenopathy, and even local invasion. It should always be performed when a thyroid nodule or goiter is identified, even if the patient has already had other neck imaging studies (CT, MRI, etc.).[1-3]

Thyroid function tests have utility in determining the functional status of a thyroid nodule. If the TSH level is suppressed and ultrasound demonstrates a single nodule with no other concerning findings, the most likely diagnosis is an autonomously functioning thyroid nodule. Also termed "hot nodules," they are rarely malignant and can be safely observed with repeat imaging to confirm that they remain stable in size. They should not undergo fine-needle aspiration (FNA) as the results are often misleading and do not alter the management strategy. Occasionally, it can be unclear if a thyroid nodule is "hot" or "cold" when the TSH level is borderline low or when there are multiple nodules on imaging.[1-3]

FNA should be performed if the lesion is not clearly benign. Studies have shown that FNA is about 95% accurate in determining the malignancy when compared to final surgical pathology. About 5 to 10% of thyroid lesions that undergo FNA will be found to be malignant on cytology. This typically cited risk does vary depending on the individual patient's age and gender, and it is important to consider the pre-test probability that an individual patient may have when counseling patients prior to FNA. FNA can be limited in its ability to distinguish certain benign and malignant follicular lesions as their malignant potential can only be confirmed by identification of invasion. About 20 to 30% of cases classified as suspicious or indeterminate by FNA are found to be malignant after surgery, with significant variation between institutional pathology departments.[6] Recent advancements in the understanding of the genetic changes behind thyroid carcinogenesis have led to enhancement of the accuracy of FNA using molecular markers. Using molecular markers, tumor cells can be analyzed for the presence of protein biomarkers as well as tested for *BRAF* and *RAS* mutations, *RET/PTC* and *PAX8/PPAR* gene fusions, and other genetic alterations common in thyroid cancer.[2,6,7]

Patients with FNA findings that prove to be malignant or indeterminate should be referred to a thyroid surgeon. Surgery remains the mainstay of treatment of non-metastatic thyroid cancer and offers a good chance at a cure, particularly for well-differentiated thyroid cancers. Total thyroidectomy with or without cervical lymph node dissection is the definitive procedure for most patients with a confirmed diagnosis of thyroid cancer. It has been suggested that thyroid lobectomy may be sufficient for small and low-risk papillary thyroid cancers (PTC) and that observation may be appropriate for micro-PTC, but this remains controversial.[8,9] If there is tumor extension into extrathyroidal tissue, an *en bloc* resection should be performed when possible. Tracheal and esophageal resections are rarely indicated in WDTC but can be performed with reconstruction in few appropriate scenarios. Evidence of metastatic disease to the cervical lymph nodes based on preoperative imaging or intra-operative findings warrants a thorough neck exploration and lymph node dissection. The benefit of a prophylactic central neck dissection remains a controversial topic, but it is advocated by many specialists and performed routinely at some institutions.[1-3,10] Prognosis in WDTC is generally excellent after surgery, though local or lymph node recurrences are not uncommon.

Patients with indeterminate follicular lesions based on FNA results can choose to undergo total thyroidectomy or opt for thyroid lobectomy knowing that a complete thyroidectomy might later be necessary if the lesion turns out to be cancer. Frozen sections analysis has not been shown to be helpful in altering the course of management.[1-3]

Patients who present with unresectable primary tumors should be managed via a multidisciplinary approach with palliation as the main goal. Thyroid cancer with distant metastasis has a poor prognosis. Surgical resection may still play a role to provide definitive histologic diagnosis, more accurate staging, and palliative benefits such as preserving the airway and swallowing functions.[1–3]

Post-operative management should include a follow-up neck ultrasound within 6 months to a year and serum Tg and TSH every 3 to 6 months for the first year and then at 3- to 5-year intervals. Radioactive iodine ablation (RAI) is often used post-operatively in patients with high-risk lesions. The American Thyroid Association (ATA) has recommended RAI for patients with stage III and IV disease, stage II disease younger than 45 years, certain patients with stage II disease older than 45, and patients with stage I disease but with large tumors, multifocality, lymph node metastases, vascular invasion, or intermediate differentiated histology. Patients with high-risk lesions will also benefit from more frequent imaging, and recurrences may require reoperation.[1–3]

Disease-Specific Epidemiology

Thyroid nodules are relatively common with a prevalence of nearly 50% by age 65 in the general population. Thyroid cancers are the most common endocrine malignancy with an estimated 44,280 new cases in the United States in 2021 according to the NIH. They make up 96% of all new endocrine cancers and about two-thirds of all deaths due to endocrine cancers. Their incidence has been increasing by roughly 3% per year over the last 10 years. Although there is certainly an element of increased detection of small indolent micro-PTC, this alone is unlikely to fully account for the rise in incidence.[7,11,12] Familial association is seen in 3 to 9% of all NMTC and includes non-syndromic cases as well as those related to known cancer syndromes such as familial adenomatous polyposis, Carney complex and DICER1 syndrome. Known hereditary cancer syndromes account for only about 5% of familial cases—most do not have an identifiable inherited gene mutation.[4]

At least 95% of thyroid cancers arise from the thyroid follicular cells and are further categorized into well-differentiated (WDTC), poorly differentiated (PDTC), and anaplastic thyroid cancer (ATC). There are two main histological subtypes of WDTC: PTC and follicular thyroid carcinoma (FTC). PTC is by far the most common form of thyroid malignancy, accounting for 80 to 85% of cases. FTC accounts for 10 to 15% of all thyroid cancer cases. There are also unique subtypes of intermediate differentiation such as tall cell variant, columnar cell variant, diffuse sclerosing variant, hobnail variant, insular carcinoma, and Hürthle cell carcinoma. PDTC and ATC are much rarer than WDTC, each accounting for less than 2% of thyroid cancer cases.[1,2,12]

WDTC has a very favorable prognosis. The 5-year survival rate of patients with PTC is around 98%; FTC sits only slightly lower. While up to 66% of patients with thyroid cancer may have regional lymph node metastases at the time of primary diagnosis, only a small minority will have distant metastasis. The presence of cervical lymph node metastasis increases the risk of local recurrence but has not always been shown to have a negative effect on overall mortality. The presence of distant metastases at the time of diagnosis, on the other hand, is a strong predictor of poor outcome. The mortality rate among patients with metastasis outside the neck or mediastinum is 43 to 90%.[1,2]

PDTC and ATC behave much more aggressively than WDTC. Most patients who are diagnosed with PDTC and ATC have unresectable primary tumors at diagnosis. PDTC carries a

5-year survival rate anywhere from 60 to 85%. ATC has a less favorable prognosis with few long-term survivors.[1,2,13–17]

Research has identified many somatic aberrations that are thought to contribute to the tumorigenesis of thyroid cancers. Among these, the most common mutations affect the MAPK and PI3K-AKT pathways. The single most commonly mutated gene in non-medullary thyroid cancers is *BRAF*. One mutation, *BRAF* V600E, occurs in about 45% of PTCs, 10 to 20% of PDTCs, and 20 to 40% of ATCs.[18] It is associated with a more aggressive phenotype, increased risk of recurrence, and decreased response to RAI treatment.

Disease-Specific Approach to Risk Assessment, Counseling, and Testing

Patients diagnosed with non-medullary thyroid cancer or thyroid adenomas without family history of thyroid cancer or cancer syndromes typically do not need in-depth investigations into their pedigrees nor genetic testing as they most likely have sporadic disease. A familial syndrome should be suspected when a patient presents with two or more first-degree relatives with histories of thyroid cancer or thyroid disorders.

Familial thyroid cancer remains an evolving field without a consensus method of classification but can traditionally be divided into two groups: syndromic and non-syndromic. The "syndromic" group is associated with cancer syndromes including Cowden syndrome, familial adenomatous polyposis (FAP), Carney complex, Werner syndrome, and DICER1 syndrome, which account for only about 5% of all familial cases of non-medullary thyroid cancer. They are also associated with benign and malignant tumors of non-thyroid origins; rarely is thyroid cancer the only manifestation. The "non-syndromic" group, sometimes referred to simply as familial non-medullary thyroid cancer, includes all familial thyroid cancers without a known heritable genetic defect. Studies thus far have not identified any useful markers to identify these cases and it remains a diagnosis of exclusion.[4,5]

Sporadic NMTC is generally not associated with an elevated risk for other tumors or diseases, and most patients who are cured can enjoy a normal life.[1] Commercial genomic-driven diagnostic assays for somatic mutations are used for assisting with risk-stratification of thyroid nodules with indeterminate cytology, but the role of genomic approaches in determining post-thyroidectomy management is still limited. However, as thyroid cancer research continues to advance, management decisions may one day be based on tumor genetic profiles.[7,11]

Hereditary Cancer Syndromes

Familial Non-Medullary Thyroid Cancer Familial non-medullary thyroid cancer (FNMTC) is defined in a family when two or more diagnoses of non-medullary thyroid cancer in first-degree relatives are made in the absence of other associated tumor susceptibility syndromes. It is a catch-all diagnosis whose criteria will almost certainly continue to evolve—up to 70% of patients diagnosed by the above criteria will actually have sporadic thyroid cancer. No definitive causative gene defects have been identified, and no confirmatory testing is available. The understanding of this disease is limited as kindreds tend to be small and various studies have used inconsistent definitions for the syndrome. A few putative causative gene loci have been discovered but have yet to be validated. The exact mechanism of inheritance is not known: some authors have suggested that it is autosomal dominantly inherited with incomplete penetrance while others feel it is likely to be polygenic.[19] One study suggests an element of anticipation, a genetic phenomenon where affected members of subsequent generations are afflicted with more aggressive disease and earlier onset.[4,5]

Some studies have suggested that FNMTC tends to be multifocal and more aggressive than sporadic NMTC, although this hypothesis remains up for debate. FNMTC also appears to be associated with other benign thyroid abnormalities including adenomas, autoimmune thyroiditis, multinodular goiter, and hyper/hypothyroidism—recognizing these associations is essential while taking a detailed family history.[4,5]

Familial Adenomatous Polyposis Familial adenomatous polyposis (FAP) is most known for its association with colon cancer; several variants are caused by mutations in the *APC* tumor suppressor gene. Extra-colonic manifestations of FAP include extracolonic neoplasms such as desmoid tumors, fibromas, osteomas, and thyroid adenomas and carcinomas. FAP is an autosomal dominant disease, but up to 25% of cases are caused by a *de novo* mutation. Most cases of FAP are diagnosed by genetic testing. In a few cases, no germline mutation is identified. Fewer than 2% of patients with Gardner's syndrome will develop thyroid cancer. However, given the increased risk of thyroid cancer, screening for thyroid cancer with annual thyroid ultrasounds is recommended. For additional details on the management of FAP, please see Chapter 6.[20]

Carney Complex Carney complex (CNC) is an autosomal dominant disorder characterized by lentigines and a range of benign and occasionally malignant tumors. It is thought to be caused by disruption to the protein kinase A signaling pathway. *PRKAR1A* is a regulatory subunit of protein kinase A and inactivating mutations in the gene cause a subset of CNC. *PRKACA, PRKACB*, and phosphodiesterase genes have also been implicated, but their roles in CNC have not been clearly demonstrated to date.[21] CNC is diagnosed by the presence of two or more major diagnostic criteria: a typical distribution of spotty skin pigmentation, cutaneous or mucosal myxoma, cardiac myxoma, breast myxomatosis, primary pigmented nodular adrenocortical disease (PPNAD), growth hormone-producing adenoma, large-cell calcifying Sertoli cell tumors, thyroid cancer or multiple thyroid nodules discovered before age 18, blue nevus, breast ductal adenoma, and osteochondromyxoma; or the presence of one of the above criteria along with either the presence of a germline mutation in the *PRKAR1A* gene or a first-degree relative with CNC.[22]

Thyroid abnormalities occur in up to 75% of patients with CNC, most of whom have non-functioning adenomas. However, patients are at higher risk to develop both papillary and follicular thyroid carcinomas. Adrenal disease in CNC is usually in the form of PPNAD (see the section on adrenocortical tumors later in the chapter). GH-producing adenomas are another hormonally active tumor frequently associated with CNC. About 10% of adult patients diagnosed with CNC will have some degree of acromegaly caused by a GH-producing adenoma. Evaluation of acromegaly involves measurement of IGF-1 levels, brain MRI, and an oral glucose tolerance test.[21,22]

Management of CNC revolves around the medical and surgical treatment of its manifestations when discovered. Once identified, patients with CNC are recommended to have routine clinical surveillance based on their age. For pre-pubertal children, growth rate should be monitored, and annual echocardiogram and testicular ultrasounds are recommended. If growth abnormalities arise, appropriate testing for GH or cortisol excess should be performed. For post-pubertal and adult patients, annual echocardiogram, testicular and thyroid ultrasound, urine cortisol, and serum IGF-1 levels are recommended.[21,22]

DICER1 *DICER1* is an endoribonuclease that regulates processing of micro-RNAs and plays a role in DNA repair. Defects in the gene predisposes to several tumor types and causes the syndrome known as *DICER1*-pleuropulmonary blastoma familial tumor predisposition syndrome, also known as *DICER1* syndrome. *DICER1* syndrome is inherited in an autosomal dominant fashion with *de novo* mutations causing about 20% of cases. The hallmark tumor of this disorder is pleuropulmonary blastoma, which typically presents in childhood. Other associated tumors also tend to present early in life and include ovarian sex-cord stromal tumors, cystic nephroma, thyroid tumors, ciliary body medulloepithelioma, Botryoid-type embryonal rhabdomyosarcoma, nasal chondromesenchymal hamartoma, pituitary blastoma, and pineoblastoma. The thyroid tumors in *DICER1* syndrome can be benign nodular goiters, adenomas, or differentiated thyroid cancer and can be approached similarly to sporadic thyroid nodules.[23,24]

There are no thyroid cancer screening or surveillance guidelines for patients with *DICER1* syndrome; however, annual clinical evaluation with targeted imaging and biochemical evaluation is recommended for each tumor based partly on clinical suspicion.[24]

Clinical Management of Patients at Increased Risk

While routine thyroid cancer screening in the general population is not recommended due to the risks of overdiagnosis, it is reasonable to screen those at an elevated risk based on family history. Patients who have predisposing syndromes or a hereditary pattern of thyroid cancer should receive yearly history and physical examinations starting 5 to 10 years before the youngest age of diagnosis within the family followed by a focused thyroid ultrasound should concerning findings be noted. Screening cervical ultrasounds can also be considered.[4,5,19]

Some specialists have advocated for prophylactic thyroidectomy in patients with a known hereditary syndrome or at very high risk of FNTMC (three or more first-degree relatives with NMTC), though this remains controversial. However, most experts agree that patients with a known or high risk of a hereditary disease with newly diagnosed thyroid cancer should undergo prophylactic central neck dissection at the time of surgery and consider post-operative radioactive iodine ablation given the increased risk for multifocality and recurrence.[4,5,19]

Patients with thyroid cancer and a known or suspected tumor susceptibility syndrome should be referred to a specialist experienced with these relatively rare syndromes. Thyroid cancer is usually still curable in these syndromes and mortality and morbidity more often result from complications involving other tumors that occur concurrently or later. Accurate identification of patients and appropriate screening are essential. As the types of tumors syndromic patients may develop can be very distinct and require multiple different specialists to manage, they will benefit most from a multidisciplinary and coordinated approach to care.[4,5,19]

▦ MEDULLARY THYROID CANCER

Risk Assessment and Management

Most medullary thyroid cancer (MTC) cases present as a new thyroid nodule. The workup proceeds similarly to that of non-medullary thyroid cancers. Detailed assessment of personal and family histories and a physical examination is followed up with thyroid ultrasound and FNA. FNA has a good diagnostic yield for MTC of around 90% based on cytological analysis alone, and it can be improved further with analysis of additional markers. MTC arises from the C cells of the thyroid gland and secretes several hormones including calcitonin, CEA, chromogranin, neurotensin, and histaminase. These secretory products can be measured in fine needle aspirates or analyzed using immunohistochemistry. High levels of these markers along with absence of thyroglobulin (the product of thyroid follicular cells) indicate the presence of MTC.[25]

All patients with thyroid nodules confirmed to be or suspicious for MTC should undergo germline DNA analysis for a *RET* mutation. The presence of that mutation will alter the management of the patient and necessitate evaluation for pheochromocytoma and hyperparathyroidism. Patients who test negative for *RET* mutations do not routinely need evaluation for other MEN2-asscociated tumors, except in rare cases of patients with highly indicative features of hereditary MTC but negative genetic testing. Pheochromocytoma can be ruled out by obtaining plasma free metanephrines and/or confirmatory 24-hour urine fractionated metanephrines and catecholamines. The presence of hyperparathyroidism is assessed with serum calcium and intact parathyroid hormone levels. Pheochromocytomas must be surgically resected prior to treatment for MTC while parathyroidectomy can be performed concurrently with surgery for MTC.[25,26]

All patients with confirmed or suspected MTC should also have measurements of serum calcitonin and CEA. Calcitonin (CT) is not only useful for detection of MTC but prognostication as well since very high CT levels correlate with a higher stage of disease. Both CEA and CT are followed post-treatment to determine the success of treatment and to monitor for recurrence. Routine CT testing as part of the workup for thyroid nodules without suggestive features of MTC is controversial. Serum CT may be elevated in certain medical conditions such as chronic renal insufficiency, multinodular goiter, and benign C-cell hyperplasia resulting in false positives. Provocative tests such as intravenous calcium or pentagastrin stimulation can help to differentiate elevated CT due to MTC from other disorders but is not available in most centers in the United States. Many European and Asian centers do routinely perform both basal and stimulated serum CT testing as part of the workup of a thyroid nodule. The ATA guidelines task force recommends that individual clinicians use their own clinical judgment when deciding whether to perform serum CT testing in patients with thyroid nodules.[25,27]

The definitive surgical procedure for non-metastatic MTC is total thyroidectomy with dissection of at least the central neck lymph nodes. Studies have shown metastasis to the central and ipsilateral lymph nodes occurs with a 50 to 75% frequency in patients with MTC, regardless of tumor size. Evidence of locally advanced disease or cervical lymph node metastases on pre-operative imaging, high pre-operative serum calcitonin levels, and intraoperative findings may warrant further dissection of the lateral neck compartments. Pre-operative serum CT can be helpful in determining the risk for lymph node metastasis; levels less than 20 pg/mL are associated with almost no risk of lymph node metastasis, while higher levels correlate with the extent of metastasis. MTC may occasionally be diagnosed on pathology review from a thyroid lobectomy. In these cases, patients should be tested for a germline *RET* mutation and serum CT levels and undergo post-operative imaging to determine if there is residual disease. A complete thyroidectomy should be considered versus watchful waiting but is indicated if genetic testing is positive for a *RET* germline mutation, serum CT level remains elevated, or residual disease is present.[25,27]

Post-operative locoregional therapy (EBRT) should be considered if there is extensive nodal disease, extra-thyroidal extension, or residual MTC on follow-up imaging. Reoperation or further lymph node dissection may be indicated if the primary surgery is deemed inadequate. Particularly, patients with incomplete lymph node dissections are most likely to benefit from re-operation. Radioactive iodine ablation (RAI), while common following NMTC resections, is not indicated following surgery for MTC as it has not been shown to be of benefit. Exceptions to this include rare cases where tumors contain MTC mixed with PTC or FTC.[25]

Advanced and metastatic disease usually cannot be cured by surgery and most patients with advanced MTC succumb to the disease. The goal of management is palliative, and EBRT, systemic chemotherapy, and other non-surgical treatments are the primary components. Debulking surgery should be considered if speech, swallowing, and respiratory functions are threatened but only to minimize complications.[25]

Post-operative patients should have a neck ultrasound and undergo measurements of serum CT and CEA 2 to 3 months after surgery and then yearly if normal. Elevated CT level after treatment is concerning for residual disease and should be followed carefully. The degree of elevation can give a clue as to the location of disease: calcitonin <150 pg/ml often indicates locoregional disease and should be followed by repeat measurements of serum calcitonin and CEA every 3 to 6 months; calcitonin >150 indicates the possibility of distant metastases and should prompt further imaging workup.[25]

Disease-Specific Epidemiology

Medullary thyroid cancer comprises 3 to 5% of all thyroid cancer cases. Hereditary MTC accounts for 25 to 30% of MTC cases and is caused by two multiple endocrine neoplasia syndromes: MEN2A (including familial MTC) and MEN2B. Together they have a prevalence estimated at 1 in 35,000. Causative mutations have been identified in many different *RET* codons and are associated with slightly different phenotypes. The *RET* mutations in hereditary MTC seem to cause a predictable development of C-cell hyperplasia progressing to MTC and then to loco-regional and subsequently distant metastasis. Patients with MEN2A have a 95% chance of developing MTC while the risk of MTC with MEN2B approaches 100%.[25,26,28–30]

MTC is relatively aggressive compared to well-differentiated thyroid cancer. Patients with sporadic MTC usually present in middle age and with locally advanced disease at presentation. The 10-year survival rate is estimated to be 80%. Older age, higher disease stage, and serum calcitonin >10 ng/mL are associated with poorer prognosis.[25]

One of the distinguishing features of MTC is its association with *RET* mutations. Almost all patients with hereditary MTC will be found to have a germline *RET* mutation while about 50% of sporadic MTCs will have somatic *RET* mutations. *RET* is a proto-oncogene located on chromosome 10q11.2 that encodes for a receptor tyrosine kinase involved in many cell-signaling pathways. Mutations or alterations causing constitutive activation of the *RET* protein can lead to development of tumors of many different types.[30]

MTC patients without a family history of MEN2, 1 to 7% have a *de novo* germline *RET* mutation. Truly sporadic MTC usually occurs later in life than hereditary forms, is less often multifocal, and typically lacks C-cell hyperplasia. *RET* mutations in sporadic MTC are not thought to be driver mutations but rather secondary mutations that contribute to tumor progression. The *RET* M918T codon mutation is the most common *RET* mutation in sporadic MTC. Sporadic MTCs that do not harbor a *RET* mutation are often found to have *RAS* mutations. *RET* and *RAS* mutations are mutually exclusive and thought to represent two distinct pathways to MTC tumorigenesis.[30]

Other epigenetic and post-transcriptional changes have also been found to play a role in the development of MTC. Certain microRNAs (miRNAs) such as miR-21, miR-183, and miR-375 have been found to be associated with worse clinical outcome, recurrences, and metastases. Other miRNAs such as miR-224 are associated with better rates of cure. In addition, sporadic and hereditary MTC appears to have different miRNA profiles. The exact roles of miRNAs are still being explored but dysregulation of their oncogenic and tumor suppressor properties may contribute to the tumorigenesis of MTC.[30]

Disease-Specific Approach to Risk Assessment, Counseling, and Testing

All patients diagnosed with MTC should undergo germline genetic testing for a *RET* mutation given the high prevalence of hereditary MTC as well as *de novo* germline mutations. The pathogenic variants of *RET* that cause the MEN2 syndromes are inherited in an autosomal dominant fashion and can occur without a family history in about 5% of MEN2A cases and 50% of MEN2B cases. Both MEN2A and MEN2B usually present early in life and identification of the syndromes in the pediatric age group is essential to early screening and treatment. Children with a parent affected by MEN2A are recommended to undergo *RET* genetic testing as early as possible. MEN2B can manifest in the first few months of life and children at risk for MEN2B should have prenatal genetic testing or testing performed as soon as possible after birth.[25]

Germline *RET* testing is also recommended for parents of children who are diagnosed with MEN2B regardless of prior family history and all first-degree relatives of patients. Some *RET* mutations that cause MEN2A are also associated with cutaneous lichen amyloidosis and Hirschsprung's disease. Therefore, individuals with cutaneous lichen amyloidosis or Hirschsprung's disease with a *RET* exon 10 mutation should also undergo testing for MEN2A.[25,26,30]

Germline genetic testing can be performed using select exon testing, single-gene testing, or the use of a multigene panel. When the pathogenic variant of *RET* within a family is known, screening of selected individuals can proceed with a straightforward targeted approach to test if an at-risk member carries the specific allele. In newly diagnosed families where the *RET* mutation is unknown, the strategy is usually multi-tiered with select exon testing for high-frequency pathogenic variants initially, then moving on to less frequent variants if the first-tier testing is negative. Initial testing for MEN2A should evaluate for *RET* mutations in exon 10 (codons 609, 611, 618, 620), exon 11 (codons 630, 634), and exons 8, 13, 14, 15, 16. Patients with suspected MEN2B should be tested for RET exon 16 codon M918T mutation and exon 15 codon A883F mutation. This strategy may miss rarer variants; therefore, if no mutations are detected or if the detected variant is discordant with the phenotype, sequencing of the entire coding region is indicated. As the expense for genetic testing continues to decrease, recommendations for initial testing may change in the coming years.[25]

There is currently no indication to test for tumor somatic mutations, micro-RNAs, or other genetic abnormalities in sporadic or hereditary MTC outside the research setting.

Hereditary Cancer Syndromes

MEN2 The MEN2 syndromes were originally known as Sipple syndrome when the tumor constellation comprising pheochromocytoma, MTC, and parathyroid adenoma was first described in 1961. As understanding of this syndrome increased, distinct variants of MEN2: MEN2A and MEN2B were recognized. Both are caused by pathogenic activating mutations of the proto-oncogene *RET*, which is located on chromosome 10q11.2 and codes for a transmembrane receptor tyrosine kinase involved in many cell-signaling pathways. Mutations causing constitutive activation of this kinase promote cell proliferation, survival, and migration, often leading to tumorigenesis. The distinct differences between the different variants of MEN2 are largely determined by the location of the mutation.[25,28–30]

MEN2A Based on the ATA recommendations on MTC, there are four variants of MEN2A: classical MEN2A, MEN2A with cutaneous lichen amyloidosis (MEN2A with CLA), MEN2A with Hirschsprung's disease (MEN2A with HD), and familial medullary thyroid cancer (FMTC).[25]

Classical MEN2A This most common variant of MEN2A represents the phenotype originally described by Sipple. It most often involves *RET* mutations in exons 10 or 11. Nearly 100% of patients will develop MTC while rates of pheochromocytoma and primary hyperparathyroidism vary based on the specific *RET* mutation. Codon 634 mutations in exon 11 are associated with higher rates of pheochromocytoma and hyperparathyroidism. Overall, about 50% of patients with classical MEN2A will develop pheochromocytoma and 20 to 30% will have parathyroid disease.[28]

The parathyroid disease in MEN2A is usually in the form of benign parathyroid adenomas and less often multi-gland hyperplasia. Patients are often asymptomatic or have mild symptoms. Severe clinical hyperparathyroidism is rare in MEN2A. If detected prior to or concurrently with MTC, most cases of hyperthyroidism can be treated with parathyroidectomy at the time of surgery for MTC.[25,28]

The pheochromocytomas of MEN2A are usually benign and bilateral, though about 4% are malignant. Pheochromocytoma can be the first expression of MEN2 syndromes, and diagnosis of a pheochromocytoma should prompt evaluation for a *RET* mutation. If discovered concurrently with MTC, pheochromocytomas must be treated first. Symptomatic blood pressure control is initially achieved with alpha-blockers such as phenoxybenzamine. Occasionally beta-blockade is required to treat the reflex tachycardia caused by alpha-blockade. Surgical resection of the pheochromocytoma is performed after blood pressure has been normalized.[25,28]

MEN2A Associated with Cutaneous Lichen Amyloidosis Cutaneous lichen amyloidosis (CLA) is a dermatologic condition characterized by scaly, pruritic skin lesions occurring over the interscapular region of the back. This rare disorder can occur as an isolated condition but has long been associated with MEN2A. It may be the first clinically apparent symptom for patients with MEN2A presenting prior to MTC; thus, patients with CLA should undergo testing for a *RET* germline mutation in order to rule out MEN2A. CLA is most often associated with *RET* codon 634 mutations. MTC, pheochromocytoma, and hyperparathyroidism develop with similar frequencies as in classical MEN2A.[25,28]

MEN2A Associated with Hirschsprung's Disease (HD) Although both MEN2A and HD are caused by *RET* mutations, the role of the *RET* protein is likely different in endocrine cells and neuronal precursor cells. However, some pathogenic *RET* variants, especially those involving exon 10, are associated with both MEN2A and HD. Therefore, patients with HD and a known exon 10 *RET* mutation should be evaluated and screened for MEN2A. Likewise, patients with MEN2A and suspicious GI symptoms such as constipation and dysmotility should receive a workup to exclude HD.[25,28]

FMTC Familial medullary thyroid cancer is defined as hereditary MTC in the presence of a pathogenic *RET* germline mutation but without development of pheochromocytoma or hyperparathyroidism. It was historically a separate disease entity but has recently been accepted as a part of the MEN2A spectrum. A germline mutation involving codons 609, 618, and 620 in exon 10 is present in over 50% of FMTC. Patients should undergo the same screening algorithm as MEN2A regardless of family history of pheochromocytoma or hyperparathyroidism.[25,28]

MEN2B MEN2B was originally known as MEN3. In contrast to MEN2A, MEN2B manifests early, usually within the first year of life. MTC can develop in infancy and is typically highly aggressive with early metastasis. About 50 to 75% of MEN2B cases are caused by *de novo* mutations, and only 25 to 50% of cases occur within families with established histories of hereditary MTC. Ninety-five percent of MEN2B cases are caused by the M918T mutation in exon 16. The rarer exon 15 (A883F) mutation is found in the other 5% of MEN2B patients and is thought to cause a less aggressive form of the syndrome. About half of MEN2B patients will develop pheochromocytoma. MEN2B has characteristic non-endocrine features not found in MEN2A. Patients have long and narrow faces and develop lip and tongue mucosal neuromas. Skeletal abnormalities are common and result in Marfanoid body habitus, chest malformations, scoliosis, and joint deformities. Patients are also prone to ganglioneuromas of the gastrointestinal tract that may cause constipation, diarrhea, nausea, and even bowel obstructions that require surgery. Most mortalities result from advanced MTC and establishing the diagnosis early is essential to timely treatment. However, most patients with MEN2B will present too late with unresectable MTC.[25,28,29]

Clinical Management of Patients at Increased Risk

Given that nearly 100% of MEN2 patients will develop MTC, the management strategy revolves around preventing the mortality and morbidity of the cancer. Prophylactic thyroidectomy has been shown to be safe and can prevent the complications of MTC in patients with MEN2. Although surgery is often referred to as "prophylactic thyroidectomy," a more appropriate term may be "early thyroidectomy" as C-cell hyperplasia and even undiagnosed MTC will already be present in most cases at the time of surgery. Infants and young children do experience higher complication rates with thyroidectomy when compared to adults. The most significant complication is hypoparathyroidism as the parathyroid glands are often small and difficult to identify early in life. Therefore, the risks of surgical complications must be carefully weighed against the benefits.[25]

The ATA Guidelines Task Force has recommended that the timing of thyroidectomy be guided by the risk level of the patient as determined by the specific *RET* mutation. The recommendations were revised in 2015 and divide patients into three risk categories: the highest-risk (HST) group includes patients with MEN2B codon M918T mutation; the high-risk (H) group includes patients with codons C634 and A883 mutations; and the moderate-risk (MOD) group includes patients with all other *RET* mutations (Table 13.1).[25]

TABLE 13.1: American Thyroid Association Risk Levels						
ATA risk category	**MEN2 syndrome and associated mutation**	**Risk of MTC**	**Risk of pheochromo-cytoma**	**Risk of HPT**	**Timing of prophylactic thyroidectomy**	**Post-thyroidectomy surveillance recommendations**
ATA-HST (highest risk)	MEN2B (codon M918T)	Highest	~50%	~20%	Months to 1 year after birth	Physical exam, neck ultrasound, serum calcitonin and Carcinoembryonic Antigen levels every 6 months for 1 year, then annually. Begin screening for pheo. at age 11
ATA-H (high risk)	MEN2B (codon A883F) and MEN2A (C634)	High	~50%	20 to 30%	Before 5 years of age, based on calcitonin level	Clinical follow-up and pheo. screening as above
ATA-MOD (moderate risk)	MEN2A (all other codons except C634)	Moderate	10 to 30%	~20%	Based on calcitonin level, or before adulthood	Clinical follow-up as above. Begin screening for pheo. at age 16

Data from Wells SA Jr, Asa SL, Dralle H, et al: Revised American Thyroid Association guidelines for the management of medullary thyroid carcinoma, Thyroid 2015 Jun;25(6):567–610.

Children who are in the ATA-HST category often develop MTC within the first year of life, and the MTC that develops is usually highly aggressive. Infants who are at risk should undergo genetic testing soon after birth. Total thyroidectomy should be performed in the first year, if possible, and with or without central neck dissection based on ability to identify and preserve the parathyroid glands. Serum calcitonin levels are elevated during the first few months of life and are of limited utility in determining the timing of surgery. Patients should be evaluated with physical exam, neck ultrasound, and serum calcitonin and CEA measurements every 6 months for one year and then annually and begin screening for pheochromocytoma with annual plasma metanephrine levels at age 11. Patients with *de novo* M918T mutations are more difficult to identify early in life. Studies have shown that those diagnosed upon recognition of non-endocrine features of the disorder have better outcomes than those diagnosed upon onset of clinically evident MTC or pheochromocytoma. Therefore, it is vital for clinicians to be aware of the non-endocrine characteristics of MEN2B.[25]

Children in the ATA-H category generally develop MTC in the early years of childhood. They should be evaluated with an annual physical examination, cervical ultrasound, and serum calcitonin measurements starting at age 3. Prophylactic total thyroidectomy should be performed when serum calcitonin elevation is detected or before age 5. Patients in this risk category should begin screening for pheochromocytoma with annual plasma metanephrine levels at age 11.[25]

Children who are in the ATA-MOD category typically develop MTC in adolescence or later in life, though there is significant variance among this patient population. It is also recommended that they a physical examination and serum calcitonin measurements start at age 3, though their parents may defer to have total thyroidectomy only after the serum calcitonin level becomes elevated. This may necessitate an extended length of high-intensity follow-up, and some parents who do not wish to undergo this evaluation for their children may elect to have prophylactic thyroidectomy at an earlier date. For patients in the ATA-MOD category, screening for pheochromocytoma with annual plasma free metanephrines begins at age 16.[25]

Adults who have confirmed pathogenic *RET* mutations and normal initial testing should still be considered for prophylactic thyroidectomy. Those who have not had a thyroidectomy should undergo yearly calcitonin testing and a neck ultrasound.[25]

◼ PRIMARY HYPERPARATHYROIDISM AND PARATHYROID TUMORS

Risk Assessment and Management

Neoplasms of the parathyroid are most often encountered during the workup for hypercalcemia. There are usually four parathyroid glands that secrete parathyroid hormone (PTH) responsible for regulating serum calcium levels. Primary hyperparathyroidism (PHPT) is the disorder caused by overactive and inappropriate secretion of PTH by one or more parathyroid glands. PHPT can be caused by benign parathyroid adenomas, parathyroid hyperplasia, or, rarely, parathyroid cancer. Most cases are idiopathic and sporadic. Risk factors include radiation exposure to the neck, lithium therapy, and the female sex (women are twice as likely to be affected). Occasionally, PHPT can be a component of a familial syndrome such as MEN1, MEN2A, calcium sensing receptor (CaSR)-related disorders, or CDC73-related disorders.[31-34]

Symptoms of PHPT are usually due to the resulting hypercalcemia and can be vague and nonspecific; weakness, fatigue, abdominal pain, nausea, polyuria, neurocognitive symptoms, osteoporosis, nephrolithiasis, and nephrocalcinosis can all occur. The diagnosis of PHPT is made based on biochemical evidence of elevated serum calcium and PTH levels. Most patients with PHPT will have elevation of both levels, but some may only have an elevated calcium level with a normal or borderline elevated PTH. PTH that is inappropriately elevated in the setting of hypercalcemia should be interpreted as evidence of PHPT. When PHPT is discovered either as part of a workup of a symptomatic patient or incidentally on routine labs, additional evaluation for complications should be performed. including bone density and kidney function testing as these are frequently not clinically evident.[34,35]

Parathyroidectomy is indicated in patients with symptomatic hyperparathyroidism. Mild asymptomatic forms can be treated conservatively, but surgery has been shown to have a benefit even in normocalcemic PHPT and is increasingly favored, especially for younger patients, to prevent long-term effects of hypercalcemia and hyperparathyroidism. The current indications for parathyroidectomy in asymptomatic patients are age <50, serum calcium >1 mg/dL above the upper limit of normal, and any evidence of skeletal or renal effects (osteoporosis, pathologic fracture, decreased creatinine clearance, nephrolithiasis, etc.).[35] Resection of the hyperfunctioning gland(s) is usually curative.

Pre-operative imaging most commonly involves sestamibi-technetium 99m parathyroid scintigraphy or 4DCT to localize enlarged glands. Ultrasound can also be an effective imaging modality and provide good localization but is somewhat limited by operator dependence and the inability to image the mediastinum where ectopic parathyroid tissue may be located. Mild cases of HPT may not be associated with markedly enlarged glands and can be more difficult to localize with imaging. Selective parathyroid venous sampling is a more invasive technique but is highly sensitive and useful when other imaging is negative or when recurrence or persistent HPT occur.[35,36]

Hyperparathyroidism was traditionally treated surgically by bilateral neck exploration in order to identify and remove the enlarged gland(s). As accuracy of preoperative imaging localization improved, minimally invasive parathyroidectomy (MIP) has emerged as the procedure of choice as it minimizes operative time, surgical trauma, length of stay, and post-operative pain. Both MIP and conventional bilateral neck exploration have similarly excellent rates of cure (95 to 100%). Patients with HPT caused by hyperplasia of multiple glands will need to be treated with partial or total parathyroidectomy with or without parathyroid autotransplantation. Total parathyroidectomy is associated with a higher risk of post-operative hypoparathyroidism than subtotal parathyroidectomy. Intra-operative monitoring of serum PTH is routinely performed in some centers and improves the success rate.[31,34,35]

Occasionally, patients may have residual or recurrent HPT after surgery. Residual disease is usually the result of additional parathyroid adenoma(s) missed by surgery or inadequate resection of parathyroid tissue in partial parathyroidectomies. Recurrence may occur due to new development of adenomas or hyperplasia and can even occur in autotransplanted parathyroid tissue after a total parathyroidectomy. Both residual and recurrent disease can be treated with reoperation. The risk of surgical complications such as recurrent laryngeal nerve injury is higher in reoperation; preoperative localization with imaging and/or selective parathyroid venous sampling is essential to maximize the probability of a cure while minimizing risks. Patients at an elevated risk for recurrence, such as those with MEN1 and MEN2A, will need lifelong follow-up of serum calcium and PTH levels.[31,34]

Parathyroid cancers are incredibly rare, however. Excessively elevated calcium and PTH levels can indicate the presence of a parathyroid cancer. If it is suspected, FNA or excisional biopsy should not be performed as the biopsy tract could become seeded with malignant cells. Given the rarity of parathyroid cancers, there is insufficient data to aid the creation of management guidelines. However, most sources agree that suspected parathyroid cancers should be resected *en bloc*. Recurrence is common and occurs in up to 49 to 60% of cases. Mortality and morbidity of advanced parathyroid cancers usually result from the metabolic consequences of hyperparathyroidism and hypercalcemia and less frequently from mass effect. Hypercalcemic crisis can occur and is a medical emergency requiring immediate treatment with aggressive intravenous fluid resuscitation, diuretics, and calcimimetics. Severe cases may need to be treated with intravenous calcitonin and/or dialysis.[36,37]

Reoperation for parathyroid cancer recurrence has a low success rate of cure and higher risk of recurrent laryngeal nerve injury but can palliate symptoms and improve hypercalcemia. Neither radiation nor chemotherapy has been shown to have significant benefit in the treatment of parathyroid cancer, but some success has been reported with combination cytotoxic chemotherapy.[36–38]

Disease-Specific Epidemiology

Primary hyperparathyroidism is estimated to affect about 0.1% of the population in the United States and is most often diagnosed from 50 to 65 years of age. Women are about twice as likely to be affected. Single adenomas are the cause of 80 to 85% of cases while multi-gland hyperplasia account for about 6% of cases. Parathyroid cancers represent less than 1 to 2% of cases. Familial syndromes are rarely the cause of hyperparathyroidism and thought to only account for about 2 to 5% of PHPT cases. Well-known syndromes associated with hyperparathyroidism include MEN1, MEN2A, MEN4, hyperparathyroidism-jaw tumor syndrome (HPT-JT), familial isolated hyperparathyroidism (FIHPT), familial hypocalciuric hypercalcemia (FHH), and neonatal severe hyperparathyroidism (NSHPT).[32,33,35,39]

In contrast to parathyroid adenoma, parathyroid cancer is one of the rarest forms of cancer; it accounts for only 0.005% of all cancer cases. Risk factors for parathyroid cancer include the HRPT2/CDC73 mutation and radiation. Parathyroid cancers can be sporadic or associated with a hereditary HPT syndrome. Patients with HRPT2/CDC73 mutations have an approximate risk of parathyroid cancer of 15%. Additionally, somatic inactivation of HRPT2/CDC73 is common in sporadic parathyroid cancers.[41]

A study from 2007 based on data derived from the SEER cancer database that included 224 cases of parathyroid cancer diagnosed between 1988 and 2003 suggests that parathyroid cancer has a 10-year overall survival rate of 50 to 70%. Recurrences occurred 40 of 60% of the time after surgery. Overall, there are limited data regarding the prognostic factors in parathyroid cancers.[36–38]

Disease-Specific Approach to Risk Assessment, Counseling, and Testing

Although 95% of PHPT cases occur sporadically, ones that represent a familial disorder may need to be approached differently. Some forms of hereditary HPT such as MEN1 are associated with a higher risk of recurrence. As the prevalence of hereditary HPT is relatively small, routine genetic testing for a familial syndrome is not recommended as part of the workup for hyperparathyroidism. Careful assessment of family history and identification of other features of a hereditary syndrome will help to identify patients who will benefit from further genetic workup. Patients presenting with HPT with one or more first-degree relatives with multiple endocrine, neuroendocrine, or jaw tumors should be evaluated for a hereditary syndrome. Germline genetic testing of the following genes can be performed to detect the suspected syndrome: *MEN1* mutations for MEN1, *RET* mutations for MEN2A, *CDKN1B* mutations for MEN4, and *HRPT2/CDC73* mutations for HPT-JT. The utility of genetic testing for FHH has not been studied as it is a benign, often asymptomatic disease and not associated with any risk for other tumors. NSHPT is a rare disorder and typically diagnosed in affected neonates clinically; the indications for germline testing for *CASR* mutations are still unclear.[32,33,35]

Hereditary Syndromes

MEN1 Multiple endocrine neoplasia syndrome 1 (MEN1), as originally described by Wermer, is an autosomal dominant inherited disorder characterized by several endocrine and non-endocrine tumors, namely parathyroid tumors, pituitary tumors, neuroendocrine tumors of the gastroenteropancreatic tract (GEP-NET), carcinoid tumors, and rarely thyroid and adrenocortical tumors.[42]

MEN1 syndrome is caused by mutations in the *MEN1/Menin* gene. This gene encodes a transcriptional regulator that is involved in regulation of cell proliferation, chromatin remodeling, and possibly DNA repair. About 10% of MEN1 cases are caused by mutations without prior family history.[26,29,42]

Hyperparathyroidism (HPT) is the dominant feature of MEN1 and develops in virtually all MEN1 patients. It is the first endocrine manifestation of MEN1 in about 90% of patients and typically presents before age 50. In MEN1, HPT is caused by asymmetric hyperplasia of multiple glands and has a very high rate of recurrence.[42]

Tumors of the anterior pituitary gland (prolactinomas, GH, TSH, or ACTH-secreting) occur in 30 to 40% of cases. The pituitary tumors of MEN1 are usually macroadenomas but do carry an increased risk of being invasive. Prolactinomas are usually treated with dopamine agonists while other pituitary adenomas can be resected with transsphenoidal surgery. (Table 13.2).[42]

TABLE 13.2: Hereditary Syndromes Associated with Hyperparathyroidism

Hereditary disorder	Responsible genes	Cause of HPT	Other associated features
MEN1	MEN1/Menin	Multiglandular	GEP-NET[1], pituitary adenoma, adrenocortical tumors, pheochromocytoma (rare), carcinoid tumors, thyroid tumors
MEN2A	RET	Adenoma or multiglandular	MTC[2], pheochromocytoma
MEN4	CDKN1B	Adenoma or multiglandular	GEP-NET[1], pituitary adenoma, adrenal tumors, thyroid tumors, gonadal tumors
HPT-JT	HRPT2/CDC73	Single or multiple adenomas, parathyroid carcinoma	Ossifying fibromas of the mandible and maxilla, renal cysts and hamartomas, uterine tumors
FIHPT	MEN1, HRPT2/CDC73, CASR, GCM2, CDKN1B	Adenoma or multiglandular	None
FHH	CASR	Mild hyperplasia	Low urinary calcium
NSHPT	CASR, GNA11, AP2S1	Severe hyperplasia	Rib and other bone fractures, hypotonia

[1]GEP-NET = gastroenteropancreatic neuroendocrine tumor.
[2]MTC = medullary thyroid cancer.[31-33,39,40]

Gastroenteropancreatic neuroendocrine tumors (GEP-NETs) occur in ~50% of cases. The most common GEP-NET in MEN1 is gastrinoma, occurring in about 40% of patients. Zollinger-Ellison syndrome results from the excess of gastrin secretion and can usually be managed with proton-pump inhibitors and medical therapy. However, the gastrinomas associated with MEN1 are often multifocal and about half are metastatic by the time of diagnosis. Similarly, glucagonomas and VIPomas associated with MEN1 carry high risks of malignancy. Insulinomas, on the other hand, are almost always benign. The surgical management and approach for these tumors is best determined by an experienced surgeon.[26,29,42]

Carcinoid tumors occur in ~14% of MEN1 cases. Carcinoids in MEN1 are most frequently gastric, thymic, or bronchial in origin. While most carcinoids are indolent in nature, thymic carcinoids can be especially aggressive and often present at late invasive stages. Carcinoids should be treated surgically if deemed to be resectable.[26,29,42]

Adrenocortical abnormalities occur in MEN1 in 20 to 70% of cases. These abnormalities are most often benign adenomas, hyperplasia, or cysts. Only about 10% of these adrenal tumors are hormonally active; those that are usually secrete cortisol and less often aldosterone. Although not typically associated with MEN1, pheochromocytoma have been reported. Tumors >1 cm have been reported to have a risk for adrenocortical carcinoma as high as 13%. All adrenal tumors should receive a full workup and be treated appropriately (see the section on adrenocortical tumors and pheochromocytoma).[26,29,42]

Thyroid tumors including adenomas, goiters, and carcinomas have also been reported in MEN1. These are generally approached the same way as sporadic thyroid abnormalities (see the section on non-medullary thyroid cancers).[26,29,42]

MEN4 MEN4 was originally classified as a variant of MEN1 and was only recently added as a distinct member of the MEN family after the discovery that it was caused by mutations in the *CDKN1B* gene. Its original status as a variant MEN1 is a result of their phenotypic similarity. Like MEN1, the most prominent features of MEN4 are parathyroid and pituitary tumors with rare occurrences of GEP-NETs. Adrenal, thyroid, and gonadal tumors have also been reported. The unique manifestations of MEN4 and extent of phenotypic overlap with MEN1 are not yet entirely known. MEN4 should be suspected in patients who have features suggestive of MEN1 but with negative *MEN1* gene testing.[32,39]

MEN2A Hyperparathyroidism affects 20 to 30% of all patients with MEN2A, though the exact risk of an individual is correlated to his or her pathologic variant of *RET*. Specifically, mutations of codon 634 in exon 11 are associated with a higher incidence of hyperparathyroidism. While most patients with MEN1 present with PHPT as their initial manifestation, patients with MEN2A more often present initially with MTC. (See the section on MEN2A under MTC).[28,32]

HPT-JT Familial hyperparathyroidism-jaw tumor syndrome (HPT-JT) is a rare disorder caused by inactivating mutations in the *HRPT2/CDC73* gene. A case of HPT-JT caused by a large-scale deletion of a segment of chromosome 1q31 containing the *HRPT2/CDC73* gene has also been reported.[43] It carries a high risk for hyperparathyroidism, parathyroid carcinoma, and benign, ossifying fibromas of the mandible or maxillary bone. About 20% of patients also have renal lesions including cysts and hamartomas. The risk of parathyroid carcinoma can be as high as 10 to 15% in HPT-JT. Hyperparathyroidism develops early, usually in the 30s, and is typically marked by severe hypercalcemia. Young patients with severe hyperparathyroidism, suspicious family history, or any patient with a diagnosis of parathyroid cancer should be evaluated for HPT-JT and germline *HRPT2* mutations.[31-33,40,43]

Familial Isolated Hyperparathyroidism (FIHP) FIHP has traditionally been a catch-all diagnosis for familial cases of PHPT. Some cases have been found to have *MEN1, HRPT2/ CDC73, CDKN1B,* and *CASR* mutations but without other syndromic non-parathyroid manifestations. Recently, mutations in the gene *GCM2* were detected in 20% of FIHP cases. *GCM2* mutations have been associated with larger than average parathyroid tumors with one case report of a potentially malignant parathyroid tumor. It is likely that the diagnosis of FIHP will evolve as understanding of the underlying genetics of hereditary HPT increases.[32,35]

FHH and NSHPT Familial hypocalciuric hypercalcemia (FHH) and neonatal severe hyperparathyroidism (NSHPT) are both hereditary disorders caused by inactivating mutations in the *CASR* gene. *CASR* encodes for a trans-membrane receptor that senses extracellular calcium and determines the set-point for the serum calcium regulation axis. Inactivating mutations cause the set-point to be inappropriately elevated resulting in PTH secretion and calcium retention. FHH is a benign disorder that is generally asymptomatic and does not increase the risk for nephrolithiasis or osteoporosis.[31,32,35]

NSHPT, on the other hand, causes life-threatening hypercalcemia shortly after birth, usually as the result of four-gland parathyroid hyperplasia. Affected neonates may suffer from respiratory distress, fractures, and hypotonia.[31,32,35]

Clinical Management of Patients at Increased Risk

MEN1 Patients with PHPT in the setting MEN1 should undergo either subtotal parathyroidectomy or total parathyroidectomy with heterotopic parathyroid autotransplantation as the initial procedure. Dissection should be meticulous and include transcervical thymectomy to exclude ectopic parathyroid tissue. Recurrences still often occur and can involve autotransplanted parathyroid tissue.

MEN1 patients need lifelong, yearly biochemical surveillance: serum calcium, glucagon, VIP, chromogranin-A, and pancreatic polypeptide starting at age 8; serum gastrin starting at age 20; and serum prolactin, IGF-1, fasting glucose, and insulin starting at age 5. Imaging should be obtained every 3 to 5 years: a head MRI starting at age 5 and abdominal CT or MRI starting at age 20. Yearly chest CT and somatostatin receptor scintigraphy can also be considered. Patients who are at risk of having MEN1 but who have not undergone genetic testing should also be monitored with yearly serum prolactin levels starting at age 5, serum calcium and PTH starting at age 10, and serum gastrin starting at age 20 if having symptoms of Zollinger-Ellison syndrome.[26,42]

MEN4 While no guidelines and recommendations have yet been established for MEN4, it is reasonable to manage and follow patients in a similar manner to those with MEN1.[26,39,42]

MEN2A The parathyroid abnormalities in MEN2A more often involve only one gland, and as a result, are usually milder than that of MEN1 and can be asymptomatic. MEN2A patients with hyperparathyroidism can be approached similarly to those with sporadic PHPT, and parathyroidectomy can be performed at the same time as thyroidectomy should it be indicated. All MEN2A patients should undergo screening for MTC and pheochromocytoma as per the ATA recommendations detailed in the sections on MTC and pheochromocytoma.[25,28]

HPT-JT Resection of enlarged parathyroid glands should be performed when discovered with additional exploration and identification of all four parathyroid glands. If parathyroid cancer is detected or suspected, *en bloc* resection of the tumor with ipsilateral thyroid lobectomy is recommended. There are currently no surveillance guidelines for patients with HPT-JT, but it is reasonable to follow patients with yearly measurements of serum calcium and PTH starting at age 5. Dental X-rays every 5 years to evaluate for mandibular and maxillary tumors and periodic cervical and renal ultrasounds can also be considered.[40,44]

FHH and NSHPT It is thought that FHH is caused by abnormal PTH secretion rather than abnormal parathyroid growth, and thus it generally causes only mild enlargement of the parathyroid glands. Most patients are asymptomatic and do not need intervention. Those who do develop symptoms can be treated with calcimimetics. Subtotal parathyroidectomy is associated with a high recurrence and is generally avoided.[31,32]

Few neonates with NSHPT survive to adulthood without treatment. There have been reports of milder variants that respond well to calcimimetics, but most patients will need total parathyroidectomy within the first few months of life. Total parathyroidectomy is curative but will leave patients with lifelong hypoparathyroidism.[31,32]

ADRENOCORTICAL TUMORS

Risk Assessment and Management

Tumors that arise from adrenocortical cells are often benign adrenocortical adenomas (ACA), but adrenocortical carcinomas (ACC) can occur, though rarely. No clear environmental risk factors have been identified for either ACA or ACCs. Both are associated with tumor susceptibility syndromes including MEN1, Carney complex, McCune-Albright syndrome, Gardner's syndrome, Beckwith-Wiedemann syndrome, and neurofibromatosis type 1. Adrenal masses presenting in children, adolescents, and young adults have a higher chance of having one of these syndromes and carry a higher risk for malignancy.[45,46]

Most ACAs and ACCs are non-functional, meaning they do not cause detectable hormone excess. Most adrenal lesions are discovered incidentally on imaging obtained for another reason. These have been termed adrenal "incidentalomas." Adrenal lesions may also be discovered during the workup of an endocrine disorder. Patients with biochemical evidence of hypercortisolism, hyperaldosteronism, and catecholamine excess should have the adrenal glands imaged with either thin-slice abdominal CT with and without IV contrast or multiplanar MRI.[45,47–49]

All patients with a newly discovered adrenal incidentaloma should undergo biochemical screening for clinical and subclinical Cushing's syndrome as they are the most commonly associated endocrine abnormalities. Testing for Cushing's syndrome begins with a 1 mg overnight dexamethasone suppression test. Different cutoffs for morning cortisol levels have been suggested to represent a positive test. Generally, morning cortisol levels >5 mcg/dL indicate ACTH-independent cortisol secretion and levels below 1.8 mcg/dL exclude autonomous ACTH secretion. Morning cortisol levels between 1.8 and 5 mcg/dL may indicate hypercortisolism but should be confirmed with serum ACTH level or DHEA-S measurement (suppressed ACTH and low DHEA-S levels support the diagnosis of hypercortisolism). If the diagnosis remains inconclusive, two-day or high-dose dexamethasone suppression tests can be performed. Patients with any level of autonomous cortisol production should be screened for hypertension and diabetes.[47,50]

Patients with incidentalomas who also have known hypertension or hypokalemia should be evaluated for an aldosteronoma by measuring plasma aldosterone against renin activity. If a pheochromocytoma is suspected, plasma free metanephrines and normetanephrines should be measured. Elevated levels should be confirmed with 24-hour collection of urine fractionated metanephrines and catecholamines. Testing for sex hormone excess is typically not indicated, although the European Society of Endocrinology recommends testing for DHEA-S, androstenedione, 17-hydroxyprogesterone, testosterone for women, and estradiol for men and postmenopausal women if there are clinical signs of virilization or suspicion for ACC. ACC is associated with over half of cases with elevated sex hormone or sex hormone-precursor levels. Biopsy of an adrenal lesion is not recommended unless there is suspicion that it may be a metastasis from another primary cancer. In this case, pheochromocytoma must be ruled out prior to the biopsy.[47,50]

Most adrenal lesions are benign; the risk of an incidentaloma being cancerous increases with its size and certain radiologic findings. Features that suggest a benign lesion include size <4 cm, attenuation on CT <10 Hounsfield units, smooth borders, and rapid contrast washout. Findings of size >4 cm, irregular borders, heterogeneous density, delayed washout, and presence of calcifications increase the suspicion for cancer.[45,47–51]

Lesions <4 cm with a benign appearance and not associated with any endocrine disturbance can be followed by repeat imaging at 3- to 6-month intervals for the first year, then annually for another year or two. Repeat biochemical evaluations should be performed annually for 5 years.[50]

Lesions that are >4 cm or with growth of more than 1 cm over a follow-up period are suspicious for cancer and should be surgically removed. Functional adrenal tumors causing clinically significant hormone excess are also treated by surgical resection, which cures the endocrine disorder if it is due to a unilateral tumor. Patients with subclinical Cushing's disease (biochemical evidence of hypercortisolism without overt clinical signs) should still consider adrenalectomy as it has been shown to be beneficial in reducing long-term complications of hypercortisolism.[50,52]

Surgery can typically be performed in a minimally invasive fashion via a laparoscopic or retroperitoneoscopic approach, although an open approach is still recommended for large tumors and those that are known cancers or at high risk of malignancy. Patients with overt or subclinical Cushing's syndrome will need steroid replacement at least in the perioperative period, although the total length of time exogenous glucocorticoids will be needed may extend past a year.[47–50,52]

Patients with bilateral adrenal incidentalomas should be managed similarly as those with unilateral lesions, except for inclusion of serum 17-hydroxyprogesterone measurements to exclude congenital adrenal hyperplasia. Bilateral adrenalectomy is typically not warranted in cases of subclinical Cushing's, although some cases with a dominant lesion can be treated with unilateral adrenalectomy.[47,50]

ACC, in contrast to ACA, is an aggressive disease that often presents at a locally advanced or metastatic stage. Given the rarity of ACC, there has been a lack of prospective randomized clinical trials to guide recommendations on management and surveillance strategies. For patients with resectable tumors, an R0 resection provides the best chance at cure though recurrence rates remain high. Radical surgery can be considered in some cases of metastatic disease along with resection of metastases if feasible. Chemotherapy generally includes mitotane with or without other cytotoxic agents and has been shown to have some benefit in the adjuvant setting for patients with locally advanced disease and as primary therapy for those with metastatic disease. Occasionally, initially unresectable tumors may regress with systemic therapy enough to consider surgical resection, but the use of neoadjuvant therapy has not been adequately studied in ACC. All patients must be followed closely post-operatively. Those with steroid-producing ACC should have steroid markers monitored at 3-month intervals for at least 2 years.[48–50,53]

Disease-Specific Epidemiology

The reported incidence of adrenal incidentalomas varies ranges from 2 to 3% of the general population based on the inclusion criteria of the study and whether it was a surgical or nonsurgical series. The true incidence of adrenal adenomas is unclear as screening for such masses is not routine. Extrapolation from autopsy studies indicates about a 2% incidence of adrenal masses while radiological studies have reported up to 10% frequency in the elderly population. Most incidentalomas will be found to be benign ACAs—ACC is a rare disease with only one or two cases per million patients per year.[47–50]

Among ACA, 70 to 85% are nonfunctioning (NFA), about 12% are cortisol-producing (CPA), and about 2.5% are aldosterone-secreting (APA). Sex hormone-producing ACAs are rare, and the true incidence is unclear. Most ACAs are sporadic, but they can rarely be associated with hereditary syndromes such as MEN1 and familial hyperaldosteronism. The exact prevalence of these syndromes within ACAs is not known but is likely very low.

However, as many as 5 to 10% of ACCs harbor germline mutations and are part of hereditary syndromes. Fifty to eighty percent of children with ACC will be found to have a germline *TP53* mutation and be diagnosed with Li-Fraumeni syndrome. Up to 3% of ACCs are associated with DNA mismatch repair mutations and Lynch syndrome. One to two percent of ACCs are associated with MEN1. Syndromes less often associated with ACC include familial adenomatous polyposis, Beckwith-Wiedemann, neurofibromatosis type 1, and Carney complex.[45,46,54–58]

Disease-Specific Approach to Risk Assessment, Counseling, and Testing

ACA is rarely associated with hereditary syndromes and the discovery of one does not typically require further genetic investigation. ACAs are often found in patients with MEN1 (27 to 36%) but are almost never the initial or only manifestation.

ACC, on the other hand, can be the presenting tumor of certain cancer syndromes and it is important to identify syndromic patients in order to screen them for other associated tumors. ACC presenting in childhood is highly suspicious for a genetic syndrome. The high prevalence of germline *TP53* mutations in patients with ACC has led to the recommendation that all patients diagnosed with ACC undergo testing for a *TP53* mutation regardless of family history. Similarly, it has been suggested that ACC patients be screened for DNA mismatch repair mutations. Some authors advocate for multigene panels to evaluate for germline mutations in all patients diagnosed with ACC. The discovery of a germline mutation in a patient with ACC should prompt evaluation of at least all first-degree relatives.[45,46,48,49,54–57,59–61]

Hereditary Cancer Syndromes

Li-Fraumeni Syndrome Li-Fraumeni syndrome (LFS) is caused by pathogenic mutations in the tumor suppressor gene *TP53* that predisposes to sarcomas, leukemias, brain cancers, breast cancers, lung cancers, and choroid plexus tumors in addition to adrenocortical cancers. It is estimated to have a prevalence of 1 in 20,000 to 1 in 1,000,000 and is higher in certain areas such as Southern Brazil due to founder's effect. Fifty to eighty percent of all children with ACC will be found to have LFS but only 3 to 10% of children with LFS will develop ACC. The risk for ACC in LFS appears to decrease with age. Affected children are also at risk for developing precocious puberty and Cushing's syndrome secondary to hormone excess.[57–59]

Classic Li-Fraumeni syndrome is diagnosed by molecular genetic testing for a pathogenic *TP53* mutation or clinically by the presence of all three diagnostic criteria: sarcoma diagnosed before age 45, first-degree relative with any cancer before age 45, and first- or second-degree relative with any cancer before age 45 or sarcoma at any age. LFS should also be suspected in women with early-onset breast cancer who tested negative for *BRCA1* and *BRCA2* pathogenic variants and any individual who meets the Chompret criteria for *TP53* testing. Patients who meet any one of the three Chompret criteria has at least a 20% chance of testing positive for a *TP53* mutation: diagnosis of a tumor belonging to the LFS tumor spectrum before age 46 with a first- or second-degree relative also with a LFS tumor (except breast) diagnosed before age 56; diagnosis of multiple tumors (except breast), two of which belong to the LFS tumor spectrum, the first of which presented before age 46; and diagnosis of ACC or choroid plexus tumor.[57–59]

Lynch Syndrome Lynch syndrome is due to defects in the DNA mismatch repair proteins *PMS2, MSH2, MSH6,* and *MLH1.* It has an estimated prevalence of 1 in 440 among the general population and is most often associated with colorectal cancers and endometrial cancers. While ACC has been associated with Lynch syndrome, the risk that a patient with Lynch syndrome will develop ACC remains very low.[56,59]

Beckwith-Wiedemann Syndrome Beckwith-Wiedemann syndrome (BWS) is associated with abnormal IGF2 signaling caused by alteration of gene transcription in the "BWS critical region" on chromosome 11p15.5. About 85% of cases are sporadic. BWS may be caused by gene mutations or methylation and imprinting abnormalities within the BWS critical region. When the specific genetic or genomic abnormality is not known, investigational testing can involve DNA methylation studies, single-gene testing, copy number analysis, karyotyping, and multigene panels.[55]

There are no consensus clinical diagnostic criteria for BWS. It is characterized by macrosomia, macroglossia, hemihyperplasia, metabolic abnormalities, visceromegaly, and renal abnormalities. Individual phenotypes vary, and a patient may have many or only a few of the possible features. BWS is associated with several types of neoplasia, most commonly Wilms tumor, hepatoblastoma, neuroblastoma, rhabdomyosarcoma, and adrenocortical tumors. Up to 1% of children with BWS develop ACC, but the adrenal tumors in BWS may also be benign adenomas and cysts. The risk of developing any BWS tumor ranges from 4 to 21% and is highest in early childhood. This risk decreases with age and tumors are rarely diagnosed after the age of 8.[55,59]

MEN1 MEN1 is rarely associated with adrenocortical tumors. Adrenal manifestations can occur in the form of benign enlargement for ACA or ACC. About 1 to 2% of ACC cases are associated with *MEN1* gene mutations. Most MEN1 patients with ACC will already have other signs and symptoms such as hyperparathyroidism, pituitary, or gastroenteropancreatic tumors. Adrenal tumors in MEN1 are most frequently non-functioning. There have been case reports of MEN1 patients with benign adrenal tumors who later developed ACC, suggesting an adenoma to carcinoma transformation.[42,59]

Carney Complex Primary pigmented nodular adrenal disease is common in patients with CNC and causes clinically evident Cushing's syndrome in about 70% of affected females and 45% of affected males before age 45. Cushing's syndrome may be atypical in these patients due to only intermittent production of cortisol, and it is recommended that patients be evaluated with diurnal cortisol levels or dexamethasone-stimulation test and adrenal imaging rather than urine cortisol levels alone. For additional information on CNC-associated tumors, see the section on non-medullary thyroid cancer.

Clinical Management of Patients at Increased Risk

Li-Fraumeni Syndrome There are no consensus guidelines for screening of ACC in LFS, but some have advocated for abdominal ultrasounds and biochemical testing (17-OH-progesterone, androstenedione, testosterone, DHEA-S, 24-hour urine cortisol) every 3 to 4 months from birth until age 40. Any tumors discovered should be managed according to the usual guidelines. However, adjuvant radiation should be avoided if the benefit is unclear as it may increase the risk for developing other malignancies.[57,59]

MEN1 Screening for adrenal tumors can be performed concurrently with GEP-NETs with cross-sectional abdominal imaging every 3 to 5 years. Adrenal tumors detected in MEN1 patients should be managed similarly to an incidentaloma and undergo complete endocrine workup with a higher baseline suspicion for malignancy. Additional guidelines for the management of patients with MEN1 syndrome can be found under the section on the parathyroid.[42,59]

Beckwith-Wiedemann Syndrome Patients with BWS should undergo routine surveillance following diagnosis. A baseline whole-body MRI or CT should be obtained at the time of diagnosis. Abdominal ultrasounds should be obtained every 3 to 4 months until age 4 to evaluate for any visceral tumors. Serum AFP should be measured every 6 to 16 weeks until age 4. Kidney and adrenal ultrasounds should be continued every 3 to 4 months until age 8 to evaluate for Wilms and adrenal tumors.[55]

Lynch Syndrome and FAP Although patients with Lynch syndrome or FAP may have higher than average risk for developing adrenal tumors, their risk remains sufficiently low that no dedicated screening recommendations exist for adrenal tumors.[20,56]

◼ PHEOCHROMOCYTOMAS AND PARAGANGLIOMAS

Risk Assessment and Management

Pheochromocytomas (PCC) and paragangliomas (PGL) are neuroendocrine tumors that secrete the catecholamines epinephrine, norepinephrine, and, rarely, dopamine. Both arise from neural crest-derived cells. PCCs develop in the chromaffin cells of the adrenal medulla, adjacent to but functionally a distinct organ from the adrenal cortex. PGLs, sometimes referred to as extra-adrenal pheochromocytomas, develop from sympathetic and parasympathetic ganglia cells of the autonomic nervous system. They most commonly occur along the paravertebral sympathetic trunk and in the organ of Zuckerkandl, a cluster of chromaffin cells near the aortic bifurcation, but can also develop in the head and neck in the form of carotid body, vagal, and jugulotympanic PGLs. Given their similarity, they are often jointly referred to as pheochromocytoma-paragangliomas (PPGLs).[62,63]

PPGLs are rare tumors. Classic symptoms such as hypertension, diaphoresis, headaches, palpitations, arrhythmias, nausea/vomiting, and anxiety will only occur with catecholamine-releasing PPGLs that arise from sympathetic tissue. These symptoms may be intermittent or triggered by positional changes, certain medications, induction of anesthesia, and exercise. Parasympathetic PPGL, such as most head and neck PGLs, are usually non-secretory and clinically silent. Rarely, PGL in the upper thorax or neck may cause Horner syndrome or cranial nerve symptoms due to mass effect.[50,64]

When a PPGL is suspected, biochemical evaluation begins with measurement of plasma free metanephrines and normetanephrines, which have a sensitivity of 97 to 100% and a specificity of 85 to 89%. Plasma free metanephrine levels 3 to 4 times above normal almost always indicate the presence of pheochromocytoma. A 24-hour collection of urine fractionated metanephrines also has a high sensitivity and specificity and can be used for confirmatory testing or in lieu of plasma testing. A variety of imaging modalities can be used to identify PCC and PGL. CT is recommended as the initial imaging of choice and has a sensitivity of 85 to 100% and specificity of 70 to 100%. MRI has a sensitivity and specificity of 95 to 100% and is preferred in patients with known germline mutations for better detection of metastases and head and neck PGLs. Malignancy can only be definitively established by the detection of metastases. If suspicion is high, functional imaging such as FDG- or 68-Ga-DOTATATE-PET, and ^{123}I-metaiodobenzylguanidine scintigraphy can be performed to evaluate for metastatic PPGL.[63–66]

The initial treatment of catecholamine excess caused by PPGL is with alpha-adrenergic blockade using agents such as phenoxybenzamine. Calcium channel blockers can also be used as second-line agents. Beta-blockers may be added in conjunction to control reflex tachycardia or arrhythmias only after adequate alpha-blockade, to avoid unopposed alpha-adrenergic activity. Stable normotension should be demonstrated for 1 to 3 weeks prior to surgery.[47,50,66]

The definitive treatment of PPGL is surgical resection. Surgery for most PCCs can be minimally invasive by being done laparoscopically or retroperitoneoscopically. Head and neck PGLs can also be resected safely but some non-secretory tumors may be managed with radiation therapy and watchful waiting. Close intra-operative blood pressure monitoring and support is essential as patients can experience hemodynamic instability ranging from severe hypertension to hypotension.[50]

Post-operative normalization of 24-hour urine metanephrines and/or plasma free metanephrines usually indicate complete resection. Patients should be followed at least annually. Even in benign cases, 16% of PCC recur. Metastatic PPGLs are usually managed symptomatically with alpha-blockade, radiation, systemic chemotherapy, and/or tumor debulking.[50]

Disease-Specific Epidemiology

The incidence of PCC in the general population is about 0.6 cases/100,000 per year. Historical teaching has been that 10% of PCC are hereditary, but with the discovery of PPGL syndromes caused by mutations in *SDHx, TMEM127,* and *MAX* genes, it is now thought that at least 25% of PCC and an even higher percentage of PGLs can be attributed to a hereditary syndrome.[62,67]

The risk of malignancy varies based on the study and ranges from 2 to 23%. Most metastatic PCC are functional and cause catecholamine excess. Reported mortality rates for metastatic PPGL also vary, but overall 5-year mortality is 50 to 60%.[68]

A total of 10 pheochromocytoma susceptibility genes have been identified to date: *RET, VHL, NF1, SDHA, SDHAF2, SDHB, SDHC, SDCD, TMEM127,* and *MAX.* Germline mutations in one of these 10 genes have been found in most hereditary cases and 10 to 20% of cases without family history. *MAX* mutations account for about 1% of PPGL syndromes, *SDHA* 0.6 to 3%, *SDHAF2* <0.1%, *SDHB* 10 to 25%, *SDHC* 2 to 8%, *SDHD* 8 to 9%, and *TMEM127* ~2%. Of note, MEN1 syndrome has also been very rarely associated with pheochromocytoma; it is more typically linked to adrenocortical tumors.[62,67]

Hereditary PCC phenotypes are correlated with the causative germline gene mutation. The pheochromocytomas of MEN2, for example, are nearly always adrenal in location, often bilateral, and carry a low risk of metastasis.[28] PCCs in VHL also tend to be benign but are associated with other tumors such as retinal angiomas, CNS hemangioblastomas, renal cell carcinoma, and pancreatic neuroendocrine tumors. On the other hand, *SDHD* mutations are associated with head and neck PGLs, and up to 50% of metastatic PPGL can be attributed to an *SDHB* mutation.[62,67,69]

Disease-Specific Approach to Risk Assessment, Counseling, and Testing

Any patient diagnosed with PCC or PGL should be evaluated for an inherited syndrome given the high prevalence of hereditary PPGL. PGLs are more often associated with an inherited disorder than PCCs. Early onset of disease, multiple synchronous tumors, recurrence, metastases, and positive family history are strongly suggestive of a hereditary syndrome (Table 13.3).[62,69]

Detailed personal and family history notes should focus on the presence of syndrome-associated features such as history of medullary thyroid cancer and hyperparathyroidism

TABLE 13.3: Hereditary Pheochromocytoma/Paraganglioma Syndromes

Affected gene	Risk of PPGL	Associated tumors and features
RET	10 to 50% depending on affected codon	MTC[1], HPT[2]
VHL	10 to 25%	Retinal angiomas, CNS hemangioblastomas, renal clear cell carcinoma and cysts, endolymphatic sac tumors, pancreatic neuroendocrine tumors
NF1	0.1 to 5.7%	Café-au-lait spots, cutaneous neurofibromas, Lisch nodules, CNS gliomas, peripheral nerve sheath tumors
SDHA	~10%	GIST[3]
SDHB	12 to 42%	RCC[4], GIST[3], possible pituitary and thyroid tumors
SDHC	~25%	GIST[3], RCC[4]
SDHD	18 to 86%, likely paternally inherited	GIST[3], RCC[4], possible pituitary and thyroid tumors
SDHAF2	Unknown; likely paternally inherited	None
TMEM127	Unknown	RCC[4]
MAX	Unknown	Possible RCC[4]

[1]MTC = medullary thyroid cancer
[2]HPT = hyperparathyroidism
[3]GIST = gastrointestinal stromal tumor
[4]RCC = renal cell carcinoma[28,29,62,64,67,69,71–74]

(MEN2); history of CNS hemangioblastomas and renal cell carcinomas (VHL), and history of gastrointestinal stromal tumor, papillary thyroid cancer, pituitary adenomas, and other neuroendocrine tumors (hereditary PPGL syndromes). Suspicion of a specific syndrome may be increased or decreased based on the presence of these associated features, and genetic testing can be targeted accordingly. Mutations in *RET* and *VHL* can be detected by single-gene testing. Testing for neurofibromatosis 1 typically involves chromosomal microarray analysis. Genetic testing for hereditary PPGL syndromes can be performed with multigene panels that include all the known causative genes (*SDHA, SDHAF2, SDHB, SDHC, SDCD, TMEM127, MAX*).[62,68–70]

Hereditary Cancer Syndromes

MEN2 MEN2 patients have about a 50% chance for developing pheochromocytoma; the exact risk correlates with the location of their *RET* mutation; those involving codon 634 appear to have the highest risk. Pheochromocytomas in MEN2 are almost always limited to the adrenal glands, often bilateral, and rarely malignant. MEN2B is most often diagnosed in childhood due to the early onset of MTC, but 13 to 27% of MEN2A patients present with PCC as the initial diagnosis. It is important to identify this group of patients as they may benefit from prophylactic thyroidectomy and/or medullary thyroid cancer screening. (See the information on MEN2 under the section on medullary thyroid cancer.)[28]

Von Hippel-Lindau VHL is caused by pathogenic mutations in the *VHL* gene and is inherited in an autosomal dominant manner. About 20% of cases are caused by *de novo* mutations. In addition to PPGLs, patients with VHL are predisposed to developing retinal angiomas, CNS hemangioblastomas, renal clear cell carcinoma and cysts, endolymphatic sac tumors, and other neuroendocrine tumors. The lifetime risk of developing PCC in VHL is 10 to 25%, and tumors are generally benign. There are two major sub-types of VHL: type I and type II. Type I is associated with truncating mutations and deletions of exons or the entire VHL gene. It carries a high risk for retinal angiomas and CNS hemangioblastomas but a relatively low risk for PPGL. Type II is associated with missense variants and carries a relatively high risk for PPGL.[67,69]

Neurofibromatosis 1 Neurofibromatosis 1 is a genetic disorder commonly associated with café-au-lait spots, cutaneous neurofibromas, Lisch nodules, CNS gliomas, and peripheral nerve sheath tumors. It is caused by loss-of-function mutations of the *NF1* tumor suppressor gene. While PPGL is not a typical tumor of neurofibromatosis 1 syndrome, 0.1 to 5.7% of patients with NF1 will develop PCC, a frequency higher than that of the general population. Up to 12% of PPGL in NF1 are malignant. Interestingly, many sporadic PCCs have been found to have somatic *NF1* gene mutations, supporting the hypothesis that the *NF1* gene plays a role in PCC tumorigenesis.[67]

Hereditary PPGL Syndromes Hereditary PPGL syndromes are a group of disorders caused by germline mutations in the *SDHx, TMEM127,* and *MAX* genes that predisposes to development of PGLs and PCCs as well as certain other tumors such as gastrointestinal stromal tumors (GIST), renal cell carcinoma (RCC), and possibly thyroid and pituitary tumors. Most mutations are inherited in an autosomal dominant manner except for *MAX, SDHAF2, and SDHD,* which may have a parent-of-origin effect and appear to only be paternally inherited.[62,67]

SDHA pathogenic variants are associated with both PCCs and PGLs in the head, neck, and thorax. Tumors are often benign and rarely bilateral. They also appear to be associated with GIST and *SDHA* mutations.[72]

SDHB pathogenic variants are associated with the highest risk for malignancy. Patients with these mutations can develop PGLs and PCCs and often have multiple and bilateral tumors. Up to 50% of patients with metastatic PGL have a germline mutation of *SDHB.* In addition, patients have a higher risk of developing renal tumors including renal clear cell carcinoma, GIST, papillary thyroid cancer, and pituitary adenomas.[62,67]

SDHC pathogenic variants display a phenotype like *SDHAF2* variants and are mainly associated with head and neck PGLs. However, thoracic PGLs do occur up to 10% of the time. Patients may also be at increased risk for developing GIST.[62,67]

SDHD pathogenic variants are most frequently associated with head and neck PGLs. PCC may also occur as well as PGLs in other locations. They are also associated with GIST, RCC, pituitary and thyroid tumors.[62,67]

SDHAF2 pathogenic variants have only been associated with benign head and neck PGLs. They do not appear to carry a risk for other tumors.[62,67,72]

TMEM127 pathogenic variants are associated with PCC and PGLs and may also increase the risk of renal cell carcinoma.[62,67,72]

MAX pathogenic variants are associated with PCC and rarely PGLs.[62,67,72]

Clinical Management of Patients at Increased Risk

MEN2 Patients with MEN2 should undergo screening for pheochromocytoma, MTC, and hyperparathyroidism based on ATA recommendations. The highest-risk patients and those in high-risk categories should have yearly biochemical screening for pheochromocytoma beginning at age 11. Patients in the moderate-risk category should have yearly biochemical screening for pheochromocytoma beginning at age 16.

VHL Several groups have proposed recommendations for tumor screening in VHL. Most advocate for annual history-taking and a physical examination including blood pressure and neurologic evaluation, eye and retinal exams every 1 to 2 years, annual plasma free metanephrines, audiology evaluation every 2 to 3 years, brain MRI every 1 to 2 years, and annual abdominal ultrasound or CT/MRI. The age at which to start screening is also debated with most recommending retinal exams start at birth, pheochromocytoma screening from age 2, audiology exams from age 5, brain imaging from age 8, and abdominal imaging from age 10.[69]

Neurofibromatosis 1 There are no recommended screening algorithms for patients with neurofibromatosis 1. Clinicians should be aware of the higher prevalence of PPGL in NF1. PPGL should be suspected based on clinical signs and symptoms, and testing proceeds according to the usual practice of plasma free metanephrines and/or 24-hour urine catecholamines.[75]

Hereditary PPGL Syndromes There are no consensus recommendations regarding management and screening of patients with *SDHx*, *TMEM127*, and *MAX* gene mutations. It is reasonable to perform screening with annual history and physical examination, blood pressure measurement, plasma free metanephrines or 24-hour urine fractionated metanephrines, and cross-sectional whole-body imaging every 1 to 2 years. Pediatric patients should be started on lifelong surveillance after age 6. An MRI can be used for pediatric or pregnant patients to minimize radiation exposure. Routine surveillance for GIST has not been recommended, but patients with unexplained gastrointestinal symptoms should undergo evaluation for it.[64,69,72]

References

1. Cooper DSD, Haugen GM, Kloos BR, et al. Revised American Thyroid Association management guidelines for patients with thyroid nodules and differentiated thyroid cancer. *Thyroid*. 2009;19(11):1167–1214.

2. Carling T, Udelsman R. Thyroid cancer. *Annu Rev Med*. 2014;65:125–137.

3. Callender GG, et al. Surgery for thyroid cancer. *Endocrinol Metab Clin North Am*. 2014;43(2):443–458.

4. Khan AS, Nutting C, Harrington K, et al. Familial nonmedullary thyroid cancer: a review of the genetics. *Thyroid*. 2010;20(7).

5. Sippel RS, Caron NR, Clark OH. An evidence-based approach to familial nonmedullary thyroid cancer: screening, clinical management, and follow-up. *World J Surg*. 2007;31(5):924–933.

6. Carling TU. Follicular neoplasms of the thyroid: what to recommend. *Thyroid*. 2005;15(6).

7. Nicolson NG, et al. Comprehensive genetic analysis of follicular thyroid carcinoma predicts prognosis independent of histology. *J Clin Endocrinol Metab*. 2018;103(7):2640–2650.

8. Ito Y, et al. An observational trial for papillary thyroid microcarcinoma in Japanese patients. *World J Surg*. 2010;34(1):28–35.

9. Welch HGD, Saving GM. Saving thyroids: overtreatment of small papillary cancers. *N Engl J Med*. 2018;379(4):310–312.

10. Carling T, Long WD, Udelsman R. Controversy surrounding the role for routine central lymph node dissection for differentiated thyroid cancer. *Curr Opin Oncol.* 2010;22(1):30–34.

11. Xing M. Molecular pathogenesis and mechanisms of thyroid cancer. *Nat Rev Cancer.* 2013;13(3):184–199.

12. Carling TO, Udelsman R. Special variants of differentiated thyroid cancer: does it alter the extent of surgery versus well-differentiated thyroid cancer? *World J Surg.* 2007;31:916–923.

13. Patel KNS. Poorly differentiated and anaplastic thyroid cancer. *Cancer Control.* 2006;13(2).

14. Landa I, et al. Genomic and transcriptomic hallmarks of poorly differentiated and anaplastic thyroid cancers. *J Clin Invest.* 2016;126(3):1052–1066.

15. Kunstman JW, et al. Characterization of the mutational landscape of anaplastic thyroid cancer via whole-exome sequencing. *Hum Mol Genet.* 2015;24(8):2318–2329.

16. Dong W, et al. Clonal evolution analysis of paired anaplastic and well-differentiated thyroid carcinomas reveals shared common ancestor. *Genes Chromosomes Cancer.* 2018;57(12):645–652.

17. Sasanakietkul T, et al. Epigenetic modifications in poorly differentiated and anaplastic thyroid cancer. *Mol Cell Endocrinol.* 2018;469:23–37.

18. Cancer Genome Atlas Research. Integrated genomic characterization of papillary thyroid carcinoma. *Cell.* 2014;159(3):676–690.

19. Bonora E, Tallini G, Romeo G. Genetic predisposition to familial nonmedullary thyroid cancer: an update of molecular findings and state-of-the-art studies. *J Oncol.* 2010;2010:385206.

20. Jasperson KP, Ahnen D. APC-associated polyposis conditions, in *GeneReviews*, Pagon RA, Adam MP, Ardinger HH, et al. (Eds). 2017.

21. Stratakis CA. Carney complex: A familial lentiginosis predisposing to a variety of tumors. *Rev Endocr Metab Disord.* 2016;17(3):367–371.

22. Stratakis CA, Raygada M. Carney complex, in *GeneReviews*, Pagon RA, Adam MP, Ardinger HH, et al. (Eds). 2018.

23. Doros LS, Steward K, Bauer DR, et al. DICER1-related disorders, in *GeneReviews*, Pagon RA, Adam MP, Ardinger HH, et al. (Eds). 2014.

24. Schultz KAP, et al. DICER1 and associated conditions: identification of at-risk individuals and recommended surveillance strategies. *Clin Cancer Res.* 2018;24(10):2251–2261.

25. Wells SAJr., et al. Revised American Thyroid Association guidelines for the management of medullary thyroid carcinoma. *Thyroid.* 2015;25(6):567–610.

26. Norton JA, Krampitz G, Jensen RT. Multiple endocrine neoplasia: genetics and clinical management. *Surg Oncol Clin N Am.* 2015;24(4):795–832.

27. Rosario PW, Calsolari MR. Usefulness of serum calcitonin in patients without a suspicious history of medullary thyroid carcinoma and with thyroid nodules without an indication for fine-needle aspiration or with benign cytology. *Horm Metab Res.* 2016;48(6):372–276.

28. Marquard JE. Multiple endocrine neoplasia type 2, in *GeneReviews*, Pagon RA, Adam MP, Ardinger HH, et al. (Eds). 2015.

29. Khatami F, Tavangar SM. Multiple endocrine neoplasia syndromes from genetic and epigenetic perspectives. *Biomark Insights.* 2018;13: 1177271918785129.

30. Accardo G, et al. Genetics of medullary thyroid cancer: an overview. *Int J Surg.* 2017;41(Suppl.1):S2–S6.

31. Carling TU. Parathyroid surgery in familial hyperparathyroid disorders. *J Int Med.* 2005;257:27–37.

32. Marx SJ, Lourenco DM Jr. Familial hyperparathyroidism: disorders of growth and secretion in hormone-secretory tissue. *Horm Metab Res.* 2017;49(11):805–815.

33. Li Y, Simonds WF. Endocrine neoplasms in familial syndromes of hyperparathyroidism. *Endocr Relat Cancer.* 2016;23(6):R229–247.

34. Starker LF, et al. Minimally invasive parathyroidectomy. *Int J Endocrinol.* 2011;2011:206502.

35. Silva BC, Cusano NE, Bilezikian JP. Primary hyperparathyroidism. *Best Pract Res Clin Endocrinol Metab.* 2018.

36. Sharretts JM, Kebebew E, Simonds WF. Parathyroid cancer. *Semin Oncol.* 2010;37(6):580–590.

37. Wei CH, Harari A. Parathyroid carcinoma: update and guidelines for management. *Curr Treat Options Oncol.* 2012;13(1):11–23.

38. Lee PK, et al. Trends in the incidence and treatment of parathyroid cancer in the United States. *Cancer.* 2007;109(9):1736–1741.

39. Alrezk R, Hannah-Shmouni F, Stratakis, CA. MEN4 and CDKN1B mutations: the latest of the MEN syndromes. *Endocr Relat Cancer.* 2017;24(10):T195–T208.

40. Howell VM, Khoo SK, Petilo D, et al. HRPT2 mutations are associated with malignancy in sporadic parathyroid tumours. *J Med Genet.* 2003;40:657–663.

41. Shattuck TV, Obara T, Gaz, RD, et al. Somatic and germ-line mutations of the HRPT2 gene in sporadic parathyroid carcinoma. *N Engl J Med.* 2003;349(18):1722–1729.

42. Giusti FIM, Brandi ML. Multiple endocrine neoplasia type 1, in *GeneReviews*, Pagon RA, Adam MP, Ardinger HH, et al. (Eds). 2017.

43. Rubinstein JC, et al. Hyperparathyroidism: jaw tumor syndrome associated with large-scale 1q31 deletion. *J Endocr Soc.* 2017;1(7):926–930.

44. Hyde SMR, Waguespack SG, Perrier ND, et al. CDC73-related disorders, in *GeneReviews*, Pagon RA, Adam MP, Ardinger HH, et al. (Eds). 2018.

45. Lerario AM, Moraitis A, Hammer GD. Genetics and epigenetics of adrenocortical tumors. *Mol Cell Endocrinol.* 2014;386(1–2):67–84.

46. Nicolson NG, Man J, Carling T. Advances in understanding the molecular underpinnings of adrenocortical tumors. *Curr Opin Oncol.* 2018;30(1):16–22.

47. Fassnacht M, et al. Management of adrenal incidentalomas: European Society of Endocrinology Clinical Practice Guideline in collaboration with the European Network for the Study of Adrenal Tumors. *Eur J Endocrinol.* 2016;175(2):G1–G34.

48. Fassnacht M, et al. Adrenocortical carcinoma: a clinician's update. *Nat Rev Endocrinol.* 2011;7(6):323–335.

49. Allolio B, Fassnacht M. Clinical review: adrenocortical carcinoma: clinical update. *J Clin Endocrinol Metab.* 2006;91(6):2027–2037.

50. Zeiger MA, Thompson GB, Duh Q, et al. The American Association of Clinical Endocrinologists and American Association of Endocrine Surgeons medical guidelines for the management of adrenal incidentalomas. Endocr Pract. Jul-Aug 2009; 15 Suppl 1:1–20.

51. Mendiratta-Lala M, et al. Adrenal imaging. *Endocrinol Metab Clin North Am.* 2017;46(3):741–759.

52. Starker LF, Kunstman JW, Carling T. Subclinical Cushing syndrome: a review. *Surg Clin North Am.* 2014;94(3):657–668.

53. Dickson PV, et al. Adjuvant and neoadjuvant therapy, treatment for advanced disease, and genetic considerations for adrenocortical carcinoma: an update from the SSO Endocrine and Head and Neck Disease Site Working Group. *Ann Surg Oncol.* 2018;25(12):3453–3459.

54. Akerstrom T, et al. Genetics of adrenocortical tumours. *J Intern Med.* 2016;280(6):540–550.

55. Shuman CB, Weksberg R. Beckwith-Wiedemann syndrome, in *GeneReviews*, Pagon RA, Adam MP, Ardinger HH, et al. (Eds). 2016.

56. Kohlmann WG. Lynch syndrome, in *GeneReviews*, Pagon RA, Adam MP, Ardinger HH, et al. (Eds). 2018.

57. Schneider KZ, Nichols KE, Garber J. Li-Fraumeni syndrome, in *GeneReviews*, Pagon RA, Adam MP, Ardinger HH, et al. (Eds). 2013.

58. Juhlin CC, et al. Whole-exome sequencing characterizes the landscape of somatic mutations and copy number alterations in adrenocortical carcinoma. *J Clin Endocrinol Metab.* 2015;100(3):E493–502.

59. Petr EJ, Else T. Adrenocortical carcinoma (ACC): when and why should we consider germline testing? *Presse Med.* 2018;47(7-8 Pt. 2):e119–e125.

60. Assie G, et al. Integrated genomic characterization of adrenocortical carcinoma. *Nat Genet.* 2014;46(6):607–612.

61. Zheng S, et al. Comprehensive pan-genomic characterization of adrenocortical carcinoma. *Cancer Cell.* 2016;29(5):723–736.

62. Else TG, Fishbein L. Hereditary paraganglioma-pheochromocytoma syndromes, in *GeneReviews*, Pagon RA, Adam MP, Ardinger HH, et al. (Eds). 2008.

63. Pacak KL, Eisenhofer G, Walther MM et al. Recent advances in genetics, diagnosis, localization, and treatment of pheochromocytoma. *Ann Intern Med.* 2001;134(4):345–329.

64. Alrezk R, et al. Update of pheochromocytoma syndromes: genetics, biochemical rvaluation, and imaging. *Front Endocrinol (Lausanne).* 2018;9:515.

65. Dhir ML, Hogg ME, Bartlett DL, et al. Clinical predictors of malignancy in patients with pheochromocytoma and paraganglioma. *Ann Surg Oncol.* 2017;24(12):3624–3630.

66. Lenders JW, et al. Pheochromocytoma and paraganglioma: an endocrine society clinical practice guideline. *J Clin Endocrinol Metab.* 2014;99(6):1915–1942.

67. Gimenez-Roqueplo AP, Dahia PL, Robledo M. An update on the genetics of paraganglioma, pheochromocytoma, and associated hereditary syndromes. *Horm Metab Res.* 2012;44(5):328–333.

68. Hamidi O, et al. Outcomes of patients with metastatic phaeochromocytoma and paraganglioma: A systematic review and meta-analysis. *Clin Endocrinol (Oxf).* 2017;87(5):440–450.

69. Rednam SP, et al. Von Hippel-Lindau and hereditary pheochromocytoma/paraganglioma syndromes: clinical features, genetics, and surveillance recommendations in childhood. *Clin Cancer Res.* 2017;23(12):e68–e75.

70. NGSnPPGL Study Group, et al. Consensus statement on next-generation-sequencing-based diagnostic testing of hereditary phaeochromocytomas and paragangliomas. *Nat Rev Endocrinol.* 2017;13(4):233–247.

71. Casey RT, et al. Clinical and molecular features of renal and pheochromocytoma/paraganglioma tumor association syndrome (RAPTAS): case series and literature review. *J Clin Endocrinol Metab.* 2017;102(11):4013–4022.

72. Bausch B, et al. Clinical characterization of the pheochromocytoma and paraganglioma susceptibility genes SDHA, TMEM127, MAX, and SDHAF2 for gene-informed prevention. *JAMA Oncol.* 2017;3(9):1204–1212.

73. Fishbein L, et al., Comprehensive molecular characterization of pheochromocytoma and paraganglioma. *Cancer Cell.* 2017;31(2):181–193.

74. Kavinga Gunawardane PT, Grossman A. The clinical genetics of phaeochromocytoma and paraganglioma. *Arch Endocrinol Metab.* 2017;61(5):490–500.

75. Ferner, RE, et al. Guidelines for the diagnosis and management of individuals with neurofibromatosis 1. *J Med Genet.* 2007;44(2):81–88.

CHAPTER 14

Risk Assessment and Clinical Management – Skin Cancer

Katherine Given Ligtenberg, Jake X. Wang, and David J. Leffell

RISK ASSESSMENT AND CLINICAL MANAGEMENT

Background

Skin cancer is the most common type of cancer in the United States, with one in five Americans predicted to develop some form of cutaneous malignancy in their lifetime.[1-4] The most common skin cancers are basal cell carcinoma, squamous cell carcinoma, and melanoma. The vast majority of cutaneous malignancies are derived from cellular components that comprise the outermost layer of the skin, or epidermis, the most abundant of which are keratinocytes and melanocytes (Figure 14.1). Malignant transformation of keratinocytes (basal cell keratinocytes and squamous epithelial keratinocytes) leads to the development of basal cell and squamous cell carcinomas, while mutations in neural-crest derived melanocytes, which are interspersed in regular intervals throughout the basal layer of the epidermis, give rise to melanoma.[5]

The skin is comprised of a wide range of cell types so it is not surprising that skin cancer genetics itself is a broad topic. The epidermis, dermis, adnexal structures, and subcutis can develop malignant transformation at different stages of differentiation. The etiology of most skin cancers is multifactorial, often requiring environmental exposure. The impact is magnified in patients with an underlying genetic predisposition. Identification of skin cancer risk factors have resulted in general risk avoidance principles and screening recommendations.[5-7]

In general, patients with increased genetic susceptibility tend to develop skin cancers at an earlier age, in greater number, and may develop tumors that behave more aggressively compared to patients who develop sporadic tumors. Despite this, results of studies that inquire whether patients with familial melanoma practice risk-reducing and early-detection behaviors suggest inconsistent adoption and maintenance of risk-avoidance behaviors.[8,9] Thus, current recommendations for exposure avoidance and risk modification are the same for higher-risk populations and the general population.[5,6] Overall assessment of risk, both genetic and environmental, is critical so that the proper screening recommendations can be made for each individual patient and family. Selection of the correct patient cohort is

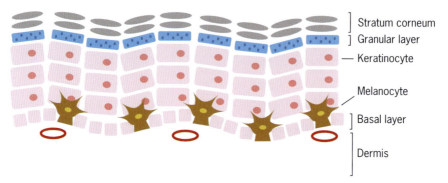

FIGURE 14.1: Components of the epidermis.

important to avoid unnecessary procedures, false positive results, and to best allocate finite resources in a productive and cost-effective manner.

The fundamental principles of risk assessment in general also apply to dermatology. They include a thorough patient history and physical examination.[10] Patients should be asked about their history of sun exposure, personal and family history of prior skin cancers, pre-cancers, or abnormal or congenital moles, sun protective behaviors, occupational exposures, tobacco use, exposure to HPV or HIV, and whether they have noticed any lesions that are changing, painful, bleeding, or not healing. Additional relevant history includes a patient's gender and age, immunosuppression status, and medications, as some may promote or accelerate the development of skin cancers. Other risk factors specific to the most common types of skin cancer are listed in Table 14.1. Patients should be examined for Fitzpatrick skin type, signs of chronic sun damage, presence of freckles, and number, size, and location of moles[10] (Figure 14.2). These risk factors vary in importance for each skin cancer type, the most common of which will be discussed in the remainder of the chapter. Those at increased risk for the development of skin cancer should have regular total body skin screening examinations by a dermatologist or trained physician, though the frequency of these exams will depend on the overall assessment of risk. Dermoscopy can enhance the dermatologist's exam when used properly by employing polarized light to better visualize pigmented structures and vessel shape and size. It has been demonstrated that early detection and treatment of skin cancers, especially melanoma, directly correlate with survival.[4,11] Specifically, 5-year survival for early stage, thin melanomas (up to 0.8 mm in depth) is ~98%, while survival for those with locally advanced disease is ~80%. If the melanoma has metastasized to local nodes or distant sites, survival drops to ~64% and 23%, respectively.[4,11]

In recent years, many attempts have been made to develop melanoma risk predictor tools or calculators, including at the National Cancer Institute (https://mrisktool.cancer.gov). Many of them seek to predict melanoma risk in patients without a personal history of melanoma based on a variety of risk factors, such as gender, age, family history, sun exposure, complexion, etc. The majority of these calculators are freely available for patient and provider use and generate recommendations for frequency of total body skin examination screening, among other outputs. Two models have been developed for research purposes to predict the probability of germline *CDKN2A* pathogenic variants, one of the most commonly implicated mutations in cases of familial melanoma (MelPREDICT, MelaPRO). While these may be

TABLE 14.1: Risk factors of skin cancer

	Basal Cell Carcinoma	Squamous Cell Carcinoma	Melanoma
Genetic Factors or Genetic Syndromes	• Fair skin, freckling, red hair • Xenoderma pigmentosum • Rothmund-Thomson syndrome • Gorlin syndrome • Bazer-Dupré-Christol syndrome • Rombo syndrome • BAP-1 mutation syndrome	• Fair skin, freckling, red hair • Xenoderma pigmentosum • Rothmund-Thomson syndrome • Oculocutaneous albinism • Bloom syndrome • Muir-Torre syndrome • Epidermodysplasia verruciformis • Epidermolysis bullosa • Ferguson-Smith syndrome	• Fair skin, red hair • Family history of cutaneous melanoma • Xenoderma pigmentosum and DNA repair defects • Familial atypical multiple mole melanoma syndrome • BAP-1 mutation syndrome • Cowden syndrome
Environmental Exposures	• Intermittent, recreational sun exposure • Tanning beds • Ionizing radiation	• Cumulative, occupational sun exposure • Tanning beds • Ionizing radiation • Chemical (arsenic) • HPV • Cigarette smoking	• Intense intermittent and chronic sun exposure • Tanning beds • Location of residence (equatorial latitudes)
Other Predisposing Factors	• Immunosuppression (e.g., organ transplantation)	• Immunosuppression (e.g., organ transplantation)	• Increased total number of acquired melanocytic nevi ($>$100, relative risk ~8–10 times) • A typical melanocytic nevi ($>$5, relative risk ~4–6 times) • Multiple solar lentigines, relative risk 3–4 times • Immunosuppression (e.g., organ transplantation)

Skin phototype	Skin color	Reaction to UV irradiation
I	White	Always burns, never tans
II	White	Burns easily, tans with difficulty
III	Beige	Burns easily, tans gradually
IV	Brown	Burns minimally, tans easily
V	Dark Brown	Rarely burns, tans very easily
VI	Black	Never burns, always tans

FIGURE 14.2: Fitzpatrick skin phototype features.

valuable adjuncts in the future, these tools have yet to be rigorously validated, their level of accuracy is currently unclear, and they are not recommended for widespread use at this time.

Clinical Management

For all types of skin cancer, prevention is key. It has been argued that the vast majority of skin cancers, including melanoma, and subsequent melanoma-related deaths, are potentially preventable. This prompted "The Surgeon General's Call to Action to Prevent Skin Cancer," which was published in 2014, to raise awareness about the connection of ultraviolet (UV) damage and development of skin cancer.[7] This initiative recommends minimizing exposure to UV radiation by wearing protective clothing (including long sleeves, pants, wide-brimmed hats), wearing sunglasses, applying broad-spectrum (UVA and UVB blocking), water-resistant sunscreen with SPF $\geq$30, seeking shade whenever possible, avoiding the sun between the hours of 10 a.m. and 4 p.m., and not sunbathing or indoor tanning. Additionally, particularly rigorous sun protection is recommended in children, as severe sunburns in childhood are thought to be related to the development of future melanomas.[4] Even one blistering sunburn during childhood can double the chance of developing melanoma in the future, and $\geq$5 blistering sunburns between 15 to 20 years of age can increase a patient's risk of developing melanoma and nonmelanoma skin cancer (NMSC) by 80% and 68%, respectively.[12,13] These recommendations are echoed by formal statements from the American Academy of Dermatology (AAD), the National Cancer Institute, the Centers for Disease Control and Prevention, U.S. Environmental Protection Agency, U.S. Food and Drug Administration, Occupational Safety and Health Administration, American Academy of Pediatrics, and the American Cancer Society.[4,6,7,14] Importantly, these behavior modification recommendations can be made and reinforced by non-dermatologist providers, which may help improve compliance.

Once skin cancers do develop, early detection of these tumors is important, and in the case of melanoma, can dramatically affect mortality. Patients should be encouraged to regularly monitor their own skin to increase personal awareness of new or changing cutaneous growths, prompting earlier evaluation by a dermatologist. Notably, about half of all melanomas are self-detected.[15] When evaluating moles, the AAD recommends the use of the ABCDEs—Asymmetry (the two halves of the mole do no match), Borders (irregular edges that are ragged, notched, or blurred), Color (multiple colors or non-uniform distribution), Diameter (larger than pencil eraser, >5 mm), Evolution (change over time) to help identify concerning lesions (Figure 14.3). Other important features include moles that look different than the majority of a patient's other moles (the "ugly duckling"), or lesions that are bleeding, painful, or not healing as would be expected normally. Despite this, lesions do not always follow the textbook and may not present with any of these typical warning signs.

As a general rule, changes that occur or progress over $\geq$1 month should be evaluated.[4] Basal cell carcinomas often appear as flat, or slightly raised, pink, translucent, somewhat shiny lesions with arborizing blood vessels on dermoscopy. Certain basal cell cancers may even appear like a scar. These lesions tend to enlarge slowly and bleed with minimal trauma or are asymptomatic. Squamous cell carcinoma also exhibits a range of clinical presentations. It may present as flat rough patches, thickened hyperkeratotic bumps, cutaneous horns, or large crateriform lesions with a central keratotic plug, among other morphologies (Figure 14.4). Dermatologists are adept at diagnosing lesions. They use augmented visual examination and information about lesion morphology, anatomic site, genetic risk factors, and clinical history to make a clinical diagnosis. If there is uncertainty, lesions can

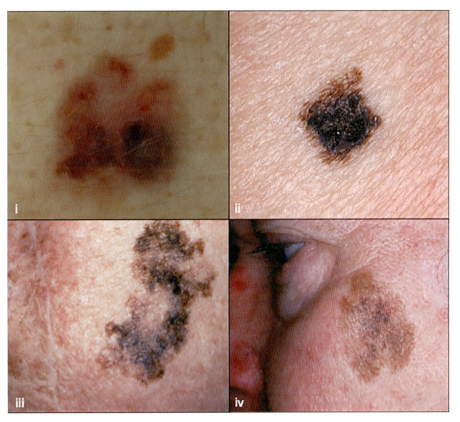

FIGURE 14.3: ABCDEs of melanoma. Asymmetry (i), **B**order irregularity or notched borders (ii), **C**olor variegation (iii), and **D**iameter >5 mm (iv) are concerning features for melanoma. The addition of **E** for evolving has also been included to raise suspicion for changing lesions. Used with permission from Suguru Imaeda, MD.

be biopsied for histopathologic diagnosis or confirmation. Once detected and diagnosed by biopsy, lesions are definitively treated, though the details of treatment are beyond the scope of this review. Importantly, nearly all cases of NMSCs can be cured with early detection and intervention, with >99% survival at 5 years.[4] In contrast, survival rate for melanoma varies widely depending on the depth of tumor at diagnosis.

Formal Screening Recommendations have been Established

The U.S. Preventative Services Task Force does not recommend regular interval screenings for early detection of any cutaneous malignancies. However, the AAD recommends routine skin self-exams and empowers dermatologists to make personalized recommendations regarding frequency of skin exams based on each patient's risk factors. Once a NMSC is detected, the National Comprehensive Cancer Network (NCCN) recommends a total body skin examination every 6 to 12 months for the first 5 years after diagnosis, and then at least annually for the remainder of the patient's life.[14,16,17] Those with genetic syndromes often require more frequent surveillance, and some disease-specific organizations have proposed formal recommendations, such as the Basal Cell Nevus Syndrome (BCNS) Colloquium Group. Factors, especially when in combination, that increase suspicion for a genetic

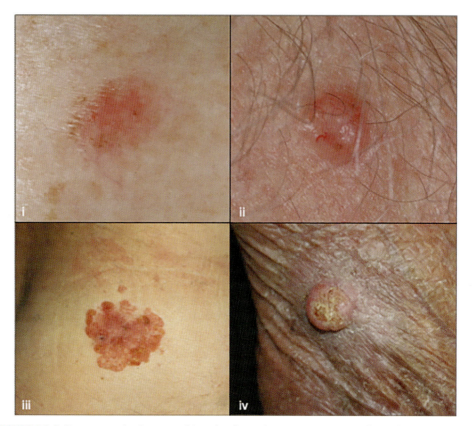

FIGURE 14.4: Representative images of basal cell carcinoma, squamous cell carcinoma in situ, and squamous cell carcinoma. Superficial basal cell carcinoma presenting as a pink macule with foci of brown pigment at the borders (i); nodular basal cell carcinoma with characteristic pearly appearance and arborizing telangiectasia (ii); squamous cell carcinoma in situ presenting as a pink plaque with scale (iii); exophytic scaly nodule on sun-damaged skin found to be invasive squamous cell carcinoma (iv). Used with permission from Suguru Imaeda, MD.

syndrome in skin cancer and should prompt consideration of a referral to a specialist (dermatology, genetics), include

- Early age of onset of the skin cancer
- Aggressive course of the tumor(s)
- Other known paired malignancies or findings (e.g., pancreatic cancer and melanoma)
- Suggestive family history

▪ DISEASE-SPECIFIC CANCER EPIDEMIOLOGY

Nonmelanoma Skin Cancer

There are over 100 different kinds of cutaneous tumors, some of which have known associations with familial syndromes.[14] The most common malignant tumor types are basal cell carcinoma (BCC), squamous cell carcinoma (SCC), and melanoma, which together comprise more than 99% of skin cancer diagnoses each year.[1-4] The most common of these, BCCs, comprise ~75 to 85% of all cutaneous tumor diagnoses. SCCs account for ~20%, making them the second most commonly diagnosed cutaneous malignancy. It is not possible to determine the exact annual incidence of NMSCs, since these diagnoses are not reportable to cancer registries. However, recent estimates predict ~5.4 million cases of NMSC were diagnosed among 3.3 million individuals in 2012.[4] The number of cases of BCC and SCC has risen by 145% and 263%, respectively, between the 1970s and 2010, with the greatest increase seen in women between 30 and 59 years of age.[18] This is attributed, in part, to increased skin cancer awareness, more screening exams and biopsies, the general aging of the population, and longer average lifespan. The associated lifetime risk of developing a BCC or SCC in those of European descent is ~30% or ~9%, respectively.[14,16,19] There are ~200,000 to 400,000 new cases of SCC each year, with ~3,000 deaths annually.[19]

While the majority of these keratinocyte-derived tumors arise spontaneously, they have also been found in association with various genetic aberrations and hereditary syndromes. The most well-known syndrome leading to development of BCCs is basal cell nevus syndrome, while syndromes predisposed to the development of SCCs include xeroderma pigmentosum and oculocutaneous albinism, among others. These will all be discussed in subsequent sections.

Melanoma

Although melanoma accounts for about only 1% of skin cancer diagnoses, it is responsible for the majority of skin cancer-related deaths. In 2020, there will be about 95,710 new cases of noninvasive melanoma and about 100,350 new cases of invasive melanoma diagnosed, 6,850 of which will result in death (>18 deaths per day).[4,20] Additionally, invasive melanoma ranks as the fifth most common malignancy for men and sixth most common for women in the United States. Among men and women aged 15 to 29, melanoma is the third and fourth most common cancer diagnosis, respectively.[21] The lifetime risk estimates for developing melanoma is 1 in 33 for men, and 1 in 52 for women (or 2 to 3% of the general population). Interestingly, while the incidence of melanoma in Caucasian men and women has continued to increase (3 to 7% per year) steadily over the last 30 years, mortality has remained stable or even declined in certain age groups. This observation is largely attributed to increased aware-ness, which prompts more frequent screenings, both by professionals and self-examinations, (earlier) detection of thinner melanomas, and recent significant advances in treatments available for later stage disease.[2,4,5,21] The incidence of familial melanoma, or melanoma aris-ing in multiple family members, is between 5 to 10% of all diagnosed melanomas.[22]

Additional Considerations While skin cancer can develop in any skin type, there are notable epidemiological differences when tumors occur in darker Fitzpatrick skin types. First, melanomas in skin phototypes III–VI (Asians, Hispanics, Africans) tend to occur in sun-protected areas of the body, such as palms, soles, nails, groin, and oral mucosa. Second, SCC, rather than BCC, is the most common form of skin cancer in African Americans (in the United States and parts of Africa).[14] Third, and most importantly, skin cancers in these populations are often diagnosed at later stages, and patients have poorer outcomes.[23]

Economic Impact From 2007 to 2011, approximately 4.9 million Americans were treated for their skin cancers. The average annual cost for their treatment was ~$8.1 billion.[1] More than half of this cost was for the treatment of NMSC. In 2006, the predicted annual average treatment cost for all skin cancers was $3.6 billion. Diagnosis and treatment of skin cancers account for about 0.53% of American healthcare system expenditures.

▦ DISEASE-SPECIFIC APPROACH TO RISK ASSESSMENT, COUNSELING, AND TESTING

For all skin cancer types, risk assessment and stratification begin with patient history. Major risk categories include (1) environmental exposure, (2) phenotypic traits, and (3) genetic predisposition. In general, individuals with more risk factors have an increased risk for developing skin cancers, and risk is often multifactorial.[10] Although there are many shared risk factors for BCC, SCC, and melanoma, there are also subtleties that tend to favor development of each of these lesions over the others.

For basal cell carcinoma, important risk factors include[14]

- A personal history of BCC or *any* other skin cancer
- A family history of BCC or *any* other skin cancer; genetic syndrome that predisposes someone to develop skin cancer
- Intermittent intense exposure to UV radiation (natural sunlight or tanning bed use)
- Exposure to ionizing radiation
- Chronic arsenic ingestion
- Fitzpatrick skin type I–II
- Immunosuppression

For squamous cell carcinoma, important risk factors include[14]

- A personal history of SCC or *any* other skin cancer
- A family history of SCC; genetic syndrome that predisposes someone to develop skin cancer
- Chronic, cumulative sun exposure (often associated with occupational exposures)
- Therapeutic radiation (e.g., psoralen and UVA therapy for psoriasis)
- Exposure to ionizing radiation
- Chronic arsenic ingestion
- Chronic scars and wounds (e.g., Marjolin's ulcers, which can develop up to decades later); HPV infections
- Fitzpatrick skin type I–II, but also darker Fitzpatrick skin types
- Degree of freckling corresponds to SCC risk
- Immunosuppression

For melanoma, important risk factors include[4,14]

- A personal history of melanoma or dysplastic nevi
- A family history of melanoma (first-degree relatives); genetic syndrome that predisposes someone to develop skin cancer
- Nevi [several large (>6 mm), atypical, or numerous small (>50 moles)]
- Intermittent, acute sun exposure leading to sunburn (indoor tanning beds, natural sunlight, history of >5 blistering sunburns in lifetime), especially in childhood and adolescence
- Chronic, cumulative sun exposure
- Fitzpatrick skin type I–II (sunburn easily, natural blond or red hair, lightly pigmented irides, moderate freckling)

- Immunosuppression (solid-organ transplant recipients, chronic lymphocytic leukemia, poorly controlled HIV)

As seen above, family history is a major contributor to risk. Studies comparing incidence of NMSCs among twins have found 43% heritability, suggesting that nearly half of the risk of development of NMSC may be due to inherited factors. Further, the cumulative risk of development of NMSC was almost 2-fold higher for monozygotic twins, compared to their dizygotic counterparts.[24] Similarly, the presence of any skin cancer is a strong predictor of development of another skin cancer. A prospective cohort study from 2015 found that in the first 5 years after diagnosis of a NMSC, the risk of developing another NMSC is 40.7% and 82% if the patient has >1 NMSC.[17] These probabilities increase at 10 years, with a 59.6% chance of developing a second lesion after the first, and 91.2% after diagnosis of >1 lesion.[16,17,19]

A number of studies have evaluated the risk of skin cancer development in the setting of different forms of immunosuppression.[14] In solid-organ transplant recipients (SOTR), the risk of BCC is 10 times that of the general population, while the risk of SCC is 65 to 250 times higher than the general population. Notably, this varies with the type of transplant and immunosuppressive agent used. Studies have also revealed that SOTR and chronic lymphocytic leukemia patients develop NMSCs at a younger age, and the tumors tend to behave more aggressively, with increased rates of recurrence and metastasis.

For BCC, primary prevention is critical. As with other skin cancer prevention, patients should be instructed to avoid excess cumulative or sporadic sun exposure. In those with BCC, and especially those with BCNS, patients need to avoid or minimize their exposure to ionizing radiation to minimize future tumor burden.[25] For SCC, primary prevention is also critical. Patients should be instructed to avoid excess sun exposure, including wearing protective eyewear. In those with certain underlying conditions, such as epidermodysplasia verruciformis (EDV), patients should avoid X-ray therapies.[14]

In the case of melanoma, if patients have a personal history of melanoma or dysplastic nevi, they should be asked about a family history of melanoma or other cancers including pancreatic cancer, which, if present, may suggest an underlying familial syndrome or predisposition. If available, the age of diagnosis and pathologic confirmation of melanoma in family members should be ascertained. It is important to determine the number of primary melanomas diagnosed in the proband. Only 4 to 5% of patients with sporadic melanomas will develop >1 primary (male, elderly); however, ~30% of kindreds of hereditary melanoma syndromes will develop >1 primary. It is important that family history is updated regularly in the setting of or concern for hereditary melanoma. Individuals with pigmented lesions (large, numerous, etc.), have a 2- to 3-fold increased risk of developing melanoma, whereas individuals with familial dysplastic nevus syndrome have about a 5-fold risk.[14] A family history of melanoma alone increases the risk of melanoma about 2-fold, but varies based on the number of family members with melanoma and by the total number of primary lesions in each family member. As with NMSC, concordance studies in twins have been performed. The heritability of melanoma is about 58%, and, interestingly, melanoma in these settings is more likely to occur on sun-protected sites compared to sporadic melanoma.[24] It is unclear whether the presence of BCC/SCC are independent risk factors for melanoma or if the relationship exists due to shared risk factors, such as sun exposure. However, two large prospective cohort studies reported that the initial diagnosis of NMSC increases the risk for a subsequent melanoma, with a relative risk of 1.99 and 2.58 for men and women, respectively. One smaller study reports a greater relative risk of 3.62 for development of melanoma after diagnosis of SCC, specifically.[19,26]

Those at higher risk for developing skin cancer should be followed clinically at regular intervals by a dermatologist. Regardless of risk category, patients should be counseled about avoiding high-risk behaviors by primary care and specialist providers. The role of genetic testing in skin cancer is still equivocal.

▥ HEREDITARY CANCER SYNDROMES

There are many hereditary cancer syndromes, though most are quite rare. We discuss the more common or well-known disease syndromes, while the less common ones are detailed in Table 14.2.[27] The hereditary cancer syndromes can be divided into four broad categories: (1) interruption of key molecular pathways involved in pathogenesis, (2) association with

TABLE 14.2: Genetic syndromes with increased skin cancer risk

Mutations in key molecular pathways	Skin cancer predisposition	Presentation	Genetic mutation(s)
BAP-1 Tumor Syndrome	MM (cutaneous and uveal), BCC	Multiple melanocytic BAP-1 mutated atypical intradermal tumors, mesotheliomas, renal cell carcinoma	BAP-1
Basal Cell Nevus (Gorlin) Syndrome	BCC	Palmar pits, ondontogenic keratocysts, bifid ribs	PTCH1, PTCH2, SUFU
Bazex-Dupré-Christol Syndrome	BCC	Vermiculate atrophoderma, multiple facial milia, hypotrichosis, trichoepitheliomas, hypohidrosis, facial hyperpigmentation, cyanosis	ARCT1 (suspected)
Brooke-Spiegler Syndrome	BCC	Cylindromas, trichoepitheliomas, spiradenomas	CYLD
Cowden Syndrome	MM	Tricholemmomas, sclerotic fibromas, acral keratosis, breast/thyroid/endometrial/renal malignancy	PTEN
Familal A typical Multiple Mole Melanoma Syndrome (FAMMM)	MM	>50 melanocytic nevi, atypical melanocytic nevi, increased risk of pancreatic cancer	CDKN2A, CDK4
Ferguson-Smith Syndrome	SCC	Multiple self-healing squamous epitheliomas	TGFBR1, TGFBR2
Keratitis-Ichthyosis-Deafness Syndrome	SCC	Transient erythroderma, hyperkeratotic plaques, palmoplantar keratoderma, congenital sensorineural hearing loss, vascularizing keratitis, mucocutaneous infections	GJB2
Muir-Torre Syndrome	SCC (keratoacanthoma), BCC	Sebaceous neoplasms, gastrointestinal/genitourinary tract malignancies	MLH1, MSH2, MSH6
Schöpf-Schulz-Passarge Syndrome	BCC	Hidrocystomas, palmoplantar kerato derma, ectodermal dysplasia (hypotrichosis, hypodontia, nail dystrophy)	WNT10A
Werner Syndrome	MM, SCC	Mottled hyperpigmentation, sclerodermoid changes, ulcerations, micrognatia, beaked nose, premature aging	RECQL2
Xeroderma Pigmentosum	SCC, BCC, MM	Photosensitivity, xerosis, premature skin aging, pigmentary changes, photophobia, keratitis, corneal opacification, hyporeflexia, deafness	XPA, XPB, XPC, XPD, XPE, XPF, XPG, POLH

TABLE 14.2: Genetic syndromes with increased skin cancer risk (*Continued*)

Mutations in key molecular pathways	Skin cancer predisposition	Presentation	Genetic mutation(s)
Immunodeficiencies			
Chédiak-Higashi Syndrome	SCC	Mild diffuse pigmentary dilution, silver hair, photo-distributed hyper/hypopigmentation, photophobia, nystagmus, strabismus, recurrent pyogenic infections, hemophagocytic syndrome	*LYST*
Epidemodysplasia Verruciformis	SCC	Widespread papules that resemble flat warts	*EVER1/TMC6, EVER2/TMC8*
Griscelli Syndrome (Type 1, 2, 3)	SCC	Pigmentary dilution, silver hair, neurologic impairment (GS1), hemophagocytic syndrome (GS2)	*MYO5A, RAB27A, MLPH*
Hermansky-Pudlak Syndrome	SCC	Pigmentary dilution, ocular albinism, bleeding diathesis, interstitial pulmonary fibrosis, granulomatous colitis, recurrent bacterial infections (HSP2, HSP10), hemophagocytic syndrome (HSP2)	*BLOC1, BLOC2, BLO3, AP3B1, AP3D1*
Disorders of pigmentation			
Bloom Syndrome	SCC	Erythema, poikiloderma, telangiectasia over the face, dorsal hands, cheilitis, café-au-lait macules, growth retardation, high-pitched voices, gastrointestinal malignancies, leukemia, lymphoma	*BLM*
Dyskeratosis Congenita	SCC (cutaneous & mucosal)	Reticulated hyperpigmentation, nail dystrophy, leukoplakia, pancytopenia	*DKC1, TINF2, TERC, TERT, RTEL1, CTC1, WRAP53, NHP2, NOP10, PARN, ACD*
Fanconi Anemia	SCC	Diffuse hyperpigmentation, pancytopenia, malignancy (leukemia > solid tumors)	*FANCA, FANCB, FANCD1, FANCD2, FANCE, FANCF, FANCG, FANCI, FANCJ, FANCL, CANCM, CANCN, CANCO, CANCP, FANCQ, FANCS*
Oculocutaneous Albinism Type 1	SCC	White skin/hair or pigmentary dilution, photosensivitiy, blue-gray eyes, iris translucency, reduced visual acuity	*TYR*
Oculocutaneous Albinism Type 2	SCC	Skin/hair/iris pigmentary dilution	*OCA2*
Rothmund-Thomson Syndrome (Types I and II)	SCC, BCC	Facial erythema, poikiloderma, dyspigmentarion, telangiectasia, growth retardation, juvenile cataract, dental dysplasia, osteosarcoma	*REFQL4*
Disorders of skin fragility			
Junctional Epidermolysis Bullosa	SCC	Erosions, blisters, atrophic scarring, nail dystrophy, tracheolaryngeal stenosis	*LAMA3, LAMB3, LAMC2, COL17A1*
Recessive Dystrophic Epidermolysis Bullosa	SCC	Erosions, blisters, atrophic scarring, nail dystrophy, esophageal strictures, pseudosyndactyly	*COL7A1*
Unknown mutations			
Rombo syndrome	BCC	Vermiculate atrophoderma, hypotrichosis, trichoepitheliomas, cyanosis	*Unknown*

Data from PDQ® Cancer Genetics Editorial Board. PDQ Genetics of Skin Cancer. National Cancer Institute. Updated February 14, 2019.

immunodeficiencies, (3) disorders of skin pigmentation, and (4) disorders of skin fragility.[27] Skin cancers arising in the setting of these syndromes are often numerous and the tumors, as well as their treatment, can be disfiguring over time. Importantly, these skin cancer syndromes are often associated with serious extracutaneous manifestations, including other malignancies. Management requires a multidisciplinary care approach, including a dermatologist, oncologist, and medical geneticist. Cutaneous malignancies are visible and proper identification may lead to earlier diagnosis of these syndromes. This highlights the importance of general practitioners and dermatologists, who are likely to see these lesions first, and can facilitate further genetic investigation and clinical workup.

Basal Cell Nevus Syndrome

See (Figure 14.5A) for three images described in the caption.

Other names: Gorlin-Goltz syndrome

Skin cancer predisposition: BCC

Mode of inheritance: autosomal dominant with complete penetrance

Epidemiology: 1 in 60,000[25]

Age of onset of skin cancer: puberty to ~35 years old

Genetic mutation(s):

PTCH1 on 9q22

PTCH2 on 1p32

SUFU on 10q24-q25

Affected pathway: hedgehog signaling pathway

Other cutaneous findings: palmar pits, milia

Extracutaneous manifestations:

Brain/neural: calcification of the falx cerebri, medulloblastoma

Ocular: lateral displacement of inner canthus, hypertelorism

Oral/palatal: ondontogenic keratocysts (jaw/dental cysts), cleft lip or palate

Musculoskeletal: mandibular prognathia, frontal and biparietal bossing, kyphoscholisosis, bifid ribs (and other rib anomalies), syndactyly

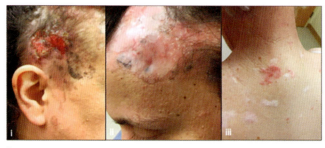

A

FIGURE 14.5A: Classic images of genetic syndromes associated with skin cancer. Basal cell nevus syndrome. Basal cell carcinomas presenting as an eroded plaque on the right parietal scalp (i), irregular pink-brown patch with telangiectasias on the left temporal scalp (ii) and pink, pearly plaque on the posterior neck (iii) in patients with Gorlin syndrome.

TABLE 14.3: Diagnosis of basal cell nevus syndrome	
Major criteria	**Minor criteria**
• BCC before age 20 or excessive numbers of BCCs out of proportion to prior sun exposure and skin type	• Rib anomalies
	• Other skeletal malformations and radiologic changes (e.g., vertebral anomalies, kyphoscoliosis, short fourth metacarpals, postaxial polydactyly)
• Odontogenic keratocyst of the jaw before age 20	• Macrocephaly
• Palmar or plantar pitting	• Cleft lip or palate
• Lamellar calcification of the falx cerebri	• Ovarian or cardiac fibroma
• Medulloblastoma, typically desmoplastic	• Lymphomesenteric cysts
• First-degree relative with BCNS	• Ocular abnormalities (e.g., strabismus, hyper-telorism, congenital cataracts, glaucoma, coloboma)

Diagnosis of basal cell nevus syndrome (BCNS) should be suspected with (1) one major criterion and molecular confirmation, (2) two major criteria, or (3) one major and two minor criteria.

Other: ovarian or cardiac fibromas

Other: Diagnosis can be made by satisfaction of major and or minor criteria (Table 14.3). Some patients will develop few BCCs, while others will develop hundreds in their lifetime.

Rombo Syndrome

Skin cancer predisposition: BCC

Mode of inheritance: autosomal dominant (suspected)

Age of onset of skin cancer: third to fourth decade

Genetic mutation(s): unknown

Other cutaneous findings: vermiculate atrophoderma, hypotrichosis (missing eyelashes and eyebrows), trichoepitheliomas

Extracutaneous manifestations: peripheral vasodilation with cyanosis

Bazex-Dupré-Christol Syndrome

Skin cancer predisposition: BCC

Mode of inheritance: X-linked dominant

Epidemiology: ~20 families reported total; 2:1 (F:M)[27]

Age of onset of skin cancer: as young as 3 years old; second to third decade more typical

Genetic mutation(s): *ARCT1* (suspected)

Affected pathway: hedgehog signaling pathway

Other cutaneous findings: vermiculate atrophoderma, multiple facial milia, hypotrichosis, trichoepitheliomas, hypohidrosis, facial hyperpigmentation

Extracutaneous manifestations: peripheral vasodilation with cyanosis

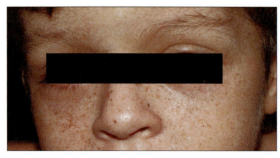

B

FIGURE 14.5B: Classic images of genetic syndromes associated with skin cancer. Xeroderma pigmentosum. Solar lentigines develop from an early age in patients with xeroderma pigmentosum. Used with permission from Julie V. Schaffer, MD.

Xeroderma Pigmentosum

See (Figure 14.5B) for the image described in the caption.

Skin cancer predisposition: SCC, BCC, MM

Mode of inheritance: autosomal recessive

Epidemiology: 1 in 250,000 (U.S.)[5]

Age of onset of skin cancer: 8 years old

Genetic mutation(s): *XPA, XPB, XPC, XPD, XPE, XPF, XPG, POLH*

Affected pathway: nucleotide excision repair (NER)

Other cutaneous findings: severe photosensitivity (severe sunburns with delayed healing), premature skin aging, pigmentary changes; increased risk of SCC, BCC, and MM; later develop hypopigmented spots, telangiectasias

Extracutaneous manifestations:

Ocular: optical photophobia, keratitis, corneal opacification, ectropion

Neurologic: hyporeflexia, progressive deafness

Other: These patients develop SCCs about 50 years before the general population. These patients have a 10,000-fold increased risk of NMSC and 2,000-fold increased risk of melanoma before age 20.

Ferguson-Smith Syndrome

Skin cancer predisposition: SCC

Mode of inheritance: autosomal dominant

Age of onset of skin cancer: puberty to ~35 years old

Genetic mutation(s): *TGFBR1, TGFBR2*

Affected pathway: TGFb-pathway

Other cutaneous findings: multiple self-healing squamous epitheliomas (MSSE)

Other: clinically MSSE resemble keratoacanthomas; histologically cannot differentiate MSSE and SCC; tumors grow over 3 to 4 weeks and will self-resolve in 2 to 3 months with residual scar; MSSEs may be locally invasive but do not metastasize

Muir-Torre Syndrome

Skin cancer predisposition: Keratoacanthomas (SCC)

Mode of inheritance: autosomal dominant with high penetrance, variable expression

Epidemiology: 200 cases reported; 2:3 (F:M)[27]

Age of onset of skin cancer: 21 years old (mean age 53)

Genetic mutation(s): *MLH1*, *MSH2*, *MSH6*

Affected pathway: DNA mismatch repair

Other cutaneous findings: keratoacanthomas (multiple), sebaceous neoplasms (sebaceous adenomas, sebaceous epitheliomas, sebaceous carcinomas)

Extracutaneous manifestations: visceral malignancies: colon, genito-urinary

Other: Thought to be a subtype of hereditary nonpolyposis colorectal cancer (HNPCC); patients with Muir-Torre syndrome should be offered same strict screenings as those with HNPCC (frequent and early colonoscopies, mammograms, dermatologic screening, abdomen/pelvic imaging).

Rothmund-Thomson Syndrome (Types I and II)

Skin cancer predisposition: SCC > BCC

Mode of inheritance: autosomal recessive

Epidemiology: >300 reported cases[5]

Genetic mutation(s): *RECQL4* (RTS-I is heterogenous; RTS II is homozygous or compound heterozygous)

Affected pathway: encodes RECQ helicase; involved in double-stranded DNA break repair

Other cutaneous findings:

Skin: erythematous, edematous, blistering facial rash at 3 to 6 months old, later involving buttocks and extremities (diagnostic hallmark); chronic phase leads to poikiloderma, dyspigmentation (hypo- and hyper-pigmentation), telangiectasias, punctate atrophy

Hair: thin, brittle, sparse

Nails: dystrophic, pachyonychia

Extracutaneous manifestations:

General: growth retardation

Ocular: juvenile cataract

Dental: microdontia, rudimentary or hypoplastic teeth

MSK: increased risk of osteosarcoma

Other: RTS-I is milder (poikiloderma, juvenile cataract, ectodermal dysplasia); RTS-II presents with poikiloderma, congenital bone defects, increased risk of childhood osteosarcoma; patients require multidisciplinary management (dermatology, oncology, ophthalmology, orthopedic surgery); same life expectancy compared to general population

Bloom Syndrome

Skin cancer predisposition: SCC

Mode of inheritance: autosomal recessive

Epidemiology: Unknown overall prevalence; 1 in 48,000 in Ashkenazi Jewish population[28]

Age of onset of skin cancer: mean 31.8 years old

Genetic mutation(s): *BLM*

Affected pathway: encodes RecQL, which restores malfunctioning replication forks in DNA replication

Other cutaneous findings: severe photosensitivity, poikiloderma, telangiectasia

Extracutaneous manifestations: Severe growth retardation, high-pitched voices, prominent appearing muscles due to smaller subcutaneous fat layer, recurrent infections, diabetes, chronic pulmonary disease, predisposition to cancer development

Other: 14% of tumors in Bloom syndrome are SCC; patients are sensitive to DNA damaging therapies so radiation therapy and alkylating drugs should be avoided.

Epidermodysplasia Verruciformis

Skin cancer predisposition: SCC

Mode of inheritance: autosomal recessive

Epidemiology: <1 in 1,000,000[27]

Age of onset of skin cancer: second or third decade

Genetic mutation(s): *EVER1/TMC6, EVER2/TMC8*

Affected pathway: encode transmembrane channel

Other cutaneous findings:

Infancy: scaly red lesions similar to verruca plana; red-brown plaques and lesions resembling tinea versicolor

Adolescence and adulthood: pre-cancerous lesions on sun-exposed sites, may progress to invasive SCC

Other: these mutations make patients highly susceptible to HPV infections; ~90% of cSCCs are positive for HPV 5 or 8 (not included in currently available HPV vaccines)

Junctional Epidermolysis Bullosa

Skin cancer predisposition: SCC

Mode of inheritance: autosomal recessive

Epidemiology: 0.49 per million (prevalence); 2.68 per million (incidence)[14]

Genetic mutation(s): *LAMA3, LAMB3, LAMC2, COL17A1*

Other cutaneous findings: erosions, blisters, atrophic scarring, nail dystrophy

Extracutaneous manifestations: corneal blisters, tracheolaryngeal stenosis, urethral meatal stenosis, dilated cardiomyopathy, osteoporosis

Recessive Dystrophic Epidermolysis Bullosa

See (Figure 14.5C) for two images described in the caption.

Skin cancer predisposition: SCC, MM

Mode of inheritance: autosomal recessive

Epidemiology: 1.4 per million (prevalence); 3.0 per million (incidence)[5]

Genetic mutation(s): *COL7A1*

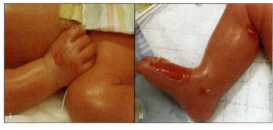

C

FIGURE 14.5C: Classic images of genetic syndromes associated with skin cancer. Epidermolysis bullosa. Intact bullae and erosions on acral surfaces in a neonate diagnosed with recessive dystrophic epidermolysis bullosa with mutations in type VII collagen.

Other cutaneous findings: erosions, blisters, atrophic scarring, nail dystrophy, pseudosyndactyly

Extracutaneous manifestations: corneal blisters, esophageal strictures, urethral meatal stenosis, dilated cardiomyopathy, osteoporosis

Oculocutaneous Albinism Type 1

Skin cancer predisposition: SCC

Mode of inheritance: autosomal recessive

Epidemiology: 1 in 40,000[27]

Genetic mutation: *TYR*

Affected pathway: absent (OCA1A) or reduced (OCA1B) tyrosinase activity

Other cutaneous findings: white skin/hair or pigmentary dilution, photosensitivity

Extracutaneous manifestations: blue-gray eyes, iris translucency, reduced visual acuity

Oculocutaneous Albinism Type 2

See (Figure 14.5D) for the image described in the caption.

Skin cancer predisposition: SCC

Mode of inheritance: autosomal recessive

Epidemiology: 1 in 36,000[27]

Genetic mutation: *OCA2*

Affected pathway: melanosomal transmembrane protein that may regulate organelle pH and processing/trafficking of tyrosinase

Other cutaneous findings: skin/hair pigmentary dilution

Extracutaneous manifestations: iris pigmentary dilution

Cowden Syndrome

Skin cancer predisposition: MM

Mode of inheritance: autosomal dominant

Genetic mutation: PTEN

Epidemiology: 1 in 200,000[5]

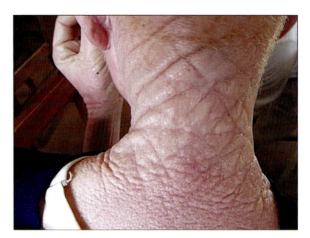

FIGURE 14.5D: Classic images of genetic syndromes associated with skin cancer.
Oculocutaneous albinism. Prominent solar elastosis on the posterior neck of this African patient with oculocutaneous albinism type 2. Used with permission from Rosemarie Mosher, MD.

Affected pathway: Phosphatidylinositol 3-kinase (PI3K)/AKT/mammalian target of rapamycin (mTOR) pathway, cell-cycle regulation and apoptosis

Other cutaneous findings: tricholemmomas, sclerotic fibromas, acral keratoses, oral papillomas

Extracutaneous manifestations: breast, thyroid, endometrial, renal malignancy, gastrointestinal hamartomas

Other: Screening recommendations: annual skin, thyroid, breast examination beginning at age 18. Annual thyroid ultrasound. Colonoscopy every 5 years beginning at age 35 or earlier (symptomatic or family history of colon cancer before age 40). In women, biannual breast examinations beginning at age 25 and monthly self-examinations, annual mammogram and breast MRI beginning at age 30 to 35 or earlier (5 to 10 years before youngest breast cancer diagnosis in family).

Familial Atypical Multiple Mole Melanoma Syndrome (FAMMM)

Skin cancer predisposition: Melanoma

Mode of inheritance: autosomal dominant, reduced penetrance and geographically variable expressivity

Epidemiology: 5 to 10% of all malignant melanomas are hereditary, 40% of them caused by mutations in *CDKN2A*; majority are caused by unknown mutations[29]

Age of onset of skin cancer: second and third decades of life

Genetic mutation(s):

P16/P16INK4A (also called *CDKN2A*) on 9p21.3sfasdffs

CDK4 (cyclin-dependent kinase 4)

Other pathogenic variants – *CDK6, BAP1, BRCA2*

Affected pathway:

Encodes for P16 and P14ARF; TP53 tumor-suppressor pathway

CDK4 insensitive to inhibition by protein P16

Other cutaneous findings: multiple melanocytic nevi (>50); often >1 mm

Extracutaneous manifestations: increased risk of pancreatic cancer

Other:

Diagnostic criteria:

1. Malignant melanoma in ≥1 first- or second-degree relatives
2. High total-body nevi count, some must be atypical (ABCDEs)
3. Nevi with specific histological features including architectural disorder with asymmetry, subepidermal fibroplasia, among others

In familial cases, mutations in *CDKN2A* are commonly implicated. However, a major population-based study suggested that *CDKN2A* may not actually contribute meaningfully to the overall incidence of melanoma. A large portion of familial cases do not have pathogenic variants in known susceptibility genes.[22]

BAP-1 Mutation Syndrome

Skin cancer predisposition: Melanoma, melanocytic *BAP-1* mutated atypical intradermal tumors (MBAITs), basal cell carcinoma

Mode of inheritance: autosomal dominant, high penetrance, in cases with multiple affected family members

Epidemiology: unknown

Age of onset of skin cancer: second decade of life (BAPomas); uveal melanomas ~50 years old (mean), as young as 16 years old reported

Genetic mutation(s): *BAP-1* (BRCA-1 associated protein-1)

Affected pathway: proposed role in DNA damage response, regulation of apoptosis, senescence, and cell cycle

Other cutaneous findings: uveal melanomas; BAPomas are often skin color or tan, elevated lesions

Extracutaneous manifestations: malignant mesothelioma, renal cell carcinoma

Other: Recommend biannual dermatology, annual ophthalmology evaluation and annual abdominal ultrasounds; q2 year MRI; annual physical exams focusing on risk of mesothelioma

Other Conditions with Increased Melanoma Risk

Genetic mutation(s): *MITF* (microphthalmia-associated transcription factor); *POT-1* (protection of telomeres 1), *ACD* (adrenocortical dysplasia protein homolog), *TERF2IP* (telomeric repeat binding factor 2 interacting protein), *TERT* (telomerase reverse transcriptase)

Affected pathway:

MITF: transcription factor in melanocytic lineage

POT-1: controls telomerase (shelterin complex)

ACD: controls telomerase (shelterin complex)

TERF2IP: controls telomerase (shelterin complex)

TERT: controls telomerase

▓ CLINICAL MANAGEMENT OF PATIENTS AT INCREASED RISK

The management of cutaneous malignancies relies on the interdisciplinary efforts of multiple providers including primary care physicians, dermatologists, oncologists, and surgeons. The following management recommendations are intended to provide a framework to approach a patient with a diagnosed, treated, or potential skin cancer. These recommendations are not inclusive of all appropriate methods of ongoing care and should be tailored to each patient's needs. We do not address specific lesion treatment.

Management of Melanoma

Patients at higher risk of developing melanoma, such as those with lightly pigmented skin (phototypes I-II), high nevi count (>100 melanocytic nevi), history of intense intermittent sun exposure or chronic sun exposure, positive family history, or tanning bed use, should be referred to dermatology for screening. Patients with lesions concerning for melanoma, guided by the ABCDE criteria or ugly duckling sign or other indicators, should also be referred for dermatologic evaluation.

Since 5 to 10% of melanomas are hereditary, genetic screening for familial melanomas has generated significant interest.[29] However, genetic testing remains controversial, even for high probability loci such as *CDKN2A*, the gene that accounts for approximately 20% of familial melanoma. Currently, clinical testing for *CDKN2A* is not recommended as most patients, even those with robust family history, will not be identified as having a pathogenic variant. Further, a positive test does not actually change clinical management and recommendations. There is substantial variation in the documented penetrance of the *CDKN2A* pathogenic variants (28 to 91%), thus a negative test result in a high-risk family is not particularly informative. These patients may still be at increased risk due to unknown factors (still with two-fold increased risk based on family history alone) and a false screening exam may provide false reassurance.[30] There are also potential harms associated with overdiagnosis or detection of biologically benign disease, including cosmetic or functional complications from potentially unnecessary diagnostic or treatment interventions, and long-lasting psychological effects for patients labeled with a serious or potentially life-threatening illness. Experts in support of genetic testing believe positive results may improve compliance with prevention strategies; however, studies suggest this may not be the case.

In medium-to-high melanoma incidence countries, including the United States, some have proposed that genetic testing should be offered to patients with three or more primary invasive melanomas or families with at least one invasive melanoma and two or more cases of melanoma or pancreatic cancer in first- and second-degree relatives.[29] Families identified by genetic testing should be referred for total body skin examinations, in an attempt to detect melanomas at earlier and thinner stages.[31] Although families with a CDKN2A mutation are at higher risk for pancreatic cancer (28% in affected families versus 6% of families without the mutation), guidelines for pancreatic cancer screening are not established.[32]

Management of Squamous Cell Carcinoma

The AAD recommends that patients with at least one cSCC should be evaluated with a total body skin examination by a dermatologist at least annually.[19] Additionally, for high-risk lesions, it is recommended that regional lymph nodes be palpated at these visits. Notably, the diagnosis of a nonmelanoma skin cancer increases the risk for malignant melanoma by 1.99 for men and 2.58 for women.[33]

Patients with a history of SCC should be instructed about the importance of daily sun protection, including wearing sun-protective clothing, wide-brimmed head coverings, and using broad-spectrum chemical and physical sunscreens. Compelling studies on the efficacy of other topical and oral agents in reducing risk of squamous cell carcinomas are limited. However, one phase-3, double-blind, randomized controlled trial showed that the rate of new NMSCs was reduced by 23% with nicotinamide 500 mg twice daily for 12 months. Patients included in this study had at least two NMSCs within the previous 5 years.[34] In renal transplant recipients with high burden of disease, acitretin (30 mg daily for 6 months) significantly reduced the occurrence of new squamous cell carcinomas compared to placebo.[35]

In xeroderma pigmentosum, aggressive sun avoidance from a young age is recommended. It is recommended that these patients have full-body photography of their skin, conjunctivae, and eyelids to aid in monitoring. Dermatologic and ophthalmologic screenings should be conducted every 6 months and 12 months, respectively. Finally, in the case of epidermolysis bullosa, skin screening exams are recommended as often as every 3 to 6 months starting at 10 years old for recessive dystrophic EB (severe subtype) or every 6 to 12 months starting at 20 years old in the absence of prior SCC diagnosis. These patients also need dental exams every 6 months.[14]

Management of Basal Cell Carcinoma

Once a basal cell carcinoma has been diagnosed, the patient should receive a total body skin examination conducted by a dermatologist at least annually.[16] The AAD strongly recommends counseling these patients on the need for regular sun protection. However, due to insufficient evidence regarding efficacy, the AAD has not published formal recommendations regarding the use of topical and oral agents, such as retinoids, for risk reduction in this patient population.

Genetic Testing in Hereditary Cancer Syndromes

According to the First International Colloquium on Basal Cell Nevus Syndrome, diagnosis of Gorlin syndrome should be suspected based on major and minor criteria (Table 14.3).[36] To avoid delays in diagnosis, triggers for early screening include the presence of BCC or odontogenic keratocysts in patients younger than 20 years of age, palmar or plantar pits, lamellar calcification of the falx cerebri, or medulloblastoma with desmoplastic histology (in addition to any major or minor criteria). Since clinical criteria are often sufficient to confirm the diagnosis, genetic testing is not always warranted. However, molecular confirmation of a *PTCH1* mutation is indicated for prenatal testing with a known familial mutation, for predictive testing in individuals with an affected family member, and for confirmatory diagnosis when clinical signs are not sufficient to meet criteria. Finally, children diagnosed with BCNS should be followed by a medical geneticist annually and undergo total body skin examinations every 6 to 12 months after developing the first BCC. Adults require more frequent dermatologic total body skin examinations; a minimum of every four months is recommended.

Clinical genetic testing for other hereditary cancer syndromes may be found at the NIH Genetic Testing Registry. Available tests exist for BAP-1 tumor syndrome (*BAP1*), Bloom syndrome (*BLM*), Brook-Spiegler syndrome (*CYLD*), Chediak-Higashi syndrome (*LYST*), Cowden syndrome (*PTEN*), dyskeratosis congenita (*DKC1, TERC, TINF2, NHP2, NOP10, TERT*), dystrophic epidermolysis bullosa (*COL7A1*), Fanconi anemia (*BRIP1, FANCA, FANCC, FANCE, FANCF, FANCG, PALB2, BRCA1, BRCA2, ERCC4, RAD51C, SLX4*), Gricelli syndrome (*RAB27A*), Hermansky-Pudlak syndrome (*HPS1, HPS3, HPS4, HPS7*), junctional epidermolysis bullosa (*LAMA3, LAMB3, LAMC2, COL17A1*), keratitis-ichthyosis-deafness syndrome (*GJB2*), Muir-Torre syndrome (*MLH1, MSH2*), oculocutaneous albinism (*TYR, TYRP1, OCA2*), Rothmund-Thomson syndrome (*RECQL4*), Schöpf-Schulz-Passarge syndrome (WNT10A), and Xeroderma pigmentosum (*XPA, XPC*) (adapted from the National Cancer Institute, https://www.cancer.gov/types/skin/hp/skin-genetics-pdq).[14]

Although genetic testing in these patients remains of uncertain clinical value at this time, it will likely become more useful in the future as genome-wide and exome sequencing become the standard of care and more pathogenic variants, including low-penetrance susceptibility alleles, are identified.

References

1. Guy GP Jr., Machlin SR, Ekwueme DU, et al. Prevalence and costs of skin cancer treatment in the U.S., 2002–2006 and 2007–2011. *Am J Prev Med.* 2015;48(2):183–187.

2. Guy GP Jr., Thomas CC, Thompson T, et al. Vital signs: melanoma incidence and mortality trends and projections: United States, 1982–2030. *MMWR Morb Mortal Wkly Rep.* 2015;64(21):591–596.

3. Stern RS. Prevalence of a history of skin cancer in 2007: results of an incidence-based model. *Arch Dermatol.* 2010;146(3):279–282.

4. American Cancer Society. Cancer Facts & Figures 2020.

5. Bolognia JL, Schaffer JV, Cerroni L. *Dermatology.* Fourth Edition. 2018.

6. American Academy of Dermatology. *Prevent Skin Cancer.* 2020.

7. U.S. Department of Health and Human Services. In *The Surgeon General's Call to Action to Prevent Skin Cancer.* Washington, DC; 2014.

8. Bergenmar M, Brandberg Y. Sunbathing and sun-protection behaviors and attitudes of young Swedish adults with hereditary risk for malignant melanoma. *Cancer Nurs.* 2001;24(5):341–350.

9. Manne S, Fasanella N, Connors J, et al. Sun protection and skin surveillance practices among relatives of patients with malignant melanoma: prevalence and predictors. *Prev Med.* 2004;39(1):36–47.

10. Maguire-Eisen M. Risk assessment and early detection of skin cancers. *Semin Oncol Nurs.* 2003;19(1):43–51.

11. Swetter SM, Tsao H, Bichakjian CK, et al. Guidelines of care for the management of primary cutaneous melanoma. *J Am Acad Dermatol.* 2019;80(1):208–250.

12. Dennis LK, Vanbeek MJ, Beane Freeman LE, et al. Sunburns and risk of cutaneous melanoma: does age matter? A comprehensive meta-analysis. *Ann Epidemiol.* 2008;18(8):614–627.

13. Wu S, Han J, Laden F, et al. Long-term ultraviolet flux, other potential risk factors, and skin cancer risk: a cohort study. *Cancer Epidemiol Biomarkers Prev.* 2014;23(6):1080–1089.

14. PDQ® Cancer Genetics Editorial Board. PDQ Genetics of Skin Cancer. *National Cancer Institute.* Updated Feburary 14, 2019.

15. Koh HK, Miller DR, Geller AC, et al. Who discovers melanoma? Patterns from a population-based survey. *J Am Acad Dermatol.* 1992;26(6):914–919.

16. Work G, Invited R, Kim JYS, et al. Guidelines of care for the management of basal cell carcinoma. *J Am Acad Dermatol.* 2018;78(3):540–559.

17. Wehner MR, Linos E, Parvataneni R, et al. Timing of subsequent new tumors in patients who present with basal cell carcinoma or cutaneous squamous cell carcinoma. *JAMA Dermatol.* 2015;151(4):382–388.

18. Muzic JG, Schmitt AR, Wright AC, et al. Incidence and Trends of Basal Cell Carcinoma and Cutaneous Squamous Cell Carcinoma: A Population-Based Study in Olmsted County, Minnesota, 2000 to 2010. *Mayo Clin Proc.* 2017;92(6):890–898.

19. Work G, Invited R, Kim JYS, et al. Guidelines of care for the management of cutaneous squamous cell carcinoma. *J Am Acad Dermatol.* 2018;78(3):560–578.

20. Siegel RL, Miller KD, Jemal A. Cancer statistics, 2020. *CA Cancer J Clin.* 2020;70(1):7–30.

21. Noone A, Howlader N, Krapcho M, et al. SEER Cancer Statistics Review, 1975–2015. *National Cancer Institute.* 2018.

22. Berwick M, Orlow I, Hummer AJ, et al. The prevalence of CDKN2A germ-line mutations and relative risk for cutaneous malignant melanoma: an international population-based study. *Cancer Epidemiol Biomarkers Prev.* 2006;15(8):1520–1525.

23. Agbai ON, Buster K, Sanchez M, et al. Skin cancer and photoprotection in people of color: a review and recommendations for physicians and the public. *J Am Acad Dermatol.* 2014;70(4):748–762.

24. Mucci LA, Hjelmborg JB, Harris JR, et al. Familial risk and heritability of cancer among twins in Nordic countries. *JAMA.* 2016;315(1):68–76.

25. High A, Zedan W. Basal cell nevus syndrome. *Curr Opin Oncol.* 2005;17(2):160–166.

26. Rees JR, Zens MS, Gui J, et al. Non melanoma skin cancer and subsequent cancer risk. *PLoS One.* 2014;9(6):e99674.

27. Jaju PD, Ransohoff KJ, Tang JY, et al. Familial skin cancer syndromes: Increased risk of nonmelanotic skin cancers and extracutaneous tumors. *J Am Acad Dermatol.* 2016;74(3):437–451; quiz 452–434.

28. Shahrabani-Gargir L, Shomrat R, Yaron Y, et al. High frequency of a common Bloom syndrome Ashkenazi mutation among Jews of Polish origin. *Genet Test.* 1998;2(4):293–296.

29. Leachman SA, Carucci J, Kohlmann W, et al. Selection criteria for genetic assessment of patients with familial melanoma. *J Am Acad Dermatol.* 2009;61(4):677 e671–614.

30. Badenas C, Aguilera P, Puig-Butille JA, et al. Genetic counseling in melanoma. *Dermatol Ther.* 2012; 25(5):397–402.

31. Carli P, De Giorgi V, Palli D, et al. Dermatologist detection and skin self-examination are associated with thinner melanomas: results from a survey of the Italian Multidisciplinary Group on Melanoma. *Arch Dermatol.* 2003;139(5):607–612.

32. Goldstein AM, Chan M, Harland M, et al. High-risk melanoma susceptibility genes and pancreatic cancer, neural system tumors, and uveal melanoma across GenoMEL. *Cancer Res.* 2006;66(20):9818–9828.

33. Song F, Qureshi AA, Giovannucci EL, et al. Risk of a second primary cancer after non-melanoma skin cancer in white men and women: a prospective cohort study. *PLoS Med.* 2013;10(4):e1001433.

34. Chen AC, Martin AJ, Choy B, et al. A phase 3 randomized trial of nicotinamide for skin-cancer chemoprevention. *N Engl J Med.* 2015;373(17):1618–1626.

35. Bavinck JN, Tieben LM, Van der Woude FJ, et al. Prevention of skin cancer and reduction of keratotic skin lesions during acitretin therapy in renal transplant recipients: a double-blind, placebo-controlled study. *J Clin Oncol.* 1995;13(8):1933–1938.

36. Bree AF, Shah MR, Group BC. Consensus statement from the first international colloquium on basal cell nevus syndrome (BCNS). *Am J Med Genet A.* 2011;155A(9):2091–2097.

CHAPTER 15

Risk Assessment and Clinical Management – Pediatric and Other Cancers

Stephanie Prozora and Gary M. Kupfer

INTRODUCTION

Great strides have been made to improve outcomes for pediatric patients suffering from cancer, decreasing mortality by over 50% in the last half century. Despite these advancements in care, cancer remains a leading cause of mortality for children across the world. In the United States alone, approximately 15,800 children under age 20 are diagnosed with cancer annually, and nearly 2,000 are expected to die from the disease. Leukemia, lymphoma, and central nervous system tumors are the most common new cancer diagnoses in the pediatric age group. While many patients and families search for an explanation of why they have been afflicted by such a devastating illness, most pediatric cancers occur without known cause. Until recent years, a very small percentage of pediatric cancer was felt to be related to a genetic predisposition. With the advancement of modern techniques in molecular analysis, more cancer predisposition syndromes have been identified, and an estimated 10% of pediatric patients with cancer have a heritable cause. Early identification of these patients and initiation of cancer surveillance protocols is essential for reducing cancer-related mortality.[1-4]

Heritable cancer predisposition syndromes in the pediatric population are a heterogenous group of disorders with a broad array of genotypic and phenotypic characteristics. In the simplest terms, a change in a child's genetic makeup results in an imbalance in the system that regulates a cell's ability to grow, differentiate, proliferate, and die. The mechanisms by which this imbalance and instability results in the development of malignancy can be used to characterize cancer predisposition syndromes into the following groups of defects: (1) DNA repair, (2) tumor suppressor genes, (3) proto-oncogenes, (4) transcription factors, (5) telomeres and RNA metabolism, (6) constitutional chromosomal abnormalities, and (7) primary immunodeficiency (Table 15.1).

DISORDERS OF DNA REPAIR

Ataxia Telangiectasia

Syndrome Overview Ataxia telangiectasia (AT) is a rare autosomal recessive genetic disorder with an estimated incidence of 1:40,000 to 1:100,000. A loss-of-function variant

TABLE 15.1: Heritable Cancer Predisposition Syndromes by Category

Defect Category	Syndrome	Commonly Associated Pediatric Cancers
DNA Repair	Ataxia Telangiectasia	NHL, HD, ALL
	Bloom Syndrome	NHL, ALL, AML, Wilms, Carcinomas (GI, Breast)
	Congenital Mismatch Repair Deficiency Syndrome	Gliomas, NHL (T-cell), ALL (T-cell), Carcinomas (GI)
	Fanconi Anemia	AML, Carcinomas (Head/Neck, Breast), CNS Tumors
	Nijmegen Breakage Syndrome	NHL (DLBCL, T-cell lymphoblastic lymphoma)
	Rothmund-Thomson Syndrome	Osteosarcoma
	Xeroderma Pigmentosum	Non-melanoma Skin Cancer, Melanoma
Tumor Suppressor Genes	Bohring-Opitz Syndrome	Wilms
	Familial Adenomatous Polyposis	Carcinoma (GI), Hepatoblastoma, Medulloblastoma
	Gorlin Syndrome	Basal Cell Carcinoma, Medulloblastoma
	Hereditary Leiomyomatosis and Renal Cell Cancer	Renal Cell Carcinoma
	Hereditary Paraganglioma-Pheochromocytoma Syndrome	Paraganglioma, Pheochromocytoma
	Hereditary Retinoblastoma	Retinoblastoma, Sarcomas (Osteosarcoma)
	Li-Fraumeni	Sarcomas (Osteosarcoma, Soft Tissue), CNS Tumors, Adrenocortical Carcinoma
	Juvenile Polyposis Syndrome	Carcinomas (GI)
	Multiple Endocrine Neoplasia Type 1	Anterior Pituitary Adenomas, Pancreatic Islet Tumors, Parathyroid Adenomas
	Neurofibromatosis 1	Glioma (Optic, CNS), MPNST, JMML
	Neurofibromatosis 2	Schwannomas, Meningiomas, Ependymomas
	Peutz-Jeghers Syndrome	GI Tumors, Pancreatic Tumors, and Gonadal Tumors
	PTEN Hamartoma-Tumor Syndrome	Epithelioid Differentiated Thyroid Cancer
	RASopathies (Non-NF1)	Rhabdomyosarcoma, Neuroblastoma, Bladder Neoplasms, JMML
	Rhabdoid Tumor Predisposition Syndrome	Rhabdoid Tumors (Brain, Kidney)
	Simpson-Golabi-Behmel Syndrome	Wilms, Neuroblastoma
	Tuberous Sclerosis	Subependymal Giant Cell Astrocytoma
	Von Hippel-Lindau Disease	Hemangioblastoma, Pheochromocytoma
Proto-oncogenes	Hereditary Neuroblastoma	Neuroblastoma
	Mulibrey Nanism	Wilms
	Multiple Endocrine Neoplasia Type 2	Medullary Thyroid Carcinoma, Pheochromocytoma
Transcription Factor Genes	Beckwith-Weidemann Syndrome	Wilms, Hepatoblastoma, Neuroblastoma
	WT1 Related Syndromes	Wilms
Telomeres and RNA	Diamond-Blackfan Anemia	Myelodysplastic Syndrome, AML
	DICER1 Syndrome	Pleuropulmonary Blastoma, Gonadal Tumors, Rhabdomyosarcoma
	Dyskeratosis Congenita	Myelodysplastic Syndrome, AML, Squamous Cell Carcinoma
	Perlman Syndrome	Wilms
	Schwachman-Diamond Syndrome	Myelodysplastic Syndrome, AML

TABLE 15.1: Heritable Cancer Predisposition Syndromes by Category *(Continued)*

Defect Category	Syndrome	Commonly Associated Pediatric Cancers
Constitutional Chromosomal Abnormalities	Trisomy 18 (Edwards Syndrome)	Wilms, Hepatoblastoma
	Trisomy 21 (Down Syndrome)	ALL, AML, AMKL
Primary Immunodeficiency Disorders	Common Variable Immunodeficiency Syndrome	NHL
	DiGeorge Syndrome	ALL, NHL
	Hyper-Immunoglobulin M Syndrome	Carcinoma (GI, Liver), HD
	Severe Combined Immunodeficiency	NHL, HD
	Severe Congenital Neutropenia	AML
	Wiskott-Aldrich Syndrome	NHL, ALL
	X-Linked Lymphoproliferative Disease	NHL

Abbreviations: ALL = acute lymphocytic leukemia; AMKL = acute megakaryocytic leukemia; AML = acute myeloid leukemia; CNS = central nervous system; DLBCL = diffuse large B-cell lymphoma; GI = gastrointestinal; HD = Hodgkin disease; JMML = juvenile myelomonocytic leukemia; MPNST = malignant peripheral nerve sheath tumor; NF1 = neurofibromatosis 1; NHL = non-Hodgkin lymphoma.

of the ataxia-telangiectasia mutated (*ATM*) gene is implicated in the pathogenesis of this childhood disorder. The *ATM* gene typically encodes a cell-cycle checkpoint kinase in the phosphatidylinositol-3 kinase protein family that is activated by DNA damage and regulates multiple tumor suppressor genes, including *p53* and *BRCA1*. With genotoxic stress, cells develop double-stranded DNA breaks; mutations in *ATM* prevent the appropriate response to this DNA damage creating genomic instability. This genomic instability often leads to cell death, specifically in neuronal cells, resulting in the progressive cerebellar ataxia that is the hallmark of AT. Other clinical features of this multisystem disorder include chorea, oculomotor apraxia, telangiectasias, and sinopulmonary infections related to immunodeficiency.[5–7]

Diagnosis AT can be diagnosed on newborn screening. T-cell receptor excision circle testing, typically used to diagnose severe combined immunodeficiency, can also identify infants with lymphocytopenia secondary to AT. For patients not identified with newborn screening, the diagnosis should be suspected in patients with typical clinical presentation in early childhood with elevated alpha-fetoprotein levels or abnormal brain MRI. For all patients, confirmatory testing with *ATM* gene sequencing is required.[5,7,8]

Cancer Risk Given their deficiencies in DNA repair and susceptibility to genomic instability, patients with AT are at significantly increased risk for malignancy. There is an approximate 25% lifetime malignancy risk with non-Hodgkin lymphoma accounting for most cases, although lymphoblastic leukemia and Hodgkin lymphoma are also common. Carcinomas occur but typically present at older ages. These patients show significant sensitivity to ionizing radiation resulting in increased malignancy risk.[5,7,9,10]

Management and Cancer Surveillance AT is a complex disorder requiring a multi-disciplinary team including neurologists, immunologists, pulmonologists, and physical therapists. Basic management strategies include IVIG repletion to reduce infectious complications and avoidance of ionizing radiation to mitigate malignancy risk. There are no evidence-based guidelines specific to cancer screening. An annual exam by an oncologist with laboratory evaluation (complete blood count, comprehensive metabolic panel, lactate dehydrogenase) to surveil for leukemia and lymphoma has been suggested. Special consideration is needed in choosing chemotherapeutic regimens for patients who do develop malignancy as deficient DNA repair puts them at increased risk of treatment-related toxicity.[5-7]

Bloom Syndrome

Syndrome Overview Bloom syndrome is a rare autosomal recessive disorder afflicting a few hundred identified patients. People of Ashkenazi Jewish descent are more commonly affected. The *BLM* gene encodes a DNA helicase responsible for unwinding DNA and limiting sister chromatid exchange. In patients with Bloom syndrome, biallelic mutations in the *BLM* gene result in deficient protein production causing high rates of sister chromatid exchange and subsequent genomic instability. Significant clinical features include growth deficiency, recurrent infections, decreased fertility, and sensitivity to sun exposure.[5,11,12]

Diagnosis Single-gene sequencing is available for diagnostic testing but may yield unclear results with variants of uncertain significance (VUS). Follow-up functional testing can be performed using a sister chromatid exchange assay to assess gene function, which demonstrates a 10- to 20-fold higher rate above baseline.[5,11]

Cancer Risk The exact risk of malignancy in this population is unclear given the small number of affected patients. Approximately 212 cancers have been reported in the 136 identified patients with Bloom syndrome. While leukemia and lymphoma are the most common pediatric malignancies associated with this syndrome, the spectrum of malignancies is broad and includes colorectal cancers, carcinomas, sarcomas, Wilms, retinoblastoma, and medulloblastoma. There is a higher incidence of multiple malignancies within the same patient.[5,11,12]

Management and Cancer Surveillance Given their significantly increased potential for diverse malignancies, patients would likely benefit from physician counseling and multiple screening modalities. Families should be made aware of generalized symptoms of cancer and be counseled to inform their doctor of any persistent symptoms. Consensus guidelines recommend screening for leukemia and myelodysplasia with complete blood counts every 3 to 4 months from time of diagnosis. Wilms tumor screening should begin at diagnosis with renal ultrasound every 3 months until age 8. For colorectal cancer screening, annual colonoscopy and fecal immunochemical testing is recommended every 6 months starting at age 15. Early breast cancer surveillance should begin with an annual breast MRI at age 18. Ionizing radiation should be avoided, given the likely increased malignancy risk.[5,11]

Congenital Mismatch Repair Deficiency Syndrome

Syndrome Overview Congenital mismatch repair deficiency syndrome (CMMRD) is an autosomal recessive disorder of unclear incidence. Since its recognition in 1999, less than 200 cases have been reported. In healthy individuals, the mismatch repair system is integral for correction of base pair mismatch during replication. Mutations in several identified genes (*MSH2, MLH1, PMS2, MSH6*) and associated promotors (i.e., *EPCAM*) have been associated with cancer syndromes. Heterozygous mutations result in Lynch syndrome, which has been associated most frequently with adult onset colorectal cancers. Homozygous mutations, most commonly of *MSH6* and *PMS2*, result in CMMRD. In addition to early onset childhood cancers, the clinical presentation of this disease can include skin lesions (i.e., café au lait macules and pilomatricomas), venous malformations, and mild immune deficiency.[13]

Diagnosis Patients with CMMRD can be difficult to diagnose as many have unaffected parents due to varying penetrance of the involved genes. The Care for CMMRD Consortium has developed a scoring system that can be used to identify patients at risk and in need of testing. Gene testing for biallelic mutations in the four mismatch repair genes is necessary for diagnosis. Staining for mismatch repair proteins by immunohistochemistry can also aid in diagnosis and will typically be absent in both normal and tumor tissue in patients with CMMRD. Because of variations in protein expression with VUS, the presence of a mismatch repair protein via immunohistochemistry does not preclude the diagnosis of CMMRD, and gene testing is necessary for confirmation.[13,14]

Cancer Risk Most patients with CMMRD will develop childhood cancer and are at increased risk of developing multiple malignancies simultaneously. The most common cancers associated with the syndrome include central nervous system tumors (i.e., gliomas) and non-Hodgkin lymphoma (i.e., T-lymphoblastic lymphoma). Other malignancies experienced in the first two decades of life by patients with CMMRD are leukemia, sarcomas, Wilms tumor, neuroblastoma, and genito-urinary cancers. Polyposis and malignancies typical of Lynch syndrome, including colorectal cancer, are also common.[13]

Management and Cancer Surveillance Diagnosis of malignancy in CMMRD portends a very poor prognosis. While germline sensitivity to chemotherapy and radiation has not been identified in CMMRD, special considerations must be made in designing chemotherapy plans for these patients, and medications that require adequate mismatch repair should be avoided (i.e., mercaptopurine). Management strategies utilizing immune checkpoint inhibitors for treatment and, potentially, tumor prevention have shown some benefit and require further investigation. Screening protocols for early tumor identification are paramount for allowing prompt initiation of therapy. Brain tumor screening at time of diagnosis and every 6 months is recommended. Additional imaging recommendations include annual colonoscopy beginning at 6 years and annual endoscopy beginning at 8 years. If polyps are identified the screening interval should decrease to 6 months. Screening CBCs and abdominal ultrasounds are recommended twice a year beginning at age 1. Recent guidelines suggest additional screening should include annual whole-body MRI beginning at age 6.[13,15]

Fanconi Anemia

Syndrome Overview Fanconi anemia (FA) is a rare disorder with an estimated incidence of 1:40,000 to 1:100,000. Inheritance of FA is typically autosomal recessive; however, autosomal dominant and X-linked mutations have also been identified. At least 22 genes have been identified in the FA pathway. When intact, the proteins transcribed from these genes are responsible for repair of DNA crosslinks. Mutations affecting the pathway cause genomic instability, and, as a result, bone marrow failure and predisposition to cancer. In two-thirds of patients, additional clinical features can be identified, including abnormal or absent thumbs, abnormal or absent radii, short stature, and microcephaly.[5,16,17]

Diagnosis FA often presents with signs and symptoms of bone marrow failure. In these cases, bone marrow aspiration and biopsy are performed. Additionally, functional testing of lymphocytes in peripheral blood through a chromosomal breakage assay with diepoxybutane or mitomycin C is indicated to screen for FA. Confirmatory testing with gene sequencing should also be obtained.[5,16]

Cancer Risk Patients with FA are at significantly increased risk of malignancy beginning in childhood. By age 50, approximately 10% of patients will develop AML, and 30% will develop a solid tumor (i.e., squamous cell carcinomas of head and neck, breast cancers, brain tumors). While patients who develop FA almost always display autosomal recessive genetics (FA-B is X-linked), heterozygous carriers of mutations of several FA genes including *FANCS* (*BRCA1*) and *FANCD1* (*BRCA2*) portend significant breast and ovarian cancer risk. Heterozygous mutations in *FANCJ* (*BRIP1*), *FANCN* (*PALB2*), and *FANCO* (*RAD51C*) are also associated with increased cancer risk. Additionally, exposure to ionizing radiation and chemotherapeutic agents that cause DNA damage increases cancer risk in patients with FA.[5,16–18]

Management and Cancer Surveillance Because AML in patients with FA is significantly difficult to treat, current management strategies center around hematopoietic stem cell transplant prior to the development of AML. Early referral to a stem cell transplant center is crucial. While this strategy has been effective in preventing AML, it does not decrease the risk for future solid tumors, and post-transplant patients may display an even increased risk of squamous cell carcinomas. Therefore, regular screening is essential for all patients, especially for those who are post-transplant. Screening for bone marrow failure and hematologic malignancies with annual bone marrow biopsies and frequent CBCs is recommended. Because of the high risk of developing head and neck squamous cell carcinomas, it is also recommended that patients do monthly oral self-exams in addition to annual ENT exams beginning in adolescence. In addition to surveillance for children with FA, family members with heterozygous mutations known to increase cancer risk may also benefit from early screening including breast cancer surveillance as adults.[5,16]

Nijmegen Breakage Syndrome

Syndrome Overview Nijmegen breakage syndrome (NBS) is an autosomal recessive condition with an approximate incidence of 1:100,000 and increased prevalence in people of Eastern and Central European descent. The *NBN* gene encodes nibrin, a necessary protein component of a DNA repair complex. Biallelic mutations in the *NBN* gene result in a loss of function allowing for accumulation of double-stranded DNA breaks. In addition to an increased risk for malignancy, clinical features of NBS include immunodeficiency with recurrent sinopulmonary infections, microcephaly, and abnormal "bird-like" facies. Patients with NBS typically have intellectual decline after the first two years of life.[5,19]

Diagnosis Evaluation for NBS should occur in patients with the primary clinical features: microcephaly, recurrent sinopulmonary infection, and malignancy. Chromosomal breakage assays will be positive in patients with NBS. Definitive diagnosis requires confirmatory *NBN* gene sequencing.[5,19]

Cancer Risk For patients with NBS, malignancy is a significant cause of mortality. An estimated 40% of patients will develop cancer in their first two decades of life. The most common malignancies are non-Hodgkin lymphomas of either B- or T-cell lineages; however, the spectrum includes leukemias, central nervous system tumors (i.e., medulloblastoma, glioma) and sarcomas (i.e., rhabdomyosarcoma). Like most disorders of DNA repair, patients with NBS who are exposed to ionizing radiation are at increased risk of malignancy.[5,19]

Management and Cancer Surveillance Because of their disease complexity, patients with NBS benefit from a multidisciplinary approach with input from immunology, pulmonology, and endocrinology, as well as oncology. Management strategies to reduce infectious complications include regular IVIG repletion. From a malignancy screening perspective, annual CBC, CMP, and LDH are appropriate.[5]

Rothmund-Thomson Syndrome

Syndrome Overview Rothmund-Thomson syndrome (RTS) is a rare autosomal recessive disorder with only a few hundred identified cases reported. There are two identified types of RTS. The genetic cause of Type 1 has not been identified. Clinically, patients with Type 1 RTS present with the characteristic skin finding of poikiloderma (changes in pigmentation with telangiectasias and atrophy) in infancy along with other associated findings of hair changes, short stature, skeletal/dental anomalies, and cataracts. Type 2 RTS is caused by a mutation in the *RECQL4* DNA helicase gene causing deficiencies in DNA repair and maintenance of telomeres. In addition to the feature described for Type 1 patients, patients with Type 2 RTS are at increased risk for malignancy.[5,20]

Diagnosis Patients with the clinical features of RTS, especially skin findings, should have confirmatory testing with *RECQL4* gene sequencing. This testing is important for discerning which patients have Type 2 RTS and are at increased risk of malignancy.[5,20]

Cancer Risk The incidence of cancer in patients with Type 2 RTS is unclear because of the small number of reported cases, but it appears to be much higher than the general population. *RECQL4* mutation type appears to convey different malignancy risk and genotyping may improve understanding of individual patient risk. The most common presentation is early onset osteosarcoma occurring in about 7 to 32% of patients. Basal and squamous cell skin cancers and hematologic malignancies have also been described. Malignancy risk is increased with exposure to ionizing radiation.[5,20,21]

Management and Cancer Surveillance Patients with RTS require management by dermatology, ophthalmology, and oncology. Annual skin exams for cancer screening and ophthalmology exams for cataracts are recommended. For patients at increased risk of osteosarcoma, the utility of routine screening is unclear. Currently a baseline skeletal survey to identify skeletal abnormalities is recommended by age 5. Patients should be counseled regarding cancer risk and evaluated for any concerning symptoms.[5]

Xeroderma Pigmentosum

Syndrome Overview Xeroderma pigmentosum (XP) is a rare autosomal recessive disorder affecting approximately 1:1,000,000. Mutations in several different nucleotide excision repair genes have been associated with XP. These mutations result in genomic instability due to nucleotide excision repair defects with extreme sensitivity to ultraviolet light. Sun sensitivity with freckling and increased risk of skin cancer is the hallmark of the disorder. Other clinical features may include cognitive impairment, keratitis, and sensorineural hearing loss.[5,22]

Diagnosis The diagnosis of XP requires identification of the clinical manifestations of the disorder. Confirmatory gene sequencing is available for patients where there is a high clinical suspicion.[5]

Cancer Risk Patients with XP are at greatest risk for the development of skin cancers; they have a 10,000-fold increased risk of developing basal or squamous cell carcinoma and a

2,000-fold increased risk of developing melanoma in the first two decades of life. Risk of skin cancer is increased with light exposure, especially UVA and UVB. Other malignancy types such as leukemia and CNS tumors have been reported.[5,23]

Management and Surveillance For patients with XP, the primary management strategy is prevention through limitation of sun exposure to the skin and eyes. Screening recommendations include dermatology evaluations every 3 months. Additional evaluations by ENT and ophthalmology every 6 months are recommended for cancer screening and hearing/vision testing.[5]

▓ DISORDERS OF TUMOR SUPPRESSOR GENES

Bohring-Opitz Syndrome

Syndrome Overview Bohring-Opitz syndrome (BOS) is an autosomal dominant condition with nearly all cases representing *de novo* mutations and a very small proportion related to parental gonadal mosaicism. BOS is exceedingly rare with less than 50 cases reported in literature. The syndrome has been linked to mutations in *ASXL-1*, a tumor suppressor that regulates Hox genes. Clinical features of BOS are severe developmental delay, abnormal facies with microcephaly and cleft lip/palate, retinal anomalies, upper/lower limb osseous abnormalities (radial head dislocation, ulnar deviation of fingers), structural brain abnormalities, and seizures. Nearly half of affected children die in early childhood.[24,25]

Diagnosis Genetic testing should be obtained in patients with clinical features of the syndrome.

Cancer Risk Given the rarity of BOS and the high-incidence of early mortality for affected patients, cancer risk is likely an underestimate. The primary malignancy seen in these patient is Wilms tumor with an estimated incidence in reported cases of 7%.[24,25]

Management and Screening BOS patients have complex symptomatology requiring care from multiple subspecialties. From a cancer surveillance perspective, renal ultrasounds are recommended every 3 months until age 7.[24]

Familial Adenomatous Polyposis

Syndrome Overview Familial adenomatous polyposis (FAP) is an autosomal dominant inherited genetic disorder with an estimated incidence of 1:9,000 to 1:18,000. A mutation in the *APC* gene, a tumor suppressor in the WNT pathway, causes a loss of function resulting in increased cellular proliferation. The primary resultant clinical manifestation is gastrointestinal polyps. Extracolonic features may include soft tissue tumors, ophthalmologic abnormalities, dental anomalies, and osteomas.[26,27]

Diagnosis Patients with concerning clinical findings for FAP including polyposis (>100 polyps), ocular findings, or Gardner-associated fibromas should have gene sequencing of the *APC* gene. Testing for patients from affected families is controversial but should be considered prior to the start of screening (~10 years old).[26,27]

Cancer Risk For patients with FAP, malignancies of the gastrointestinal tract are most common. Without colectomy, virtually all patients will develop colorectal cancer in adulthood. In addition to colorectal cancer, children with FAP have a 1 to 2% risk of hepatoblastoma and a less than 1% risk of WNT-activated medulloblastoma. In general patients, are at an increased risk for papillary thyroid carcinoma, but this is less common in the pediatric age group.[26,27]

Management and Surveillance Current medical management and well-established screening protocols for FAP have improved survival. Current recommendations include flexible sigmoidoscopy or colonoscopy annually starting at age 10 until colectomy. Upper endoscopy is recommended beginning at age 20. Annual physical exams should include assessment of the thyroid to detect potential malignancy. Regarding hepatoblastoma, no consensus guidelines exist. Consideration can be given to screening with abdominal ultrasounds and laboratory evaluation of AFP every 3 months from birth until age 4 to 7.[26,27]

Gorlin Syndrome

Syndrome Overview Gorlin syndrome (GS) is a rare autosomal dominant condition with an incidence of 1:15,000. Mutations in the *PTCH1* and *SUFU* genes have been implicated in GS pathogenesis. Both genes encode tumor suppressors in the sonic hedgehog pathway. With loss of heterozygosity, mutations in these genes result in cellular proliferation and tumor development. When first described, three primary clinical features were associated with GS: basal cell carcinomas, jaw cysts, and bifid ribs. Additional features common to patients with GS are plantar/palmar pits, calcification of the falx cerebri, hypertelorism, and macrocephaly.[28,29]

Diagnosis Established clinical criteria for diagnosing GS include (1) multiple basal cell carcinoma or basal cell carcinoma at age less than 30, (2) jaw keratocysts, (3) palmar/plantar pits, (4) lamellar calcification of the falx, or (5) first-degree relative with GS. Gene sequencing of *PTCH1* and *SUFU* is recommended for all patients meeting clinical criteria. Gene testing is also recommended in infancy for patients with a family history. Moreover, patients with neuroblastoma should undergo gene testing if they have a family member meeting any criteria for GS or they develop neuroblastoma before age 3 with somatic sonic hedgehog abnormalities, desmoplastic histology, or nodular histology.[28,29]

Cancer Risk Basal cell carcinoma is the primary malignancy identified in patients with GS. In the pediatric age group, there is also an increased risk of medulloblastoma, specifically desmoplastic subtype, occurring in about 5% of patients. Risk for development of medulloblastoma is greater in patients with *SUFU* mutations compared to those with *PTCH1* mutations. Additional rare malignancies, such as rhabdomyosarcomas, have also been reported in patients with GS, although their incidence is unclear.[28,29]

Management and Surveillance Surveillance strategies for GS vary based on genetic mutation. For patients with variants of *SUFU* or *PTCH1*, basal cell screening is recommended annually beginning at age 10. For patients with *SUFU* mutations, medulloblastoma surveillance with brain MRI every 4 months through age 3 and every 6 months through age 5 is recommended. Routine screening for medulloblastoma in patients with *PTCH1* mutations is not indicated. Regardless of their genetic variant, all patients with GS who develop medulloblastoma should receive radiation sparing therapy when possible to reduce skin cancer risk.[28]

Hereditary Leiomyomatosis and Renal Cell Cancer

Syndrome Overview Hereditary leiomyomatosis and renal cell cancer (HLRCC) is a rare autosomal dominant disorder. The fumarate hydratase gene is affected, causing fumarate increase due to its role in the Krebs cycle, with subsequent activation of pathways causing cell proliferation. The resulting clinical features of HLRCC include cutaneous piloleiomyomas, multiple uterine leiomyomas, and early onset of papillary renal cell cancer (Type 2).[30,31]

Diagnosis Clinical criteria for diagnosis of HLRCC include multiple cutaneous piloleiomyomas or two of the following: (1) surgical removal of leiomyomas before age 40, (2) papillary renal cell carcinoma (Type 2) before age 40, or (3) first-degree relative meeting criteria. Molecular testing for patients meeting clinical criteria will identify mutations in the fumarate hydratase gene in most cases. Functional immunohistochemical testing of tumor cells is also available for patients for whom a germline mutation cannot be identified. For children with affected relatives, germline testing is recommended at age 8 to allow for early screening.[31]

Cancer Risk The lifetime incidence of developing renal cell carcinoma (Type 2) is approximately 15% for patients with HLRCC. For pediatric patients, this risk is about 1 to 2%. There are rarely reported cases of pheochromocytoma and paraganglioma in this population as well.[30]

Management and Surveillance Management of children with HLRCC includes annual skin exams as well as renal MRI beginning as early as age 8. Given the low risk of tumors prior to age 20, screening decisions should be discussed with families of affected children. Gynecological exams can be deferred until adulthood.[30,31]

Hereditary Paraganglioma-Pheochromocytoma Syndrome

Syndrome Overview Hereditary paraganglioma-pheochromocytoma syndrome (HPP) is primarily an autosomal dominant inherited disorder with an approximate incidence of 1:1,000,000. In some cases, genetic imprinting can affect the penetrance of the disease. A variety of different gene mutations have been implicated in the pathogenesis of HPP. Most commonly, mutations in the succinate dehydrogenase (SDH) family of genes (*SDHA, SDHB, SDHC, SDHD, SDHAF2*) disrupt their role as tumor suppressors. SDH converts succinate to fumarate; its dysfunction results in succinate accumulation contributing to pseudo-hypoxia with decreased breakdown of hypoxia inducible factor 1 (HIF1). This results in unregulated cell growth and angiogenesis. Mutations in other tumor suppressors including *TMEM127* and *MAX* have also been identified in patients with HPP. The primary clinical feature of HPP is tumor development of paragangliomas and pheochromocytomas as well as other rare tumors (i.e., gastrointestinal stromal tumors, pituitary adenomas and renal cancer).[32,33]

Diagnosis Given the high incidence of a heritable cause in patients with paraganglioma or pheochromocytoma, all patients with these diagnoses should be offered genetic testing for HPP.[32]

Cancer Risk Paraganglioma and pheochromocytoma are the primary tumors diagnosed in HPP. These tumors are typically benign but can be life threatening secondary to mass-effect and catecholamine-effect. Multiple studies of cancer risk in patients with HPP suggest that penetrance is incomplete, and the risk of tumor development is ranges from 14 to 90%. Patients who develop paraganglioma and pheochromocytoma in the setting of HPP have an increased risk of treatment-resistant and aggressive metastatic disease. Of note, gastrointestinal stromal tumors also occur in this population and typically present in a gastric location with gastrointestinal bleeding.[32,33]

Management and Surveillance Surveillance of patients with HPP is recommended beginning at age 6 to 8. Screening includes annual blood pressures, plasma methoxytyramine, and plasma/urine metanephrines. Chromogranin A can also be considered to increase detection rates. Whole body MRI is also recommended every other year but its efficacy in detecting small gastrointestinal tumors is unclear. Annual complete blood counts to identify anemia have been suggested as a mechanism for monitoring for gastrointestinal stromal tumors in this population.[32]

Hereditary Retinoblastoma

Syndrome Overview Retinoblastoma (RB) is a malignant eye tumor, and in 40% of cases, is part of a hereditary genetic disorder. Hereditary RB is a rare disease with an estimated incidence of 3 to 5 out of 1,000,000 children. It has an autosomal dominant inheritance pattern with 80% of cases from *de novo* mutations. The *RB1* gene normally encodes a nuclear phosphoprotein (pRB1) that acts as a tumor suppressor preventing progression through the cell cycle. The *RB1* gene is the model for the "two-hit hypothesis" of tumor suppressors, as described originally by Knudson. Patients with a germline *RB1* mutation require an acquired loss of heterozygosity (second hit) for tumor development. In general, cancer predisposition is the major feature of hereditary RB, although a small proportion of patients with full gene deletions may have other clinical findings (abnormal facies, cognitive impairment).[34,35]

Diagnosis *RB1* gene sequencing is appropriate in patients presenting with RB or those with a family history of hereditary RB. Prenatal testing is available for patients with a family history.[36]

Cancer Risk Hereditary RB is highly penetrant with 90 to 95% of children developing RB before age 5. These children predominately present with bilateral disease; however, patients may also present with unilateral disease (15%) or pineoblastoma (trilateral RB). Patients with unilateral disease who have germline RB1 mutations are also at increased risk of developing RB in the unaffected eye within 2 to 3 years following diagnosis. Additionally, there is a significantly increased risk of secondary malignancies in approximately 40 to 50% of patients who receive radiation and 20% of patients who do not receive radiation. Secondary malignancies include sarcomas, especially osteosarcoma, melanoma, and other CNS tumors.[34,37,38]

Management and Surveillance Early identification and treatment of patients with RB is essential for vision preservation and survival. The basis of surveillance protocol is frequent ophthalmologic examination from birth until at least age 5. An initial ophthalmologic exam should take place within 24 hours of birth and should be repeated at 2-week intervals until 2 months of age. Exams under anesthesia should then be commenced monthly at first and then at slowly increased intervals. MRI should be completed at diagnosis to evaluate for trilateral retinoblastoma and can be considered every 6 months until age 5. For secondary cancers, patients should be screened with annual dermatologic exam for melanoma. Whole-body MRI is under investigation for older children as a means for evaluating for secondary sarcomas.[34]

Li-Fraumeni Syndrome

Syndrome Overview Li-Fraumeni syndrome (LFS) is an autosomal dominant cancer predisposition syndrome. Its prevalence is difficult to estimate given its incomplete penetrance. LFS is caused by germline mutations in the *TP53* tumor suppressor gene.

Normally, *TP53* encodes a transcription factor (p53) responsible for upregulating the transcription of proteins necessary for cell cycle arrest and control of apoptosis. Over 250 mutations in *TP53* have been identified in LFS. An estimated 25% of mutations are likely *de novo*. These mutations result in increased risk of cancer at an early age without any other clinical features. One specific mutation, TP53 (R337H), is more prevalent among Brazilians and is specifically associated with adrenal cortical tumors in pediatric patients.[39–41]

Diagnosis The modified "Chompret criteria" are used diagnostically to identify patients at high risk of having *TP53* mutations. These criteria include (1) a proband with an LFS tumor (i.e., breast cancer, soft tissue sarcoma, CNS tumor, adrenocortical carcinoma, osteosarcoma) before age 46 and a first- or second-degree relative with an LFS tumor (excluding breast cancer if present in proband) before age 56; (2) a proband with multiple tumors (at least two LFS tumors) before age 46; (3) a proband with rare cancers (i.e., adrenocortical carcinoma, choroid plexus carcinoma, or embryonal anaplastic rhabdomyosarcoma); and (4) a proband with early-onset breast cancer before age 31. Patients who meet clinical criteria should be screened for *TP53* mutation with germline sequencing.[40–42]

Cancer Risk It is estimated that approximately 41% of patients with LFS develop malignancy by age 18 with high rates even in small children under 5 years (22%). The most commonly identified tumors in the pediatric age group are osteosarcomas, adrenocortical carcinomas, CNS tumors, and soft tissue sarcomas. To a lesser extent, pediatric patients with LFS have also been diagnosed with leukemia (especially hypodiploid acute lymphoblastic leukemia), lymphoma, Wilms, and neuroblastoma.[39,40]

Management and Surveillance Surveillance to promote early detection of tumors is crucial and can improve overall survival of patients with LFS from 60% to nearly 90%. Surveillance is recommended for all patients who meet clinical criteria for LFS with or without identification of a pathogenic LFS variant. Current surveillance strategies in the pediatric age group include physical exams every 3 to 4 months with abdominal ultrasound to monitor for adrenocortical carcinoma until age 18. Lifelong annual brain MRIs and annual whole-body MRI are also recommended to monitor for CNS tumors and soft tissue sarcomas, respectively. Additional screening guidelines exist for adults (i.e., Toronto protocol) and include annual breast imaging, biennial colonoscopies, and frequent blood count monitoring.[40,42]

Juvenile Polyposis Syndrome

Syndrome Overview Juvenile polyposis syndrome (JPS) is a genetic disorder with an autosomal dominant inheritance pattern and estimated incidence of 1:100,000. The pathogenesis of JPS is not entirely understood, but approximately 75% of cases have a family history. Mutations in two tumor suppressor genes, *SMAD4* and *BMPR1A*, have been identified in up to 40% of people with JPS. In addition to juvenile polyps for which the syndrome is named, patients with JPS can also present with vascular anomalies. Patients with *SMAD4* mutations can also have features of hereditary hemorrhagic telangiectasia syndrome with mucocutaneous telangiectasias and arteriovenous malformations in the brain, lung, and abdomen.[26,43]

Diagnosis JPS is a clinical diagnosis made based on the presence of one of the following three criteria: (1) five or more juvenile polyps in the colon, (2) juvenile polyps in the extracolonic gastrointestinal tract, or (3) juvenile polyps in the colon and a family history of JPS. Patients who meet clinical criteria should have gene sequencing for *SMAD4* and *BMPR1A*.[26,43]

Cancer Risk Patients with JPS are primarily at an increased risk of gastrointestinal cancers; however, cancer of the breast and thyroid have also been reported. Lifetime risk is increased 40 to 70% for colon cancer and 20 to 30% for gastric cancer. In the Japanese population with JPS, the gastric cancer risk has been estimated to be as high as 73%.[26,40,43]

Management and Surveillance Cancer risk in JPS can be mitigated by early identification of polyps with polypectomy. Patients with known JPS should have annual physical exams with complete blood counts to evaluate for anemia. Colonoscopy is also indicated for surveillance beginning between ages 12 to 15. Colonoscopy should be repeated annually if polyps are found or every 3 years if normal. Endoscopy with small bowel follow through can also be initiated for ages 12 to 15. Patients with *SMAD4* mutations require additional screening for arteriovenous malformations prior to and after puberty and every 5 to 10 years throughout life. Screening should consist of a brain MRI to evaluate CNS vasculature and oxygen saturation to assess for thoracic malformations.[26,43]

Multiple Endocrine Neoplasia Type 1

Syndrome Overview Multiple endocrine neoplasia type 1 (MEN1) is an autosomal dominant disorder affecting 1:30,000. MEN1 is one of a group of distinct syndromes that result in the development of hormone-secreting tumors. MEN1 results from mutations in the *MEN1* tumor suppressor gene. The *MEN1* gene normally encodes menin protein, and inactivating mutations result in dysregulation of the cell cycle and increased proliferation. MEN1 manifests clinically with anterior pituitary adenomas, pancreatic islet tumors, and parathyroid adenomas with resultant primary hyperparathyroidism. Patients can have additional findings including lipomas, angiofibromas, adrenocortical adenomas, and, more rarely, other CNS tumors.[45,46]

Diagnosis Clinical diagnostic criteria for MEN1 include the presence of at least two of the three typical MEN1 tumors or one tumor and a family history of MEN1. These patients should have confirmatory molecular testing. Additionally, patients with any pancreatic islet tumor or with pancreatic precursor lesions and primary hyperparathyroidism diagnosed before 30 years of age should receive genetic testing. As many as 10 to 30% of patients with clinical MEN1 will not have an identifiable mutation in the *MEN1* gene.[45,47]

Cancer Risk MEN1 is highly penetrant, and patients are likely to develop one of the major tumors associated with disease (anterior pituitary adenomas, pancreatic islet tumors, parathyroid adenomas). Approximately 17% of these tumors are diagnosed in childhood and adolescence.[45,46]

Management and Surveillance All patients with MEN1 should have regular physical exams with a detailed physician assessment of signs and symptoms related to hormonal disturbances. Pediatric patients with MEN1 should have surveillance initiated at age 5 with annual labs to include prolactin and fasting insulin/glucose. Imaging in this age group should include a brain MRI every 3 years to evaluate for pituitary adenoma. Annual calcium testing is recommended starting at age 8. Chromogranin A, glucagon, proinsulin, pancreatic polypeptide, and VIP screening should be considered as early as age 10. Abdominal MRI to evaluate for pancreatic and adrenal tumors should be performed annually starting at age 10. As patients approach adulthood, surveillance guidelines also include gastrin screening and imaging of the chest.[45,46]

Neurofibromatosis 1

Syndrome Overview Neurofibromatosis 1 (NF1) is an autosomal dominant disorder with half of cases representing *de novo* mutations. It is a relatively common disorder with an estimated incidence of 1:1,900 to 1:2,800. Broadly categorized, NF1 is one of a group of disorders termed RASopathies. The gene affected in this disorder is the *NF1* gene, which encodes neurofibromin, a GTPase that serves to suppress RAS signaling. Mutations in NF1 result in dysregulation of the RAS pathway and increased cell proliferation especially in neural crest cells. As outlined below, patients with NF1 can present with a myriad of dermatologic, ophthalmologic, and osseous findings, in addition to predisposition to cancer.[48–51]

Diagnosis Patients who meet any one of the following clinical diagnostic criteria should have genetic testing for NF1 mutations: (1) café au lait macules (six or more, greater than or equal to 5 mm in size if prepubertal and 15 mm if postpubertal); (2) neurofibromas (two or more or one plexiform); (3) axillary or inguinal freckling; (4) optic glioma; (5) Lisch nodules (two or more); (6) distinct skeletal abnormalities (i.e., sphenoid dysplasia, pseudoarthrosis); or (7) first-degree relative with NF1. Patients who have negative NF1 testing but meet clinical criteria should have further exome sequencing to look for syndromes with similar presentation, including CMMRD, RASopathies, Leigus syndrome, and McCune-Albright.[48,49]

Cancer Risk Patients with NF1 are at increased risk for developing a large spectrum of malignancies. Optic glioma is the most common malignancy, presenting during childhood in as many as 15% of patients. Other tumors present in 1% or less of children with NF and include malignant peripheral nerve sheath tumors (MPNST), high-grade gliomas, juvenile myelomonocytic leukemia, embryonal rhabdomyosarcoma, pheochromocytoma, GI carcinoid, and GI stromal tumors.[49,51]

Management and Surveillance Patients with NF1 are at greatest risk for developing optic gliomas in childhood, and as such, require routine ophthalmologic screening, recommended every 6 to 12 months until age 8 and then every 1 to 2 years until age 20. For patients with a change in visual acuity, repeat testing at two weeks is recommended. Persistent vision loss should be evaluated with MRI. It is important to note that routine MRI surveillance for optic glioma is not recommended as asymptomatic optic gliomas do not require therapy and do not affect patient survival. Surveillance for other tumors in this patient population includes an annual physical exam with a thorough neurological assessment. Blood pressure should be assessed given the increased risk for developing pheochromocytoma. A complete history including any changes to neurofibromas (i.e., growth, pain) is necessary to evaluate for MPNST. Additional imaging for MPNST is not required during childhood; however, a whole-body MRI can be used to assess total body tumor burden between ages 16 to 20, as increased tumor burden is associated with future development of MPNST.[49]

Neurofibromatosis 2

Syndrome Overview Neurofibromatosis 2 (NF2) is an autosomal dominant genetic disorder with an approximate incidence of 1:25,000 to 1:33,000. A large proportion of cases are mosaics or represent *de novo* mutations. The pathogenesis of NF2 involves mutations in the NF2 gene that typically encodes merlin, a regulator of cell growth. As with other disorders of tumor suppressors, loss of heterozygosity results in clinical manifestations including the development of schwannomas, meningiomas, glioma (ependymoma), and cataracts. Severity of the disease has been correlated with mutation type with more severe presentations associated with truncating mutations.[48,52,53]

Diagnosis A set of diagnostic criteria have been developed to identify patients with NF2; these criteria are known as the Manchester criteria. A clinical diagnosis of NF2 can be made for patients with a family history of NF2 if they also have a unilateral vestibular schwannoma or two other characteristic findings (i.e., meningioma, glioma, neurofibroma, schwannoma, posterior subcapsular lenticular opacities). For patients without a family history, a clinical diagnosis can be made for patients with (1) bilateral vestibular schwannomas, (2) unilateral vestibular schwannoma and two other characteristic findings, or (3) multiple meningiomas with either a unilateral vestibular schwannoma or two other characteristic findings. Gene sequencing should be performed on patients who meet clinical criteria or on children with any meningioma or schwannoma. Blood and tumor sequencing should be performed to help detect patients with mosaicism. Additional testing for other schwannomatosis may also be indicated for patients with isolated schwannoma (SMARCB1, LZTR1) or isolated meningioma (SMARCE1).[52,53]

Cancer Risk The clinical hallmark of NF2 is tumor development, being at increased risk for schwannoma, meningioma, and ependymoma.[52,53]

Management and Surveillance A multidisciplinary team is paramount to effective management of patients with NF2. In addition to oncology care, patients benefit from neurology, surgery, audiology, ophthalmology, and genetics follow-up. Patients should receive annual physical exams. Surveillance recommendations include neuroimaging beginning at age 10. A brain MRI should be obtained annually with closer follow-up if positive findings, and a spinal MRI should be obtained every 2 to 3 years.[52,53]

Peutz-Jeghers Syndrome

Syndrome Overview Peutz-Jeghers syndrome (PJS) is an autosomal dominant disorder with approximately 25% of cases being *de novo*. The incidence is unclear, and estimates vary from 1:8500 to 1:200,000. Mutations in the *STK11* gene have been identified as the cause of PJS. *STK11* encodes the LKB1 protein, a serine/threonine kinase that acts as a tumor suppressor ultimately downregulating the mTOR pathway. Clinical feature of PJS include hamartomatous polyps (gastrointestinal and extraintestinal) and freckling around the vermillion border of the lip.[26,43,54,55]

Diagnosis Clinical diagnosis of PJS requires meeting one of the following criteria: (1) two or more PJS polyps, (2) any PJS polyp and PJS in close relative, (3) characteristic pigmentation changes and PJS in close relative, or (4) any PJS polyp with characteristic pigmentation. Sequencing of *STK11* will identify mutations in 90% of patients.[26,43]

Cancer Risk The risk for malignancy in patient with PJS increases with age. For patients under age 20, malignancy is identified in 1 to 2%; by age 50 this increases to 30%. The spectrum of malignancies diagnosed is broad and it includes gastrointestinal tumors, pancreatic tumors, and gonadal tumors.[26,55]

Management and Surveillance Current guidelines for surveillance in patients with PJS recommend active screening for gastrointestinal tumors/polyps starting at age 8 or earlier if there are symptoms. Screening should consist of endoscopy with video capsule and colonoscopy. For patients with polyps, repeat imaging should occur every 3 years; otherwise imaging can be repeated at age 18. Given the increased risk of gonadal tumors, patients should also receive a thorough physical exam with special attention to changes associated with hormonal abnormalities. Adult patients require additional screening for breast cancer, ovarian cancer, cervical cancer, and endometrial cancer.[26,43,55]

PTEN Hamartoma Tumor Syndrome

Syndrome Overview PTEN hamartoma tumor syndrome (PHTS) is a spectrum of rare syndromes of autosomal dominant inheritance. Cowden syndrome, Bannayan-Riley-Ruvalcaba syndrome, and PTEN-related Proteus-like syndrome fall in the general category of PHTS. These syndromes all entail mutations in the *PTEN* gene, which normally acts as a tumor suppressor downregulating cell proliferation through the mTOR pathway. Clinical features among patients with PHTS are syndrome-dependent but commonly include autism, macrocephaly, vascular malformations, lipomas, and polyposis.[30,43,56]

Diagnosis PHTS diagnosis requires molecular genetic testing with sequencing of the *PTEN* gene. Clinical criteria have been developed and are available to guide testing.[43]

Cancer Risk Cancer risk for patients with PHTS varies with age and likely specific mutation type. For pediatric patients with PHTS, epitheliod-differentiated thyroid cancer is the most commonly seen malignancy with an incidence of 5% in patients younger than age 20. This cancer typically spares younger children with the earliest reported case occurring at age 7. Recent work has demonstrated a broader range of malignancies associated with PHTS in adults including breast cancer, endometrial cancer, colorectal cancer, and melanoma; these cancers have not been associated with the pediatric age group.[30,56,57]

Management and Surveillance Because the spectrum of malignancy is limited to thyroid cancer in pediatric patients with PHTS, surveillance involves thyroid ultrasounds. Guidelines vary regarding the onset and interval of screening. The most recent guidelines recommended by the American Association for Cancer Research are for ultrasounds beginning at age 7 and repeated every 2 years if normal.[30,43,56]

RASopathies (Non-NF1)

Syndrome Overview The term RASopathies applies to a set of genetic disorders that affect the RAS cell signaling pathway. In addition to NF1 (which is discussed separately), these disorders include Noonan syndrome, cardiofaciocutaneous syndrome, Leigus syndrome, Costello syndrome, and CBL syndrome, among others. The genes affected in these syndromes vary but all result in RAS pathway dysregulation. Clinical features also vary by specific disorder; however, patients will display some features of a Noonan phenotype (i.e., dysmorphism, abnormal growth, cardiac defects, dermatologic abnormalities).[50,51,58]

Diagnosis Specific RASopathies are typically diagnosed by identifying disease-specific clinical features and performing confirmatory gene sequencing.[58]

Cancer Risk In general, patients with RASopathies are at an increased risk of developing malignancy. Exact risk is specific to each disorder and mutation type. Patients with Costello syndrome are at highest risk for cancer development, with approximately 15% of children developing malignancy by age 20. The most common malignancies in patients with Costello syndrome are embryonal rhabdomyosarcoma, neuroblastoma, and bladder neoplasms.

Notably, patients with Noonan syndrome (*PTPN* and *KRAS* mutations) and CBL syndrome are at increased risk of juvenile myelomonocytic leukemia in early childhood.[50,51]

Management and Surveillance For all patients with RASopathies, counseling regarding increased malignancy risk and physician evaluation for development of new symptoms is crucial. Surveillance for patients with Costello syndrome should also include abdominal/pelvic ultrasounds from diagnosis until age 8 to 10 and urinalysis beginning at 10. Chest X-rays may be considered for neuroblastoma monitoring, but urine metanephrine testing is often not helpful as patients with Costello syndrome can have baseline elevations in urine catecholamines. For patients at increased risk of juvenile myelomonocytic leukemia, patients should receive thorough physical exams and complete blood counts from diagnosis until age 5.[34,50]

Rhabdoid Tumor Predisposition Syndrome

Syndrome Overview Rhabdoid tumor predisposition syndrome (RTPS) is an exceedingly rare autosomal dominant disorder of unclear incidence. Rhabdoid tumors are aggressive rare tumors of early childhood and seen most frequently in the first year of life, with an approximate incidence of 5:1,000,000. RTPS is thought to be the cause in approximately 35% of cases. Two tumor suppressor genes are associated with this syndrome: *SMARCB1* and *SMARCA4*. Normally these genes encode proteins that are part of a chromatin remodeling complex and regulate gene expression. Patients' germline mutations associated with RTPS develop rhabdoid tumors with loss of heterozygosity of the normal allele. Malignancy development is the primary clinical feature of RTPS, although some mutations in the involved genes can cause other rare congenital abnormalities and developmental delays.[28,59,60]

Diagnosis Gene sequencing of *SMARCB1* and *SMARCA4* should be considered in all patients with rhabdoid tumors. Testing should also be considered for immediate family members of patients found to have a germline mutation in either gene.[28,59]

Cancer Risk Given the rarity of RTPS and unclear penetrance of the disorder, the exact risk of malignancy development for these patients remains unclear. Rhabdoid tumors of the CNS (atypical teratoid/rhabdoid tumors) and extracranial sites, such as the kidneys, are the primary malignancies associated with RTPS. Patients with *SMARCB1* mutations are also at increased risk for schwannomas, malignant peripheral nerve sheath tumors, and meningiomas. In contrast, women with *SMARCA4* mutations are at increased risk for small cell carcinoma of ovary, hypercalcemic type.[28,59,60]

Management and Surveillance Suggested surveillance for patients with RTPS varies with mutation type. For patients with *SMARCB1* mutations, brain MRI and abdominal ultrasound should be considered every 3 months through age 5. Surveillance for patients with *SMARCA4* mutations is less clear. Ultrasounds can be considered for female patients during childhood to identify small cell carcinoma of the ovary. Post-pubertal women in this group may benefit from prophylactic oophorectomy, although this requires further study.[28]

Simpson-Golabi-Behmel Syndrome

Syndrome Overview Simpson-Golabi-Behmel syndrome (SGBS) is a rare X-linked genetic syndrome with approximately 250 cases reported worldwide. The syndrome is associated with mutations in the tumor suppressor gene *GPC3*, needed for regulation of the hedgehog pathway and inhibition of cell proliferation. *GPC4*, another tumor suppressor gene in the hedgehog pathway, potentially affects the pathogenesis of SGBS, but its role is less clear. Patients with SGBS suffer from a multitude of congenital abnormalities including macrocephaly, abnormal facies with coarse features, macrosomia, macroglossia, palatal defects, heart defects, genitourinary defects, diaphragmatic/umbilical/rectal hernias, bony anomalies of ribs and vertebrae, polydactyly, hip dislocation, and intellectual disability.[24,61,62]

Diagnosis Diagnosis is made by molecular sequencing of the *GPC3* gene looking for deletions, duplications, and point mutations in individuals presenting with clinical features of SGBS. In identified males with SGBS, only 20 to 30% are *de novo* mutations. As such, mothers of affected individuals should be tested. Siblings may also benefit from testing if maternal testing is positive.[61,62]

Cancer Risk Children with SGBS are at risk for Wilms tumor and neuroblastoma. There have also been reported cases of hepatoblastoma, gonadoblastoma, and medulloblastoma.[24,61]

Management and Surveillance Patients with SGBS require a multidisciplinary team for management of their multiple congenital anomalies. Monitoring from an oncologic perspective is centered around Wilms tumor surveillance. Patients should be screened with renal ultrasound every 3 months from diagnosis until age 7. Currently, there are no specific guidelines for monitoring for other malignancies, although monitoring for neuroblastoma with urine catecholamines and gonadoblastoma/hepatoblastoma with alpha fetoprotein and beta human chorionic gonadotropin concentrations has been suggested.[24,61,63]

Tuberous Sclerosis

Syndrome Overview Tuberous sclerosis (TS) is an autosomal dominant disorder with approximately 60% of cases representing *de novo* mutations. The estimated incidence of TS is 1:5800. The primary genes affected are *TSC1*-encoding hamartin and *TSC2*-encoding tuberin. Hamartin and tuberin act as tumor suppressors through inhibition of mTORC1 in the brain. Patients with TS experience a myriad of clinical manifestations including seizures, cortical dysplasia (tubers), dermatologic abnormalities (chagrin patches, hypomelanotic macules), retinal hamartomas, angiofibromas, and CNS tumors.[64–67]

Diagnosis A diagnosis of TS can be made from clinical criteria or genetic criteria. Clinical criteria include two major findings or one major finding and two minor findings. Major criteria are defined as (1) three or more angiofibromas, (2) three or more hypomelanotic macules, (3) two or more ungual fibromas, (4) chagrin patch, (5) multiple retinal hamartomas, (6) cortical dysplasia, (7) subependymal nodules, (8) subependymal giant cell astrocytoma (SEGA), (9) cardiac rhabdomyoma, (10) lymphagioleiomatosis, and (11) two or more renal angiomyolipomas. Minor criteria refer to dental enamel pits, intraoral fibromas, non-renal hamartomas, retinal acromatic patch, confetti skin lesions, and multiple renal cysts. Identification of a known pathogenic variant in *TSC1* or *TSC2* meets diagnostic genetic criteria and is sufficient to make a diagnosis of TS. Importantly, as many as 15% of patients with clinical TS will not have an identifiable mutation; negative genetic testing does not rule out the diagnosis.[64–67]

Cancer Risk TS is associated with an increased risk of SEGAs particularly during childhood. Moreover, patients have a 1 to 2% increased lifetime risk of renal cell carcinoma.[64–67]

Management and Surveillance TS is a complex syndrome requiring multidisciplinary management. A detailed management and surveillance protocol has been developed by the

International Tuberous Sclerosis Consensus Group. Most relevant to cancer surveillance in the pediatric age group are the screening protocols for SEGAs and renal cell carcinomas. Brain and abdomen MRIs are recommended every 1 to 3 years in asymptomatic patients and more frequently for patients with growing tumors. Management strategies for symptomatic or growing lesions include resection (SEGA) and embolization (renal angiomyolipomas). mTOR inhibitors have also been found to be effective at managing many of the tumors associated with TS.[64–67]

Von Hippel-Lindau Disease

Syndrome Overview Von Hippel-Lindau Disease (VHL) is a rare genetic disorder with an incidence of approximately 1:35,000. It is inherited in an autosomal dominant manner with only about 20% of cases representing *de novo* mutations. The *VHL* gene typically functions as a tumor suppressor and encodes a multi-functional protein product that plays a key role in the protein degradation of hypoxia-inducible factors that regulate cell growth and angiogenesis. Mutations in *VHL* lead to unregulated cell growth. Clinically, patients with VHL suffer from an array of benign and malignant tumors. Different subtypes of the disease are categorized by specific tumor types and correlate with specific genetic abnormalities. Generally, hemangioblastomas, renal cell carcinomas, pheochromocytomas, neuroendocrine tumors, and multiple cysts (i.e., renal, pancreatic, epididymal, broad ligament) are common in patients with VHL.[32,68,69]

Diagnosis Genetic testing of children with a first-degree relative with VHL should be performed to allow for improved surveillance and reduction of complications. For pediatric patients without a family history, molecular testing for VHL should be performed in the presence of CNS/retinal hemangioblastoma, pheochromocytoma, paraganglioma, clear cell renal carcinoma, pancreatic neuroendocrine tumors, epididymal or adnexal papillary cystadenoma, endolymphatic cell tumor, or multiple renal/pancreatic cysts.[32]

Cancer Risk Patients with VHL are at high risk for tumor development with a lifetime risk of up to 80% for hemangioblastoma, 70% for renal cell carcinoma, and 25% for pheochromocytoma. While all the tumors associated with VHL have been reported in the pediatric age group, hemangioblastomas and pheochromocytomas more commonly present in early childhood.[32,69,70]

Management and Surveillance Multiple surveillance protocols have been developed to guide the management of patients with VHL. Surveillance identifies manifestations of VHL prior to the development of clinical symptoms and reduces morbidity and mortality associated with the disease. Currently, surveillance guidelines apply to all patients with VHL regardless of clinical subtype and pathogenic genetic variant. For pediatric patients, annual screening for retinal hemangioblastoma with ophthalmologic retinal exam should be performed beginning at birth. Patients should also be monitored for pheochromocytomas with blood pressure checks and annual plasma/urine metanephrine analysis beginning at age 2. Audiology exams are recommended every other year for endolymphatic cell tumors beginning at age 5. Monitoring with MRI of the brain and spine for CNS hemangioblastomas should be performed every other year beginning at age 8. Additionally, MRI of the abdomen is recommended annually beginning at age 10 for renal cell carcinoma and pancreatic neuroendocrine tumors.[32,70]

DISORDERS OF PROTO-ONCOGENES

Hereditary Neuroblastoma

Syndrome Overview Hereditary neuroblastoma (HN) accounts for an estimated 1 to 2% of the 650 new cases of neuroblastoma diagnosed each year. There are a variety of causes of HN, many of which are discussed in other sections of this chapter (i.e., Li-Fraumeni syndrome, *CDKN1C* mutations, RASopathies). In addition to these genetic syndromes, mutations in the *ALK* and *PHOX2B* genes can contribute to the pathogenesis of HN. *ALK* encodes a tyrosine kinase thought to act as an oncogene with activating mutations inhibiting apoptosis and contributing to unregulated cell growth. *PHOX2B* plays a central role in nerve cell differentiation, and specific mutations, especially nonpolyalanine repeat mutations (NPARMs), have an increased risk of neuroblastoma development. Patients with HN secondary to *ALK* mutations are unlikely to exhibit any other clinical features. In patients with *PHOX2B* mutations, other clinical features such as congenital central hypoventilation syndrome and Hirschsprung disease may be present.[34,71–73]

Diagnosis Patients with a family history of neuroblastoma or bilateral/multifocal disease should be offered germline testing for syndromes known to cause HN.[34]

Cancer Risk The risk of neuroblastoma varies based on patient genotype. For patients with HN secondary to *ALK* or NPARMs in *PHOX2B*, the risk of neuroblastoma may be as high as 50%. HN is more likely to present at an earlier age and with multi-site disease.[34,73]

Management and Surveillance Surveillance for neuroblastoma is indicated in patients with a known diagnosis of HN as well as those with a strong family history or bilateral/multifocal disease without an identified pathogenic variant. Recommendations for surveillance include an abdominal ultrasound, urine metanephrines, and chest X-ray every 3 months from diagnosis until age 6. The surveillance interval can then be increased to every 6 months until age 10 when surveillance can be discontinued.[34]

Mulibrey Nanism

Syndrome Overview Mulibrey nanism (MN) is a very rare genetic disorder reported in approximately 130 people worldwide, with the majority of cases in the Finnish population. Autosomal recessive inheritance of biallelic mutations in *TRIM37* causing loss of gene function have been identified as the cause of MN. The exact role of *TRIM37* in tumor pathogenesis in MN patients is unclear. TRIM37 is a known oncogene, and its overexpression results in proliferation of somatic cancer cells; however, patients with MN have decreased *TRIM37* expression, yet they still have an increased risk of tumor development. From a clinical perspective, the primary features of MN include abnormalities in the muscles, liver, brain, eyes, and Mulibrey. Patients often have growth failure, hepatomegaly, dysmorphic features, metabolic derangements, and a significant predisposition to malignancy.[24,74,75]

Diagnosis In patients with concerning clinical features, diagnosis can be made with molecular analysis of the *TRIM37* gene.[24]

Cancer Risk A wide range of tumors, benign and malignant, affect up to 74% of patients with MN. In the pediatric age group, there is an increased risk of Wilms tumor estimated at

6.7%. Benign cysts, pheochromocytomas, renal papillary carcinoma, and thyroid carcinoma, among others, also occur more commonly in the adult population.[24,75]

Management and Surveillance MN is a complex condition requiring multidisciplinary management. From an oncologic perspective, surveillance for Wilms tumor is recommended for pediatric patients with this disorder. Screening should consist of renal ultrasound every 3 months from time of diagnosis until age 7. Other cancer screening is not recommended in the pediatric population, but additional surveillance guidelines are available for adults.[24]

Multiple Endocrine Neoplasia Type 2

Syndrome Overview Multiple endocrine neoplasia type 2 (MEN2) is an inherited autosomal dominant disorder categorized as a multiple endocrine neoplasia syndrome. MEN2 has an estimate prevalence of 1:40,000. Unlike MEN1, MEN2 is not related to tumor suppressor dysfunction but rather oncogene activation. Activating mutations in the *RET* gene, which encodes a receptor as tyrosine kinase, causes uncontrolled cell division characteristic of MEN2. Multiple mutations have been identified, each conveying a different risk profile for tumor development. Clinically, two distinct subtypes of MEN2 are recognized: MEN2A and MEN2B. Patients with MEN2A, the more common one, are at risk for developing medullary thyroid carcinoma, pheochromocytoma, and parathyroid adenomas resulting in primary hyperparathyroidism. MEN2B is also associated with medullary thyroid carcinoma and pheochromocytoma, as well as mucosal neuromas and intestinal ganglioneuromas. Patients with MEN2B may also have abnormal Marfanoid features.[45,46,76]

Diagnosis Patients suspected of having MEN2 with at least two characteristic tumor types or a family history should be evaluated with molecular testing of the *RET* gene.[40,77]

Cancer Risk The risk of malignancy in MEN2 is correlated with the type of genetic mutation present. The highest risk for medullary thyroid cancer is associated with abnormalities in *RET* codon 918 (MEN2B). High risk is conveyed by allelic variations in codons 634 and 883. All other mutations carry a moderate risk. In the highest-risk patients, penetrance or medullary thyroid cancer near 100%, with many cases occurring in infancy and early childhood. Pheochromocytomas can occur in up to 50% of patients with MEN2 and have been identified in some patients prior to adolescence.[40,46,76]

Management and Surveillance Surveillance for malignancy in patients with MEN2 also depends on their genetic variant. All patients should be screened starting from birth, with calcitonin and carcinoembryonic antigen measurements as well as thyroid ultrasound every 6 months for the first year and then annually. For patients in the highest risk category, prophylactic thyroidectomy is recommended prior to 1 year. Patients in the high-risk category should have thyroidectomy at age 5 or earlier if abnormalities in screening. Patients at moderate risk can have thyroidectomy deferred until calcitonin becomes abnormal or earlier at parental request. For patients who develop medullary thyroid cancer, specific *RET* inhibitors have been developed and their efficacy is being evaluated in clinical trials. Additional screening for pheochromocytoma with urine/plasma metanephrines should begin at age 11 for patients in the high and highest-risk categories and 16 years in the moderate risk category. Patients with high-risk mutations should have calcium screening for primary hyperparathyroidism starting at age 11; this can be deferred until age 16 for patients in the moderate risk category.[45,46,76]

■ DISORDERS OF TRANSCRIPTION FACTOR GENES

Beckwith-Weidemann Syndrome

Syndrome Overview Beckwith-Weidemann syndrome (BWS) is a genetic disorder with an estimated incidence of 1:10,500 that occurs due to *de novo* mutations in 85% of cases. The remaining inherited cases can be related to one of several changes on chromosome 11: gain of methylation at imprinting control center 1 (IC1), loss of methylation at imprinting control center 2 (IC2), paternal uniparental disomy, or *CDKN1C* gene mutations. These genetic changes cause altered regulation of growth genes resulting in a clinical syndrome of overgrowth with hemihyperplasia, macroglossia, abdominal wall defects (omphalocele, umbilical hernia), facial nevus flammeus, neonatal hypoglycemia, and cancer predisposition.[24,78]

Diagnosis A diagnosis of BWS is made clinically. A variety of scoring systems are available to aid diagnosis but currently there is no agreed-upon diagnostic criteria. Patients with any clinical features of the disease should be evaluated by a geneticist and have molecular testing for methylation changes in chromosome 11p15 as well as sequencing of *CDKN1C*. Of note, negative genetic testing does not exclude a diagnosis of BWS given the high rate of mosaicism in this disorder.[24,78]

Cancer Risk The incidence of developing malignancy is 5 to 10% for patients with BWS, and children under 2 years are at greatest risk. The most common malignancies associated with the disorder are Wilms tumor and hepatoblastoma. Patients with *CDKN1C* mutations are also at increased risk for developing neuroblastoma. Rarely, pheochromocytoma and rhabdomyosarcoma have also been associated with the diagnosis. Specific genotypes identified convey varying tumor risks. Risk is reportedly highest with gain of methylation in IC1 with an incidence of 28% of affected patients.[24,78]

Management and Surveillance Patients diagnosed with BWS should receive surveillance for Wilms tumor. A complete abdominal ultrasound is recommended every 3 months until age 4 followed by renal ultrasounds every 3 months until age 7. It has been suggested that, because patients with loss of methylation at IC2 have less risk of developing Wilms tumor, screening these patients may not be as beneficial. Abdominal ultrasounds are also recommended to screen patients for hepatoblastoma. Recommendations for AFP testing are controversial, given variation in infant AFP levels making results difficult to interpret. If AFP surveillance is planned, then levels should be obtained every 3 months. Patients with large increases in AFP of 50 to 100 should have testing repeated in 6 weeks. Patients with AFPs that remain high should receive an MRI. Any patient with an AFP >1000 should have MRI imaging immediately. For patients with *CDKN1C* mutations, additional screening for neuroblastoma should be obtained with abdominal US, urine metanephrines, and CXR every 3 months until age 6 and then every 6 months until age 10.[24,34,78]

WT1-Related Syndromes

Syndrome Overview WT1-related syndromes are a group of autosomal disorders with abnormalities in the *WT1* gene. These disorders include Wilms tumor with aniridia, genito-urinary abnormalities and mental retardation (WAGR) syndrome, Denys-Drash syndrome (DDS), and Frasier syndrome (FS). *WT1* encodes a transcription factor responsible for regulating cell growth in multiple organs including the kidney and gonads. Patients with

WAGR have four primary clinical manifestations: Wilms tumor, aniridia, genito-urinary abnormalities, and intellectual disability. The clinical features of DDS also include Wilms tumor, in addition to nephrotic syndrome and gonadal dysgenesis. Patients with FS may develop focal segmental glomerulosclerosis, gonadal dysgenesis, and gonadoblastoma.[24,79]

Diagnosis Molecular testing of patients with clinical features of WT1-related disorders can clarify the diagnosis. Patients with WAGR have large gene deletions of *WT1* and the adjacent gene *PAX6*. DDS is typically associated with missense mutations in *WT1* exon 8 or 9. Patients with FS commonly have single nucleotide alterations in *WT1* intron 9.[24,80]

Cancer Risk Patients with WAGR and DDS have an extremely increased risk of developing Wilms tumor: 50% and 90%, respectively. FS and DDS also convey an increased risk of approximately 40% for gonadoblastoma, especially in patients who are 46XY with gonadal dysgenesis.[24,79,80]

Surveillance and Management Patients with WT1-related syndrome require cancer surveillance at an early age. Patients with WAGR and DDS should undergo surveillance for Wilms tumor with renal ultrasound at time of diagnosis and repeat imaging every 3 months. Recommendations on a cutoff age to stop screening vary, but continuing screening until age 7 has been suggested. For patients with gonadal dysgenesis and a diagnosis of DDS and FS, gonadectomy should be considered.[24,81]

DISORDERS OF TELOMERES AND RNA

Diamond-Blackfan Anemia

Syndrome Overview Diamond-Blackfan anemia (DBA) is a very rare autosomal dominant disorder with an incidence of 1 to 4 out of 500,000. About half of patients with DBA have *de novo* mutations. Multiple ribosomal proteins have been identified in the pathogenesis of this disorder. Ribosomal instability in patients with DBA has been demonstrated to result in myeloid stress and increased cell growth and proliferation. Clinically, patients with DBA may present with a range of findings including macrocytic anemia, pancytopenia, abnormal facies (i.e., flat nasal bridge, hypertelorism), palatal anomalies, triphalangeal thumbs, cataracts, kidney abnormalities, structural heart disease, and hypospadias.[82–84]

Diagnosis DBA is a heterogenous disorder with large phenotypic variation, so a high index of suspicion is necessary to make the diagnosis. Approximately 90% of patients are diagnosed prior to age 1 with macrocytic anemia and reticulocytopenia. In a minority of cases, pancytopenia can also be observed. These patients should be evaluated for elevated erythrocyte adenosine deaminase activity and have a bone marrow aspirate with karyotyping to assess for decreased red cell precursors. For patients with a clinical picture consistent with DBA, molecular testing of known genes should be performed; however, mutations are only identified in 65% of cases. Family members of patients with DBA should also be tested.[82–84]

Cancer Risk The spectrum of malignancies afflicting patients with DBA is broad. In pediatric patients, myelodysplastic syndrome, acute myeloid leukemia, and osteosarcoma pose the greatest risk, occurring in up to 30% of patients. Other commonly identified cancers in the adult population with DBA are colorectal and genito-urinary.[85,86]

Management and Surveillance For children with DBA, anemia can often be managed with steroid therapy, chronic transfusions, or stem cell transplant. Frequent blood count monitoring is recommended at least every 3 to 4 months. If patients develop additional abnormalities on complete blood count, bone marrow evaluation for myelodysplastic syndrome and leukemia is indicated. Currently, no other routine cancer surveillance recommendations exist for children with DBA.[82,86]

DICER1 Syndrome

Syndrome Overview DICER1 syndrome is a rare disorder with an autosomal dominant inheritance pattern. The exact incidence of the disorder is unclear but is estimated to be 1:2500 to 1:10,000. The DICER1 gene is known to encode an RNAse III endonuclease responsible for processing miRNA. Mutations in this gene result in cancer predisposition and thyroid goiter. Clinically, patients may also present with macrocephaly and subsets of patients with mosaicism can have additional features of overgrowth.[87-89]

Diagnosis A diagnosis of DICER 1 should be suspected and molecular testing should be performed in pediatric patients with any of the following: (1) pleuropulmonary blastoma, (2) multinodular goiter (age <18), (3) cystic nephroma, (4) Sertoli-Leydig cell tumor of ovary, (5) embryonal rhabdomyosarcoma of the cervix, bladder, or ovary, (6) ciliary body medulloepithelioma, (7) nasal chondromesenchymal hamartoma, (8) pituitary blastoma, (9) pineoblastoma, (10) gynadroblastoma, (11) primitive neuroectodermal tumor of the cervix, (12) anaplastic sarcoma of the kidney, or (13) personal/family history suggestive of DICER1 and epithelial differentiated thyroid cancer, juvenile hamartomatous intestinal polyps, medulloblastoma, congenital phthisis bulbi, or juvenile granulosa cell tumor. In familial cases, infant testing should occur prior to age 4 months to avoid unnecessary pleuropulmonary blastoma screening.[87-89]

Cancer Risk Patients with the DICER1 mutation are at risk for developing a myriad of tumor types. More commonly presenting tumors are pleuropulmonary blastoma, Sertoli-Leydig gonadal tumors, and embryonal rhabdomyosarcoma.[87-89]

Surveillance and Management Patients with DICER 1 syndrome require complex cancer surveillance. For pleuropulmonary blastoma, patients should have a chest CT at 3 to 6 months and, if normal, a follow-up CT around age 3. Chest X-rays should be considered for patients every 6 months until age 8 and then annually until age 12. Suggested screening for Wilms tumor in this population involves renal ultrasounds every 6 months through age 8 and then annually until at least age 12. Pelvic ultrasounds at least every 12 months throughout childhood are also indicated to evaluate for gonadal tumors. Thyroid ultrasounds for goiter and malignancy should begin at age 8 and repeated every 3 years. Of note, CNS monitoring with MRI is not indicated in asymptomatic patients with DICER1 syndrome.[30-89]

Dyskeratosis Congenita

Syndrome Overview Dyskeratosis congenita (DKC) is a rare genetic disorder with an unclear prevalence currently estimated to be 1:1,000,000. More than 10 genes have been identified in the pathogenesis of DKC, and inheritance patterns (autosomal dominant, autosomal recessive, or X-linked) are dependent on the specific mutation. Mutations in affected genes in this disorder result in disruption of telomere maintenance. In addition to predisposition to cancer and bone marrow failure, common clinical features of DKC include nail dystrophy, skin pigmentation abnormalities, and leukoplakia. Patients may also suffer from eye abnormalities, dental anomalies, pulmonary fibrosis, and gastrointestinal anatomic abnormalities.[5,90]

Diagnosis The diagnosis of DKC can be made by measuring telomere length in leukocytes using flow cytometry with fluorescence in situ hybridization (FISH). Telomere lengths less than the first percentile for age are consistent with DKC. Molecular testing for specific gene abnormalities can also be obtained.[5]

Cancer Risk Patients with DKC have an increased risk of developing hematologic disorders including bone marrow failure, myelodysplastic syndrome, and leukemia. They are also at increased risk of developing solid tumors, specifically squamous cell carcinomas of the head/neck and genito-urinary cancers.[5,90]

Surveillance and Management Patients with DKC require an interdisciplinary approach to care. From a hematologic standpoint, complete blood counts and bone marrow aspiration/biopsy are recommended annually. Because of the increased risk of squamous cell carcinomas of the head and neck, dermatologic and ENT exams are also recommended annually. Patients should be encouraged to perform oral exams monthly beginning at age 16 and report new lesions or symptoms to their healthcare provider immediately.[5]

Perlman Syndrome

Syndrome Overview Perlman syndrome (PS) is a rare disorder of unknown incidence inherited in an autosomal recessive fashion. Patients with PS have a variant in the *DIS3L2* gene, which normally encodes a protein needed for miRNA degradation. Patients with PS have a poor prognosis and about half die in the neonatal period. Clinical features of the disorder include fetal overgrowth, polyhydramnios, macrosomia, abnormal facies (depressed nasal bridge, everted upper lip, deep-set eyes, low-set ears), visceromegaly, and renal dyplasia with nephroblastomatosis.[24,91]

Diagnosis Patients with clinical features of PS should have molecular evaluation to help distinguish them from other overgrowth syndromes.[24]

Cancer Risk For patients with PS surviving the newborn period, the incidence of Wilms tumor is estimated to be 64%. These patients are at increased risk for early onset and bilateral disease.[24,91]

Management and Surveillance Given the high incidence of Wilms tumor in patients with PS, surveillance should be considered for those who survive the newborn period. Monitoring should be similar to other syndromes with high risk for Wilms development and include renal ultrasounds every 3 months until age 7.[24]

Schwachman-Diamond Syndrome

Syndrome Overview Schwachman-Diamond syndrome (SDS) is a primarily autosomal recessive condition with an estimated incidence of 1:76,000. In 90% of cases, the pathogenesis has been linked to mutations in the *SBDS* gene. The protein encoded by this gene has been shown to be involved in ribosomal maturation with dysregulation resulting in cellular proliferation. Patients with SDS exhibit large variation in clinical features, which commonly include cytopenias, bone marrow failure, and pancreatic dysfunction. Additional features present in some patients include short stature, skeletal abnormalities, and neurocognitive delays.[92–94]

Diagnosis The diagnosis should be considered in the clinical in the setting of cytopenias, recurrent infections, and poor growth during infancy. Older patients may have presentations limited to bone marrow failure. Molecular analysis of the *SDBS* gene should be performed along with additional SDS-associated genes (i.e., *EFL1, DNAJC21, SRP54*). A lack of a molecular finding in a patient fitting the clinical syndrome does not exclude the diagnosis.[92,93]

Cancer Risk SDS is associated with an elevated risk of myelodysplastic syndrome and acute myeloid leukemia with as many as 20% of patients affected by age 18. Solid tumors are also reported in the adult population but are not known to affect the pediatric age group.[92,93]

Management and Surveillance SDS is a multisystem disorder requiring multidisciplinary care. Endocrinology evaluation of growth and gastroenterology management of pancreatic dysfunction are essential for patient care. From a hematologic perspective, the only curative management of bone marrow failure and prevention of acute myeloid leukemia is stem cell transplant. Patients who have not received transplant should receive surveillance for hematologic malignancies with complete blood counts every 3 months and bone marrow evaluations at least every 1 to 3 years if counts remain normal.[92,93]

▥ CONSTITUTIONAL CHROMOSOMAL ABNORMALTIES

Trisomy 18 (Edwards Syndrome)

Syndrome Overview Trisomy 18 is a constitutional chromosomal abnormality afflicting 1:6,000 to 1:8,000 newborns. Patients have a third copy of chromosome 18 resulting in a clinical syndrome of poor growth, rocker bottom feet, micrognathia, clenched hand, renal anomalies, structural cardiac defects, and developmental delays. Patients with trisomy 18 suffer significant mortality with only 10% surviving the first year of life.[24,95,96]

Diagnosis Trisomy 18 can be diagnosed pre- or postnatally by chromosome analysis that reveals an extra copy of chromosome 18.[24,96]

Cancer Risk Patients with trisomy 18 have increased rates of Wilms and hepatoblastoma. The risk of developing malignancy in these patients has been estimated at 1%; however, this is likely an underestimate of risk, given the early mortality in this patient population.[24,95]

Management and Surveillance Poor outcomes associated with trisomy 18 make surveillance for malignancy controversial. Given reports that patients with trisomy 18 have tolerated therapy and survived malignancy, early identification of malignancy may be beneficial. Surveillance plans should be individualized based on family preferences. Screening for Wilms and hepatoblastoma should be offered with abdominal ultrasounds every 3 months until age 4 and renal ultrasounds every 3 months until age 7. Monitoring of AFP should also be offered every 3 months with a management plan similar to patients with Beckwith-Wiedemann syndrome.[24,95]

Trisomy 21 (Down Syndrome)

Syndrome Overview Trisomy 21 is the most common constitutional chromosomal abnormality with an incidence of 1:1,000 births. Additional copies of genetic material on chromosome 21 manifest clinically as developmental/cognitive delays, cardiac abnormalities, hypotonia, microcephaly, abnormal facies (small mouth/nose, epicanthal folds, flat nasal bridge, upward-slanting palpebral fissures), Brushfield spots, excessive skin at the nape of the neck, single transverse palmar crease, and short fifth finger with clinodactyly. Specific genetic features associated with Trisomy 21 have been linked to the pathogenesis of malignancy. Increased risk of hematologic malignancy in this patient population has been associated with *GATA1* and *JAK2* mutations, resulting in abnormal megakaryopoiesis and increased myeloid proliferation. Interestingly, patients with trisomy 21 have a decreased risk of developing solid tumors, potentially related to increased presence of putative tumor suppressors. Patients with trisomy 21 also have increased levels of endostatin, which decreases angiogenesis, or blood vessel production, in solid tumors.[97-99]

Diagnosis Trisomy 21 can be screened for prenatally. Until recently, prenatal diagnosis was typically confirmed with amniotic fluid sampling. Currently, maternal serum can be collected to obtain fetal cell-free DNA for amplification and sequencing to provide earlier and safer diagnostic testing. Diagnosis is typically confirmed postnatally with chromosomal analysis, FISH, or PCR.[99]

Cancer Risk Patients with trisomy 21 are at a 10- to 20-fold increased risk of developing hematologic malignancies. The incidence of acute myeloid leukemia in general and acute megakaryoblastic leukemia in particular is much higher for these patients than the general population; however, they are also at increased risk for developing acute lymphoid leukemia, the most common pediatric hematologic malignancy. Approximately 10% of patients with trisomy 21 will develop transient myeloproliferative disorder (TMD) in the neonatal period. For patients without multiorgan involvement, this typically resolves on its own. About 20% of patients with TMD will develop acute myeloid leukemia later in life, often prior to age 5. Occurrence of acute myeloid leukemia after TMD is more likely in patients with *GATA1* mutations, and the risk is not modified by administration of therapy for the initial TMD.[97,98]

Management and Surveillance The American Academy of Pediatrics publishes complex guidelines for the comprehensive management of patients with trisomy 21. The current recommendation is for a complete blood count in the newborn period to screen for TMD, as well as parental education regarding the signs and symptoms of leukemia. Any patient with concerning signs or symptoms should have prompt medical evaluation; otherwise, complete blood counts can be monitored annually. There is minimal published data justifying surveillance protocols for patients with a history of TMD; however, given the high risk of developing acute myeloid leukemia in the first four years of life, surveillance with complete blood counts every 3 to 4 months should be considered. If patients do develop leukemia, protocols are specifically tailored to patients with trisomy 21 as they often have increased chemotherapy related toxicity. Overall, outcomes for young children with trisomy 21 who develop acute myeloid leukemia are better than unafflicted peers.[97-101]

■ PRIMARY IMMUNODEFICIENCY DISORDERS

Primary immunodeficiency disorders (PID) are a heterogenous group of disorders that result in altered cellular or humoral immunity. After infection, malignancy is the second leading cause of mortality in patients with PID. The pathogenesis of malignancies in these patients vary based on the specific type of immune defect. Defects in lymphocyte differenti-ation or maturation can result directly in hematologic malignancies of the type of lympho-cyte infected. For example, in combined variable immunodeficiency syndrome, impaired

B-cell differentiation can result in the development of B-cell lymphomas. Similarly, in severe combined immunodeficiency, DNA repair defects in lymphocytes can result in lymphoma or leukemia. In patients with PIDs, inherent stem cell defects such as severe congenital neutropenia can result in altered myeloid maturation and result in acute myeloid leukemia. Additionally, for patients with T-cell deficiencies, malignancy risk is increased secondary to deficient immune surveillance; the inability to detect and destroy malignant cells results in a predisposition to both hematologic malignancies and solid tumors. Moreover, environmental factors may provoke malignancy in patients with PID in the setting of a viral trigger, such as EBV or chronic inflammation.[102-104]

Common Variable Immunodeficiency Syndrome

Syndrome Overview Common variable immunodeficiency syndrome (CVID) is primarily a sporadic disorder with an incidence of 1:25,000 to 1:50,000. Many genes identified can contribute to the disorder; however, the pathogenesis of the disorder seems to involve both genetic and environmental factors. CVID is caused by impaired B-cell differentiation resulting in hypogammaglobulinemia. Malignancy in this syndrome is likely multifactorial related to inherent B-cell differentiation defects as well as chronic inflammation secondary to infection. In addition to malignancy, patients experience recurrent sinopulmonary infections as well as autoimmunity and granulomatous disease. CVID usually has an adult onset with affected pediatric patients not developing symptoms until after age 2.[102-104]

Diagnosis Because the genetics of CVID is poorly understood, diagnosis is primarily clinical. Patients with recurrent infections likely to have CVID have low or normal numbers of B-cells with decreased levels of IgG (2 standard deviations below the mean), IgA, and IgM.[104-106]

Cancer Risk Malignancy risk increases with advancing age for patients with CVID. Pediatric patients have a 2.2% risk of developing malignancy. The most common cancer in this population is non-Hodgkin lymphoma for which there is a greater than 30-fold risk increase. Gastric cancer also occurs in adults, frequently in association with *H. pylori* infection.[104,105]

Management and Surveillance The hallmark of therapy for patients with CVID is intravenous immunoglobulin repletion and prophylactic antibiotics. There are no guidelines specific to cancer surveillance in pediatric patients with CVID. Adult patients may benefit from endoscopic surveillance and *H. pylori* testing.[104,105]

DiGeorge Syndrome

Syndrome Overview DiGeorge syndrome is primarily a sporadic disorder with *de novo* mutations affecting 1:3,000 to 1:6,000 newborns. Non-sporadic cases have an autosomal dominant inheritance pattern. Patients with DiGeorge syndrome have a microdeletion at chromosome 22q11.2. This microdeletion results in immunodeficiency in about 75% of patients. Dysfunctional immune surveillance in these patients likely contributes to their increased risk of malignancy. Additional pathogenetic features contributing to malignancy associated with this microdeletion include haploinsufficiency of the *COMT* gene (carcinogen detoxification), *SMARCB1* gene (tumor suppression), and *DGCR8* gene (miRNA processing). Identifying clinical features of patients with DiGeorge syndrome include cardiac abnormalities, abnormal facies, thyroid dysfunction/aplasia, cleft palate, and hypocalcemia. Cognitive abnormalities and developmental delays are also common in this group.[107,108]

Diagnosis The diagnosis of DiGeorge syndrome is made by identifying the microdeletion on chromosome 22. Fluorescence in situ hybridization or chromosomal microarray will identify most cases.[108]

Cancer Risk The prevalence of malignancy in patients with DiGeorge syndrome remains unclear but reportedly is above that of the general population. As with many immunodeficiency syndromes, commonly occurring malignancies are hematologic; hepatoblastoma, Wilms tumor, and atypical teratoid/rhabdoid tumors have also been described.[107]

Management and Surveillance Because of the complexity of their disorder, patients with DiGeorge syndrome require care from multiple subspecialties. Management may include calcium supplementation, growth hormone therapy, speech therapy, and intravenous immunoglobulin therapy for immunocompromised patients. Given the risk of multiple hematologic and oncologic disorders associated with DiGeorge syndrome, patients should have annual surveillance complete blood counts. Other routine cancer surveillance is not recommended.[108]

Hyper-Immunoglobulin M Syndrome

Syndrome Overview Hyper-Immunoglobulin M syndrome (Hyper IgM) is an inherited X-linked immunodeficiency syndrome afflicting 1:500,000 newborn males. It is caused by alterations in the *CD40LG* gene, which encodes CD40 ligand expressed on T cells, a necessary protein for interactions with B cells. Patients typically have decreased levels of IgG and IgA with normal to increased levels of IgM. Clinically, patients with Hyper IgM suffer from recurrent sinopulmonary infections beginning before age 2. Chronic diarrhea is often present, which causes growth failure. Patients can also develop neutropenia, sclerosing cholangitis, and cirrhosis.[105,109]

Diagnosis Flow cytometry can be used to identify decreased CD40 ligand expression in patients with clinical features and immunoglobulin testing consistent with Hyper IgM. Molecular sequencing of the *CD40LG* gene can be used to confirm the diagnosis.[109]

Cancer Risk Patients with Hyper IgM are at increased risk of developing carcinomas of the gastrointestinal tract and liver occurring in as many as 80% of patients by age 20. There is also an increased incidence of lymphomas in this population.[105,109]

Surveillance and Management Infection prevention is key in managing patients with Hyper IgM. Children require prophylactic antibiotics and intravenous immunoglobulin therapy. Stem cell transplant is curative for these patients. Counseling regarding increased malignancy risk should be provided to patients and their family. Annual endoscopies are recommended to evaluate the gastrointestinal tract. Other signs of malignancy are assessed regularly by a thorough history and physical exam. Complete blood counts should be obtained to monitor for neutropenia.[109]

Severe Combined Immunodeficiency

Syndrome Overview Severe combined immunodeficiency (SCID) is the term applied to several genetic disorders that disrupt both cellular and humoral immunity. Inheritance is gene dependent, and both X-linked and autosomal recessive variants have been described.

Overall, the prevalence of SCID is approximately 1:50,000. Genetic defects in one of many genes (i.e., *IL2RG*) result in a clinical syndrome of recurrent infections (bacterial, viral, and fungal) in the first months of life with failure to thrive, diarrhea, and rashes. Patients have a high mortality rate in early childhood if the disease is left untreated. The development of malignancy in SCID is likely multifactorial. Intrinsic defects in DNA repair contribute to genomic instability and malignant transformation of lymphocytes into lymphoma/leukemia. Additionally, defects in immune surveillance reduce patients with SCIDs ability to detect and eliminate malignant cells.[102,105]

Diagnosis Newborn screening is crucial in the early diagnosis of SCID. T-cell receptor excision circle (TREC) testing can identify patients at birth with lymphopenia and is part of routine screening in most states. For patients with a positive newborn screen or suspected clinical features, further workup includes lymphocyte subset evaluation by flow cytometry and immunoglobulin levels. Definitive diagnosis is confirmed with molecular gene analysis.[110]

Cancer Risk For patients with SCID, cancer incidence is estimated to be 1.5%. Most commonly patients develop non-Hodgkin lymphoma, but Hodgkin's disease and leukemia also occur.[105]

Syndrome Overview and Management For most patients with SCID, stem cell transplant or gene therapy is necessary for survival past early childhood. Prior to curative therapy, the hallmark of patient therapy is infection prevention with intravenous immunoglobulin and prophylactic antibiotics. Currently, there are no specific surveillance guidelines for malignancy in this group.[105,110]

Severe Congenital Neutropenia

Syndrome Overview Severe congenital neutropenia (SCN) is a clinical syndrome with an estimated incidence of 1:200,000. The hallmark of SCN is the arrest of myeloid cell development leading to neutropenia. A variety of different genetic mutations have been identified in its pathogenesis. More than half of cases have mutations in the *ELA2* gene, which can be sporadic or autosomal dominantly inherited. Another common mutation is in *HAX1,* which has an autosomal recessive inheritance pattern. Patients with SCN typically present with recurrent infections in infancy and persistently low neutrophil counts. Patients can also present with cyclic neutropenia, a subtype of SCN, with oscillating neutrophil counts. The pathogenesis of malignancy in SCN is not related to lymphocyte defects or dysfunctional immune surveillance but rather inherent stem cell defects. These defects have the potential to cause abnormal myeloid proliferation and myelodysplastic syndrome/acute myeloid leukemia.[102,104,105]

Diagnosis A diagnosis of SCN should be suspected in patients with recurrent infections and persistent or cyclic neutropenia. Bone marrow biopsy and cytogenetics should be performed at diagnosis and should reveal arrest of neutrophil maturation without abnormalities in other cell lines. Molecular testing for known SCN-related genes should be performed.[101,111]

Cancer Risk Patients with SCN have an increased risk of developing leukemia. SCN is most commonly associated with acute myeloid leukemia; however, patients can also develop acute lymphocytic leukemia, bi-phenotypic leukemias, and chronic myeloid leukemia.[101,104,105]

Management and Surveillance Management of patients with SCN typically involves infection prevention using granulocyte colony-stimulating factor (G-CSF) to increase circulating neutrophil counts. Unfortunately, its use has been associated with leukemia development, and a large proportion of patients who develop leukemia have *G-CSFR* gene mutations. Frequent surveillance for leukemia is indicated with complete blood counts every 3 to 4 months. Bone marrow evaluations are recommended annually or sooner if a new cytopenia develops.[101,105]

Wiskott-Aldrich Syndrome

Syndrome Overview Wiskott-Aldrich syndrome (WAS) is an X-linked disorder affecting 1 to 10 out of 1,000,000 males; it rarely occurs in females. Mutations in the *WAS* gene result in abnormal WAS protein (WASP). WASP normally regulates cytoskeleton organization in hematopoietic cells. Aberrations in the WASP protein lead to defective adhesion, which disrupts cellular immune response. Patients with WAS often present with a triad of clinical features in infancy: recurrent infections, microthrombocytopenia, and eczema. Patients are also at increased risk for autoimmunity and malignancy. Pathogenesis of malignancy may be related to dampened immune surveillance, but a more direct effect of WASP on genomic stability has also been postulated.[104,105,112]

Diagnosis WAS should be suspected in patients with typical clinical features or those with family history of WAS. While platelet abnormalities and abnormal flow cytometry with lymphocyte abnormalities or absent WASP expression can guide diagnosis, confirmatory testing with molecular sequencing of the *WAS* gene is required.[104,105,112]

Cancer Risk Patients with WAS are at a significantly increased risk of malignancy, which occurs in 13 to 23% of patients. Non-Hodgkin lymphoma and leukemia are most common and typically present in adolescence. Malignancies are often associated with Epstein-Barr virus (EBV) in this population.[103–105,112]

Management and Surveillance Management of patients with WAS is primarily supported with antibiotic prophylaxis and intravenous immunoglobulin. Curative therapy consists of allogenic stem cell transplant to prevent early mortality from infection. There are no specific guidelines for monitoring malignancy in patients with WAS. Thorough histories and physical exams should be performed along with complete blood counts to evaluate severity of thrombocytopenia.[104,105,112]

X-Linked Lymphoproliferative Disease

Syndrome Overview X-linked lymphoproliferative disease (XLP) is an immunodeficiency disorder with X-linked inheritance. There are two types of the disease: XLP1 (altered *SH2D1A* gene) and XLP2 (altered *XIAP* gene) with an incidence of 1 in a million males and 1 in 5 million males, respectively. Patients with XLP1 have dysfunctional natural killer and T cells and impaired lymphocyte apoptosis. When exposed to EBV, patients with XLP1 have an exaggerated response that can result in hemophagocytic lymphohistiocytosis (HLH) and organ failure. Development of lymphoma is common. For patients with XLP2, HLH and colitis are common features; lymphoma is less frequently reported. Patients with either XLP1 or XLP2 may also present with hypogammaglobulinemia.[105,113]

Diagnosis Testing should be considered in all males with severe cases of EBV, HLH, recurrent lymphoma, multiple lymphoma diagnoses, or unexplained hypogammaglobulinemia. The diagnosis should also be considered in patients with a family history of a male relative with XLP related features. Flow cytometry testing for expression of SH2 domain protein1A (low in XLP1) and XIAP (low in XLP2) should be performed. Confirmatory testing with gene sequencing should be performed.[113]

Cancer Risk As many as 30% of patients with XLP1 will develop lymphoma, primarily non-Hodgkin, with a median age of onset of 6 years. These patients are more likely to have extra-nodal or intestinal disease than the general population. They are also more likely to have EBV-associated disease.[103,105]

Management and Surveillance Allogenic stem cell transplant remains the only curative option for XLP and is beneficial early in life to prevent complications. Supportive care with intravenous immunoglobulin in patients with hypogammaglobulinemia is indicated. There are no specific surveillance recommendations for patients with XLP; however, if lymphoma develops, patients should receive standard chemotherapy followed by stem cell transplant when in remission.[105,113]

References

1. Smith M, Hare ML. An overview of progress in childhood cancer survival. *J Pediatr Oncol Nurs.* 2004;21(3):160–164.

2. Siegel RL, Miller KD, Jemal A. Cancer statistics, 2018. *CA Cancer J Clin.* 2018;68(1):7–30.

3. Ward E, DeSantis C, Robbins A, et al. Childhood and adolescent cancer statistics, 2014. *CA: A Cancer Journal for Clinicians.* 2014;64(2):83–103.

4. Malkin D, Nichols KE, Schiffman JD, et al. The future of surveillance in the context of cancer predisposition: through the murky looking glass. *Clin Cancer Res.* 2017;23(21):e133–e137.

5. Walsh MF, Chang VY, Kohlmann WK, et al. Recommendations for childhood cancer screening and surveillance in DNA repair disorders. *Clinical Cancer Research.* 2017;23(11):e23–e31.

6. Spacey SD, Gatti RA, Bebb G. The molecular basis and clinical management of ataxia telangiectasia. *The Can J Neurol Sci.* 2000;27(3):184–191.

7. Rothblum-Oviatt C, Wright J, Lefton-Greif MA, et al. Ataxia telangiectasia: a review. *Orphanet J Rare Dis.* 2016;11(1):159.

8. Mallott J, Kwan A, Church J, et al. Newborn screening for SCID identifies patients with ataxia telangiectasia. *J Clin Immunol.* 2013;33(3):540–549.

9. Suarez F, Mahlaoui N, Canioni D, et al. Incidence, presentation, and prognosis of malignancies in ataxia-telangiectasia: a report from the French national registry of primary immune deficiencies. *J Clin Oncol.* 2015;33(2):202–208.

10. Suarez F, Mahlaoui N, Canioni D, et al. Incidence, presentation, and prognosis of malignancies in ataxia-telangiectasia: a report from the French national registry of primary immune deficiencies. *J Clin Oncol.* 2015;33(2):202–208.

11. Sanz MM, Cunniff C. Bloom's syndrome. GeneReviews® [Internet]. Seattle: University of Washington.

12. Cunniff C, Bassetti JA, Ellis NA. Bloom's syndrome: clinical spectrum, molecular pathogenesis, and cancer predisposition. *Mol Syndromol.* 2017;8(1):4–23.

13. Tabori U, Hansford JR, Achatz MI, et al. Clinical management and tumor surveillance recommendations of inherited mismatch repair deficiency in childhood. *Clinical Cancer Research.* 2017;23(11):e32–e37.

14. Wimmer K, Kratz CP, Vasen HF, et al. Diagnostic criteria for constitutional mismatch repair deficiency syndrome: suggestions of the European consortium "care for CMMRD" (C4CMMRD). *J Med Genet.* 2014;51(6):355–365.

15. Westdorp H, Kolders S, Hoogerbrugge N, et al. Immunotherapy holds the key to cancer treatment and prevention in constitutional mismatch repair deficiency (CMMRD) syndrome. *Cancer Lett.* 2017;403:159–164.

16. Longerich S, Li J, Xiong Y, et al. Stress and DNA repair biology of the Fanconi anemia pathway. *Blood*. 2014;124(18):2812–2819.

17. Nalepa G, Clapp DW. Fanconi anaemia and cancer: an intricate relationship. *Nat Rev Cancer*. 2018;18(3): 168–185.

18. Alter BP. Fanconi anemia and the development of leukemia. Best Pract Res *Clin Haematol*. 2014 Sep–Dec;27(3–4):214–21.

19. Chrzanowska KH, Gregorek H, Dembowska-Bagińska B, et al. Nijmegen breakage syndrome (NBS). *Orphanet Journal of Rare Diseases*. 2012;7:13.

20. Wang LL, Levy ML, Lewis RA, et al. Clinical manifestations in a cohort of 41 Rothmund-Thomson syndrome patients. *Am J Med Genet*. 2001;102(1):11–17.

21. Colombo EA, Locatelli A, Cubells Sánchez L, et al. Rothmund-Thomson syndrome: insights from new patients on the genetic variability underpinning clinical presentation and cancer outcome. *Int J Mol Sci*. 2018;19(4).

22. DiGiovanna JJ, Kraemer KH. Shining a light on xeroderma pigmentosum. *J Invest Dermatol*. 2012;132(3 Pt. 2): 785–796.

23. Bradford PT, Goldstein AM, Tamura D, et al. Cancer and neurologic degeneration in xeroderma pigmentosum: long term follow-up characterises the role of DNA repair. *Journal of Medical Genetics*. 2011;48(3):168–176.

24. Kalish JM, Doros L, Helman LJ, et al. Surveillance recommendations for children with overgrowth syndromes and predisposition to Wilms tumors and hepatoblastoma. *Clinical Cancer Research*. 2017;23(13):e115–e122.

25. Russell B, Johnston JJ, Biesecker LG, et al. Clinical management of patients with ASXL1 mutations and Bohring-Opitz syndrome, emphasizing the need for Wilms tumor surveillance. *American Journal of Medical Genetics, Part A*. 2015;167a(9):2122–2131.

26. Achatz MI, Porter CC, Brugières L, et al. Cancer screening recommendations and clinical management of inherited gastrointestinal cancer syndromes in childhood. *Clinical Cancer Research*. 2017;23(13):e107–e114.

27. Aihara H, Kumar N, Thompson CC. Diagnosis, surveillance, and treatment strategies for familial adenomatous polyposis: rationale and update. *Eur J Gastroenterol Hepatol*. 2014;26(3):255–262.

28. Foulkes WD, Kamihara J, Evans DGR, et al. Cancer Surveillance in Gorlin Syndrome and Rhabdoid Tumor Predisposition Syndrome. *Clinical Cancer Research*. 2017;23(12):e62–e7.

29. Bresler SC, Padwa BL, Granter SR. Nevoid basal cell carcinoma syndrome (Gorlin syndrome). *Head Neck Pathol*. 2016;10(2):119–124.

30. Schultz KAP, Rednam SP, Kamihara J, et al. PTEN, DICER1, FH, and their associated tumor susceptibility syndromes: clinical features, genetics, and surveillance recommendations in childhood. *Clinical Cancer Research*. 2017;23(12):e76–e82.

31. Menko FH, Maher ER, Schmidt LS, et al. Hereditary leiomyomatosis and renal cell cancer (HLRCC): renal cancer risk, surveillance and treatment. *Fam Cancer*. 2014;13(4):637–644.

32. Rednam SP, Erez A, Druker H, et al. Von Hippel–Lindau and hereditary pheochromocytoma/paraganglioma syndromes: clinical features, genetics, and surveillance recommendations in childhood. *Clinical Cancer Research*. 2017;23(12):e68–e75.

33. Henegan JC Jr., Gomez CR. Heritable cancer syndromes related to the hypoxia pathway. *Front Oncol*. 2016;6:68.

34. Kamihara J, Bourdeaut F, Foulkes WD, et al. Retinoblastoma and neuroblastoma predisposition and surveillance. *Clinical Cancer Research*. 2017;23(13):e98–e106.

35. Alfred GK. Mutation and cancer: statistical study of retinoblastoma. *Proc Natl Acad Sci U S A*. 1971; 68(4):820–823.

36. Rao R, Honavar SG. Retinoblastoma. *Indian J Pediatr*. 2017;84(12):937–944.

37. Soliman SE, Racher H, Zhang C, et al. Genetics and molecular fiagnostics in tetinoblastoma: an update. *Asia Pac J Ophthalmol*. 2017;6(2):197–207.

38. Temming P, Viehmann A, Biewald E, et al. Sporadic unilateral retinoblastoma or first sign of bilateral disease? *Br J Ophthalmol*. 2013;97(4):475–480.

39. Bougeard G, Renaux-Petel M, Flaman JM, et al. Revisiting Li-Fraumeni syndrome from TP53 mutation carriers. *J Clin Oncol*. 2015;33(21):2345–2352.

40. Kratz CP, Achatz MI, Brugières L, et al. Cancer screening recommendations for individuals with Li-Fraumeni syndrome. *Clinical Cancer Research*. 2017;23(11):e38–e45.

41. Ferreira AM, Brondani VB, Helena VP, et al. Clinical spectrum of Li-Fraumeni syndrome/Li-Fraumeni-like syndrome in Brazilian individuals with the TP53 p.R337H mutation. *J Steroid Biochem Mol Biol*. 2019;190:250–255.

42. Guha T, Malkin D. Inherited TP53 mutations and the Li-Fraumeni syndrome. *Cold Spring Harb Perspect Med*. 2017;7(4).

43. Syngal S, Brand RE, Church JM, et al. ACG clinical guideline: Genetic testing and management of hereditary gastrointestinal cancer syndromes. *Am J Gastroenterol*. 2015;110(2):223–262; quiz 63.

44. Ishida H, Ishibashi K, Iwama T. Malignant tumors associated with juvenile polyposis syndrome in Japan. *Surg Today*. 2018;48(3):253–263.

45. Wasserman JD, Tomlinson GE, Druker H, et al. Multiple endocrine neoplasia and hyperparathyroid-jaw tumor syndromes: clinical features, genetics, and surveillance recommendations in childhood. *Clinical Cancer Research*. 2017;23(13):e123–e132.

46. Al-Salameh A, Baudry C, Cohen R. Update on multiple endocrine neoplasia Type 1 and 2. *Presse Med (Paris, France: 1983)*. 2018;47(9):722–731.

47. Agarwal SK. The future: genetics advances in MEN1 therapeutic approaches and management strategies. *Endocr Relat Cancer*. 2017;24(10):T119–T134.

48. Yohay KH. The genetic and molecular pathogenesis of NF1 and NF2. *Semin Pediatr Neurol*. 2006;13(1): 21–26.

49. Evans DGR, Salvador H, Chang VY, et al. Cancer and central nervous system tumor surveillance in pediatric neurofibromatosis 1. *Clinical Cancer Research*. 2017;23(12):e46–e53.

50. Villani A, Greer M-LC, Kalish JM, et al. Recommendations for cancer surveillance in individuals with RASopathies and other rare genetic conditions with increased cancer risk. *Clinical Cancer Research*. 2017;23(12):e83–e90.

51. Niemeyer CM. RAS diseases in children. *Haematologica*. 2014;99(11):1653–1662.

52. Evans DGR, Salvador H, Chang VY, et al. Cancer and central nervous system tumor surveillance in pediatric neurofibromatosis 2 and related disorders. *Clinical Cancer Research*. 2017;23(12):e54–e61.

53. Ardern-Holmes S, Fisher G, North K. Neurofibromatosis type 2:presentation, major complications, and management, with a focus on the pediatric age group. *J Child Neurol*. 2017;32(1):9–22.

54. Riegert-Johnson D, Westra W, et al. Peutz-Jeghers syndrome. In: Riegert-Johnson DL, Hefferon T, et al. (Eds). *Cancer Syndromes* [Internet]. Bethesda, MD: National Center for Biotechnology Information; 2008.

55. Beggs AD, Latchford AR, Vasen HF, et al. Peutz-Jeghers syndrome: a systematic review and recommendations for management. *Gut*. 2010;59(7):975–86.

56. Mester J, Charis E. PTEN hamartoma tumor syndrome. *Handb Clin Neurol*. 2015;132:129–137.

57. Tan MH, Mester JL, Ngeow J, et al. Lifetime cancer risks in individuals with germline PTEN mutations. *Clinical Cancer Research*. 2012;18(2):400–407.

58. Rauen KA. The RASopathies. *Annu Rev Genomics Hum Genet*. 2013;14:355–369.

59. Sredni ST, Tomita T. Rhabdoid tumor predisposition syndrome. *Pediatr Dev Pathol*. 2015;18(1):49–58.

60. Fitzhugh VA. Rhabdoid tumor predisposition syndrome and pleuropulmonary blastoma syndrome. *J Pediatr Genet*. 2016;5(2):124–128.

61. Tenorio J, Arias P, Martínez-Glez V, et al. Simpson-Golabi-Behmel syndrome types I and II. *Orphanet Journal of Rare Diseases*. 2014;9:138.

62. Vuillaume ML, Moizard MP, Baumer A, et al. CUGC for Simpson-Golabi-Behmel syndrome (SGBS). *European Journal of Human Genetics*. 2019;27(4):663–668.

63. Scott RH, Walker L, Olsen ØE, et al. Surveillance for Wilms tumour in at-risk children: pragmatic recommendations for best practice. *Arch Dis Child*. 2006;91(12):995–999.

64. Krueger DA, Northrup H. Tuberous sclerosis complex surveillance and management: recommendations of the 2012 International Tuberous Sclerosis Complex Consensus Conference. *Pediatr Neurol.* 2013; 49(4):255–265.

65. Northrup H, Krueger DA. Tuberous sclerosis complex diagnostic criteria update: recommendations of the 2012 International Tuberous Sclerosis Complex Consensus Conference. *Pediatric Neurology.* 2013;49(4):243–254.

66. Samueli S, Abraham K, Dressler A, et al. Tuberous Sclerosis Complex: new criteria for diagnostic work-up and management. *Wien Klin Wochenschr.* 2015;127(15-16):619–630.

67. Wataya-Kaneda M, Uemura M, Fujita K, et al. Tuberous sclerosis complex: Recent advances in manifestations and therapy. *Int J Urol.* 2017;24(9):681–691.

68. Gossage L, Eisen T, Maher ER. VHL, the story of a tumour suppressor gene. *Nature Reviews Cancer.* 2014;15:55.

69. Chittiboina P, Lonser RR. Von Hippel-Lindau disease. *Handbook of Clinical Neurology.* 2015;132:139–156.

70. Poulsen M, Budtz-Jørgensen E, Bisgaard M. Surveillance in von Hippel-Lindau disease (VHL). *Clin Genet.* 2010;77(1):49–59.

71. Liu Z, Thiele CJ. ALK and MYCN: when two oncogenes are better than one. *Cancer Cell.* 2012;21(3):325–326.

72. Mossé YP, Laudenslager M, Longo L, et al. Identification of ALK as a major familial neuroblastoma predisposition gene. *Nature.* 2008;455(7215):930–935.

73. Tolbert VP, Coggins GE, Maris JM. Genetic susceptibility to neuroblastoma. *Curr Opin Genet Dev.* 2017;42:81–90.

74. Tang SL, Gao YL, Wen-Zhong H. Knockdown of TRIM37 suppresses the proliferation, migration and invasion of glioma cells through the inactivation of PI3K/Akt signaling pathway. *Biomed Pharmacother.* 2018;99:59–64.

75. Brigant B, Metzinger-Le Meuth V, Rochette J, et al. TRIMming down to TRIM37: relevance to inflammation, cardiovascular disorders, and cancer in MULIBREY nanism. *Int J Mol Sci.* 2018;20(1).

76. Wells SA Jr. Advances in the management of MEN2: from improved surgical and medical treatment to novel kinase inhibitors. *Endocr Relat Cancer.* 2018;25(2):T1–T13.

77. Marquard JEC. Multiple endocrine neoplasia type 2. In: Adam MP, Ardinger HH, Pagon RA, et al. (Eds). *GeneReviews® [Internet].* Seattle: University of Washington; 1999 [Updated 2015].

78. Brioude F, Kalish JM, Mussa A, et al. Expert consensus document: Clinical and molecular diagnosis, screening and management of Beckwith-Wiedemann syndrome: an international consensus statement. *Nat Rev Endocrinol.* 2018;14(4):229–249.

79. Charlton J, Irtan S, Bergeron C, et al. Bilateral Wilms tumour: a review of clinical and molecular features. *Expert Rev Mol Med.* 2017;19:e8.

80. Dome JS. Wilms tumor predisposition. In: Adam MP, Ardinger HH, Pagon RA, et al. (Eds). *GeneReviews® [Internet].* Seattle: University of Washington; 2003.

81. McCann-Crosby B, Mansouri R, Dietrich JE, et al. State of the art review in gonadal dysgenesis: challenges in diagnosis and management. *International Journal of Pediatric Endocrinology.* 2014;2014(1):4.

82. Vlachos A, Muir E. How I treat Diamond-Blackfan anemia. *Blood.* 2010;116(19):3715–3723.

83. Lipton JM, Ellis SR. Diamond-Blackfan anemia: diagnosis, treatment, and molecular pathogenesis. *Hematol Oncol Clin North Am.* 2009;23(2):261–282.

84. Engidaye G, Melku M, Enawgaw B. Diamond Blackfan anemia: genetics, pathogenesis, diagnosis and treatment. *EJIFCC.* 2019;30(1):67–81.

85. Vlachos A, Rosenberg PS, Atsidaftos E, et al. Incidence of neoplasia in Diamond Blackfan anemia: a report from the Diamond Blackfan Anemia Registry. *Blood.* 2012;119(16):3815–3819.

86. Bartels M, Bierings M. How I manage children with Diamond-Blackfan anaemia. *Br J Haematol.* 2019;184(2):123–133.

87. Schultz KAP, Rednam SP, Kamihara J, et al. PTEN, DICER1, FH, and their associated tumor susceptibility syndromes: Clinical features, genetics, and surveillance recommendations in childhood. *Clinical Cancer Research.* 2017;23(12):e76–e82.

88. Robertson JC, Jorcyk CL, Oxford JT. DICER1 syndrome: DICER1 mutations in rare cancers. *Cancers.* 2018;10(5).

89. Schultz KAP, Williams GM, Kamihara J, et al. DICER1 and associated conditions: identification of at-risk individuals and recommended surveillance strategies. *Clinical Cancer Research.* 2018;24(10):2251–2261.

90. Dokal I. Dyskeratosis congenita. *Hematology Am Soc Hematol Educ Program.* 2011;2011:480–486.

91. Astuti D, Morris MR, Cooper WN, et al. Germline mutations in DIS3L2 cause the Perlman syndrome of overgrowth and Wilms tumor susceptibility. *Nature Genetics.* 2012;44(3):277–284.

92. Nelson AS, Myers KC. Diagnosis, treatment, and molecular pathology of Shwachman-Diamond syndrome. *Hematology/oncology Clinics of North America.* 2018;32(4):687–700.

93. Dror Y, Donadieu J, Koglmeier J, et al. Draft consensus guidelines for diagnosis and treatment of Shwachman-Diamond syndrome. *Ann N Y Acad Sci.* 2011;1242:40–55.

94. Nakhoul H, Ke J, Zhou X, et al. Ribosomopathies: mechanisms of disease. *Clin Med Insights Blood Disord.* 2014;7:7–16.

95. Satgé D, Nishi M, Sirvent N, et al. A tumor profile in Edwards syndrome (trisomy 18). *Am J Med Genet C Semin Med Genet.* 2016;172(3):296–306.

96. Cereda A, Carey JC. The trisomy 18 syndrome. *Orphanet Journal of Rare Diseases.* 2012;7:81.

97. Rabin KR, Whitlock JA. Malignancy in children with trisomy 21. *Oncologist.* 2009;14(2):164–173.

98. Gamis AS, Alonzo TA, Gerbing RB, et al. Natural history of transient myeloproliferative disorder clinically diagnosed in Down syndrome neonates: a report from the Children's Oncology Group Study A2971. *Blood.* 2011;118(26):6752–6759; quiz 996.

99. Asim A, Kumar A, Muthuswamy S, et al. Down syndrome: an insight of the disease. *J Biomed Sci.* 2015;22(1):41.

100. Bull MJ. Health supervision for children with Down syndrome. *Pediatrics.* 2011;128(2):393–406.

101. Porter CC, Druley TE, Erez A, et al. Recommendations for surveillance for children with leukemia-predisposing conditions. *Clinical Cancer Research.* 2017;23(11):e14–e22.

102. Hauck F, Voss R, Urban C, et al. Intrinsic and extrinsic causes of malignancies in patients with primary immunodeficiency disorders. *J Allergy Clin Immunol.* 2018;141(1):59–68.

103. Riaz IB, Faridi W, Patnaik MM, et al. A systematic review on predisposition to lymphoid (B and T cell) neoplasias in patients with primary immunodeficiencies and immune dysregulatory disorders (inborn errors of immunity). *Front Immunol.* 2019;10:777.

104. Mortaz E, Tabarsi P, Mansouri D, et al. Cancers related to immunodeficiencies: update and perspectives. *Frontiers in Immunology.* 2016;7:365.

105. Shapiro RS. Malignancies in the setting of primary immunodeficiency: implications for hematologists/oncologists. *Am J Hematol.* 2011;86(1):48–55.

106. Ameratunga R, Brewerton M, Slade C, et al. Comparison of diagnostic criteria for common variable immunodeficiency disorder. *Frontiers in Immunology.* 2014;5:415.

107. Lambert MP, Arulselvan A, Schott A, et al. The 22q11.2 deletion syndrome: Cancer predisposition, platelet abnormalities and cytopenias. *AM J Med Genet A.* 2017.

108. McDonald-McGinn DM, Zackai EH. 22q11.2 deletion syndrome. In: Adam MP, Ardinger HH, Pagon RA, et al. (Eds). *GeneReviews® [Internet].* Seattle: University of Washington; 1999.

109. Johnson J, Zhang K. X-linked hyper IgM syndrome. In: Adam MP, Ardinger HH, Pagon RA, et al. (Eds). *GeneReviews® [Internet]* Seattle: University of Washington; 2007.

110. Allenspach E, Scharenberg AM. X-linked severe combined immunodeficiency. In: Adam MP, Ardinger HH, Pagon RA, et al. (Eds). *GeneReviews® [Internet].* Seattle: University of Washington; 2003.

111. Dale DC. ELANE-related neutropenia. In: Adam MP, Ardinger HH, Pagon RA, et al. (Eds). *GeneReviews® [Internet].* Seattle: University of Washington; 2002 (Updated 2018).

112. Candotti F. Clinical manifestations and pathophysiological mechanisms of the Wiskott-Aldrich syndrome. *J Clin Immunol.* 2018;38(1):13–27.

113. Zhang K, Marsh R. Lymphoproliferative Disease, X-Linked. In: Adam MP, Ardinger HH, Pagon RA, et al. (Eds). *GeneReviews® [Internet].* Seattle: University of Washington; 2004.

16

Ethical, Legal, and Psychosocial Issues in Cancer Genetic Assessment and Genetic Testing

Jennifer Scalia Wilbur, Jessica Haddad, Marcina Beaston, and Katherine Crawford

With excitement, we embrace the exponential growth of cancer genetics and risk assessment as it yields an increase in the identification of high-risk families and provides a more personalized approach to cancer treatment. However, this rapid growth of knowledge brings developments that have impacted important principles of ethics, legal issues, and psychosocial concerns, which in turn have directly affected the clinical care of this high-risk population. This chapter will address topics that include the healthcare practitioners' duty to recontact; legal clarity surrounding the obligation to warn at-risk family members; and the identification of vulnerable patient groups who could benefit from added support during this revolutionary era of medicine.

ETHICAL AND LEGAL ISSUES

Though there are many ethical theories debated within the biomedical field, the two most relevant to genetic testing are *ethics of care* and *principle-based ethics*.[1,2] The focus of ethics of care is to meet the needs of, and act on behalf of, those for whom the caregiver takes responsibility for.[2,3] This theory arose in response to the rights-based theories that can overlook the realities of human dependence and thus emphasize relationships.[2–4] Principle-based ethics has been derived from broad moral principles to provide guidelines that serve as an analytic framework to resolve ethical issues. These guidelines can be used to help determine the actions that result in the greatest overall good.[1,4,5] These guidelines are broadly defined as autonomy, beneficence, nonmaleficence, and justice.[1,5]

Autonomy is the understanding that each individual has a unique viewpoint and a respect for their personal decision-making.[2] Autonomy, in the context of biomedical ethics, focuses less on the autonomous person—a person capable of self-governance—and more on the principle of autonomous choice. Beauchamp and Childress assert that the autonomous chooser should act with (1) intent, (2) understanding, (3) and without controlling influence in their decision-making. Intent represents the most straightforward of these criteria, since one's acts are either intentional or unintentional; however, the presence of controlling influences presents a spectrum of autonomous consent.[1] For example, children are not able to make decisions independent of parental input, but they are able to provide assent from as early as 7 years old. Children are not considered autonomous, but they are able to express intent and many Institutional Review Boards require assent for studies with child participants. Understanding is closely tied to informed consent and is based on the chooser having a full and clear understanding of the benefits, consequences, and limitations of medical care. Similarly, Uhlmann presents obligations derived from autonomy that are relevant to bioethics in the genetics field: truth-telling, confidentiality, and informed consent. Truth-telling is an important part of fidelity and promise-keeping to the patient but also pertains to the patient's understanding of their medical care. Consent can only be valid if the communication of information is truthful.[2] Confidentiality and informed consent will be discussed in greater detail later in the chapter, but it is important to note that these tenets also fall under the umbrella of autonomy.

Beneficence is defined as the act of producing or promoting the well-being of others.[6] There should be a net benefit of an action that ultimately benefits society's general welfare. In a clinical context, it is important to note that the principle of beneficence assumes that both provider and patient have similar views of what constitutes a benefit. Practically, beneficence dictates the provider act in good faith as an advocate for their patient. Sometimes beneficence can be interpreted as paternalism when a provider's perception of beneficent behavior violates a patient's autonomy. An attempt to be beneficent should not supersede a patient's autonomy and a provider must still respect a patient's choices.[2]

Nonmaleficence can be seen as being derived from beneficence; it is most commonly framed as "do no harm."[2] Nonmaleficence is both an ethical and a legal duty within the medical system to not inflict harm on patients.[1] It is an important principle in genetics in regard to research as well as other ethical issues, such as duty to warn and incidental findings that will be discussed in detail later in the chapter.

Justice is a principle shared across ethical theories and relates to treating people equitably and with fairness.[2] What this most readily applies to in biomedical ethics is the distribution of resources and care.[7] Four values are derived from justice in the healthcare field: equality, liberty, excellence, and efficiency. Equality is also referred to as distributive justice; it is the principle that resources of the healthcare system should be distributed equally across a society.[2,8] While conceptually this may be simple, the limited nature of healthcare resources and the market economy of the U.S. healthcare system can make this a very complex ethical issue.[2,8] Liberty is the freedom to choose within the healthcare system for both the provider and patient. Excellence represents the best possible care for all while efficiency is also known as stewardship, which refers to the management of healthcare costs.[2]

Examples of ethical principles and the applications to cancer genetics can be found in Table 16.1.[9]

The genetic conditions are often discussed in broad categories that may be useful for the reader to consider for ethical decision-making. Note that not every genetic condition falls neatly into a category; they are meant to provide a basic framework (see Table 16.2 for examples). The first major distinction is childhood-onset versus adult-onset conditions. Many

TABLE 16.1: Definitions of Tenets of Principle-based Ethics		
Ethical Principle	**Definition**	**Example**
Autonomy	An individual's right to make decisions and act in a way free from manipulation of outside forces.	Allowing patients to make their own decisions regarding genetic testing after providing them with the relevant information.
Beneficence	The moral obligation to act in a way that benefits others.	The return of clinically actionable results to a deceased person's family.
Nonmaleficence	The obligation to not cause harm.	Recontacting patients after a variant of uncertain significance (VUS) reclassification to pathogenic as it will meaningfully alter their care.
Justice	The principle guiding equal distribution of and access to care and services.	Access to genetic testing being offered to all individuals meeting NCCN guidelines for testing regardless of socioeconomic status.

TABLE 16.2: Intervention Framework for Genetic Syndrome Evaluation		
	Childhood-onset	**Adult-onset**
Intervention available	Beckwith-Wiedemann syndrome	*BRCA1/BRCA2*
No intervention available	Duchenne's Muscular Dystrophy	Huntington's disease

inherited cancer syndromes do not onset until adulthood, with few notable exceptions, which is why testing is often delayed until the information is pertinent and the individual can make an informed decision about testing. The second major distinction is treatment and whether or not there is a medical intervention that is curative or would greatly improve quality of life. Conditions for which there is an intervention, such as breast screening for carriers of pathogenic *BRCA1* or *BRCA2* variants, can have a greater moral imperative to test.

With this framework in mind, we will explore the ethical and legal issues that arise within the field of genetic testing with a specific focus on those issues especially pertinent to oncology.

Informed Consent

Informed consent is primarily a manifestation of autonomy; it is the authorization to do something with understanding, intention, and free from the control of others.[2,10] However, this cornerstone of the therapeutic alliance can be more difficult to achieve when the subject matter is related to genetic testing.[11-13] The complexity of genetic mechanisms as well as the important choices often made as a result of these tests warrant special consideration in regards to informed consent.[11] Both accuracy and amount of information provided should be tailored to the setting. The information should always be truthful as veracity is paramount to the patient-provider relationship. The information should include both risks and benefits, as well as alternative options available to the patient. The provider should assess the patient's comprehension of the information and try to overcome any barrier to understanding, such as language barriers, unscientific beliefs, or fear or confusion due to illness or low numeracy.[2] Without the patient's understanding of this information, informed consent cannot be obtained. It is important that a patient gives consent *voluntarily* and that their authorization is an active agreement and not simply complying with the suggestion of a provider. Furthermore, a patient must have the *capacity* to make these choices, meaning they must be able to understand the information and the consequences as well as communicate their desired choice.[2,14] *Competency* is the legal term referring to someone with the capacity and legal ability to make decisions regarding their care.[14,15] Someone is considered competent at the age of 18, but if the issue of competency is of concern it can be determined by a court, who can assign a guardian to make decisions on the individual's behalf.[15] Informed consent is both an ethical and legal issue, especially in regard to research in which informed consent must include disclosure of information, competency of the patient (or surrogate), and voluntary consent. Without these three elements, informed consent is not obtained under the regulations of the FDA.[16] Exceptions to informed consent do arise in clinical care with notable instances being low-risk interventions with obvious risk and benefit; in these instances consent is implied. Additionally, it also applies in emergency situations in which a patient may not be able to be an active participant in their own care. Under these circumstances a "reasonable person" standard is used, meaning that a reasonable person under similar circumstances would consent and thus consent is presumed.[2,17]

In terms of genetic testing, risks and benefits are not considered obvious and so consent is not implied; however, a blood draw for the purpose of genetic testing would meet the standards to have consent implied. While genetic testing is rarely considered as part of an emergency event, testing someone who is not competent or capable, without informed consent of a guardian, violates both autonomy and established legal principles. The process of obtaining informed consent should always allow for the patient to elect not to proceed with genetic testing as many "reasonable people" choose to do.[18,19] Further, the Convention on Human Rights and Biomedicine created the Universal Declaration on the Human Genome and Human Rights, which states that individuals have a right to be informed about their own genetic information and equally have a right to remain unaware, if they so choose.[11,20]

Legally, some type of consent is required for genetic testing in approximately half of all U.S. states with at least one state requiring written consent of the person being tested.[21] Laws regarding consent have mainly focused on privacy of data and disposal of sample after testing.[22] The American College of Medical Genetics and Genomics (ACMG) and the National Society of Genetic Counselors (NSGC) both have statements regarding informed consent in the context of secondary findings pertinent to return of exome, but not in response to clinical testing.[23,24] A survey done by the ACMG found that the more experience someone had in ordering exome-type tests that could include incidental findings, the less they supported the idea that patients should be able to opt out or customize the secondary finding gene list.[23] This suggests that more experienced practitioners do not always support the need for informed consent in genetic testing. The concept of genetic exceptionalism is discussed later in the chapter but applies to the conflicting views regarding whether informed consent is necessary when it is not required for other complex medical tests that can also reveal incidental findings. Of note, the most common genetic test performed in the country is the newborn screen (NBS), which includes at least 29 genetic diseases in all states with most states not having an opt-out option. Informed consent is not obtained for NBS and most parents are uninformed or misinformed about it.[25] It is important to remain up to date regarding each individual state's laws regarding informed consent. See https://www.genome.gov/about-genomics/policy-issues/Genome-Statute-Legislation-Database.

> **KEY POINTS**
>
> - Informed consent is not legally required for genetic testing but may be considered ethically virtuous. The core principles of informed consent are
>   - a. Capacity and competence
>   - b. Accuracy and amount of information
>   - c. Patient understanding
>   - d. Voluntary consent
> - Informed consent is both an ethical and legal principle.

▥ TESTING OF MINORS

The testing of minors can be an ethical quagmire. Individuals under the age of 18 are not considered competent to make decisions regarding healthcare unless emancipated. The American Medical Association (AMA), the NSGC, the American Society of Human Genetics (ASHG), the European Society of Human Genetics (ESHG), and many other governing societies have published statements on testing minors. They collectively agree that in the case of testing minors for adult-onset conditions with no intervention available or that would be provided before age 18, often referred to as *predictive testing* (see Table 16.2), genetic testing should be deferred until adulthood.[26-29] This protects patient autonomy by allowing them to decide for themselves. Additionally, this is an example of nonmaleficence and beneficence in that it attempts to protect the psychological well-being of the patient by not burdening them with potentially traumatic or life-altering information.

The majority of genetic testing in the oncology setting falls into the category of adult-onset with no interventions available until after age 18. However, some parents have argued for the testing of minors, most notably in the context of the *BRCA1/2* genes. Work examining parental attitudes toward testing of minors from *BRCA*-positive parents found that 24% of adult mutation carriers surveyed described specific scenarios in which testing of a minor could be appropriate. These scenarios included both maturity of the minor as well as perceived health benefit. However, the same study identified that the majority of these *BRCA*-positive parents were opposed to the testing of minors, citing psychological harm and lack of maturity.[30] Some have argued for earlier ages of consent to better foster autonomous decision-making, while others contend that maturity of decision-making is variable and parental decisions violate future autonomy of the child.[30-35] Overall, the perspective of *BRCA*-positive parents was mixed as far as situations in which testing might be applicable. Open and honest communication about deferment of testing, as supported by many societies, is often the supported course of action. It is important to note that in some countries minors may give valid consent at a younger age and that within the United States some states allow minors to consent for specific services, but genetic testing does not fall within those allowed services.[36,37]

However, there are notable exceptions within the field of cancer genetic testing for which the testing of minors is recommended, such as genetic mutations in the *TP53* gene or familial adenomatous polyposis (FAP) syndrome. These conditions fall into the category of childhood or near childhood onset with early interventions that do reduce risk or improve outcome. The interest of beneficence and nonmaleficence can conflict with autonomy; however, a guardian is able to give consent and act in the best interest of the minor. Still, performing tests on minors requires caution and if at all possible, it is considered best to wait until an age in which minors are more able to understand the scope and purpose of the test and to give assent. In some cases, the information is needed for medical decision-making before that point and only genetic testing can provide the information necessary for care.[11,38–40] The ACMG states a minor's expression of dissent is final in the case of genetic testing, but if the testing is in the child's best interest and the family has considered the potential psychosocial harms to the child, as well as the larger family, genetic testing can be performed[41] (more detail reviewed within the psychosocial portion of this chapter). The AAP has stated that minors should play a larger role in their own healthcare as they age, but both the AAP and ACMG lack guidelines about the return of secondary findings to minors.[41–44]

The essentials of testing minors in cancer genetics are as follows:

- Testing for conditions that have no change in management before 18 should be deferred until 18 when possible.
- For conditions with management changes before 18, testing can be performed.
- Testing of a minor requires caution and should be done only in the child's best interest with careful consideration of psychosocial implications.

DIRECT-TO-CONSUMER (DTC) TESTING

There is risk of harm in genetic testing when an individual lacks proper genetic counseling influencing the information aspect of informed consent or when inaccurate testing or interpretation of genetic information impacts clinical decision-making.[45] Direct-to-consumer tests with hereditary cancer information are widely available on the open market and raise concerns that providers must be prepared to address.[46] Arguments for DTC testing are based on greater access to information; however, there are also concerns about consumer education and informed consent with the use of these tests.[45] The 23andMe test available to consumers was authorized by the FDA to test only the *BRCA1/2* genes for three founder mutations seen in the Ashkenazi Jewish population.[46] The FDA noted that this test had limitations and should not be a substitute for seeing a physician to guide care.[47] Most notable is that 23andMe is not a CLIA-approved lab and thus does not meet the strict standards of proficiency testing of personnel and quality control of other genetic laboratories.[45] Proficiency testing of laboratory personnel is strongly associated with increased quality of results and fewer reported analytic errors.[45,48] Yet advertising of DTC testing has the potential to drive up demand for genetic testing while decreasing referrals of high-risk women to high-risk clinics demonstrating that advertising of these tests does not fully capture their limitations.[45,49] Further, a recent study found that 38% of participants had not considered the possibility of receiving unwanted information before purchasing DTC tests.[46,50] Return of higher-risk results from DTC testing raises concerns about behavioral changes, willingness to contact appropriate medical professionals, and psychological harm.[46,51] More research is required to fully understand the effect of receiving these medically actionable results through DTC.

Additional issues around this testing include other incidental findings such as autosomal recessive conditions or non-paternity. Non-paternity can arise through other genetic testing avenues. However, discussions of implications of genetic testing including discovery of unexpected familial relationships can be addressed prior to results. DTC testing can also provide a false sense of security to patients who test negative but harbor mutations other than the common Ashkenazi Jewish founder variants. These patients may be less likely to seek further testing without understanding the scope of their previous testing.

As a result, the NSGC, ACMG, ASHG, and other societies have issued position statements calling for increased transparency about the test limitations, CLIA status of the lab, and risks of testing while advising the consumer to carefully consider the implications for themselves and their families.[52-54]

KEY POINTS

- Consumers have often not considered they might receive unwanted information from DTC tests.
- The openly available 23andMe test only includes the three common Ashkenazi Jewish variants on *BRCA1/2*.
- 23andMe as well as other DTC labs are not CLIA approved and clinical management should not be altered without confirmatory testing.

Genetic Exceptionalism

"Genetic exceptionalism" is a term coined by Thomas Murray; it alleges genetic information is qualitatively different from other health information.[55] Genetic information has been argued to have distinct psychological, social, economic, and political consequences due to the vast amount of information contained within DNA and its potential use as a unique identifier.[56-58] Critics of genetic exceptionalism say that it contributes to genetic reductionism (i.e., the belief that understanding genes is sufficient to understand all aspects of human behavior) and genetic determinism (i.e., the idea that our genes conclusively shape our behavior), thus increasing the stigma associated with genetic disease.[55,57,59,60] As previously discussed, the differences in choices made by a "reasonable person" is part of what makes genetic testing unique and leads to differences in opinion about its role. Others have argued that genetic exceptionalism is unnecessary.[60] Regardless of differing opinions, it is difficult to separate genetic information from other health information in the electronic health record (EHR) in daily practice.

The ACMG provides recommendations regarding the interface of genetic information with the EHR.[61] EHR systems and their users have the legal responsibility to protect sensitive health information from inadvertent disclosure according to the aforementioned federal and state laws. The ACMG proposes that documentation of genetic information within the EHR be standardized so that provider access is streamlined. Relatedly, providers need to include their interpretation of the test result and details of genetic counseling sessions so that others unambiguously understand the implications of the patient's genetic status. Some have suggested that genetic information be limited to a designated area within the EHR for sensitive information, but current EHR systems do not have this feature. Furthermore, the Health Insurance Portability and Accountability Act (HIPAA) gives patients the right to access and amend their medical records, so healthcare providers are legally mandated to provide requested documentation. Lastly, the ACMG suggests that DTC genetic testing *not* be incorporated into the EHR until confirmatory testing is conducted by a CLIA-approved laboratory so that only quality-controlled genetic data is documented.

KEY POINTS

- Given the lack of consensus on genetic exceptionalism, healthcare providers should treat genetic information as sensitive health information within the EHR.

▉ EQUITY

Equity is not always considered in genetic testing, but it is relevant to the accessibility to genetic services and precision medicine. People of minority ethnic groups are widely underrepresented in genetic services, with measurable disparities in use of genetic testing and counseling in cancer genetics.[62-64] Studies in Europe have noted that there is an overrepresentation of upper-class white women with referrals to genetics clinics.[45] This is despite similar frequencies of mutations in cancer susceptibility genes across ethnic groups suggesting that differences in hereditary cancer risk do not explain lower referral rates.[62,64]

Studies looking into the cause of these disparities have found cultural perceptions could lead to fatalistic attitudes toward cancer and family histories of cancer.[45,62] Those with more fatalistic views are less likely to pursue genetic testing.[65] Understanding of the roles genetics can play in health care also represents an important barrier to care. African American and Hispanic patients in the United States cite lack of information from physicians and lack of knowledge as the top reasons they are unlikely to undergo genetic testing.[62,66-68] An understanding of cross-cultural communication remains an important part of providing accurate information and care for minority populations especially when genetic counseling is a field made up of primarily white providers who speak only English.[62,69] Additional barriers to genetic services can include higher socioeconomic burden and difficulty in getting access to providers based on location, public transit options, and lack of adequate childcare, all which disproportionately impact minority populations.[63,67-72] These barriers to care create a system that prevents easy access to genetic care for minority populations and furthers the lack of familiarity and understanding that can drive despondent views.

These systemic barriers also create genetic services that are not tailored to minority populations. Genome-wide association studies (GWAS) are most often conducted in populations of European descent, but more recently the diverse populations have been used to improve imputations, provide replication cohorts, identify novel variants more common in minority populations, and provide increased resolution in fine mapping.[73,74] Yet, a striking lack of minority populations are represented in GWAS, with only 19% of published GWAS participants coming from a non-European background as of 2017.[74-76] However, African and Hispanic populations contribute disproportionately large numbers of genotype-phenotype correlations, but because of the paucity of research in these populations, fewer clinically actionable findings are reported on exomes in these groups.[74,77,78] It is expected that current reference populations do not fully capture genomic variation in the Hispanic and Latino background and as a result, less actionable information can be returned.[74,79] Genetic tools are built around data that is collected from whites; for example, BRCAPRO was built using data from whites and as a result performs poorly across all minorities despite mutation prevalence being similar across populations.[67,80-83] Clinical studies of *BRCA1/2* variants report higher rates of VUS in minority patients and long-term risk reduction studies offer little data on minority carriers.[67,84-87] Thus, even if testing were equitable, results of genetic testing provide less clinically actionable information for minority populations. Equal access to services must be considered when providing referrals and information regarding genetic services.

KEY POINTS

- The majority of genetic testing is performed on those of European descent despite all populations having a similar risk of a pathogenic variant in a cancer-related gene.
- Cultural, socioeconomic, and scientific barriers all exist for minority groups; minority patients are more likely to receive inconclusive or not clinically actionable results from genetics.
- Minority patients cite lack of information or knowledge as the main reason for not pursuing genetic testing.
- Prediction models such as BRCAPRO perform poorly in minority populations.

Duty to Recontact

Duty to recontact is a particularly salient concern in cancer genetics. It refers to recontacting patients as their genetic results are updated (i.e., a VUS being reclassified as benign) or new genetic discoveries that may be relevant to their healthcare (i.e., offering a panel test to someone who previously had *BRCA* testing only). Arguments against recontact for additional genetic testing include nonmaleficence and a patient's right not to know.[88] More practical concerns have been raised about the feasibility of recontacting patients and the burden it poses on healthcare professionals for recontacting patients about amended results as well as new testing options.[88,89] In favor of recontacting is the consensus that individuals have an interest in their own genetic information as it pertains to their health.[88,89] Thus, beneficence and autonomy could support recontact of individuals. Historically and conceptually, providers have always been in favor of recontact. A 1999 survey of genetics providers reported that recontact was ethically favorable but practically difficult.[90,91] More recent literature has further addressed concerns regarding incidental findings and VUS as compounding factors. Ethical and legal concerns remained a driving force behind the case for recontact but practical and social concern remained arguments against. Legal concerns around liability are raised in older literature but have been used less frequently as there is no existing legal precedent.[89] Recent works come to the same conclusion regarding recontact, which is that, while it is ethically and morally desirable, there is no legal basis for duty to contact.[88-90] A recent study showed genetic counselors have mixed views about whether it is the patient or the provider's responsibility to ensure patients remain informed as well as when a patient should be recontacted and what lengths should be met in an attempt to reach the patient.[90]

The practical hurdles of provider time and resources become an issue of justice when considering equitable distribution of healthcare.[90] Arguments have been made that a duty to recontact could influence the number of patients seen and the quality of care provided.[90] The rapid increase in genetic testing put a strain on the number of genetic counselors and other professionals with hereditary cancer testing being the second most common type of genetic test ordered.[92] Thus, consideration must be given to the benefit of updating previously tested patients as opposed to those with no history of genetic testing.[90] This can present a burden not only to healthcare providers but also to support staff, especially in cases in which contact information is not systematically kept up to date.

KEY POINTS

- There is a moral obligation to recontact patients with amended results and new testing options that may be clinically impactful, but there is no legal precedent.
- There are practical difficulties that can strain a provider's time and resources in ways that may be impactful to other patients. The equity of healthcare availability must also be considered in regard to how a practice approaches recontact.

▣ DUTY TO DISCLOSE TO PATIENT

There is clear legal precedent establishing the physician's duty to warn the individual patient about hereditary cancer risk.[93] Ann Chadwick was a 43-year-old nurse with an extensive family history of breast and ovarian cancer; she survived bilateral breast cancer at ages 28 and 37 but subsequently died of ovarian cancer at age 43. Her family filed a malpractice suit against a Seattle, WA, medical center for failing to offer Chadwick a risk-reducing bilateral salpingo-oophorectomy and for failing to make the genetic diagnosis of a presumed hereditary cancer syndrome. In 2001, the suit settled for $1.6 million. This case highlighted healthcare providers' responsibility to identify hereditary cancer syndromes and to pursue genetic testing when the patient has a suspicious personal or family history. There is now widespread agreement that physicians have a responsibility to disclose clinically significant health information to their patients, especially if it is potentially relevant to decision-making.[94,95]

A more controversial issue is whether healthcare providers have a legal responsibility to disclose incidental or secondary findings—that is, information not directly related to the original testing indication.[96] Recently there has been an increased use of panel-based genetic testing and nontargeted whole-genome and exome sequencing due to the rising affordability and availability of these tests.[97] We can consequently expect to see a dramatic increase in the frequency of incidental and secondary findings.[96] Because patients have the right to access their medical records and test results under HIPAA, they might uncover these results independently. Thus, the ordering physician has a responsibility to warn the patient of potential incidental findings during the informed consent process.[95,98,99] The ACMG originally required healthcare providers to disclose all genetic test results to the patient, regardless of patient or provider preferences or relevance to the patient's clinical problem.[99] However, it later amended its policy to allow patients to decline to receive secondary results after pervasive criticism.[100]

The aforementioned concerns are particularly applicable to tumor sequencing, as germline sequence variants may be identified by certain laboratories during tumor sequencing.[95] Healthcare providers should honor patient preferences; if a patient declines receipt of incidental germline findings, the laboratory should only report somatic findings.[61,96,101] On the other hand, if a patient agrees to receive these results and a medically actionable finding is discovered, the American Society of Clinical Oncology (ASCO) recommends the patient undergo confirmatory germline testing to differentiate a germline predisposition versus a *de novo* mutation arising during tumor development.[95]

Further, the ACMG has set forth a list of 59 genes for which pathogenic variants, if identified on clinical exome or genome, should be returned to the patient, regardless of clinical indication.[100] This list includes genes for which clinical management would be altered if a pathogenic variant was identified. Notably, this list includes genes such as *BRCA1/2*, *TP53*, four of the genes associated with Lynch syndrome, and other highly penetrant cancer risk genes. Though the rate of incidental findings is considered low, reports indicating around 4%, secondary—or incidental—findings can lead families to further cancer genetic counseling and testing.[102,103] High-risk cancer genes can also be identified in patients younger than might otherwise be tested due to exome testing for indications other than cancer risk.

KEY POINTS

- Healthcare providers should disclose clinically significant health information to the patient, especially if it is potentially relevant to decision-making.
- Healthcare providers should warn the patient of potential incidental or secondary findings during the informed consent process. They should assess patient preferences and honor those preferences.

    If the patient agrees to receive secondary results after tumor profiling, they should subsequently undergo confirmatory germline testing.

■ DUTY TO WARN AT-RISK RELATIVES

It is not uncommon for healthcare providers to encounter patients who refuse to disclose their genetic status to an at-risk relative.[104–106] Reasons for refusal include pre-existing physical or emotional estrangement from family members, protecting personal privacy, concern for social stigma, misunderstanding health implications for relatives, reluctance to deliver bad news, or emotional difficulty discussing the topic.[104–107] There is a general consensus that healthcare providers should encourage their patients to inform their at-risk relatives of a genetically transferable condition in the family.[106,108,109] However, there is continued controversy about whether or not healthcare providers are ethically or legally obligated to warn family members if patients refuse to do so themselves. A duty to warn might discourage patients from undergoing genetic testing due to mistrust of healthcare providers, can be burdensome or infeasible, and can cause psychological harm to the recipient relatives.[57] On the contrary, disclosure to at-risk family members abides by the ethical principles of justice and beneficence.[59,60,101,107,108,110] Four landmark court cases have set precedence on the matter of duty to warn (Table 16.3).

Genetic testing raises complex ethical and legal issues.[59,101,108,111] Since genetic testing became publicly available in the mid-1990s, many legal protections related to genetic discrimination and informational privacy have been developed.[57,112] These laws were developed in response to several landmark medical malpractice cases that highlighted the need for broadly applicable legal principles for genetic privacy.[96,107] It has become increasingly difficult for legislation to balance autonomy, justice, beneficence, and confidentiality for at-risk family

TABLE 16.3: Case Laws Regarding Duty to Warn

Case	Legal precedent
Tarasoff v. Regents of the University of California (1976)	The physician has a duty to warn a third party of harm if there is a foreseeable risk of injury or death and an identifiable contact.
Pate v. Threlkel (1995)	The physician has a duty to warn the proband that risk is transmissible. Duty is fulfilled at the level of the proband.
Safer v. Pack (1996)	The physician's duty to warn is not always fulfilled at the level of the proband.
Molloy v. Meier (2004)	The physician has a duty to warn the biological parents of an afflicted child if the risk is transmissible to future children.

members in the setting of increasingly powerful genetic technologies, expansion of entities with access to protected health information (PHI), and current movements toward precision medicine.[96,111,112] The legal protections and cases are outlined here.

Case Law

In the case of *Tarasoff v. Regents of the University of California* (1976), a graduate student, Prosenjit Poddar, disclosed to his psychotherapist that he was planning on killing a fellow student, Tatiana Tarasoff, who had rejected his advances.[113] The psychotherapist informed the police, but Poddar was deemed rational and immediately released from custody. But Tarasoff and her family were not warned, and months later Poddar brutally murdered her. Her family sued the university and several of its employees. The California Supreme Court held that mental health workers have a duty to warn a third party of harm if there is a foreseeable risk of injury or death and an identifiable contact. The doctrine has since expanded to cover all medical providers.

Another landmark case is *Pate v. Threlkel*.[114] In 1987, Marianne New was treated for multiple endocrine neoplasia (MEN)—associated medullary thyroid cancer. Three years later, her adult daughter, Heidi Pate, was diagnosed with advanced medullary thyroid cancer. Pate subsequently sued New's physicians, alleging that (1) the physicians knew or should have known the condition was inheritable, (2) the physicians had a duty to warn New's children of their risk, and (3) if the physicians had warned Pate of her risk she would have been tested at that time and intervened earlier in the disease process. The Florida Supreme Court affirmed that a reasonably prudent physician has a duty to warn the patient of the genetic transferability of their disease. When faced with the question of whether a physician also has a duty to warn the patient's at-risk relatives, the court recognized that warning the patient also benefited their relatives, and that warning relatives without the patient's permission would conflict with Florida's confidentiality statute. In other words, the court held that the duty to warn was fulfilled at the level of the proband.

Only one year after *Pate v. Threlkel*, the court held in *Safer v. Pack* (1996) that the duty to warn those at risk of avoidable harm from a genetically transferable condition was not always fulfilled at the level of the proband.[115] In 1956, Robert Batkin underwent medical and surgical treatment for "multiple polyposis" of the colon under the care of his surgeon, George Pack. Batkin died of the condition in 1964 at the age of 45, when his daughter, Donna Safer, was 10 years old. In 1990, Safer, then age 36, was diagnosed with metastatic colon cancer resulting from the same condition as her father. In 1992, Safer sued Pack's estate (he had died in 1969), alleging that his failure to inform her of the genetic nature of the disease prevented her from obtaining early and potentially curative treatment. The New Jersey appellate court held that a physician has a duty to directly warn individuals at risk of a genetic disorder whether or not the patient consents. This decision was criticized as being overly broad and potentially undermining trust in the physician–patient relationship. Indeed, in 2001, the New Jersey Legislature overturned the *Safer v. Pack* decision and enacted a broad genetic privacy statute making it illegal for a physician to disclose genetic information to the patient's at-risk relatives without consent from the patient or their legal representative (N.J. Stat. Ann. § 10:5-47). Exceptions to the law include forensic identification, paternity determinations, and pursuant to a court order.

Another commonly referenced case is *Molloy v. Meier*.[116] In 2001, Kimberly Molloy sued three physicians with medical malpractice for allegedly failing to diagnose her daughter with

Fragile X syndrome and for not informing the family about the hereditary risk of this missed diagnosis. Molloy claimed that she was specifically told her daughter's condition was not genetic and that she was very unlikely to have another child with a similar affliction. She subsequently had a son with Fragile X. In 2004, the Minnesota Supreme Court held that "a physician's duty regarding genetic testing and diagnosis extends beyond the patient to biological parents who foreseeably may be harmed by a breach of that duty."

Taken together, the above cases illustrate the physician's ethical and legal obligations to warn at-risk relatives of genetically transferable conditions and are commonly referenced in discussions about the legal aspects of cancer genetics. However, the disclosure of medical information without the patient's consent is currently regulated by HIPAA, which is described in detail later in the chapter. Consequently, healthcare providers are neither required nor permitted to warn at-risk relatives without patient consent or authorization as a matter of ethics and law.[117]

Policy Statements Regarding Duty to Warn

Following Pate and Safer, the ASHG published a policy that recommended that physicians inform patients about familial implications before and after genetic testing, thus reaffirming the general rule of confidentiality.[118] The policy also describes circumstances in which disclosure by the physician is appropriate. It suggests that physicians have the discretion to inform family members when the following four factors are present: (1) Attempts to encourage disclosure on the part of the patient have failed; (2) the harm is highly likely to occur and is serious and foreseeable; (3) the at-risk relative is identifiable; and (4) the disease is preventable or treatable, or medically accepted standards indicate that early monitoring will reduce the genetic risk. Not only is this policy reminiscent of the Tarasoff case, but it is also in line with the HIPAA Privacy Rule, which allows for a breach in patient confidentiality when there is a "serious and imminent threat to the health or safety of a person of the public."[117]

Other professional societies have contrary opinions. Unlike the courts in Pate and Safer, the NSGC and the AMA both published codes of ethics that emphasize the duty to protect the patient's information. The NSGC believes it is the patient's right to decide who has access to their medical information, and that physicians should "maintain the privacy and security of their client's confidential information and individually identifiable health information, unless released by the client or disclosure is required by law." The AMA likewise underscores the physician's duty of confidentiality: "Physicians also should identify circumstances under which they would expect patients to notify biologic relatives of the availability of information related to risk of disease. In this regard, physicians should make themselves available to assist patients in communicating with relatives to discuss opportunities for counseling and testing, as appropriate."[119] Similarly, ASCO believes that the provider should encourage communication within the family and emphasize the importance of disclosure to their at-risk relatives.[56] ASCO and AMA both acknowledge the legal precedence previously reviewed but assert that the physician's duty of confidentiality usually overrides the competing duty to warn. Regardless of the intervention, physicians are encouraged to judiciously document their counseling sessions for legal purposes. Finally, the American College of Obstetricians and Gynecologists (ACOG) concurs that although a patient's health information should be kept confidential, they feel that healthcare providers should feel empowered to counsel at-risk family members if given patient consent or authorization.[94] ACOG also highlights the utility of consultation with a genetics professional, ethicist, or legal counsel in ethically or legally ambiguous situations.

Disclosure of Result if the Patient is Deceased

Ideally, healthcare providers should develop a plan with each patient for communicating genetic information upon the patient's death.[120] However, if no such conversation is documented, there are several privacy principles that healthcare providers can reference. The HIPAA privacy rule applies to both living and deceased patients. In 2013, HIPAA was modified such that it protects the identifiable health information about a decedent for 50 years following the date of death of the individual.[121] Nonetheless, disclosure of medical information, including genetic testing results, is now permitted to the decedent's family members and caretakers unless the decedent specifically expressed otherwise, or the healthcare provider is uncomfortable doing so. Before disclosure, the healthcare provider must do their due diligence to ascertain patient preferences and to ensure that the recipient is a relative or caretaker by reviewing documentation and recalling past interactions. Providers must weigh the principles of beneficence and nonmaleficence against respect for the autonomy of the deceased in order to come to a decision about disclosure of results. Institutional ethics boards can also be a resource for these types of decisions and may provide institutional guidance.

The Experience of Genetic Counselors and Medical Geneticists

Three studies explore the practical experiences of genetics professionals regarding the duty to warn. Falk et al. (2003) and Dugan et al. (2003) looked at the actions and experiences of medical geneticists and genetic counselors, respectively.[104,105] Twenty-five percent of medical geneticists and 21% of genetic counselors faced clinical scenarios in which they seriously considered notifying at-risk relatives without consent when faced with the conflict of duty to warn. Only a small proportion (4 of 31 medical geneticists and 1 of 24 genetic counselors) of those considering disclosure actually disclosed genetic information to family members without patient consent.

These studies were replicated by Perry et al. in 2020. Of 51 medical geneticists studied, 30 (59%) had a patient refuse to notify an at-risk relative. Of these, 8 (27%) considered disclosure without consent, but none actually disclosed. Of the 206 genetic counselors, 95 (46%) had a patient refuse to notify an at-risk relative. Of these, 17 (18%) considered disclosure without consent, but only two actually went forward with disclosure.[106] Thus, genetics professionals were significantly less likely to believe they had an obligation to inform in this study compared to earlier studies. One possible explanation for this discrepancy is a greater emphasis on privacy and confidentiality in the current era of social media. Notably, the providers who went forward with disclosure put themselves at risk for legal action.

KEY POINTS

- Healthcare providers should encourage communication within the family and emphasize to the patient the importance and benefit of sharing the genetic information with their at-risk relatives.
- Healthcare providers should make themselves available to assist patients in communicating with relatives to discuss opportunities for counseling and testing, as appropriate.
- In the vast majority of cases, it is inappropriate for a healthcare provider to disclose a patient's genetic information to their at-risk relatives without the patient's explicit consent.
- Healthcare providers should carefully document discussions regarding this issue as part of both the pretest and posttest counseling session.

▓ GENETIC DISCRIMINATION

Genetic discrimination occurs when an individual is treated differently by others because they have a gene mutation that causes or increases the risk of an inherited disorder.[122] An example of a social effect of genetic discrimination is reduced desirability by potential romantic partners due to the potential transmission of a genetic condition to future offspring.[59] Economic effects of genetic discrimination include discrimination in the workplace, being denied life insurance coverage due to a "pre-existing condition," or having higher life insurance premiums.[59] Although there have been very few reports of genetic discrimination, the perceived fear remains high.[59,96,108,120] As discussed, legislation at the federal and state levels helps to protect people against genetic discrimination.

Federal Law

The Americans with Disabilities Act (ADA; 42 U.S.C. § 12101)[123] of 1990 is a civil rights law that prohibits discrimination against individuals with disabilities, particularly in the workplace. It also requires employers to provide reasonable accommodations to employees with disabilities and imposes enforceable accessibility requirements for public and commercial buildings, transportation, and communication services. It provides limited genetic protections. If an individual has a genetic disease that causes significant impairment in their ability to perform one or more functions, then their disease qualifies as a disability under the ADA and they would be protected from employment discrimination providing they are able to perform their professional duties with reasonable accommodations. Most individuals with hereditary cancer syndromes do not qualify as "disabled" under the ADA, but there are some exceptions (e.g., PTEN hamartoma tumor syndrome causing cognitive impairment).

HIPAA was enacted in 1996. Its primary purpose was to ensure continuity of employer-sponsored health insurance coverage for the employee and their dependents when they change employers. HIPAA gave the U.S. Department of Health and Human Services (HHS) the jurisdiction to regulate entities that provide healthcare or pay for it (i.e., insurance companies). The HHS issued the Standards for Privacy of Individually Identifiable Health Information ("Privacy Rule"), which became operational in 2003, as a set of national standards for the protection of individuals' health information.[124] It states that the use and disclosure of protected health information beyond treatment, payment, and healthcare operations requires HIPAA-compliant written authorization signed by the patient. Of note, there are no special provisions for genetic information; rather, it is subsumed within general health information. The entities covered under the Privacy Rule include health plans (i.e., health insurer, HMO, Medicare or Medicaid program, or other entity that provides or pays the costs of medical care), most healthcare providers, healthcare clearinghouses (i.e., billing services or health information management systems), and business associates and subcontractors of covered entities. Entities that are not covered include life insurers, schools, workers compensation carriers, law enforcement, drug manufacturers, research institutions, companies that sell fitness-tracking devices, DTC genetic testing services, and many state agencies such as child protective services. Of note, many of these entities store and use health and genetic data.

The HIPAA Privacy Rule permits disclosure of protected health information without an individual's authorization or consent for the following "public" purposes: (1) required by law (45 C.F.R. § 164.512(a)); (2) for public health activities (45 C.F.R. § 164.512(b));

(3) about victims of abuse, neglect, or domestic violence (45 C.F.R. § 164.512(c)); (4) for health oversight activities (45 C.F.R. § 164.512(d)); (5) for judicial and administrative proceedings (45 C.F.R. § 164.512(e)); (6) for law enforcement (45 C.F.R. § 164.512(f)); (7) about decedents (45 C.F.R. § 164.512(g)); (8) for cadaveric organ, eye, or tissue donation (45 C.F.R. § 164.512(h)); (9) for some types of research (45 C.F.R. § 164.512(i)); (10) to avert a serious threat to health or safety (45 C.F.R. § 164.512(j)); (11) for essential government functions, including national security (45 C.F.R. § 164.512(k)); and (12) for workers' compensation (45 C.F.R. § 164.512(l)). The most applicable provision is "serious threat to health or safety," in which covered entities "may disclose protected health information that they believe is necessary to prevent or lessen a serious and imminent threat to a person or the public, when such disclosure is made to someone they believe can prevent or lessen the threat (including the target of the threat)."[124] As mentioned previously, this provision is reminiscent of the Tarasoff case. Healthcare providers might struggle with the interpretation of the words "serious" and "imminent threat" when considering the duty to warn, especially for genetic conditions with incomplete penetrance.[112]

The Genetic Information Nondiscrimination Act (GINA; Pub. L. 110–233, 122 Stat. 881 (May 21, 2008), 42 U.S.C. § 2000ff(2018)) is a federal law that was signed into law by President George W. Bush in 2008 after 13 years of deliberation in Congress to address widespread concerns about genetic discrimination. GINA has two parts: Title I prohibits genetic discrimination in health insurance and Title II prohibits genetic discrimination in employment. More specifically, Title I makes it illegal for health insurance providers to use or require genetic information for underwriting or enrollment purposes (i.e., determining eligibility or coverage), while Title II makes it illegal for employers with more than 15 employees to use or require an employee's genetic information when making decisions about hiring, promotion, placement, or termination. GINA defines genetic information broadly, including genetic test results, information on genetic assessment services pursued by the patient, or family history information up to and including fourth-degree relatives. GINA does not prohibit genetic discrimination in all circumstances. For instance, GINA does not apply to employers with fewer than 15 employees and or forms of insurance other than health insurance such as life, disability, or long-term care insurance. For a complete list of entities covered and uncovered by GINA, see Table 16.4.

In addition to the previously mentioned limitations, GINA only applies to asymptomatic individuals. Asymptomatic individuals are only at risk for developing a genetic disease, whereas symptomatic individuals have a known, existing disease. Fortunately, there are other laws, such as the Patient Protection and Affordable Care Act (ACA; 42 USC §18001), that protect symptomatic individuals.[125] The ACA, passed in 2010, prohibits health insurance discrimination based on a pre-existing health condition, such as hereditary cancer syndromes that have manifested. Through GINA's interaction with the ACA, both pre-symptomatic and symptomatic individuals are protected. Despite numerous limitations, GINA continues to play a critical role in preventing genetic discrimination.

State Law

Prior to GINA, many states had created laws prohibiting genetic discrimination.[126] These laws vary significantly depending on jurisdiction. For an up-to-date list of the state protections regarding genetic discrimination enacted before GINA, please see the list compiled by the National Conference of State Legislatures website (http://www.ncsl.org). Notably, some

TABLE 16.4: Entities Covered and Uncovered by GINA*	
Insurance providers and employers who need to comply with GINA	**Insurance providers and employers who do *not* need to comply with GINA**
Most group or individual health insurance providers Most employers	*Health insurance providers:* • Federal government employees • Military • Veteran's Administration • Indian Health Services *Employers:* • Federal government • Military • Employers with fewer than 15 employees *Other forms of insurance:* • Life insurance • Disability insurance • Short/long-term care insurance

*Data from Gammon A, Neklason DW. Confidentiality & the Risk of Genetic Discrimination: What Surgeons Need to Know, *Surg Oncol Clin N Am* 2015 Oct;24(4):667–681.

state laws provide stronger or more extensive privacy protections than GINA, including regulation regarding life insurance or disability insurance. As specified explicitly in GINA, the more comprehensive law takes precedence, whether that is GINA or a stronger local law. GINA, therefore, offers "minimum" privacy protections at the federal level, but these protections can be strengthened by state law.

KEY POINTS

- Legislation at the federal and state levels prohibits genetic discrimination, particularly as it relates to employment and health insurance.
- Genetic information is protected under HIPAA and GINA, but not all groups of individuals are currently covered.

CAN HUMAN GENES BE PATENTED?

Since the emergence of genomic technologies, the U.S. Patent Office issued patents on human genes for decades. After Myriad Genetics, a molecular diagnostic company located in Salt Lake City, filed patent applications for isolated DNA sequences for *BRCA1* and *BRCA2* in 2013, the American Civil Liberties Union (ACLU) and the Public Patent Foundation (PUBPAT) filed a lawsuit in federal court on behalf of researchers, genetic counselors, patients, and several medical professional associations (*Association for Molecular Pathology v. Myriad Genetics*).[127] The litigation was mainly in response to concerns over Myriad claiming a monopoly on genetic diagnostic tests, restricting genetics research, and demanding a high price for its genetic test (up to $4000).[128-130] In a groundbreaking Supreme Court decision, all nine justices agreed that naturally occurring human genes cannot be patented because they are products of nature (35 U.S.C. § 101). However, the Court held that complementary DNA (cDNA)—that is, laboratory reconstructions of human DNA—could be patented because these molecules do not naturally occur. Overall, the Court's decision aims to foster scientific discovery and incentivize biomedical innovation. Ethically, it prevents the human genome from being used for financial gain, setting a powerful precedent in the era of precision medicine.[131]

> **KEY POINT**
> - Human genes cannot be patented.

Healthcare providers face numerous legal issues when it comes to cancer genetic testing. First, providers have an obligation to determine patient preferences regarding disclosure of incidental or secondary findings. If the patient agrees to receive such findings, the provider should honor those preferences in addition to test results related to the primary clinical problem. Second, providers are legally prohibited from warning their patients' relatives about genetically transferable conditions without patient consent but should do their best to encourage patients to warn their at-risk relatives themselves. Third, providers should familiarize themselves with genetic discrimination legislation, particularly HIPAA, GINA, and their state's specific laws. Helpful resources for patients and providers include:

- State laws regarding genetic discrimination per the National Conference of State Legislatures:
  - Genetic employment laws: https://www.ncsl.org/research/health/genetic-employment-laws.aspx
  - Genetic health insurance laws: www.ncsl.org/research/health/genetic-nondiscrimination-in-health-insurance-laws.aspx
- Information on GINA, its protections in health insurance and employment, and its shortcomings: www.ginahelp.org/
- Information on HIPAA policies: www.hhs.gov/hipaa/index.html

▨ PSYCHOSOCIAL ISSUES

Why are Psychosocial Issues Important?

The potential for psychosocial struggles associated with cancer genetic testing is increasing due to the rapid advances of cancer genetics, and the advent of multi-gene panel testing. The national criteria for cancer genetic testing, and the number of genes available to test, broaden each year, affecting the routine medical management, and now cancer treatment, for a growing number of patients. In the past, studies unrelated to genetics have shown that inveterate psychosocial stressors can significantly impact both mental and physical health and can also be associated with risky behaviors, such as tobacco and alcohol use. For example, Cohen et al. (1998) found a significant increase in risk for development of the common cold among individuals with severe chronic stressors.[132] Another study highlighted the impact of stressful life events on depression, behavior, and health at different points in development.[133] This emphasizes the importance of understanding the potential impact of psychosocial stressors for patients undergoing genetic testing, and/or the avoidance of medical management recommendations associated with a genetic test result. Unlike the typical relationship with a cancer genetic counselor, healthcare providers such as primary care physicians, gynecologists, and gastroenterologists have regular opportunities to care for the patient before, during, and after cancer genetic testing and also at regular intervals over an extended period of time. This allows the non-genetic healthcare practitioners the opportunity to guide the at-risk patient in a healthy direction, avoiding unnecessary distress, anxiety, or depression associated, for some, with the experience of cancer genetic testing. What follows is an account of the findings from more recent studies, and justification for the ongoing involvement of healthcare providers to identify individuals who may benefit from extra support in dealing with distress, anxiety, or depression associated with genetic testing and hereditary cancer. We offer recommendations and tools that may help providers more effectively guide their patients through the process of cancer genetic testing, enable improved patient compliance of the recommended medical management changes, and disseminate potentially lifesaving information to loved ones.

Broad research into the psychosocial implications of cancer genetic testing began decades ago with the advent of clinical testing for pathogenic variants associated with hereditary breast and ovarian cancer syndrome (HBOC) and Lynch syndrome. Results were conflicting. Some found a minimal impact of genetic testing on psychosocial issues, such as distress, anxiety, and depression, while others showed a significant impact. Recently investigators began taking a more granular look at the psychosocial impact of cancer genetic testing, focusing more on factors such as age, lifestyle, gender, support system, coping style, family history, and family dynamics. Researchers are also working to delineate the impact at different points in time throughout the genetic counseling and testing process. For example, will a patient be likely to experience more distress or anxiety at the initial consultation, or during or after the result disclosure visit. The goal is targeting those more likely in need of added support and/or resources and when they might be most beneficial. This is particularly important as we enter a time when access to genetic testing is far greater due to lower test costs and the availability of direct-to-consumer testing. This can be true even for those whose personal and/or cancer family history may not warrant cancer genetic testing. With the advent of, and easy access to, multi-gene panel testing in recent years, some investigators are concerned with the psychosocial impact of these much larger and more complex tests. Although research is relatively new and emerging, existing evidence shows that while many will not require added support through their experience of cancer genetic testing, knowing when and how to offer support, resources, and guidance can lead to a healthier outcome for both the patient and his or her family. One can also argue the financial efficacy in identifying those who may need extra support in areas that potentially represent roadblocks to necessary, and sometimes lifesaving, medical management recommendations.

What are the Sources of Distress, Anxiety, and Depression?

To elucidate how to guide patients who may be dealing with increased distress, anxiety, or depression, we must first consider the various sources of those feelings in the context of cancer genetic counseling and testing. It is important to note that the act of seeking out genetic counseling for consideration of testing is itself an indication of some level of worry. Therefore, it follows that individuals seeking cancer genetic counseling, whether or not they were the first in a family to be tested, will have a higher baseline of distress, anxiety, and/or depression than seen in the general population. Cicero et al. (2017) considered two groups in their study. The first group consisted of 60 probands (those who were first to test within a family) who had been diagnosed with breast or ovarian cancer at a reportedly young age. The second group was composed of 60 family members who pursued genetic counseling and underwent testing for hereditary breast and/or ovarian cancer as a result of communication regarding familial risk from one of the 60 probands. These researchers found that both groups exhibited higher levels of anxiety and depressive symptoms than would be expected in the general population. In fact, they found the levels of anxiety and depressive symptoms to be "clinically significant" and ultimately suggested further investigation into this topic.[134]

An important aspect of the decision-making process in genetic testing, and medical management choice, involves numbers, chance, and statistics. Risk perception has been shown to impact distress, anxiety, and/or depression in individuals seeking genetic counseling and potentially testing. The discussion around cancer risk during a genetic counseling session has meaning on multiple levels. First, it is quantifiable. Through population studies, we know the risk to the general population of women for breast cancer, over the course of a lifetime, is 8 to 12%. We know the lifetime risk for breast cancer associated with a pathogenic variant in *BRCA1* or *BRCA2* can be as high as 60 to 80%.[135] However, this lifetime breast cancer risk can be adjusted based on the age of the *BRCA*-positive patient.[135] For example, the remaining lifetime risk for an unaffected 60-year-old woman found to harbor a pathogenic variant in her *BRCA1* gene may approach 20%. These numbers are specific and objective; however, their meaning is subjective for individual people. For example, to one person 20% may feel reassuring, particularly when considering it means an 80% chance of remaining free of breast cancer. To another person, perhaps someone who has lost a loved one to cancer, that 20% may be very distressing. Conversely, a 25-year-old woman facing an 80% lifetime risk for breast cancer may not realize that it means approximately 20% of *BRCA*-positive women are never diagnosed with breast cancer.

Another aspect of risk perception that comes into play during genetic counseling is genetic risk perception, or the perceived chance of having inherited a pathogenic variant in a gene associated with increased risk for cancer. In the setting of a known familial pathogenic variant, the risk is easily quantifiable. If a first-degree relative carries the known familial variant, the chance of being positive is 50%. If a second-degree relative is positive, the chance is 25%, and so on. Far more common, in the absence of a known familial pathogenic variant, many variables come into play. Ancestry and family structure can be informative. For example, is there Ashkenazi Jewish ancestry? This could represent as much as a 1 in 40 chance of having inherited one of the Ashkenazi Jewish founder mutations in *BRCA1* or *BRCA2*. A small family size could potentially mask an otherwise evident pattern of cancer within a family line yielding one false reassurance regarding inherited risk. Are there many women in the family, and how old are they? What types of cancers are seen in the family? Additionally, the patient's experience of watching or caring for a loved one affected with cancer can impact his or her perception around the chance of a positive test result. With a widely varied baseline of knowledge, individual people can have wildly differing ideas about the likelihood of having inherited a pathogenic variant; however, clinical experience consistently shows us the majority of individuals have an inflated perception of how much cancer is inherited.

Researchers have considered the possibility that ascertaining the patient's risk perception can reveal a significant barrier to testing and/or risk reducing options. Two such studies found risk perception to be predictive of increased distress among unaffected women with a significant family history of breast cancer.[36,137] Cabrera et al. (2010) and Tong et al. (2015) also published studies supporting the outcome that breast cancer family history can greatly influence feelings of worry and inflate understood risk.[138,139] Cicero et al. (2017) found a significant relationship between genetic risk perception and anxiety and/or depression in their proband group (60 individuals affected by disease), as well as in their family group (60 unaffected family members, who pursued counseling and testing in response to the proband's communication regarding familial risk). They concluded that both genetic risk perception and cancer risk perception can be used as potential predictors of the development of psychological symptoms such as distress, anxiety, and/or depression. Among probands, genetic risk perception and cancer risk perception were correlated only with depression. Anxiety and depression were higher, as one may expect, during cancer treatment. Among unaffected family members, genetic risk perception was correlated with all variables, which included anxiety, depression, and distress. A higher cancer risk perception was correlated with a higher genetic risk perception (the perceived chance of having inherited a pathogenic variant) as well as anxiety and distress. Specific concerns among family members included fear of facing medical management changes in the setting of a positive genetic test result and fear of facing treatment in the event of a diagnosis.[134]

More recently, researchers are also turning to the genetic test result to help more clearly define who may be at risk for psychosocial struggles and could therefore benefit from added support and/or resources. Voorwinden et al. considered individuals with a known familial pathogenic variant in *BRCA1, BRCA2*, or in a mismatch repair gene causing Lynch syndrome. Their subjects each had a 50% chance of having inherited a pathogenic variant, which had been previously identified in a family member. The research goal was to delineate factors predictive of psychological problems following an unfavorable test result at three points in time; at the initial genetics consultation, 2 days later, and then 4–6 weeks after receiving the test result. Compared to those not found to have inherited their family variant, researchers discovered genetically positive subjects did not have more emotional distress 4–6 weeks after assessment, but they did have significantly more cancer worries. Overall prognostic factors for cancer worries included pre-existing cancer worries, being single (support system), high risk perception, and an unfavorable test result.[140]

Several studies have explored the impact of cancer genetic testing in women newly diagnosed with breast cancer. Meiser et al. investigated the effect of the specific genetic test result on newly diagnosed women with a family history of cancer compared to those newly diagnosed women *without* a family history. Women were recruited through eight clinics across Australia. Researchers completed assessments at four intervals; at the time of recruitment, 1 week after the initial genetics consultation, 2 weeks following result disclosure, and 12 months after enrollment. Overall, carriers of pathogenic or likely pathogenic (P/LP) variants experienced a greater decrease in anxiety over time compared to noncarriers. Their study provides evidence that while explaining the cause of a cancer diagnosis, and in spite of potential increased risk for additional cancer diagnoses, a positive genetic test result can have a calming impact over time.[141]

Other studies reveal evidence of guilt among individuals found to harbor a pathogenic variant. Through their qualitative research, involving semi-structured interviews, Mahat-Shamir and Possick (2017) delved into the experiences of 13 Ashkenazi Jewish women found to be carriers of a pathogenic variant in *BRCA1* or *BRCA2*. They discovered their subjects felt empathy for their ancestors who passed on the pathogenic variant, while at the same time they felt guilt about passing on the variant to their own children. Specifically, these women expressed guilt about having their children watch them face illness, about transferring the pathogenic variant on to their children, and about putting their children in a position of having to contemplate issues around family planning.[142] One can imagine how this might impact uptake of medical management recommendations resulting from a positive genetic test result or the willingness to communicate with at-risk family members that they too may have inherited this cancer genetic variant.

Over the course of approximately 5 years, reduction in cost, changes in the NCCN guidelines, and direct-to-consumer testing translated into a significant increase in the number of people undergoing multi-gene cancer panel tests. With this increase in testing, and the concomitant growing body of knowledge, comes a need to explore the impact of these much larger tests on the psychological well-being of those who chose to pursue them. This stems from the added complexity, the potential uncertainty, and the increased chance of incidental findings associated with these larger tests. In 2018, researchers in Spain explored the psychological impact of multi-gene panel testing. One hundred and eighty-seven unrelated patients with clinical suspicion of hereditary cancer underwent a 25-gene panel test, completing questionnaires at four points in time; at the initial consultation and then 1 week, 3 months, and 12 months after result disclosure. They did find an increase in cancer worry among carriers of a moderately penetrant pathogenic variant compared to carriers of a highly penetrant variant. However, the cohorts used to draw this conclusion were quite low as there were only 34 carriers of highly penetrant P/LP variants and four carriers of moderately penetrant P/LP variants. Overall, their research suggested that, in general, patients have the capacity to cope with the increased uncertainty inherent in multi-gene cancer panel tests.[143]

Another group of researchers incorporated multi-gene panel testing into their observational prospective study published in 2019. They assessed 460 women before and after genetic testing, using psychosocial aspects of hereditary cancer (PAHC). The tool is composed of six scales, or sources of distress, anxiety, and/or depression. These include hereditary predisposition, familial and social issues, emotions, familial cancer, personal cancer, and children-related issues. Subjects completed assessments before testing and then again 2 months post-test disclosure, allowing investigators to take into account the passage of time, as well as the impact of specific test results. The study spanned three sites located in France, Germany, and Spain. Over time, concerns that remained high included personal cancer risk, familial cancer risk, and children-related issues. Regardless of the outcome of the genetic test result, there was no impact in the areas of emotions, familial cancer, personal cancer, and children-related issues. Specific test results *did* impact concerns around hereditary predisposition and familial and social issues. At the 2-month post-disclosure assessment, there was little change in concerns related to hereditary predisposition among women who tested positive or for those whose result was uninformative (negative with no known familial pathogenic variant). Surprisingly, among those who were found to harbor a VUS, researchers noted a clinically significant decrease in hereditary predisposition concerns, even though it actually represents an increase in uncertainty. Those with a VUS result were more comparable to those with a *true* negative result (negative for a known familial pathogenic variant typically reverting cancer risk back to that of the general population regardless of cancer family history) than to those with an uninformative result. Despite the reported findings, the overall study concluded that psychosocial problems were mostly unaffected by multi-gene panel testing. However, the decrease in concerns among those found to harbor a VUS is important to consider when choosing the specific language used during the result disclosure consultation.[144]

KEY POINTS

- The act of pursuing genetic counseling and testing is itself an indication of some level of worry.
- Genetic risk perception and cancer risk perception can be predictive of the development of psychological symptoms such as distress, anxiety, and/or depression.

- To date, there is no evidence of major risks for psychological dysfunction in those undergoing genetic testing or in those found to harbor a pathogenic variant. This includes research into those undergoing multi-gene panel tests.
- Close attention should be given to discussing a VUS result, as it may lead to a false sense of security related to hereditary cancer risk. While this result typically does not impact medical management, referral to an experienced practitioner, who is knowledgeable about cancer genetics, for interpretation is important.
- Family structure is important to note. For example, having children may leave a patient inclined to feel guilty about a positive test result.

Who to Consider for Added Support, Information, and/or Additional Resources?

Beyond risk perception and genetic test results, research has also addressed other factors such as gender, age, family structure, and family history. Investigators are working to better understand the psychosocial issues related to those women unaffected in the setting of cancer family history, those with a new diagnosis with or without significant cancer family history, and those with a personal history of cancer. Research into at-risk men is still burgeoning, with the most recent studies looking at unmet needs among men diagnosed with breast cancer. With ease of access to genetic testing, other topics of interest include the population of adults who chose to delay or decline genetic testing and testing of adolescents for adult-onset conditions.

Several researchers have looked at the ways in which individuals typically confront a stressful situation and how they deal with it. Ho et al. (2010) investigated factors predicting psychological resilience in adults undergoing genetic testing for hereditary colorectal cancer in Hong Kong. Their study included 71 individuals from nine families affected with familial adenomatous polyposis and 24 families affected with Lynch syndrome. Participants completed a questionnaire measuring hopefulness immediately before result disclosure. They also completed a questionnaire measuring psychological distress, anxiety, and depression before the result disclosure, and again at 2 weeks, 4 months, and 1 year after result disclosure. They found hopefulness at baseline to be a significant predictor of resilience. Specifically, those whose baseline measure of hope was higher showed lower scores in the areas of psychological distress, anxiety, and/or depression at all subsequent points in time (2 weeks, 4 months, and 1 year after disclosure).[145]

Another group found that predictors of long-term distress among unaffected women at risk for hereditary breast cancer included coping style and excessive breast self-examination. Among these women they identified a passive coping style as a risk factor, leaving the patient more likely overwhelmed, feeling helpless, and relying on others to solve problems. The study showed a palliative coping style, the tendency to distract oneself from problems, to also be a risk factor. They identified coping through reassuring thoughts as a beneficial coping style.[136]

In recent years, as genetic status is increasingly used to help guide treatment decisions, women newly diagnosed with breast cancer can find themselves introduced to cancer genetic testing with minimal time to consider the overwhelming amount of information, weighing the pros and cons for themselves, and for family members. Recent studies provide a look at the impact on these women newly diagnosed with breast cancer. One such study, published in 2018, found women newly diagnosed with breast cancer *without* cancer family history to be a particularly vulnerable group. They reported poorer adjustment up to 12 months after diagnosis, showing lower decreases in anxiety, and more regret regarding their surgical choices compared to newly diagnosed women with a cancer family history. Those women with no cancer family history also reported greater regret regarding the choice to undergo treatment-focused genetic testing (testing for the purpose of surgical decisions), and greater test-related distress. Notably, this held true regardless of test result. Newly diagnosed women with *no* family history of cancer were more likely to experience regret over having genetic testing and to experience less reduction in anxiety over time compared to those *with* a family history of cancer. One may wonder if this outcome is related to an increased familiarity and/or comfort with cancer in those women coming from families already having relatives diagnosed with cancer. Therefore, women who are contemplating cancer genetic testing at the time of their diagnosis who are without cancer family history may benefit from additional support beyond that which might otherwise be offered. For example, this population of women may benefit from additional follow-up counseling to facilitate psychological adjustment to their results, extra support in making surgical decisions, and counseling about how best to communicate results to family members.[141]

In 2017, researchers completed a qualitative study of 17 women undergoing genetic testing after being diagnosed with breast or ovarian cancer. They conducted four semi-structured focus-group interviews. Notably, they did not delineate between women with and without a cancer family history, as was later done by Meiser et al. (2018). However, they also found that personalized support and counseling may be particularly important in this group overall. The needs expressed by newly diagnosed women included more clarification about genetic testing, assistance in prioritizing information to make it more manageable, and added attention in tailoring the information to their personal situation.[146]

Research looking specifically at men undergoing cancer genetic testing is limited. One such study considered psychological distress in members of families with a known *BRCA* gene mutation. They found that men showed high levels of distress *only* when they had a sibling with a known pathogenic variant,[147] whereas women usually experienced adverse short-term psychological reactions regardless of sibling status.[147] Lodder et al. found similar outcomes reporting that men with daughters were at greater risk for distress.[148] Early in 2020, two studies exploring distress, anxiety, and depression focused on the impact of cancer genetic testing and needs specific to men. Pellini et al. found significantly higher mean scores on the Hospital Anxiety and Depression Scales (HADS-A and HADS-D) in affected men compared to unaffected men.[149] They found no evidence of distress among men undergoing genetic testing, at high risk, or affected with breast cancer.[149] They also found no difference based on result or age.[149] Through the use of focus groups and questionnaires, Bootsma et al. aimed to identify unmet needs among 107 male breast cancer patients. Patients identified information about psychological impact/coping, genetics, and family as lacking in their experience.[150] They found, in the period of time after treatment for breast cancer, men sought information regarding sexuality related to emotional and physical side effects.[150]

With easier access to genetic testing, and growing public awareness, we may see more requests by adolescents, and/or their parents, for genetic testing related to adult-onset conditions such as hereditary breast and ovarian cancer syndrome. It is important to note, over the years, different organizations have published position statements regarding the genetic testing of minors for adult-onset conditions. The American Academy of Pediatrics and the American College of Medical Genetics provide the following statements. "The AAP and

ACMG do not support routine carrier testing in minors when such testing does not provide benefits in childhood." However, their statement goes on to allow for exceptions related to psychosocial burden. "Predictive genetic testing for adult-onset conditions generally should be deferred unless an intervention initiated in childhood may reduce morbidity or mortality. An exception might be made for families for whom diagnostic uncertainty poses a significant psychosocial burden, particularly when an adolescent and his or her parents concur in their interest in predictive testing." The National Society of Genetic Counselors updated their position statement in April 2018. The organization discourages the testing of minors for adult-onset conditions, while allowing for the reality that some will pursue it. The NSGC position statement includes the following. "The decision for a minor to undergo genetic testing that could identify variants for adult-onset conditions either specifically or secondarily (e.g., through genomic sequencing) should be made cautiously, and whenever possible, with appropriate assent of the minor. If a minor undergoes genetic testing and results are not disclosed to the child, the healthcare provider should discuss strategies with the parents/guardian for sharing the results as he/she develops capacity, or by the age of majority."

For obvious reasons, there is not much available research addressing genetic testing of minors for adult-onset conditions; however, this area of interest is expanding due to the easy access of genetic testing by all age groups. Bradbury et al. (2012) found that the majority of parents do discuss their familial and/or genetic risk with their children, particularly as they age.[151] A 2013 qualitative study of nine adolescents who underwent genetic testing (six with positive results) found evidence of distress around the pretest process but no psychological harm.[152] Adult-onset conditions for which they were tested included hereditary breast and ovarian cancer syndrome (HBOC), hereditary diffuse gastric cancer syndrome (HDGC), Huntington disease, and autosomal-dominant cerebellar ataxia (ADCA).[152] Life experience prior to testing, including having cancer family history and knowledge of genetic risk within the family, may make these individuals better equipped to handle the information.[152] Bradbury et al., 2016 found that adolescent girls from *BRCA1-* or *BRCA2*-positive and/or strong breast cancer families exhibited greater breast cancer-specific distress and increased perceived risk of breast cancer when compared to those at general population risk.[153] This supports the possibility that these adolescents, although exhibiting more breast-specific distress, may be better prepared to obtain genetic testing information due to their exposure to cancer than those without a strong cancer family history.

Under very specific parameters, as stated by professional organizations, these studies all lend themselves to the testing of adolescents for adult-onset conditions. However, research is quite limited, highlighting the importance of case studies when considering the specific needs of adolescents wishing to undergo genetic testing for adult-onset conditions, such as HBOC. Through two case reports, Callard and Skirton discuss challenges with establishing rapport and engaging adolescents in discussion about feelings around genetic testing. They recommend the anticipated regret model as a useful tool.[154] This model first came into the spotlight in the 1980s when mental health researchers were exploring the specific needs of adolescents, taking into account their unique developmental limitations.[155] It was later introduced as a tool in assisting pregnant adolescents in decision-making in the genetic counseling setting.[156] The model encourages an individual to think about hypothetical results or outcomes to imagine how they might feel. As access becomes more widespread, potentially even through the growing number of individuals undergoing direct to consumer testing, larger studies will be needed to better serve this younger testing population.

In spite of the removal of prior barriers such as cost and access, and with integration into mainstream clinical care, cancer genetic testing is still being declined or delayed by some individuals at highest risk, when medical management change could be life-saving. The decision to decline or delay genetic testing can potentially leave the individual without access to important cancer risk reducing screening or even preventative surgeries. Investigations go back to the late 1990s, but recent research is again limited. In 1998, Lerman et al. published their study, which looked at families with a known pathogenic variant in *BRCA1* or *BRCA2*. They found decliners reported depressive symptoms, and all reported elevated cancer-related distress at baseline.[157] Another study, published the following year, found the same. Researchers looked at family members of patients diagnosed with Lynch syndrome. They discovered evidence supporting clinically significant levels of depression as having a negative impact on the uptake of genetic testing in both men and women.[158] Smith et al. published a longitudinal study in 2008, which reported on participants who underwent genetic testing, and completed a questionnaire at 3 months and 6 months post-test. Additionally, those who declined genetic testing were invited to complete the questionnaire. At 3-months post-test or after declining for those who did not test, participants with uninformative/ negative or VUS results reported less intrusive thoughts than decliners and carriers.[159] At 6-months post-test, decliners reported significantly more cancer related distress than those with VUS results.[159] These studies suggest an underlying psychological barrier to testing that may be overcome with time and extra support. It is also interesting to see that declining genetic testing could present more harm to individuals when compared to those testers found to carry a VUS or have an uninformative result. Primary care physicians, OB/GYNs, and gastroenterologists can play a particularly important role with this group of individuals whose personal and/or family history warrants cancer genetic testing but who choose to decline the test. Specifically, these non-genetic healthcare practitioners can help by encouraging them to explore their feelings or by guiding them to someone (i.e., cancer genetic professional) who can help explore these barriers that could be preventing access to critical and potentially life-saving medical management changes.

KEY POINTS

- Coping style can help predict development of psychological distress, anxiety, and/or depression.
  - Risk factors: passive or palliative coping styles
  - Beneficial: coping through reassuring thoughts
- Hopefulness is a predictor of resilience.
- Newly diagnosed women with *no* cancer family history are a particularly vulnerable group.
- Men with breast cancer have expressed a desire for information specific to their diagnosis.
- Position statements published by professional organizations discourage testing of minors for adult-onset conditions.
- Studies have shown that clinically significant levels of depression can have a negative impact on the uptake of genetic testing in both men and women.

When can Additional Support be Beneficial?

Being able to efficiently target individuals who may benefit from added support while going through the process of cancer genetic testing rests not only on knowing what may be the trigger, and who may be more likely to need the help, but also when, during the experience, they might benefit most from that support. As mentioned previously, Bredart et al. included individuals undergoing multi-gene panel testing in their prospective study. Their study captured information from 646 individuals, 75% of whom had a personal history of breast cancer. One goal was to examine when in the process of cancer genetic testing feelings of distress, anxiety, and depression were more likely to surface. Researchers explored changes in psychosocial issues before and after genetic testing in women for susceptibility to breast and ovarian cancers. They followed those undergoing both targeted and multi-gene panel testing between November 2016 and April 2018; their goal was to identify points in time during the process to consider the need for added support for those at greater risk for distress, anxiety, and/or depression. The Psychosocial Aspects of Hereditary Cancer (PAHC) questionnaire was administered before testing and again 2 months following result disclosure. At both assessment points, familial and social issues had the lowest mean scores, indicating people had fewer issues in these areas compared to the others, which included hereditary predisposition, emotions, familial cancer, personal cancer, and children-related issues. Two months after the result disclosure, highest scores were seen in the areas of familial cancer (concern about family members being diagnosed with cancer) and personal cancer (concern about themselves being diagnosed with cancer). These results suggest that the areas of patient support will greatly depend on where the individual is within the process of testing. The information obtained from testing can naturally increase a patient's concerns regarding a personal or family cancer diagnosis and therefore paying close attention to the time soon after a patient receives his or her results may be an important time for psychosocial evaluation.[144]

Contrasting the result from Bredart et al. (2019), Meiser et al. followed women newly diagnosed with breast cancer who underwent genetic testing. In total, subjects completed four questionnaires over 12 months, at baseline following recruitment, 1 week after genetic counseling, 2 weeks, post-result disclosure, and 12 months after initial enrollment. They found that breast cancer-specific worry decreased over time. Anxiety was significantly lower at all points compared to baseline. Over time, as mentioned previously, women newly diagnosed with breast cancer with a family history experienced less distress than those with no family history.[141] Although the Bredart et al. study described previously included a total of 646 subjects compared to 128 in the Meiser et al. study, the differences in outcome are most likely related to the fact that Meiser et al. examined only *newly* diagnosed patients and therefore their distress at baseline was likely the highest at the onset.

When examining the available research, we do have some information as to when, in the process of cancer genetic testing, an adolescent may benefit from added support. In 2013 researchers conducted a qualitative study of nine adolescents who underwent genetic testing for adult-onset conditions. They found evidence of distress around the pretest process, but no psychological harm.[152] From this study, acknowledging the very limited body of knowledge in this area, and based on position statements from professional organizations, we highlight that caution, care, and time should be given to adolescents in the period leading up to the point at which they undergo cancer genetic testing for adult-onset conditions.

When looking at the modest number of studies addressing the experience of cancer genetic testing for men, no research, so far, elucidates any specific moment in time throughout the genetic testing process that men may be more vulnerable. Bootsma et al. published early in

2020, found that men diagnosed with breast cancer tend to seek out information after treatment that regards sexuality related to emotional and physical side effects.[150] These men also expressed an absence of, and a desire for, more information specific to male breast cancer.[150] This missing information was as rudimentary as access to what breast cancer can physically look like in a man. It seems that basic information related to male breast cancer and perhaps information related to genetic testing may be helpful to men upon initial diagnosis of breast cancer.

> **KEY POINTS**
> - Individuals may be more susceptible to experience psychological worry soon after receiving results.
> - Women newly diagnosed with breast cancer who undergo genetic testing demonstrate a decrease in feelings of worry over time.
> - While testing of minors for adult-onset conditions should be the exception, if offered, some evidence suggests higher levels of distress during the time leading up to testing.
> - Men with breast cancer have expressed a need for information regarding sexuality and treatment side effects both at the time of their diagnosis and after treatment.

How can Healthcare Providers Provide Support?

While acknowledging the growing, emerging body of knowledge, the goal of this section is to assist providers in helping patients face what might otherwise be overwhelming for them. Research tells us the majority of patients can cope with the weight of information that can be unveiled through cancer genetic testing. The value in this research is in identifying the minority of people who may be in need of extra support. Once we are able to anticipate who needs the help, and when they need it, having the necessary knowledge and resources becomes paramount. Table 16.5 provides key points from available research regarding which patients may need support, when they are likely to benefit from these added resources, and recommendations for how to provide these supportive services. We include some anecdotal recommendations as well.

TABLE 16.5: Patient Populations With Potential for Increased Distress During Cancer Genetic Counseling and Testing, and Suggested Responses for Positive Outcomes

Patient Populations of Concern	Effective Responses
Patient demonstrating distortion in cancer or genetic risk perception	Communicate basic information. - "Most cancer is not hereditary." - "We all have genes and they work to protect us from cancer." - "Genetic testing helps us to accurately estimate cancer risks for you and your family, so we are able to protect you from getting cancer or detect it early." - "A positive test result does not mean a diagnosis of cancer."
Women newly diagnosed with breast cancer (particularly those without cancer family history)	- Provide clarification about genetic testing. - Prioritize information, making it more manageable. - Tailor information to the individual's personal situation. - Refer to a genetic specialist.

TABLE 16.5: Patient Populations With Potential for Increased Distress During Cancer Genetic Counseling and Testing, and Suggested Responses for Positive Outcomes (*Continued*)

Patient Populations of Concern	Effective Responses
Men diagnosed with breast cancer • with a sibling who is a carrier • with a daughter	• Provide information about psychological impact/coping and genetics, and how it affects the family. https://www.mannenmetborstkanker.nl/ • The Dutch Breast Cancer Society (BVN) and Breast Cancer Research Group (BOOG) • *The Pink Unicorns of Male Breast Cancer* by Alan F. Herbert • Refer to a genetic specialist.
Decliners of • genetic counseling • genetic testing • risk-management recommendations	• Communicate basic information. • Refer to a genetic specialist. • Decision-making tool meant specifically for unaffected *BRCA1/2*-positive women (https://www.brcadecisionaid.com).
Individuals failing to communicate positive test results to family members	• Revisiting the subject periodically can positively impact cascade testing. • Offer letters and other strategies to ease the stress of communicating complicated information. • Refer to a genetic specialist when the patient desires to communicate information but is unsure how.

Online Supportive Resources for Patients

Patients Who Are *BRCA* Positive
• Facing Our Risk of Cancer Empowered (FORCE): https://www.facingourrisk.org/
• Bright Pink: https://brightpink.org/

Patients with Lynch Syndrome
• Lynch Syndrome International: https://lynchcancers.com/

Patents with Hereditary Diffuse Gastric Cancer
• No Stomach for Cancer: https://www.nostomachforcancer.org/

Patients with Li-Fraumeni Syndrome
• Li-Fraumeni Syndrome Association: https://www.lfsassociation.org/

▨ CONCLUSION

What healthcare providers have in common is a desire to help individuals live long and healthy lives. The universal truth is that no one can be helped unless he or she is willing to accept that help. The goal of research into psychosocial issues associated with cancer genetic testing is to identify barriers to access the needed information that may improve quality of life, or even save a life, leaving the patient able to access his or her best self.

There are many limitations to the psychosocial research discussed in this review including small sample size, homogeneity among subjects, study location, and recruitment bias. Authors recommend additional research, not only to address study limitations, but because they also recognize evidence will constantly grow and change, and with that, we must evolve in our expectations and recommendations. In writing this section, we acknowledge this and welcome the evolution of information and new recommendations going forward. This is of particular importance in the setting of cancer genetics, as information is growing exponentially.

REFERENCES

1. Beauchamp TL, Childress JF. *Principles of biomedical ethics*. Oxford University Press; 2001.

2. Uhlmann WR, Schuette JL, Yashar B. *A guide to genetic counseling*. John Wiley & Sons; 2011.

3. Held V. *The ethics of care: Personal, political, and global*. Oxford University Press on Demand; 2006.

4. Balcom JR, Kotzer KE, Waltman LA, et al. The genetic counselor's role in managing ethical dilemmas arising in the laboratory setting. *J Genet Couns*. 2016;25(5):838–854.

5. Beauchamp TL. Methods and principles in biomedical ethics. *J Med Ethics*. 2003;29(5):269–274.

6. Murphy LB. The demands of beneficence. *Philosophy & Public Affairs*. 1993;22(4):267–292.

7. Twomey J. Ethical, legal, psychosocial, and cultural implications of genomics for oncology nurses. *Semin Oncol Nurs*. 2011;27(1):54–63.

8. Morrison EE. *Ethics in health administration: a practical approach for decision makers*. Jones & Bartlett Publishers; 2011.

9. Beauchamp TL. The principle of beneficence in applied ethics. In Zalta EN, ed. *The Stanford Encyclopedia of Philosophy*. 2019. https://plato.stanford.edu/archives/spr2019/entries/principle-beneficence. Metaphysics Research Lab, Stanford University.

10. McGuire AL, Beskow LM. Informed consent in genomics and genetic research. *Annu Rev Genomics Hum Genet*. 2010;11:361–381.

11. Bin P, Conti A, Capasso E, et al. Genetic testing: ethical aspects. *Open Med*. 2018;13(1):247–252.

12. Borello A, Ferrarese A, Passera R, et al. Use of a simplified consent form to facilitate patient understanding of informed consent for laparoscopic cholecystectomy. *Open Medicine*. 2016;11(1):564–573.

13. Ferrarese A, Pozzi G, Borghi F, et al. Informed consent in robotic surgery: quality of information and patient perception. *Open Medicine*. 2016;11(1):279–285.

14. Leo RJ. Competency and the capacity to make treatment decisions: a primer for primary care physicians. *Prim Care Companion J Clin Psychiatry*. 1999;1(5):131–141.

15. Black HC. Black's Law Dictionary, St. Paul, MN: West; 1990.

16. Shah PT, Turrin, D. *Informed Consent*. Treasure Island, FL: StatPearls Publishing; 2020.

17. Reasonable Person. *Wex*. Legal Information Institute: Cornell Law School.

18. Menko FH, ter Stege JA, van der Kolk LE, et al. The uptake of presymptomatic genetic testing in hereditary breast-ovarian cancer and Lynch syndrome: a systematic review of the literature and implications for clinical practice. *Fam Cancer*. 2019;18(1):127–135.

19. Ropka ME, Wenzel J, Phillips EK, et al. Uptake rates for breast cancer genetic testing: a systematic review. *Cancer Epidemiol Biomarkers Prev*. 2006;15(5):840–855.

20. Lenoir N. Universal declaration on the human genome and human rights: the first legal and ethical framework at the global level. *Colum Hum Rts L Rev*. 1998;30:537.

21. Genetic Testing: Informed Consent. 2016.

22. NHGRI. Genome Statute and Legislation Database. NIH.

23. Scheuner MT, Peredo J, Benkendorf J, et al. Reporting genomic secondary findings: ACMG members weigh in. *Genet Med*. 2015;17(1):27–35.

24. NSGC. Secondary and Incidental Findings in Genetic Testing. 2020; https://www.nsgc.org/p/bl/et/blogaid=30.

25. Tluczek A, Orland KM, Nick SW, et al. Newborn screening: an appeal for improved parent education. *J Perinat Neonatal Nurs*. 2009;23(4):326–334.

26. Botkin JR, Belmont JW, Berg JS, et al. Points to consider: ethical, legal, and psychosocial implications of genetic testing in children and adolescents. *Am J Hum Genet*. 2015;97(3):501.

27. Borry P, Evers-Kiebooms G, Cornel MC, et al. Genetic testing in asymptomatic minors: recommendations of the European Society of Human Genetics Recommendations of the European Society of Human Genetics. *Eur J Hum Genet*. 2009;17(6):720–721.

28. Counselors NSoG. Genetic Testing of Minors for Adult-Onset Conditions. *Position Statements*. NSGC Headquarters; 2018.

29. AMA. Genetic Testing of Children: Code of Medical Ethics Opinion 2.2.5. *Code of Medical Ethics: Decisions for Minors*, https://www.ama-assn.org/delivering-care/ethics/genetic-testing-children, 2020.

30. Bradbury AR, Patrock-Moller L, Pawlowski K, et al. Should genetic testing for BRCA1/2 be permitted for minors? Opinions of BRCA mutation carriers and their adult offspring. *Am J Med Genet C Semin Med Genet*. 2008;148C(1):70–77.

31. Wertz DC, Reilly PR. Laboratory policies and practices for the genetic testing of children: a survey of the helix network. *Am J Hum Genet*. 1997;61(5):1163–1168.

32. Elger BS, Harding TW. Testing adolescents for a hereditary breast cancer gene (BRCA1): respecting their autonomy is in their best interest. *Arch Pediatr Adolesc Med*. 2000;154(2):113–119.

33. Richards FH. Maturity of judgement in decision making for predictive testing for nontreatable adult-onset neurogenetic conditions: a case against predictive testing of minors. *Clin Genet*. 2006;70(5):396–401.

34. Bloch M, Hayden MR. Predictive testing for Huntington Disease in childhood— challenges and implications: opinion. *Am J Hum Genet*. 1990;46(1):1–4.

35. Clarke A. The genetic testing of children. *J Med Genet*. 1994;31(10):785–797.

36. Dickenson DL. Can children and young people consent to be tested for adult onset genetic disorders? *BMJ*. 1999;318(7190):1063–1065.

37. Boonstra H, Nash E. Minors and the right to consent to health care. *Issues Brief (Alan Guttmacher Inst)*. 2000(2):1–6.

38. Conti A. I test genetici: etica, deontologia, responsabilità. Giuffrè Editore; 2007.

39. Newson AJ. Whole genome sequencing in children: ethics, choice and deliberation. *J Med Ethics*. 2017;43(8):540–542.

40. Anderson JA, Hayeems RZ, Shuman C, et al. Predictive genetic testing for adult-onset disorders in minors: a critical analysis of the arguments for and against the 2013 ACMG guidelines. *Clinical Genetics*. 2015;87(4):301–310.

41. Ross LF, Saal HM, David KL, et al. Amer Acad Pediatrics, Amer Coll Med Genetics Genomics. Technical report: ethical and policy issues in genetic testing and screening of children. *Genet Med*. 2013;15(4):321.

42. Clayton EW. How much control do children and adolescents have over genomic testing, parental access to their results, and parental communication of those results to others? *J Law Med & Ethics*. 2015;43(3):538–544.

43. Wilfond BS, Fernandez CV, Green RC. Disclosing secondary findings from pediatric sequencing to families: considering the "benefit to families". *Journal of Law Medicine & Ethics*. 2015;43(3):552–558.

44. Committee on Bioethics; Committee on Genetics, and; American College of Medical Genetics and; Genomics Social; Ethical; Legal Issues Committee. Ethical and policy issues in genetic testing and screening of children. *Pediatrics*. 2013 Mar;131(3):620–622.

45. Pasche B. *Cancer Genetics*. Volume 155. Springer Science & Business Media; 2010.

46. Kilbride MK, Domchek SM, Bradbury AR. Ethical implications of direct-to-consumer hereditary cancer tests. *JAMA Oncol*. 2018;4(10):1327–1328.

47. FDA authorizes, with special controls, direct-to-consumer test that reports three mutations in the BRCA breast cancer genes [press release]. US FDA 2018.

48. Lapham EV, Kozma C, Weiss JO. Genetic discrimination: perspectives of consumers. *Science*. 1996;274(5287):621–624.

49. CDC. Genetic testing for breast and ovarian cancer susceptibility: evaluating direct-to-consumer marketing: Atlanta, Denver, Raleigh-Durham, and Seattle, 2003. *MMWR Morb Mortal Wkly Rep*. 2004;53(27):603–606.

50. Roberts JS, Gornick MC, Carere DA, et al. Direct-to-consumer genetic testing: user motivations, decision making, and perceived utility of results. *Public Health Genomics*. 2017;20(1):36–45.

51. Oh B. Direct-to-consumer genetic testing: advantages and pitfalls. *Genomics Inform*. 2019;17(3):e33.

52. Hudson K, Javitt G, Burke W, et al. ASHG statement on direct-to-consumer genetic testing in the United States. *Am J Hum Genet*. 2007;81(3):635–637.

53. ACMG Board of Directors. Direct-to-consumer genetic testing: a revised position statement of the American College of Medical Genetics and Genomics. *Genetics in Medicine*. 2016;18(2):207–208.

54. NSGC. At-home genetic testing position statement. In *Counselors NSoG*, Vol. 2020: NSGC; 2019.

55. Evans JP, Burke W. Genetic exceptionalism: too much of a good thing? *Genet Med*. 2008;10(7):500–501.

56. Statement of the American Society of Clinical Oncology: genetic testing for cancer susceptibility. Adopted on February 20, 1996. *J Clin Oncol*. 1996;14(5):1730–1736; discussion 1737–1740.

57. Clayton EW, Evans BJ, Hazel JW, et al. The law of genetic privacy: applications, implications, and limitations. *J Law Biosci*. 2019;6(1):1–36.

58. American Society of Clinical Oncology policy statement update: genetic testing for cancer susceptibility. *Journal of Clinical Oncology*. 2003;21(12):2397–2406.

59. Offit K, Thom P. Ethical and legal aspects of cancer genetic testing. Paper presented at: Seminars in Oncology. 2007.

60. Offit K, Thom P. Ethicolegal aspects of cancer genetics. *Cancer Treat Res*. 2010;155:1–14.

61. Grebe TA, Khushf G, Chen M, et al. The interface of genomic information with the electronic health record: a points to consider statement of the American College of Medical Genetics and Genomics (ACMG). *Genet Med*. 2020:1–6.

62. Allford A, Qureshi N, Barwell J, Lewis C, Kai J. What hinders minority ethnic access to cancer genetics services and what may help? *European Journal of Human Genetics*. 2014;22(7):866–874.

63. Armstrong K, Micco E, Carney A, et al. Racial differences in the use of BRCA1/2 testing among women with a family history of breast or ovarian cancer. *JAMA*. 2005;293(14):1729–1736.

64. Pagan JA, Su D, Li L, et al. Racial and ethnic disparities in awareness of genetic testing for cancer risk. *Am J Prev Med*. 2009;37(6):524–530.

65. Hughes C, Fasaye GA, LaSalle VH, Finch C. Sociocultural influences on participation in genetic risk assessment and testing among African American women. *Patient Educ Couns*. 2003;51(2):107–114.

66. Suther S, Kiros GE. Barriers to the use of genetic testing: A study of racial and ethnic disparities. *Genet Med*. 2009;11(9):655–662.

67. Forman AD, Hall MJ. Influence of Race/Ethnicity on Genetic Counseling and Testing for Hereditary Breast and Ovarian Cancer. *Breast J*. 2009;15:S56–S62.

68. Hamilton JG, Shuk E, Arniella G, et al. Genetic Testing Awareness and Attitudes among Latinos: Exploring Shared Perceptions and Gender-Based Differences. *Public Health Genomics*. 2016;19(1):34–46.

69. NSGC. National Society of Genetic Counselors, Inc.-Professional Status Survey 2019.

70. Penchaszadeh VB. Genetic counseling issues in Latinos. *Genet Test*. 2001;5(3):193–200.

71. Thompson HS, Valdimarsdottir HB, Jandorf L, et al. Perceived disadvantages and concerns about abuses of genetic testing for cancer risk: differences across African American, Latina and Caucasian women. *Patient Educ Couns*. 2003;51(3):217–227.

72. Susswein LR, Skrzynia C, Lange LA, et al. Increased uptake of BRCA1/2 genetic testing among African American women with a recent diagnosis of breast cancer. *J Clin Oncol*. 2008;26(1):32–36.

73. Li YR, Keating BJ. Trans-ethnic genome-wide association studies: advantages and challenges of mapping in diverse populations. *Genome Med*. 2014;6(10):91.

74. Hindorff LA, Bonham VL, Brody LC, et al. Prioritizing diversity in human genomics research. *Nat Rev Genet*. 2018;19(3):175.

75. MacArthur J, Bowler E, Cerezo M, et al. The new NHGRI-EBI Catalog of published genome-wide association studies (GWAS Catalog). *Nucleic Acids Res*. 2017;45(D1):D896–D901.

76. Popejoy AB, Fullerton SM. Genomics is failing on diversity. *Nature*. 2016;538(7624):161–164.

77. Morales J, Welter D, Bowler EH, et al. A standardized framework for representation of ancestry data in genomics studies, with application to the NHGRI-EBI GWAS Catalog. *Genome Biol*. 2018;19(1):21.

78. Amendola LM, Dorschner MO, Robertson PD, et al. Actionable exomic incidental findings in 6503 participants: challenges of variant classification. *Genome Res*. 2015;25(3):305–315.

79. Moreno-Estrada A, Gignoux CR, Fernández-López JC, et al. The genetics of Mexico recapitulates Native American substructure and affects biomedical traits. *Science*. 2014;344(6189):1280–1285.

80. Huo D, Senie RT, Daly M, et al. Prediction of BRCA mutations using the BRCAPRO model in clinic-based African American, Hispanic, and other minority families in the United States. *J Clin Oncol*. 2009;27(8):1184.

81. Kurian AW, Gong GD, John EM, et al. Performance of prediction models for BRCA mutation carriage in three racial/ethnic groups: findings from the Northern California Breast Cancer Family Registry. *Cancer Epidemiol Biomarkers Prev*. 2009;18(4):1084–1091.

82. Vogel KJ, Atchley DP, Erlichman J, et al. BRCA1 and BRCA2 genetic testing in Hispanic patients: mutation prevalence and evaluation of the BRCAPRO risk assessment model. *J Clin Oncol*. 2007;25(29): 4635–4641.

83. John EM, Miron A, Gong G, et al. Prevalence of pathogenic BRCA1 mutation carriers in 5 US racial/ethnic groups. *JAMA*. 2007;298(24):2869–2876.

84. Nanda R, Schumm LP, Cummings S, et al. Genetic testing in an ethnically diverse cohort of high-risk women: a comparative analysis of BRCA1 and BRCA2 mutations in American families of European and African ancestry. *JAMA*. 2005;294(15):1925–1933.

85. Hall MJ, Reid JE, Burbidge LA, et al. BRCA1 and BRCA2 mutations in women of different ethnicities undergoing testing for hereditary breast-ovarian cancer. *Cancer*. 2009;115(10):2222–2233.

86. Meijers-Heijboer H, van Geel B, van Putten WL, et al. Breast cancer after prophylactic bilateral mastectomy in women with a BRCA1 or BRCA2 mutation. *N Engl J Med*. 2001;345(3):159–164.

87. Eisen A, Weber BL. Prophylactic mastectomy for women with BRCA1 and BRCA2 mutations—facts and controversy. *Mass Medical Soc*. 2001.

88. Giesbertz NAA, van Harten WH, Bredenoord AL. A duty to recontact in genetics: context matters. *Nat Rev Genet*. 2019;20(7):371–372.

89. Otten E, Plantinga M, Birnie E, et al. Is there a duty to recontact in light of new genetic technologies? A systematic review of the literature. *Genet Med*. 2015;17(8):668–678.

90. Mueller A, Dalton E, Enserro D, Wang C, Flynn M. Recontact practices of cancer genetic counselors and an exploration of professional, legal, and ethical duty. *J Genet Couns*. 2019;28(4):836–846.

91. Fitzpatrick JL, Hahn C, Costa T, Huggins MJ. The duty to recontact: Attitudes of genetics service providers. *Am J Hum Genet*. 1999;64(3):852–860.

92. Phillips KA, Deverka PA, Hooker GW, Douglas MR. Genetic Test Availability And Spending: Where Are We Now? Where Are We Going? *Health Aff*. 2018;37(5):710–716.

93. Miletich SA, Mayo, J. Life or death question, but debate was hidden for years. *Seattle Times*; 2006.

94. Legal Considerations in Genetic Screening and Testing: Three Case Studies: ACOG Committee Opinion Summary, Number 805. *Obstet Gynecol*. 2020;135(4):994–995.

95. Robson ME, Storm CD, Weitzel J, Wollins DS, Offit K. American Society of Clinical Oncology policy statement update: genetic and genomic testing for cancer susceptibility. *J Clin Oncol*: *official journal of the American Society of Clinical Oncology*. 2010;28(5):893–901.

96. Braverman G, Shapiro ZE, Bernstein JA. Ethical issues in contemporary clinical genetics. *Mayo Clin Proc Innov Qual Outcomes*. 2018;2(2):81–90.

97. Nagahashi M, Shimada Y, Ichikawa H, et al. Next generation sequencing-based gene panel tests for the management of solid tumors. *Cancer Sci*. 2019;110(1):6–15.

98. Burke W, Antommaria AHM, Bennett R, et al. Recommendations for returning genomic incidental findings? We need to talk! *Genet Med*. 2013;15(11):854–859.

99. Green RC, Berg JS, Grody WW, et al. ACMG recommendations for reporting of incidental findings in clinical exome and genome sequencing. *Genet Med*. 2013;15(7):565–574.

100. Kalia SS, Adelman K, Bale SJ, et al. Recommendations for reporting of secondary findings in clinical exome and genome sequencing, 2016 update (ACMG SF v2. 0): a policy statement of the American College of Medical Genetics and Genomics. *Genet Med*. 2017;19(2):249–255.

101. Lolkema MP, Gadellaa-van Hooijdonk CG, Bredenoord AL, et al. Ethical, legal, and counseling challenges surrounding the return of genetic results in oncology. *J Clin Oncol*. 2013;31(15):1842–1848.

102. Dorschner MO, Amendola LM, Turner EH, et al. Actionable, pathogenic incidental findings in 1,000 participants' exomes. *Am J Hum Genet*. 2013;93(4):631–640.

103. Yang Y, Muzny DM, Xia F, et al. Molecular findings among patients referred for clinical whole-exome sequencing. *JAMA*. 2014;312(18):1870–1879.

104. Dugan RB, Wiesner GL, Juengst ET, O'Riordan M, Matthews AL, Robin NH. Duty to warn at-risk relatives for genetic disease: Genetic counselors' clinical experience. Paper presented at: American Journal of Medical Genetics Part C: Seminars in Medical Genetics; 2003.

105. Falk MJ, Dugan RB, O'Riordan MA, et al. Medical geneticists' duty to warn at-risk relatives for genetic disease. *Am J Med Genet A*. 2003;120(3):374–380.

106. Perry TJ, Patton SI, Farmer MB, et al. The duty to warn at-risk relatives—The experience of genetic counselors and medical geneticists. *American Journal of Medical Genetics Part A*. 2020;182(2):314–321.

107. Weaver M. The double helix: applying an ethic of care to the duty to warn genetic relatives of genetic information. *Bioethics*. 2016;30(3):181–187.

108. Aronson M. Genetic counseling for hereditary colorectal cancer: ethical, legal, and psychosocial issues. *Surg Oncol Clin N Am*. 2009;18(4):669–685.

109. Offit K, Groeger E, Turner S, Wadsworth EA, Weiser MA. The duty to warn a patient's family members about hereditary disease risks. *JAMA*. 2004;292(12):1469–1473.

110. Counselors NSoG. National society of genetic counselors code of ethics. *Journal of Genetic Counseling*. 2018;27(1):6–8.

111. Storm C, Agarwal R, Offit K. Ethical and legal implications of cancer genetic testing: do physicians have a duty to warn patients' relatives about possible genetic risks? *J Oncol Pract*. 2008;4(5):229.

112. Rothstein MA. Reconsidering the duty to warn genetically at-risk relatives. *Genet Med*. 2018;20(3):285–290.

113. *Tarasoff v. Regents of Univ. of Cal.* (1976).

114. *Pate v. Threlkel* (1995).

115. *Safer v. Estate of Pack* (1996).

116. *Molloy v. Meier* (Minn 2004).

117. Health insurance portability and accountability act of 1996. *Public law*. Vol 1041996:191.

118. ASHG statement. Professional disclosure of familial genetic information. The American Society of Human Genetics Social Issues Subcommittee on Familial Disclosure. *Am J Hum Genet*. 1998;62(2):474–483.

119. Association AM. § 2.131 Disclosure of Familial Risk in Genetic Testing, 2014–2015. *Code of Medical Ethics* 2015.

120. Gammon A, Neklason DW. Confidentiality & the Risk of Genetic Discrimination: What Surgeons Need to Know. *Surgical oncology clinics of North America*. 2015;24(4):667–681.

121. Kels CG, Kels LH. Medical privacy after death: implications of new modifications to the health insurance portability and accountability act privacy rule. Paper presented at Mayo Clinic Proceedings, 2013.

122. Ajunwa I. Genetic testing meets big data: tort and contract law issues. *Ohio St LJ*. 2014;75:1225.

123. Americans with disabilities act of 1990 In: ADA, ed. *Pub. L. 101-336 US Code 12111–12201*. https://www.ada.gov/pubs/adastatute08.htm. Accessed 6/13/20.

124. Standards for Privacy of Individually Identifiable Health Information. vol. 45, parts 160, 164 ed. Code of Federal Regulations US Department of Health and Human Services, Office for Civil Rights; 2002.

125. Patient Protection and Affordable Care Act (PPACA). Vol 42 USC §180012010.

126. Slaughter LM. The Genetic Information Nondiscrimination Act: why your personal genetics are still vulnerable to discrimination. *Surg Clin North Am*. 2008;88(4):723–738.

127. *Association for Molecular Pathology v. Myriad Genetics* (2013).

128. Cook-Deegan R. Are human genes patentable? *Ann Intern Med*. 2013;159(4):298–299.

129. Kesselheim AS, Cook-Deegan RM, Winickoff DE, et al. Gene patenting—the Supreme Court finally speaks. *The N Engl J Med*. 2013;369(9):869.

130. Kesselheim AS, Mello MM. Gene patenting—is the pendulum swinging back? *N Engl J Med*. 2010;362(20):1855–1858.

131. McCarthy M. Genes can't be patented, rules Supreme Court. *BMJ*. 2013 Jun 14;346:f3907.

132. Cohen S, Frank E, Doyle WJ, et al. Types of stressors that increase susceptibility to the common cold in healthy adults. *Health Psychol*. 1998;17(3):214–223.

133. Adkins DE, Wang V, Elder GH Jr. Structure and Stress: Trajectories of Depressive Symptoms across Adolescence and Young Adulthood. *Soc Forces; a scientific medium of social study and interpretation.* 2009; 88(1):31.

134. Cicero G, De Luca R, Dorangricchia P, et al. Risk Perception and Psychological Distress in Genetic Counselling for Hereditary Breast and/or Ovarian Cancer. *J Genet Couns.* 2017;26(5):999–1007.

135. Kuchenbaecker KB, Hopper JL, Barnes DR, et al. Risks of Breast, Ovarian, and Contralateral Breast Cancer for BRCA1 and BRCA2 Mutation Carriers. *JAMA.* 2017;317(23):2402–2416.

136. Heijer M, Seynaeve C, Vanheusden K, et al. Long-term psychological distress in women at risk for hereditary breast cancer adhering to regular surveillance: a risk profile. *Psychooncology.* 2013;22(3):598–604.

137. Bredart A, Kop JL, De Pauw A, Caron O, Fajac A, Nogues C. Effect on perceived control and psychological distress of genetic knowledge in women with breast cancer receiving a BRCA1/2 test result. *Breast.* 2016;31:121–127.

138. Cabrera E, Blanco I, Yagu C, Zabalegui A. The impact of genetic counseling on knowledge and emotional responses in Spanish population with family history of breast cancer. *Patient Educ Couns.* 2010; 78:382–388.

139. Tong A, Kelly S, Nusbaum R, et al. Intentions for risk-reducing surgery among high-risk women referred for BRCA1/BRCA2 genetic counselling. *Psychooncology.* 2015;24(1):33–39.

140. Voorwinden JS, Jaspers JP. Prognostic Factors for Distress After Genetic Testing for Hereditary Cancer. *Journal of Genetic Counseling.* 2016;25(3):495–503.

141. Meiser B, Quinn VF, Mitchell G, et al. Psychological outcomes and surgical decisions after genetic testing in women newly diagnosed with breast cancer with and without a family history. *European Journal of Human Genetics.* 2018;26(7):972–983.

142. Mahat-Shamir M, Possick C. The experience of women carriers of BRCA mutations following risk-reducing surgery: A cultural perspective. *Health Care Women Int.* 2017;38(4):344–360.

143. Esteban I, Vilaró M, Adrover E. Psychological impact of multigene cancer panel testing in patients with a clinical suspicion of hereditary cancer across Spain. *Psychooncology.* 2018;27(6):1530–1537.

144. Brédart A, Kop JL, Dick J. Psychosocial problems in women attending French, German and Spanish genetics clinics before and after targeted or multigene testing results: an observational prospective study. *BMJ Open.* 2019;9(9):e029926.

145. Ho SM, Ho JW, Bonanno GA, et al. Hopefulness predicts resilience after hereditary colorectal cancer genetic testing: a prospective outcome trajectories study. *BMC Cancer.* 2010;10:279.

146. Augestad MT, Høberg-Vetti H, Bjorvatn C, et al. Identifying Needs: a Qualitative Study of women's experiences Regarding Rapid Genetic Testing for Hereditary Breast and Ovarian Cancer in the DNA BONus Study. *Journal of Genetic Counseling.* 2017;26(1):182–189.

147. Smith KR, West JA, Croyle RT. Familial context of genetic testing for cancer susceptibility: moderating effect of siblings' test results on psychological distress one to two weeks after BRCA1 mutation testing. *Cancer Epidemiol Biomark Prev.* 1999;8(4):385–392.

148. Lodder L, Frets PG, Trijsburg RW, et al. Men at risk of being a mutation carrier for hereditary breast/ovarian cancer: an exploration of attitudes and psychological functioning during genetic testing. *Eur J Hum Genet.* 2001;9(7):492–500.

149. Pellini F, Mirandola S, Granuzzo E, Urbani S, Piccinni Leopardi G, Pollini GP. Italian Men Tested for BRCA1/2 Mutation: Psychological Distress during 6-Month Follow-Up. *J Oncol.* 2020 Jan 31;2020:3987935.

150. Bootsma TI, Duijveman P, Pijpe A, Scheelings PC, Witkamp AJ, Bleiker EMA. Unmet information needs of men with breast cancer and health professionals. *Psychooncology.* 2020. [Epub ahead of print] PMID: 32040237

151. Bradbury AR, Patrick-Miller L, Egleston BL. When parents disclose BRCA1/2 test results: Their communication and perceptions of offspring response. *Cancer.* 2012;118:3417–3425.

152. Mand C, Gillam L, Duncan RE, Delatycki MB. "It was the missing piece": adolescent experiences of predictive genetic testing for adult-onset conditions. *Genet Med.* 2013;15(8):643–649.

153. Bradbury AR, Patrick-Miller L, Schwartz LA. Psychosocial adjustment and perceived risk among adolescent girls from familieswith BRCA1/2 or breast cancer history. *J Clin Oncol.* 2016;34(28):3409–3416.

154. Callard A, Williams J, Skirton H. Counseling adolescents and the challenges for genetic counselors. *Journal of Genetic Counseling.* 2012;21(4):505–509.

155. Mills MC. Adolescents' reactions to counseling interviews. *Adolescence.* 1985;20(77):83–95.

156. Peters-Brown T, Fry-Mehltretter L. Genetic counseling for pregnant adolescents. *Journal of Genetic Counseling.* 1996;5(4):155–168.

157. Lerman C, Hughes C, Lemon SJ. What you don't know can hurt you: adverse psychologic effects in members of BRCA1-linked and BRCA2-linked families who decline genetic testing. *J Clin Oncol.* 1998;16(5):1650–1654.

158. Lerman C, Hughes C, Trock, BJ, et al. Genetic testing in families with hereditary nonpolyposis colon cancer. *JAMA.* 1999;281(17):1618–1622.

159. Smith AW, Dougall AL, Posluszny DM, et al. Psychological distress and quality of life associated with genetic testing for breast cancer risk. *Psychooncology.* 2008;17(8):767–773.

Talking to Children and Family About Hereditary Cancer Risk and Genetic Test Results

Amanda Ganzak

Upon receipt of a genetic test result identifying an inherited cancer predisposition, parents are often most focused on the potential impact of their result for their children and wonder how and when to tell them. This chapter focuses on strategies to help healthcare professionals to prepare patients to discuss genetic test results with their children and extended family members by outlining general communication guidelines, reviewing hereditary cancer communication literature, and identifying patient resources.

After patients receive their positive genetic test result, they are then tasked with the responsibility to share their results with relatives, as well as convey the results in a meaningful and motivational manner.[1] However, genetic test results are not always consistently shared within families. Some studies have shown that as many as 20 to 40% of at-risk family members are not aware that a cancer predisposing mutation has been identified in the family.[2–6] Prior studies have reported those with a *BRCA1/2* mutation were most likely to disclose results to sisters and least likely to disclose results to young children;[6,7] mothers were more likely than fathers to communicate their *BRCA1/2* test results to children;[8] and ethnicity influenced the likelihood of result disclosure, such that African Americans and Asians were less likely to disclose results than both white non-Hispanic and Hispanic patients.[9] Overall, the decision to disclose results to family members and who decides to disclose results can vary significantly from person to person and can be influenced by a myriad of compounding factors.

Adult-onset hereditary cancer predisposition syndromes, such as hereditary breast and ovarian cancer (HBOC) and Lynch syndrome, present a unique conundrum for parents since associated cancer risks and changes in medical management are not until adulthood, while inherited cancer syndromes, such as familial adenomatous polyposis (FAP) syndrome or multiple endocrine neoplasia (MEN1 and MEN2), have associated cancer risks and medical management changes starting in childhood. For this reason, predictive genetic testing for adult-onset hereditary cancer predisposition is not recommended for children; thus, some parents may not see the value of informing children about their results of genetic testing until they are older. However, genetic healthcare professionals should explore and demonstrate the importance of parents being upfront and honest with children about the genetic risk information, even though it may not have immediate medical implications. These discussions with patients may ultimately help guide and formalize parental decision-making to disclose their results and potential future implications with their children and other family members.

▥ OVERVIEW OF HEREDITARY CANCER RISK COMMUNICATION LITERATURE

Genetics providers will commonly hear parents ask, "When is the best time or age to inform my children?" A number of studies have examined parental discussions of genetic test results with their children. We provide a summary of several of these studies to highlight some of the observed patterns resulting from parental dissemination of genetic test results. While many parents are motivated to share hereditary risk information and genetic test results with children for the value of the information itself rather than the immediate clinical or medical impact, 30% of parents delay communication to at least one child, ranging from several months to 6 years post-parental receipt of the genetic test result.[10,11] Parents have reported the primary reasons for delay of disclosure included the age and maturity of the child, parental adjustment to the genetics information, the perceived utility of the information for the child, perceived vulnerability or resilience of the child, or desire to wait for an opportunity to share results in person with a child, especially those who were away at college.[6,10,11]

Parental decision to disclose a *BRCA1/2* result with children was often influenced by the older age of the child; on average, parents reported the pros of disclosure outweighed the cons by a factor of nearly 3:1.[12] Other studies reported approximately half of parents who underwent *BRCA1/2* genetic testing reported informing one or more of their children of their result status and hereditary risk information.[8,10,11] Rates of parental result disclosure to their children based on age were as follows: 6% of children less than age 10, 24% of children aged 10 to 13, 31% of children 14 to 17, and 87% of young adult children 18 to 25 were informed. The majority of young adult children were informed of the familial *BRCA1/2* mutation, whereas genetic test results were less often communicated to young children.[10,11]

Among families with children in both the teen and pre-teen age group, parents typically chose to inform both (29%) or neither (52%) groups of children. Importantly, relatively few families had instances where only older or younger children were told while their other children remained uninformed (19%); studies concluded that parental motivations to disclose results to children may be based less so on child age or age disparity between children but instead on other factors.[8] Some of these other factors included the mother being the parent who tested positive for the gene mutation, a parent's history of or upcoming prophylactic surgery, and parents with less formal education.[10,11] Conversely, factors that did not statistically impact the likelihood of result disclosure was the sex of the child or the parent's history of cancer.[10,11]

One reason parents were motivated to inform their children was as an attempt to reduce their own distress level. However, in actuality, disseminating results of genetic testing with children did not significantly improve parental distress symptoms or lighten the burden of knowing about the hereditary cancer risk in the family.[7] Therefore, some parents with high baseline distress may require their own psychosocial assessment to deal with their own unaddressed stress and needs over time. On the other hand, parents who chose to share results with children experienced significantly greater satisfaction of their decision than those parents who chose not to disclose their results to children. Additionally, parents with greater decisional conflict and psychological distress were less satisfied with their disclosure decision.[12]

Other factors influencing parental disclosure may include children being aware that genetic testing was performed and subsequently asking parents about the outcomes of testing or parents placing high value on maintaining open communication and preferring not to withhold information from their children.[7,8] These interpretations of parents assigning high value on open communication are consistent with the application of family systems theory to medical genetics, which emphasizes the role of open communication about hereditary risk information with at-risk relatives.[13]

Patenaude et al. reported parents were concerned with both protecting, as well as educating, their children about the hereditary cancer susceptibility. Parents surveyed reported confidence that they have the ability to convey genetic information to minor children; and as a result, many parents felt relief and satisfied in their sense of parental duty. As prior studies reported, parents also "advised child-specific, age-appropriate tailoring of genetic information and emphasized conveying the positive, preventive utility of genetic information to children."[14]

◾ PREPARATION FOR RESULT DISCLOSURE WITH CHILDREN

Parents should consider the following stages prior to result disclosure with their children. In the first stage, parents should work toward their own emotional stability and informational strength prior to disclosure. Children are sensitive to changes to their surroundings and emotional environment and are perceptive of the emotional state of the household and their parents. While parents may wish to hide how they are feeling, children may already be aware and able to sense subtle emotional changes subconsciously displayed by parents.[15]

Furthermore, children learn as much from what parents do as from what they say. According to the social learning theory, children observe and model their behaviors, attitudes, and emotional responses of those around them, including their parents.[16] If a parent is extremely emotional or frightened when discussing their genetic test result with children, then children may learn and internalize that genetic testing and its associated cancer risks are to be feared. One study reported that higher general anxiety in adolescent girls was associated with higher mother anxiety and poorer family communication, whereas high self-esteem in girls was associated with lower mother anxiety and better family communication. It also concluded that adolescent girls exposed to relatives with cancer in the family may foster adaptive responses and reduced cancer-specific distress but may also be influenced by the individual, mother, and other family factors.[17]

Thereby, parents should attempt to present the information in such a manner to balance the seriousness, but also the hopefulness, of being aware of the genetic risk information in order to be proactive in the future. How the information is framed by the parent and the tone of the discussion will impact how a child reacts, responds, and internalizes the meaning of the parental genetic test result. Parents should be honest and upfront with their children about their own feelings of worry or sadness but also of hope and resilience, as much as possible. Relaying a positive attitude toward the results of genetic testing is important, even if does not necessarily feel that way to parents in the moment. Hence, in preparation for disclosure, patients must first come to terms with their own feelings toward their results of genetic testing, and address the potential emotional burden it may have before notifying their children and at-risk relatives.[15]

In the next stage, parents should make a plan for disclosure with their children, ideally supported by all caregivers, and prepare what will be said to children in advance.[15] Parents should practice what they would like to say to their children in an attempt to find the right words. Healthcare providers should remind parents to keep the information simple in their initial conversations and only answer questions being asked by the child, so as to not overload them with too much detailed information.[15] Some strategies used by parents have included sharing segments of information over time by first discussing the cancer diagnoses in the family, then later introducing the concepts of hereditary risk due to the familial gene mutation and its associated cancer risks.[10,11]

In preparation, healthcare providers should have parents reflect on how other information has been previously communicated throughout the family to use as a model to plan and implement similar strategies for disclosing genetic test results with their children. As an example, did parents sit down one-on-one with each child or have a family dinner at home? In addition, parents should recall how difficult conversations were previously approached with children, such as when a new sibling was expected, they were moving and starting at a new school, or parents were getting a divorce. By analyzing how children responded in the past to emotionally difficult information, thinking about what worked well to make those discussions effective, and evaluating what was tough for each child to handle, will allow parents to use prior experiences to plan for how to inform children of their genetic test result.[15]

Healthcare professionals should inform parents to adapt the language and information presented based on the age, cognitive developmental, and maturity level of the child.[15] Parents should be reminded that there will never be the perfect words or time to tell children about hereditary cancer risk in the family, and waiting until the "right" time may delay an important conversation. Early and open communication with children creates trust and helps them feel confident that family members will support each other at every step. Children will use their memory of other moments of communication within the family to know how to react to these types of conversations.[15]

Finally, in the third stage, prior to the results disclosure, parents should assess the child's reaction to the results and be prepared to continually gauge the child's needs over time.[15] As healthcare providers, we can educate parents to observe and follow cues from their children, such as times when their children may be asking more questions or becoming more clingy than usual. Encourage parents to take time to explore their children's behaviors, questions, and attitudes, as it may be an unconscious way the child is trying to handle changes to their surroundings or picking up on something different going on in the household. Parents should be aware that by following their child's cues, it may provide an opportunity to initiate a conversation about what has been going on and potentially take a step toward disclosure of genetic testing.[15]

CHILD DEVELOPMENTAL CONSIDERATIONS PRIOR TO DISCLOSURE

Children in the family may span the developmental spectrum and have a difficult time understanding information that is biologically, numerically, and emotionally complex. Parents may need to tailor their language and explanations of their genetic test results for each of their children depending on their developmental age.[10,18] General developmental information for children in preschool, elementary school, middle school, high school, and emerging adult age are reviewed here to help parents appropriately refine these conversations

TABLE 17.1: Common Questions from Children Based on Developmental Age and Sample Parental Responses[15]

	Common questions from children	Sample responses
Preschool	Are you sad?	Everyone feels sad sometimes, and that's okay. You don't have to worry when I'm sad. You can always tell me your worries and I will take care of you.
	Are you mad at me?	No, I'm not mad at you. I wasn't here when you wanted to play because I had to go see the doctor, not because you did something naughty. I'm also sad we didn't get to play together.
Elementary	Do I have your genes?	Yes, you get half of your genes from each of your parents. That means half of your genes are the same as mine and half are the same as your [mother/father].
	What do genes do?	Genes are the instructions for how our body grows and works. Just like we have instructions for the games we play together and how to make cupcakes, our body has instructions, too.
	Why are you going to the doctor so much when you aren't sick?	When I grew up, I had my genes tested because some of our family had cancer, and I learned that I may develop cancer one day, too. I am going to the doctor because I want to take whatever steps I can to make sure I stay healthy, so that way I can take care of you.
	What is cancer?	Cancer is a sickness that causes cells, the body's building blocks, to grow faster and in different ways than they are supposed to grow. This makes it harder for parts of the body to do their job. Cancer is not contagious, and doctors treat cancer with powerful medicine.
Middle school	Did you have testing for the breast cancer gene?	Yes, I did, after much thought and discussion with my doctor and genetic counselor, and with other people in our family, I decided to have a test to see if I have a greater chance to develop cancer than other people. Now I can make good decisions about [my cancer treatment or how to reduce my risk to develop cancer or how to help the family members I care so much about].
	Do I have this gene, too?	Everyone has the gene, but in my body it is different because it does not work like it should. My gene is different because I was born with a mutation in the gene, which is like a typo. I have a higher chance of getting cancer like [grandma, aunt]. We do not yet know whether you have the same mutation, but you could find out one day.
	Since you have this mutation, can I get tested to see if I have it, too?	When you are an adult, you can choose to know your risk and get tested. There is a 50% chance that you have the same mutation as me and [grandma]. That means that there is an equal chance to you do not (show a pie chart or flip a coin to demonstrate the concept). However, even if you do have it, it doesn't mean that you will develop cancer. It means that you should work closely with your doctor to stay healthy.
High school	Can I have testing right now?	Although you may wish to know right now if you have this mutation or not, there are many more issues that we need to consider together first. Let's schedule an appointment with my [doctor or genetic counselor] to discuss this more.
	What will I do if my friends find out about this? Can I tell them?	This is your information to share. If you choose to share it, you might tell your friends that this doesn't mean you have the mutation or even that you'll develop cancer. But it may mean that your doctors will be keeping a close eye on you.
Emerging adults	When should I have genetic testing?	I recommend you speak to a genetic specialist when you decide you are ready, so that you can learn more about the timing of testing and discuss its pros and cons. It is important to remember most cancer screening does not start until you are 25 years old (or older), so we should also consider how you might use this information before that time.
	If I have this mutation, will anyone ever want to date or marry me? Will my kids have it? If so, I don't think I want to have kids.	We all have risk for something – remember that. There are many people out there who will love you and want to be with you for who you are regardless of whether you have this mutation.

with their children. In addition, common questions and sample parental responses for each age group are outlined in Table 17.1.

A preschooler's world evolves around their home and their relationship with their family, caregivers, and teachers. Children in this age group need regular reassurance they are safe and trusted adults will care for them. Young children lack basic concepts of physical distance or chronological time, are egocentric, and engage in magical thinking. An effective mode of communication with young children is through interactive play and fantasy. Thereby, it is suggested for parents to talk to their preschool-aged child in a familiar and quiet setting and consider using a book or toy to help illustrate topics or concepts being discussed. See Table 17.2 for age-appropriate resources. Any information discussed with children of this age should be followed up with reassurances, as appropriate.[15]

Elementary school-aged children have begun formal education, and egocentrism and magical thinking begin to decline as they learn about the world through mathematics, social science, and reading. At this stage, discussions about the human body may incorporate descriptions of genes as instructions or "building blocks." Children have developed skills to notice the ways people look, sound, and act, and they are able to verbalize and categorize similarities and differences in these traits. Parents can utilize these developmental changes when discussing results of genetic testing by using physical traits as examples to illustrate concepts of genetics and inheritance, such as commenting how a parent and child have the same eye color or explaining that the ability to roll the tongue is hereditary, followed by saying, "I can roll my tongue. Can you?"[15] By using these techniques and tailoring information to the developmental level of the child, parents will be able to help their children make appropriate connections for overall improved understanding.

By middle school, children have become concrete thinkers and have developed the capacity to understand the concept of inheritance, so more advanced topics about science and DNA

TABLE 17.2: Age-Specific Resources for Parents to Aid in Communication with Children[15]		
	Resource	**Annotation**
Preschool	Balkwill F, Rolph M (2002). *Enjoy Your Cells*. Cold Spring Harbor Laboratory Press, Cold Spring Harbor, NY.	First book in a series about cellular and molecular biology. Introduces cell structure. Includes colorful, engaging pictures.
	Hape Your Body 5-Layer Wooden Puzzle, by Beleduc.	Layered puzzle showing body organs and systems, including skeletal and muscular. It displays growth of plants from seed to fruit, humans from infancy through aging, and animals.
	Moore-Mallinos J, Fabrega, M (2008). *Mom Has Cancer!* (Let's Talk About It series) Barron's Educational Series.	Discusses children's worries when a parent is diagnosed with cancer, normalizes lifestyle changes, and balances reassurances with honest information.
	Par, T (2009). *It's OK to be Dfferent*. Little, Brown Book for Young Readers.	Picture book designed to increase confidence and self-esteem in preschool-aged children. Introduces children to, and embraces, human variation.
	Harris, RH, Westcott, NB (2012). *Who's in My Family? All About Our Families*. Candlewick.	Visually appealing display of varied family forms across the animal kingdom.

TABLE 17.2: Age-Specific Resources for Parents to Aid in Communication with Children[15] (Continued)

	Resource	Annotation
Elementary School	Balkwill F, Rolph M (2002). *Gene Machines*. Cold Spring Harbor Laboratory Press, Cold Spring Harbor, NY.	Authors use simple, concrete language and colorful graphics to assist young children in learning about cells, DNA, and proteins.
	Balkwill F, Rolph M (2002). *Have a Nice DNA*. Cold Spring Harbor Laboratory Press, Cold Spring Harbor, NY.	Author explains genetics in a fun and easy way for kids. Topics include cells, DNA, and proteins. Helpful illustrations.
	Balkwill F, Rolph M (2002) *Enjoy Your Cells*. Cold Spring Harbor Laboratory Press, Cold Spring Harbor, NY.	First book in a series about cellular and molecular biology. Introduces cell structure. Colorful, engaging pictures.
	Duke, S. (2011). *You Can't Wear These Genes*. Rourke Publishing: Vero Beach, FL.	Addresses mutations, inherited conditions, and mentions cancer.
	Brain Pop Video – DNA, www.brainpop.com/health/freemovies/dna	Developed by pediatrician, immunologist, and entrepreneur Dr. Avraham Kadar. Animated video explaining basic genetic and modern genetic concepts like GMOs and the Human Genome Project. Includes games, quizzes, and articles with trivia. Brief mention of familial disease.
Middle School	About Kids Health, www.aboutkidshealth.ca	From the Hospital for Sick Children in Toronto, Canada. An introduction to cells, chromosomes, DNA, inheritance, and genetic testing.
	DNA Animation, www.popsci.com/science/article/2013-03/watch-absolutely-beautiful-animated-explainer-dna	Curated and written by California-based molecular biologist Matthew Adams, this animated video about basic genetic concepts includes information about the "universal genetic code," relationships to other species, and the future of genetic engineering. Not specific to familial cancer.
	Genetics for Kids, www.neok12.com/Genetics.htm	Quizzes, interactive activities, and explanatory videos with examples and narration focuses on the basis of genetics and heredity.
	Learn Genetics™, Genetic Science Learning Center, learn.genetics.utah.edu	This animated website introduces chromosomes, genes, DNA, how a protein is made, interesting heritable traits, and fun activities for children. Information is suitable for teenagers interested in the basics and for those looking for more advanced topics.
	National Human Genome Research Institute. National Institute of Health, www.genome.gov/10506367	This website includes many links to interactive lessons about DNA, a glossary of terms, information about the Human Genome Project, tools for researching family history, and DNA experiments for the motivated student. Includes a talking glossary of genetic terms.
	Personal Genetics Education Project, www.pgED.org	From the Department of Genetics at Harvard Medical School. Complete lesson plans about controversies and novel, evolving issues in genetics and personalized medicine. Includes newspaper clippings, activities, PowerPoint slides, and discussion questions. Addresses traits and heredity but not specifically familial cancer.
	"Cracking the Code of Life" (PBS)	Tells the story of the race to decode the human genome; reviews implications for health, understanding disease, and technological innovation.

can be introduced. They have also become information seekers. Pictures and diagrams can be useful among this age group to further support genetics discussions and help children visualize concepts such as DNA. When discussing autosomal dominant inheritance, it can be helpful for parents to draw a pie chart or flip a coin to illustrate the concept of 50% odds of inheriting a familial mutation. Another consideration for children in this age group is the development of secondary sexual characteristics and children being more aware of their changing body. Parents may thereby wish to use these conversations about puberty as an opportunity to educate children about potential cancer risks to these developing parts of their body, but should still keep the discussion simple to continue facilitating ongoing, open discussions together.[15]

When a middle schooler feels like a parent is withholding information, the child may draw their own inaccurate conclusions or seek information elsewhere, such as the internet. However, when a parent initiates an open and honest conversation with accurate information, especially pertaining to the results of genetic testing or associated cancer risks, it sends the message to the child that the information is important and acceptable to discuss together. During this developmental age, if a parent does not know the answer to a specific question or is not ready to address a particular question, it is best for the parent to validate the children's curiosity and arrange a time to address the questions at a later time without the presence of distractions or after more information can be obtained.[15]

In the transition to high school, adolescents become more independent from their family, take on more responsibility outside the home, and develop more meaningful social connections and relationships. It is also a period of time of rapid sexual development. In addition, many teens learn about genetics and inheritance in science class, which may use specific examples including hereditary breast and ovarian cancer caused by an inherited *BRCA1/2* mutation. As a result, children may inquire about the possibility of a hereditary cancer predisposition in their family and apply these concepts to their own observed patterns of cancer in their family. Rather than parents being surprised when these questions are raised, they should instead use these inquiries as a springboard to discuss the results of genetic testing and potential future impact on the child. Hereditary cancer risk conversations with teens may also be beneficial in fostering and supporting healthy life choices and behaviors.[19]

In the era of social media, numerous online support groups and resources are at a teen's fingertips. While they may be more comfortable seeking information online rather than asking their parents follow-up questions, many teens may be unable to synthesize and discern credible, reliable resources and information on the internet. Thus, parents may wish to provide them with trustworthy websites and information about specific syndrome patient advocacy groups to ensure accurate information is being consulted; they can encourage their children to ask questions if they are unsure about any information read online. See Table 17.3 for patient resources, support, information, and advocacy for hereditary cancer predisposition syndromes. This promotes the continued independence of the teenager while also providing the child with parental support and oversight.[15]

If parents decide to delay these discussions, they may lose some control over how and when these conversations occur. For example, a child may overhear a conversation between a parent and health professional or family member, leading to unanticipated questions at an inopportune time. This may force a parent to either dismiss these important questions or feel unprepared to handle the discussion at that moment.[15]

▪ THE "FIVE Ws" FOR RESULT DISCLOSURE

When preparing parents to disclose their genetic test results with children, encourage parents to think about the "five Ws" (who, what, where, when, why) as they get ready for a

TABLE 17.3: Resources for Support, Information, and Patient Advocacy for Hereditary Cancer Predisposition Syndromes[31]

Hereditary Cancer Syndrome	Resources	
Familial Adenomatous Polyposis	"FAP & Me, A Kid's Guide to Familial Adenomatous Polyposis"	Booklet
	Hereditary Colon Cancer Foundation	www.hcctakesguts.org
Hereditary Breast and Ovarian Cancer	Basser Center for BRCA	www.basser.org
	Bright Pink	www.brightpink.org
	Facing Our Risk Cancer Empowered (FORCE)	www.facingourrisk.org 1-866-288-RISK(7475)
	HIS Breast Cancer Awareness	www.hisbreastcancer.org
	Sharesheret	www.sharsheret.org 1-866-474-2774
Hereditary Diffuse Gastric Cancer	No Stomach for Cancer	www.nostomachforcancer.org
Hereditary Leiomyomatosis and Renal Cell Cancer	HLRCC Family Alliance	www.hlrccinfo.org
Hereditary Pheochromocytoma and Paraganglioma Syndrome	PheoParatroopers	www.pheoparatroopers.org
Li-Fraumeni Syndrome	Li-Fraumeni Syndrome Association	www.lfsassociation.org
Lynch Syndrome	AliveandKickn	www.aliveandkickn.org
	Hereditary Colon Cancer Foundation	www.hcctakesguts.org
Multiple Endocrine Neoplasia	American Multiple Endocrine Neoplasia (AMEN)	www.amensupport.org
***PTEN* Hamartoma Tumor Syndrome (PHTS) or Cowden Syndrome**	*PTEN* Hamartoma Tumor Syndrome Foundation	www.ptenfoundation.org
Tuberous Sclerosis (TSC)	TSC Alliance	www.tsalliance.org
Von Hippel-Lindau (VHL)	VHL Alliance	www.vhl.org

result dissemination. Much of this advice and parental considerations are further detailed in "Talking About BRCA in Your Family Tree,"[20] a helpful resource to provide parents in advance of these discussions with their children and family members, and the principles can be adapted to other hereditary cancer predisposition syndromes.

The first question parents should address is *who* they plan to tell about their genetic testing results and *who* will be present during these conversations. As parents consider informing their children of a hereditary cancer predisposition in the family, they should consider the similarities and differences in ages, maturity, and level of comprehension and understanding among the children. The level of informational content and amount of detail may need to be adjusted depending on each child. In order to tailor the conversation appropriately, parents should examine the coping skills of each child and how they previously responded to and dealt with other important life events. It may also be crucial for parents to contemplate who else should be included in the result disclosure conversation with children, such as one or both parents, step-parents, or other important family members or caregivers.

Furthermore, parents should determine if they plan on talking to all of their children together or whether a one-on-one approach would be more effective. For example, some siblings have very close relationships and would turn to one another for emotional support, while others could push each other's buttons and derail that important conversation. There may be potential harms of telling only select children, as these children may experience distress from having to keep the "family secret" until other siblings are made aware of it, or they may lack the support of their uninformed siblings during this difficult time. Therefore, parents should scrutinize all of these factors in advance of result dissemination.

The next element to consider is *what* parents plan on telling their children about the result. It is helpful for parents to practice the conversation with a trusted individual before attempting to tell their children; it will help them organize their thoughts and become more comfortable with the information, which will increase their confidence heading into the disclosure. It also enables parents to help find the best wording during a potentially difficult conversation.

These first conversations with children may be easier than parents were expecting; however, they may not be the optimal time to expand on all details related to the genetic test results, associated cancer risks, and long-term implications. The initial discussion should build the foundation slowly by simply introducing the concept of a hereditary predisposition. It can be used to introduce the parent's or relative's cancer history and help to explain why the parent needs to go to the doctor more often or have surgery. It is important for parents to not dismiss or overly reassure children; they should be as honest as they can be. Over time, parents should encourage their children to ask questions and allow the child to guide future conversations, even if it's not the best time the parents had pictured for disclosure or discussion of the information.

Subsequently, parents should determine *where* they plan on having the conversation. They should ponder where other important conversations with their children have taken place, such as in bed at the end of the day, at the kitchen table during dinner, or on a walk. The time of day may also be important to consider; some children do best in the morning while others are more attentive at night. It may be more effective to have these conversations on the weekend when there may be more time to provide additional support to children rather than during the week. Having enough time to process the information could influence the child's response to the information. In any case, parents must create a comfortable and safe environment for children when they plan to have these potentially difficult, emotional conversations.

One of the most asked questions by parents is, "*When* should I tell my child about my result?" There are no current guidelines or an "ideal" age when children should be informed about their parent's genetic test result. Parents should be encouraged to consider the age, maturity, and development of each child when making decisions about when to inform them of the familial cancer susceptibility. These discussions may also be influenced by the need to explain a parent's upcoming surgery or recent cancer diagnosis. For hereditary cancer syndromes that alter medical management of children, disclosing the results of genetic testing with young children may help to explain why certain tests, procedures, and surgeries need to be performed.

Parents should understand the reasons *why* informing their children of genetic test results can be beneficial, as it may help to prepare a child for a parent's upcoming surgery or recent cancer diagnosis, but it could also clarify why a parent may have been upset or distracted.

This could provide a platform to explain why genetic testing was performed, explore the parent's personal and/or extended family history of cancer (if children are old enough), and emphasize the future relevance and importance for the children.

As mentioned previously, many children from an early age are perceptive and aware of emotional or stressful issues in their environment and home life. Moreover, children value being included in important conversations and prefer to learn information firsthand from their parents. These discussions may help to comfort a child if they have been worried the parent is dying or very ill based on their recent observed behavior, when in fact the parent may have just been distracted or upset about the outcomes of genetic testing. These conversations can give context as to what has been going on around the child rather than the child picturing the worst possible outcome and coming to their own inaccurate conclusions.[15]

Various studies have demonstrated open and honest conversations regarding risk information and results of genetic testing have been associated with better long-term outcomes.[6,19,21–25] It can also foster honesty and truthfulness beyond the immediate discussion of results of genetic testing with a parent. Once children feel their parents are being honest and entrust them with difficult information, it can create a conduit that children can use in the future, particularly if they are nervous about their own genetic testing, fear of cancer risks, or need for increased cancer surveillance.

POST-RESULT DISCLOSURE WITH CHILDREN

By having parents complete the exercise of addressing each of the "five Ws" and assessing their children's ability to process and understand information based on their stage of development, the initial steps in preparing parents to inform their children have begun. After the initial disclosure, parents should have their children put the conversation in their own words. By having children repeat what they learned and what it means to them, the parents can assess their children's understanding, emotional reaction, and well-being, as well as create an opportunity to correct any inaccuracies or misperceptions.

Healthcare providers should instruct parents to observe any changes in their child's behavior to actively gauge how the child is doing and coping post-disclosure. Parents should check in with their children over time to see if they have any follow-up questions, worries, or concerns, so they can be addressed together. By leaving the conversation open-ended, it will reinforce to children that their parents are available for any follow-up questions or concerns that may arise over time. However, some questions asked by children may not have answers or the question can wait until later. For most people, it is uncomfortable when there is no answer to a question, but emphasize to patients that it is completely acceptable to answer "I don't know" or "Nobody knows" to some of the questions children ask. This once again demonstrates to children that their parents are being as honest as possible, and not withholding information, with the goal to make the child feel involved throughout the whole process.[15]

While there may be limited data assessing long-term impact of genetic test result disclosure on children, one potential impact could include significant consequences for a child's sense of security and socioemotional well-being in becoming aware of parent's elevated risk for developing cancer.[8] These children may become withdrawn or depressed, which may warrant clinical attention. Consequently, families may benefit from continued psychosocial monitoring to assist parents in managing their children's thoughts and feelings post-disclosure.[8] Prior studies have demonstrated the importance of disclosure and accurate risk perception as a significant motivator of positive health behaviors and plan for future choices.[21-25] Bradbury et al. reported the majority of children and young adults reported a good understanding of the information shared, no negative aspects for learning parental BRCA status, and health behaviors even improved post-disclosure including many tobacco users who stopped smoking.[19]

Parents who disclosed results to children were surveyed to learn more about their offspring's initial reaction to the genetic test result information and subsequent impact of result disclosure on their relationship. The most frequently described response from children was neutral and/or happiness or relief.[11] Adverse reactions reported by parents in almost half of their children ranged from concern, distress, or anxiety to more severe reactions, such as crying or fear. Of note, parents most frequently reported concern as a common response among their older offspring.[11] In addition, parents reported almost half of offspring did not appear to understand the importance or significance of the information; but some children had been aware of the hereditary risk in the family, so parental result disclosure may not have added much significance to information already known or assumed. Lastly, the majority of parents (65%) reported no change in parental-child relationship post-disclosure, whereas 22% reported a strengthening of their relationship, and only two parents reported an "area of sensitivity" that was not addressed or discussed often post-disclosure.[10,11] Additional studies have also suggested that result disclosure may have the potential to strengthen family relationships and cohesion.[26,27]

A subsequent study evaluating the psychosocial adjustment and perception of risk among girls (ages 11 to 19) in families with a *BRCA1/2* mutation or breast cancer reported all girls accurately reported their mother's history of breast cancer and 55% of girls with a BRCA-positive mother reported knowledge of their mother's BRCA status. Of those daughters aware of their mother's *BRCA* mutation, they did not experience significantly different outcome scores using either the behavioral assessment system for children (BASC-2) or breast cancer-specific distress assessment compared to those who did not report knowledge of their mother's genetic test result. This study reported no significant differences in associations between age and self-esteem, depression, or breast cancer-specific distress.[17] These findings suggest girls with a mother diagnosed with breast cancer, regardless of mutation status, experience minimal negative outcomes when informed of the family history of breast cancer and/or results of genetic testing.

ROLE OF THE HEALTHCARE PROVIDER

Due to privacy laws, genetic healthcare professionals are unable to directly warn at-risk relatives of the familial gene mutation associated with a hereditary cancer predisposition. When asked, parents favored more active involvement by genetic counselors around the topic of delivery of genetic information to children.[14] Therefore, health professionals should take a more directive role to encourage and support patients to disclose genetic test results to family members.[28] As healthcare providers, it is imperative to identify at-risk relatives within the family to make patients aware of who needs to be informed of the familial mutation. They should also identify resources to educate and strategies to empower patients in order for them to accurately and successfully share their genetic test results with relatives.

This responsibility can begin during the initial genetics consultation when discussing genetic testing and its potential impact for the patient and their relatives but can be reiterated when reviewing inheritance risks and the inevitability of informing relatives of their results. Ultimately, this better prepares patients regarding the importance of and need to inform relatives. Genetic healthcare providers should explicitly explain that the test results are to the benefit of the whole family, not just the patient.[28] During the informed consent process, there may be a section dedicated to family member disclosure authorization for patients to specify who within the family has or does not have permission to obtain the result information in the future. This is another opportunity for healthcare providers to emphasize the relevancy of genetic test results for relatives.[28]

During the results disclosure, genetic healthcare professionals can help to explore patients' plans for disclosure of their results with relatives, as well as how and when they plan on telling relatives. Patients should be encouraged to practice these difficult conversations ahead of time, thereby enabling patients to plan for these potentially burdensome conversations and determine timing of discussion to improve follow-through with these difficult discussions. Providers can also question patients on who they plan to share results with in the family. These conversations may reveal there are at-risk relatives the patients have not yet thought about or plan to inform within the family (i.e., cousins) or patients may even disclose they have no intention of telling their children or certain relatives. As an example, a patient may report, "I don't want to tell my children until they are much older. Why would I want to worry them now?" Genetic healthcare professionals should respond by validating the patient's feelings about wanting to protect their children from the burden of learning about a hereditary cancer predisposition in the family. However, providers should also take the opportunity to reinforce the importance of notifying their children, provide patients with resources and literature demonstrating the benefit of informing offspring, and further illuminate the benefits of being honest with children about the familial mutation.

Follow-up visits are another occasion to inquire about how dissemination of results has been going for the patient and, once again, echo the importance of family disclosure. During these times, reassess what the patient may need to support them in continuing to inform their children and at-risk relatives. In the end, providers should continually stress and readdress the importance and implications of genetic test results for their children and relatives as many times as possible throughout the initial consultation, result disclosure, and follow-up appointments. It is the responsibility of healthcare providers to offer advice, feedback, and recommendations to help adjust and improve the patient's disclosure plans to enable a more seamless and timely disclosure.

Interestingly, one study reported few patients (5%) identified their healthcare professional as the most important person in assisting in their decision to disclose genetic test results to children, whereas the majority of patients reported themselves (45%) and their spouses (43%) were the most influential people. However, when patients were specifically asked if a healthcare professional was involved in the decision at any point, they responded that a genetic counselor (21%) and a physician (14%) were involved. This may be the result of the lack of established guidelines for healthcare providers to help guide parents as to the best time to inform offspring, but parents may not have been offered or understood about the existence of support from their healthcare providers.[10] Prior studies have also suggested there may be a risk of inaccurate information or misconceptions during the result communication process with children without professional assistance.[29] Therefore, these studies highlight that healthcare professionals should offer their expertise, advice, and communication strategies to continually extend their support to patients in order to promote effective communication of genetic test results to children and relatives.

When a positive result is disclosed to patients, informational resources should be provided to the patient. Genetic healthcare professionals can give patients a detailed summary letter overviewing results of genetic testing, associated cancer risks, and medical management recommendations, as well as identify at-risk relatives who would benefit from being notified of the genetic test results in the family. Therefore, the patient can use the summary letter as a guide for discussions with family members.[28] In addition, a family notification letter can also be given to use as an aid in dissemination of their genetic test results. Then, this letter can be used by relatives to share the familial genetic information with their physician or genetic healthcare professional for personalized risk discussions.[28] Lastly, genetic healthcare providers can identify resources for patients' relatives, such as a local genetic counselor, to make it easier for family members to schedule a genetic consultation to initiate their own education and genetic testing.

There are hereditary cancer patient advocacy groups and websites with information about family disclosure, gene-specific information, webinars, and message boards to connect with other individuals who also have a hereditary cancer predisposition. See Table 17.3 for a list of specific hereditary cancer predisposition syndrome resources. Encourage patients to have these resources available when disseminating results to their children and at-risk family members. They may even serve as a safeguard for patients.

The healthcare provider should aim not to have patients force their children and family members to have genetic testing but rather to inform their children and at-risk relatives of the option of genetic testing and potential impact of results on cancer risks and medical management recommendations.[28] It is important to be cognizant of and sensitive to cultural differences, such as patients' own feelings about cancer, family relationships, and inheritance. As an example, a patient's belief of fatalism surrounding a cancer diagnosis or shame about a cancer gene mutation may inhibit an open discussion, and conversely, principles of familialism and collectivism emphasized in some cultures may motivate communication of information to family members.[1]

Remember, each patient and family is unique, and the patient's decisions to inform their children and family members may be impacted by a host of factors. MacKenzie et al. stated that "optimal outcomes of communication of genetic test results … requires not only the effective communication of risk information, but also an understanding of the consumers' translation of that information into personalized perceptions of risk of disease, benefits of interventions, and the bio-psychosocial factors that mediate the process."[30] The duty and responsibility of healthcare providers is to provide appropriate education, guidance, and continued support to patients. This has benefits reaching far beyond the single patient being seen in clinic, as it extends to all of their at-risk relatives. Healthcare providers should equip their patients with the tools to successfully inform their children and relatives, since the interpretation of results, risk perception, and adherence to screening recommendations among children and at-risk relatives is dependent upon the efficacy of these initial disclosure conversations.

References

1. Ricker C, Koff RB, Qu C, et al. Patient communication of cancer genetic test results in a diverse population. *TBM*. 2018;8(1):85–94.

2. Gaff CL, Collins VC, Symes, Halliday J. Facilitating family communication about predictive genetic testing: probands' perceptions. *J Genet Couns*. 2005;14(2):133–140.

3. Landsbergen K, Verhaak C, Kraaimaat F, et al. Genetic update in BRCA-mutation families is related to emotional and behavioral communication characteristics of index patients. *Fam Cancer*. 2005;4(2):115–119.

4. Sharaf RN, Myer P, Stave CD, et al. Uptake of genetic testing by relatives of Lynch syndrome probands: A systematic review. *Clin Gastroenterol Hepatol*. 2013;11:1093–1100.

5. Lerman C, Hughes C, Trock BJ, et al. Genetic testing in families with hereditary nonpolyposis colon cancer. *JAMA*. 1999;281(17):1618–1622.

6. Daly MB, Montgomery S, Bingler R, et al. Communicating genetic test results within the family: Is it lost in translation? A survey of relatives in the randomized six-step study. *Fam Cancer*. 2016;15(4):697–706.

7. Hughes C, Lynch H, Durham C, et al. Communication of BRCA1/2 test results in hereditary breast cancer families. *Cancer Res Ther Control*. 1999;8:51–59.

8. Tercyak KP, Hughes C, Main D, et al. Parental communication of BRCA1/2 genetic test results to children. *Patient Educ Couns*. 2001;42(3):213–224.

9. Cheung EL, Olson AD, Yu TM, Han PZ, Beattie MS. Communication of BRCA results and family testing in 1,103 high-risk women. *Cancer Epidemiol Biomarkers Prev*. 2010;19(9):2211–2219.

10. Bradbury AR, Dignam JJ, Ibe CN, et al. How often do BRCA mutation carriers tell their young children of the family's risk for cancer? A study of parental disclosure of BRCA mutations to minors and young adults. *J Clin Oncol*. 2007;25(24):3705–3711.

11. Bradbury AR, Patrick-Miller L, Egleston BL, et al. When parents disclose BRCA1/2 test results: their communication and perceptions of offspring response. *Cancer*. 2012;118(13):3417–3425.

12. Tercyak KP, Mays D, DeMarco TA, et al. Decisional outcomes of maternal disclosure of BRCA1/2 genetic test results to children. *Cancer Epidemiol Biomarkers Prev*. 2013;22(7):1260–1266.

13. Rolland JS. Families and genetic fate: A millennial challenge. *Fam Sys Health*. 1999;17(1):123–132.

14. Patenaude AF, DeMarco TA, Peshkin BN, et al. Talking to children about maternal BRCA1/2 genetic test results: a qualitative study of parental perceptions and advice. *J Genet Couns*. 2013;22(3):303–314.

15. Werner-Lin A, Merrill SL, Brandt AC, et al. Talking with children about adult-onset hereditary cancer risk: A developmental approach for parents. *J Genet Couns*. 2018;27(3):533–548.

16. Bandura A. *Social Learning Theory*. Englewood Cliffs, NJ: Prentice Hall; 1977.

17. Bradbury AR, Patrick-Miller L, Schwartz LA, et al. Psychosocial adjustment and perceived risk among adolescent girls from families with BRCA1/2 or breast cancer history. *J Clin Oncol*. 2016;34(28):3409–3416.

18. Tercyak KP, Peshkin BN, DeMarco TA, et al. Parent-child factors and their effect on communicating BRCA1/2 test results to children. *Patient Educ Couns*. 2002;47(2):145–153.

19. Bradbury AR, Patrick-Miller L, Pawlowski K, et al. Learning of your parent's BRCA mutation during adolescence or early adulthood: a study of offspring experiences. *Psychooncology*. 2009;18(2):200–208.

20. Castonguay C, Friedman S, Leininger A, et al. Talking about *BRCA* in your family tree. 2014. Available at http://www.facingourrisk.org/understanding-brca-and-hboc/publications/documents/booklet-talking-about-brca-family.pdf.

21. Klein WM, Stefanek ME. Cancer risk elicitation and communication: Lessons from the psychology of risk perception. *CA Cancer J Clin*. 2007;57(3):147–167.

22. Etchegary H, Fowler K. They had the right to know. Genetic risk and perceptions of responsibility. *Psychol Health*. 2008;23(6):707–727.

23. Forrest LE, Curnow L, Delatycki MB, et al. Health first, genetics second: Exploring families' experiences of communicating genetic information. *Eur J Hum Genet*. 2008;16(11):1329–1335.

24. Metcalfe A, Plumridge G, Coad J, et al. Parents' and children's communication about genetic risk: A qualitative study, learning from families' experiences. *Eur J Hum Genet*. 2011;19(6):640–646.

25. Plumridge G, Metcalfe A, Coad J, et al. Parents' communication with siblings of children affected by an inherited genetic condition. *J Genet Couns.* 2011;20(4):374–383.

26. McConkie-Rosell A, Heise EM, Spiridigliozzi GA. Genetic risk communication: experiences of adolescent girls and young women from families with fragile X syndrome. *J Genet Couns.* 2009;18(4):313–325.

27. Forrest Keenan F, van Teijlingen E, McKee L, et al. How young people find out about their family history of Huntington's disease. *Soc Sci Med.* 2009;68(10):1892–1900.

28. Derbez B, de Pauw A, Stoppa-Lyonnet D, et al. Supporting disclosure of genetic information to family members: professional practice and timelines in cancer genetics. *Fam Cancer.* 2017;16(3):447–457.

29. Fanos JH. Developmental tasks of childhood and adolescence: implications for genetic testing. *Am J Med Genet.* 1997;71(1):22–28.

30. Mackenzie A, Patrick-Miller L, Bradbury AR. Controversies in communication of genetic risk for hereditary breast cancer. *Breast J.* 2009;15(Suppl. 1):S25–32.

31. Powers JM, Long JM, Mendonca W. Psychosocial, Ethical, and Legal Implications for Mutation Carriers. In Chagpar AB (ed.), *Managing BRCA Mutation Carriers.* Cham, Switzerland: Springer International Publishing AG; 2017. 205–234.

CHAPTER 18

Future Challenges and Opportunities in Clinical Cancer Genomics

Kyle A. Glose, Monica A. Giovanni, and Michael F. Murray

▓ INTRODUCTION

Cancer is the second-leading cause of death in the United States.[1] We can imagine a future where both germline and somatic genomics play an ever-increasing role in decreasing cancer deaths through (1) preemptive identification of germline cancer risk, (2) early-stage genomic cancer diagnoses, and (3) genome-based individually tailored therapeutics.

The term "precision medicine" was coined by U.S. President Barack Obama in the 2015 State of the Union address.[2] The "All of Us" research program is a key NIH Precision Medicine initiative that seeks to enroll at least one million persons in the United States in an observational cohort complete with DNA sequencing that both accelerates biomedical research and improves health.[3] Precision medicine, like "individualized medicine" or "personalized medicine," seeks to shift from a "one-size-fits-all" approach to one that takes into account differences in an individual's "genes, environments, and lifestyles." With advances in genomic sequencing technologies, the promise of care that is routinely informed by an individual's genetic code appears within reach. In the era of genomic medicine, sequence data will be used as both a screening and a diagnostic tool. Implementation of genome-based care, fueled by both falling costs and growing evidence, will continue to become increasingly accessible to patients and clinicians.[4-6]

Genomics will be a key tool but not the only tool in the advancing application of precision medicine in oncology. While cancer genomics focuses on variations in human DNA, other tools focus on other data sources: transcriptomics (RNA), proteomics (proteins), metabolomics (bioactive molecules), epigenomics (DNA modifications), as well as commensal bacterial communities (microbiomics). The clinical implementation of these other tools will advance both separately and in combination with genomics in the decades ahead.[7,8] In addition to the three key roles for genomics already listed, these other tools are also important areas to expect advances in the management of cancer.

▧ PREEMPTIVE IDENTIFICATION OF GERMLINE CANCER RISK

Identifying Germline Cancer Risk

The capacity of clinical laboratories to interpret an individual's germline DNA variants has improved significantly in the last decade. This improved interpretation builds on (1) the extraordinary amount of sequence data that is being generated, (2) the development of a framework for clinical interpretation of variants, and (3) the availability of public-facing resources that make consensus variant interpretations broadly available.

The standards and guidelines for the interpretation of sequence variants published in 2015 established a framework for the clinical interpretation of variants.[9] This framework, a joint consensus recommendation of the American College of Medical Genetics and Genomics and the Association for Molecular Pathology, is criteria-based and has been widely accepted by clinical laboratories to categorize variants using standard terminology, namely pathogenic, likely pathogenic, uncertain significance, likely benign, and benign. It is clear that these categorizations, while incredibly useful for care, are made based on evidence at a single point in time and can in some cases change categories as more data accumulates.[10]

ClinVar is a publicly available database that aggregates information about genomic variation and its relationship to human health.[11] ClinVar (https://www.ncbi.nlm.nih.gov/clinvar/) was created by the National Center for Biotechnology Information (NCBI) as a freely available archive for interpretations of clinical significance of variants. While this database collects evidence-based variant interpretation submission from clinical laboratories and research groups on any genetic variant, it is highly enriched for data on syndromic cancer genes given the amount of clinical evidence that has been generated for those genes over the last two to three decades.

Categories of Risk Modifying Germline Variants

Monogenic Risk for Cancer Syndromes In 1994, sequence variants in the *BRCA1* gene were causally associated with hereditary breast and ovarian cancer syndrome.[12,13] In 1995, the *BRCA2* gene was also linked to this same syndrome.[14] These discoveries soon allowed for the identification of pathogenic variants in these genes within highly burdened families; this included the ability to identify individuals within these families who had the pathogenic risk variant but had not yet had a personal history of cancer.[15] The capacity to identify presymptomatic risk through cascade testing within families has now been explored and studied for over 20 years and provides insights into the potential use of DNA-based strategies to identify and address elevated monogenic risk for a cancer syndrome in the general population.

There are more than a dozen monogenic cancer syndromes (see Table 18.1). These syndromes vary widely in the types of cancers they are associated with and the frequency of syndrome diagnoses in the population. Lynch syndrome and hereditary breast and ovarian cancer syndrome are the most common and best studied of these syndromes.[16] There is the potential to identify risk variants for these syndromes in individuals who do not have cancer but have an increased risk for developing it.[17]

Copy Number Variants, Structural Variants, and Risk for Cancer The presence of structural variants was underappreciated at the time of the announcement of the Human Genome Project.[18] In 2006, the inclusion of this category of pathogenic variants for syndromic cancer risk was found in 12% of families with familial breast cancer who had tested negative for sequence variants in the *BRCA1* and *BRCA2* genes; this led clinical testing companies to extend testing to include assessment for these variants in addition to sequence variants.[19,20]

Polygenic Risk for Cancer The clinical utility of genome wide associations identified through genome wide association studies (GWAS) has been debated for some time. In general, the GWAS approach has identified many disease associations with single nucleotide polymorphisms (SNPs), each with highly significant p values but small effect sizes. There were early attempts to aggregate SNPs into scoring that could be marketed directly to consumers; however, such attempts were fraught with disparate analytical interpretations from the same SNP data sets, and the scores had limited predictive value.[21,22]

More recently, new polygenic risk scoring (PRS) has been revisited and this time the number of GWAS loci and new statistical approaches have led to more robust predictions. Since 2018 there is a growing literature that suggests a potential clinical utility for PRS to inform both increased individual risk for cancer in the absence of monogenic risk, and increased risk for penetrant disease in the presence of monogenic risk.[23,24]

Protective Variants Against Cancer Among the genetic variants that can currently be clinically interpreted is a relatively small percentage that has been demonstrated to confer protection. There are, however, some specific variants that confer protection from specific cancers; for example, rs140068132 and reduced risk for breast cancer in Latin American women.[25] In addition, the methodology that elucidates PRS simultaneously elucidates polygenic protection scores (PPS).[23] There has not been sufficient research on these findings to define a model for clinical implementation. However, one could conceive of a strategy where an individual's screening schedule for things like colonoscopy would be adjusted based on both risk and protection scores, starting at either a younger or older age than the population average.

The clinical utility of protective variants remains uncertain and will require an evidence base that offers sufficient confidence in the predictive value of the result. There is the chance, for instance, that the assessed data in an individual suggests strong polygenic protection but misses an unassessed monogenic risk. In addition, the potential exists for data suggesting strong genomic protection, which could be irrelevant if an individual has a strong environmental risk. Currently, protective variants are not usually reported clinically, though some have advocated for change.[26]

Methods of Germline Risk Identification

Family History for Cancer Risk Identification Family health history has been used for decades to assist healthcare providers in efforts to assess risk for disease. Patterns of family history have been successfully used to discern Mendelian patterns within heavily burdened families. Through these strategies, family health history has proven itself useful as (1) a proxy for DNA-based information and (2) a strategy for increasing the pretest probability for a positive result in a diagnostic genetic test.

Recommendations for primary screening of adults for monogenic cancer syndromes via comprehensive family history ascertainment and analysis have been difficult to operationalize. In the case of HBOC, the USPSTF made recommendations for family history based HBOC screening for adult women since 2005.[27] Universal uptake of these recommendations has not occurred in part because they compete for provider attention within the busy agenda of primary care delivery where a multitude of screenings are recommended.

The workflow problems presented to healthcare providers who may aspire to ascertain and analyze comprehensive family health history has prompted a search for alternative solutions.

TABLE 18.1: Monogenic Cancer Syndromes

Syndrome	Associated Genes	Estimated Prevalence	# of Known Pathogenic Variants[1,2]	Inheritance Pattern	Primary Associated Cancers	Lifetime Cancer Risk			Populations with Increased Prevalence	References
							BRCA1	BRCA2		
Hereditary Breast and Ovarian Cancer Syndrome (HBOC)	BRCA1 BRCA2	1:190	1. BRCA1: 2821 2. BRCA2: 3244	AD	Breast Male Breast Ovarian Prostate Pancreatic	Breast 2nd Primary Breast Male Breast Ovarian Prostate Pancreatic	46–87% 83% 1.2% 39–63% 8.6% 1–3%	38–84% 62% 8.9% 16.5–27% 15% by age 65 2–7%	Ashkenazi Jewish 1:40	3,4
Hereditary Non-polyposis Colon Cancer (HNPCC) Syndrome (Lynch Syndrome)	MLH1 MSH2 MSH6 PMS2 EPCAM	1:440	MLH1: 696 MSH2: 761 MSH6: 631 PMS2: 248 EPCAM: 42	AD	Colorectal Endometrial Gastric Ovarian	Colorectal: 52–82% Endometrial: 25–60% Gastric: 6–13% Ovarian: 4–12%			N/A	5,6
Neurofibromatosis Type 1	NF1	1:4,000	NF1: 1027	AD	Neurofibroma (benign) Malignant peripheral nerve sheath tumors Glioma Leukemia Breast cancer Other neuroendocrine tumor	Neurofibroma: Glioma: 20% Other: 5%			N/A	7,8
Familial Retinoblastoma	RB1	1:15,000–1:20,000	RB1: 244	AD	Retinoblastoma	~100%			N/A	9
Multiple Endocrine Neoplasia Type 1	MEN	1:10,000–1:100,000	MEN: 3855	AD	Parathyroid Pituitary Pancreatic Gastric endocrine	95% by age 40			N/A	10,11

Syndrome	Associated Genes	Estimated Prevalence	# of Known Pathogenic Variants[1,2]	Inheritance Pattern	Primary Associated Cancers	Lifetime Cancer Risk	Populations with Increased Prevalence	References
Multiple Endocrine Neoplasia Type 2	RET	1:35,000	RET: 75	AD	Medullary thyroid Parathyroid Pheochromocytoma	MTC: 95–100% Parathyroid: 0–30% Pheochromocytoma: 0–50%	N/A	12
Familial Adenomatous Polyposis	APC	1:6850–31,250	APC: 679	AD	Colorectal Duodenum Papillary thyroid	Colorectal: 7% by age 21, 87% by age 45, ~100% lifetime Duodenum: 4–12% Thyroid: 1–12%	N/A	13
Von Hippel-Lindau Syndrome	VHL	1:36,000	VHL: 176	AD	Pheochromocytoma Renal cell carcinoma Hemangioblastoma Retinal angioma	Total: ~100% by age 65 RCC: 70% by age 60 Pheochromocytoma: Varies	N/A	14
Li-Fraumeni Syndrome	TP53	1: 3555–1:5476	TP53: 286	AD	Primarily: Adrenocortical carcinoma Breast CNS Osteosarcoma Soft tissue sarcoma Also multiple other types	Men: >70% Women: >90%	Southern Brazil, 1:375	15,16
MUTYH-Associated Polyposis	MUTYH	1:20,000–1:60,000	MUTYH: 66	AR	Colorectal (mostly) Duodenal Ovarian Bladder	CRC: 80–90% lifetime Duodenum: 4% Ovary: 6–14% Bladder: 6–25%	N/A	17
PTEN-Hamartomata Syndrome (Cowden Syndrome)	PTEN	Unknown, possibly 1:200,000	PTEN: 344	AD	Colorectal Hamartomas/ Cancer Breast Thyroid Endometrium	CRC: 9% Breast: 85% Thyroid 25% Endometrial: 28%	N/A	18,19

(Continued)

435

TABLE 18.1: Monogenic Cancer Syndromes *(Continued)*

Syndrome	Associated Genes	Estimated Prevalence	# of Known Pathogenic Variants[1,2]	Inheritance Pattern	Primary Associated Cancers	Lifetime Cancer Risk	Populations with Increased Prevalence	References
DICER1 Tumor Predisposition	DICER1	1:4600	DICER1: 185	AD	Pleuropulmonary blastoma (PPB) Multinodular goiter Sex-cord stromal tumor Cystic nephroma Ciliary body medulloepithelioma	Pleuropulmonary blastoma: 25–40% Multinodular goiter: 75% women, 17% men Sex-cord stromal tumor: ~10% Cystic nephroma: ~10% Ciliary body medulloepithelioma: ~3%	N/A	20
Familial Acute Myeloid Leukemia with Mutated CEBPA	CEBPA	11 families	CEBPA: 15	AD	Acute myeloid leukemia	80%	N/A	21
Hereditary Diffuse Gastric Cancer	CDH1	1:400,000–1:1,200,000	CDH1: 129	AD	Diffuse gastric cancer Lobular breast cancer	Gastric: 70% males, 56% females Lobular Breast: 42% females	N/A	22,23
Peutz-Jeghers Syndrome	STK11	Variable, estimated 1:25,000–1:280,000	STK11: 131	AD	Colorectal Stomach Small intestine Breast Ovarian (sex-cord stromal) Cervi Uterus Pancreas Testicular (Sertoli) Lung	Colorectal: 39% Stomach: 29% Small intestine: 13% Breast: 32–54% Ovarian (Sex-cord stromal): 21% Cervix: 10% Uterus: 9% Pancreas: 11–36% Testicular (Sertoli): 9% Lung: 7–17%	N/A	24

TABLE 18.1: Monogenic Cancer Syndromes

1. Perez-Palma E, Gramm M, Nürnberg P, et al. Simple ClinVar. http://simple-clinvar.broadinstitute.org/

2. Pérez-Palma E, Gramm M, Nürnberg P, et al. Simple ClinVar: an interactive web server to explore and retrieve gene and disease variants aggregated in ClinVar database. *Nucleic Acids Res.* 2019;47(W1):W99–W105.

3. Petrucelli N, Daly MB, Pal T. BRCA1- and BRCA2-associated hereditary breast and ovarian cancer. In Adam MP, Ardinger HH, Pagon RA, et al. (Eds). GeneReviews®. Seattle: University of Washington; 1993. Accessed July 7, 2020. http://www.ncbi.nlm.nih.gov/books/NBK1247/

4. Manickam K, Buchanan AH, Schwartz MLB, et al. Exome sequencing–based screening for BRCA1/2 expected pathogenic variants among adult biobank participants. *JAMA Netw Open.* 2018;1(5):e182140–e182140.

5. Kohlmann W, Gruber SB. Lynch syndrome. In Adam MP, Ardinger HH, Pagon RA, et al. (Eds). GeneReviews®. Seattle: University of Washington; 1993. Accessed July 7, 2020. http://www.ncbi.nlm.nih.gov/books/NBK1211/

6. Møller P, Seppälä T, Bernstein I, et al. Cancer incidence and survival in Lynch syndrome patients receiving colonoscopic and gynaecological surveillance: first report from the prospective Lynch syndrome database. *Gut.* 2017;66(3):464.

7. Friedman JM. Neurofibromatosis 1. In Adam MP, Ardinger HH, Pagon RA, et al. (Eds). GeneReviews®. Seattle: University of Washington; 1993. Accessed July 13, 2020. http://www.ncbi.nlm.nih.gov/books/NBK1109/

8. Varan A, şen H, Aydin B, et al. Neurofibromatosis type 1 and malignancy in childhood. *Clin Genet.* 2016;89(3):341–345.

9. Lohmann DR, Gallie BL. Retinoblastoma. In Adam MP, Ardinger HH, Pagon RA, et al. (Eds). GeneReviews®. Seattle: University of Washington; 1993. Accessed July 14, 2020. http://www.ncbi.nlm.nih.gov/books/NBK1452/

10. Giusti F, Marini F, Brandi ML. Multiple endocrine neoplasia type 1. In Adam MP, Ardinger HH, Pagon RA, et al. (Eds). GeneReviews®. Seattle: University of Washington; 1993. Accessed July 15, 2020. http://www.ncbi.nlm.nih.gov/books/NBK1538/

11. Carroll RW. Multiple endocrine neoplasia type 2. In Adam MP, Ardinger HH, Pagon RA, et al. (Eds). GeneReviews®. Seattle: University of Washington; 1993. Accessed July 14, 2020. http://www.ncbi.nlm.nih.gov/books/NBK1257/

12. Eng C. Multiple endocrine neoplasia type 2. In Adam MP, Ardinger HH, Pagon RA, et al. (Eds). GeneReviews®. Seattle: University of Washington; 1993. Accessed July 14, 2020. http://www.ncbi.nlm.nih.gov/books/NBK1257/

13. Jasperson KW, Patel SG, Ahnen DJ. APC-associated polyposis conditions. In Adam MP, Ardinger HH, Pagon RA, et al. (Eds). GeneReviews®. Seattle: University of Washington; 1993. Accessed July 14, 2020. http://www.ncbi.nlm.nih.gov/books/NBK1345/

14. van Leeuwaarde RS, Ahmad S, Links TP, et al. Von Hippel-Lindau syndrome. In: Adam MP, Ardinger HH, Pagon RA, et al. (Eds). GeneReviews®. Seattle: University of Washington; 1993. Accessed July 14, 2020. http://www.ncbi.nlm.nih.gov/books/NBK1463/PMID: 20301636

15. Schneider K, Zelley K, Nichols KE, et al. Li-Fraumeni syndrome. In Adam MP, Ardinger HH, Pagon RA, et al. (Eds). GeneReviews®. Seattle: University of Washington; 1993. Accessed July 14, 2020. http://www.ncbi.nlm.nih.gov/books/NBK1311/PMID: 20301488

16. de Andrade KC, Frone MN, Wegman-Ostrosky T, et al. Variable population prevalence estimates of germline TP53 variants: a gnomAD-based analysis. *Hum Mutat.* 2019;40(1):97–105.

17. Nielsen M, Infante E, Brand R. MUTYH polyposis. In Adam MP, Ardinger HH, Pagon RA, et al. (Eds). GeneReviews®. Seattle: University of Washington; 1993. Accessed July 14, 2020. http://www.ncbi.nlm.nih.gov/books/NBK107219/

18. Eng C. PTEN Hamartoma Tumor Syndrome. In: Adam MP, Ardinger HH, Pagon RA, et al. (Eds). GeneReviews®. Seattle: University of Washington; 1993. Accessed July 14, 2020. http://www.ncbi.nlm.nih.gov/books/NBK1488/

19. Heald B, Mester J, Rybicki L, et al. Frequent gastrointestinal polyps and colorectal adenocarcinomas in prospective series of PTEN mutation carriers. *Gastroenterology.* 2010;139(6):1927–1933.

20. Schultz KAP, Stewart DR, Kamihara J, et al. DICER1 tumor predisposition. In Adam MP, Ardinger HH, Pagon RA, et al. (Eds). GeneReviews®. Seattle: University of Washington; 1993. Accessed July 15, 2020. http://www.ncbi.nlm.nih.gov/books/NBK196157/

21. Tawana K, Fitzgibbon J. CEBPA-associated familial acute myeloid leukemia (AML). In Adam MP, Ardinger HH, Pagon RA, et al. (Eds). GeneReviews®. Seattle: University of Washington; 1993. Accessed July 15, 2020. http://www.ncbi.nlm.nih.gov/books/NBK47457/

22. Kaurah P, Huntsman DG. Hereditary diffuse gastric cancer. In Adam MP, Ardinger HH, Pagon RA, et al. (Eds). GeneReviews®. Seattle: University of Washington; 1993. Accessed July 15, 2020. http://www.ncbi.nlm.nih.gov/books/NBK1139/

23. Corso G, Marrelli D, Roviello F. Familial gastric cancer and germline mutations of E-cadherin. *Ann Ital Chir.* 2012;83(3):177–182.

24. McGarrity TJ, Amos CI, Baker MJ. Peutz-Jeghers syndrome. In Adam MP, Ardinger HH, Pagon RA, et al. (Eds). GeneReviews®. Seattle: University of Washington; 1993. Accessed July 15, 2020. http://www.ncbi.nlm.nih.gov/books/NBK1266/

Platforms to promote and organize patient self-reported family history have included the U.S. Surgeon General's online tool for self-reporting of family history.[28] Other tools and strategies have been built and tested, many of which show promise for increased detection of individuals who meet criteria for DNA-based screening.[29]

Recent studies have examined the use of DNA-based screening of large cohorts of adult volunteers and have demonstrated that current family health history-based healthcare strategies miss 80 to 90% of individuals with monogenic risk for HBOC and Lynch syndrome.[30,31] These screening failures are attributable to both failures in implementation of recommended screening and failures of the established strategies to detect risk.[17]

DNA-based Screening for Cancer Risk Identification Population-based genomic screening offers opportunities for early, presymptomatic detection and proactive risk management when the conditions and associated genomic variants meet three specific criteria: (1) a pathogenic variant in the gene of interest is associated with a high risk for a disorder associated with serious morbidity and/or mortality; (2) well-established preventive interventions are available for those identified as high risk; and (3) there exists an established knowledge base regarding the gene and the condition(s) associated with pathogenic variants.[32]

An important distinction must be drawn between genomic sequencing for the purpose of confirming a suspected diagnosis (diagnostic testing) and that performed with the intention of uncovering previously unknown genomic risks (screening). Diagnostic genomic testing has been utilized in clinical cancer care for decades. These highly specific tests are offered to individuals with a personal or family history of cancer suggestive of an underlying monogenic etiology. Conversely, screening is the process of proactively identifying disease risk, a mainstay of preventive medical care of adults. Genomic sequencing for the purpose of screening is done with no prior indication for the testing, and the results must be delivered in a careful manner to appropriately address risks discovered. While diagnostic testing requires a distinct indication for testing, population-based genomic screening is offered irrespective of personal or family history of disease. Rather than attempting to confirm a diagnosis, following the development of disease, population screening provides the opportunity to detect a pathogenic, disease-associated genomic variant in an otherwise healthy individual prior to the development of symptoms.

Data from large scale genomic sequencing programs suggest that 1 to 2% of the U.S. population has a pathogenic genomic variant conferring a substantially elevated risk of a serious, preventable disease such as cancer or heart disease.[33,34] The fact that only a small percentage of people would benefit is counterbalanced by growing evidence that the benefit could be significant, perhaps even life-saving.[4] There are well-established management recommendations for individuals identified as elevated risk through a personal or family history of such conditions. Building upon generations of clinical genetics practice, there is an opportunity to use genomic screening to identify otherwise healthy individuals, offer proactive management, and thereby reduce the morbidity and potentially early mortality of these conditions.

Challenges to Population-Based Genomic Screening The task of offering the entire population germline DNA sequencing and periodic re-screening does not have an established infrastructure to support this type of lifelong screening. Currently health screening is mostly carried out by providers and health systems (e.g., blood pressure, mammograms, colonoscopy). For newborn screening (NBS), however, there is a collaborative infrastructure involving departments of public health and health systems. The NBS infrastructure allows for inclusion of the entire population and may be the best model for the type of DNA-based screening that would support germline risk identification and management in the years ahead. Like NBS, population screening for cancer risk will carry ethical, technical, and organizational challenges.[35]

Due to the rapid pace of discovery in the arena of genomic medicine, the symptomatology and pathophysiology of many genomic conditions are well understood. The causes of variable disease penetrance and clinical severity remain unclear. These crucial questions must be better understood for the effective population use of genomic data for health screening since the presence of a pathogenic genetic variant alone may not be sufficient to lead to disease.

PREVENTIVE ACTION TO ADDRESS GERMLINE RISK

When germline evidence of elevated cancer risk is identified, the two types of response are clinical screening to identify early stage cancer (e.g., mammography and colonoscopy) and preventive measures to ameliorate risk. It is reasonable to anticipate that the numbers and types of evidence-based preventive strategies will increase with time. We also anticipate that the molecular targeting of the preventive measures will improve. The current categories of preventive action include chemoprevention, risk-reducing surgery, and measures that seek to avoid secondary risk in genetically at-risk individuals.

The best studied chemoprevention strategy is the use of estrogen inhibitors in individuals at elevated risk for breast cancer. The U.S. Preventive Services Task Force (USPSTF) recommended tamoxifen and raloxifene for women with elevated risk for breast cancer and without elevated risk for adverse side effects in 2013 and an updated USPSTF recommendation in 2019 added aromatase inhibitors.[36,37] Other cancer chemoprevention strategies have been studied, including aspirin to inhibit colorectal cancer and nicotinamide to prevent skin cancer, but the evidence base for these measures is not as strong.[38,39]

Risk-reducing surgery is well supported by evidence in the setting of *BRCA1* and *BRCA2* related cancer risk.[40] This includes the removal of the at-risk organ specifically through prophylactic mastectomy and bilateral salpingo-oophorectomy. In the setting of familial adenomatous polyposis (FAP) colectomy is routinely recommended since the lifetime colorectal cancer risk in FAP is 100%.[16]

Lastly there is evidence to support strategies to avoid specific secondary risks in susceptible individuals such as diagnostic radiation in younger women with *BRCA1* and *BRCA2*.[41] There is less direct evidence for other reasonable risk avoidance strategies such as the avoidance of smoking, sun exposure, and others.

EARLY STAGE GENOMIC CANCER DIAGNOSES

Liquid Biopsy Strategy and Potential Utility

The concept of a "liquid biopsy" (LB) is that circulating tumor DNA obtained through a simple blood draw can provide essential diagnostic and prognostic information in a less invasive manner than the traditional options of solid tumor or fine-needle aspiration biopsies.[42,43] The hope is that through genomics LB can not only be less invasive but might ultimately be more robust than traditional methods. In aggregate, the genomic material circulating tumor cells and cell free DNA, which originates from tumor cells, is referred to as circulating tumor DNA (ctDNA), and this can be analyzed to provide a picture of whole-body tumor genetic makeup. LB samples can provide information about both primary and metastatic tumors, as well as information about variant heterogeneity within a single tumor. LB opens the door to more frequent longitudinal profiling of tumor characteristics throughout the course of therapy and disease. Importantly, LB also represents a platform for future surveillance strategies wherein if the sensitivity of these methods increases with time, then individuals without a cancer diagnosis could undergo LB sampling for genomic evidence of very early stage cancer prior to the emergence of signs, symptoms, or a detectable tumor mass.

Circulating Tumor Cells (CTCs) These cells have migrated into the bloodstream or broken away from the primary tumor to circulate in the bloodstream. CTCs were first described in the nineteenth century.[44] They enter the bloodstream intact as individual cells or clustered as micro emboli. Individual cells that have undergone epithelial-to-mesenchymal transition migrate through the extracellular matrix and into the bloodstream. Micro emboli break off from a primary tumor that has invaded adjacent vasculature. CTCs have been found in patients with both early and late stage disease, and their role in the establishment of metastatic disease is under investigation.[45]

Cell-free DNA (cfDNA) This DNA has a predominant size distribution of 130 to 170 base pairs, consistent with the amount of DNA present around nuclease-cleaved nucleosomes. Thus, most cfDNA likely originates from apoptotic cells. However, the existence of some larger cell free DNA molecules also suggests varied origins for cfDNA. Increased levels of cell-free DNA in blood specimens of cancer patients was first described in 1977, though it was not until some years later that the clinical potential of this was recognized in 1994.[46] ctDNA can provide insight into specific DNA mutations present in cancer patients as well as to track tumor burden. Interestingly, the use of cell-free DNA in noninvasive prenatal testing for aneuploidy has in some cases revealed underlying maternal malignancy.[47]

Circulating Tumor DNA (ctDNA) This DNA is present in the bloodstreams of most patients with stage III and IV cancer, with the notable exception of tumors confined to the CNS.[45] The half-life of ctDNA is variable in circulation but on average is around 15 minutes, making it a powerful indicator of current tumor status. Additionally, tumors regularly release their DNA into circulation, with spikes occurring during moments of increased cell turnover, such as after treatment with chemotherapeutics. As such, ctDNA yields have been proposed as a measure of chemotherapeutic effectiveness and longitudinal tracking of tumor burden.

▩ GENOME-BASED INDIVIDUALLY TAILORED THERAPEUTICS

Therapeutics Based on Somatic Variants

Driver Mutations The changes in DNA that give a cell the required growth advantage that drives neoplastic transformation are referred to as driver mutations. It is estimated that 80 to 90% of these genomic variants are somatic or acquired changes, and 10 to 20% are germline or inborn changes.[48] The number of genes that have the potential to include a driver mutation are between 500 and 600.[49] Driver mutations can act in concert with one another and can increase in number over the course of an individual's cancer. The somatic changes in tumor molecular profiles over the course of the disease are attributable to both selective pressures instituted by therapy and genomic instability of tumor cells.

Liquid biopsy combined with serial genomic sequencing holds great promise for improving the diagnosis, management, and treatment of cancer. It has the potential to be used to provide non-invasive screening, tumor-specific molecular profiling, treatment-related monitoring, and detection of residual disease in post-surgical patients. As laboratory methodologies improve and standards of practice are developed through larger clinical studies, liquid biopsy is expected to be a highly useful tool in monitoring somatic variants and adjusting therapeutic solutions for cancer.[50,51]

Therapeutics Based on Germline Variants

Pharmacogenomics (PGx) The field of pharmacogenomics grew out of clinical observations in the 1950s of inherited differences in drug effects.[52] More than 60 years of research have yielded an approach to therapeutic decision-making that uses easily ascertained common genetic variants to predict an individual's drug response. The Clinical Pharmacogenetics Implementation Consortium (CPIC) is an expert organization that makes recommendations on the clinical implementing of pharmacogenomics. CPIC maintains a curated list of gene-drug pairs wherein a given variant in the specific gene results in a recommendation to change dose or change drug in order to improve its efficacy or avoid adverse drug reactions. Relevant to clinical cancer genetics, CPIC has an evidence-based recommendation for tamoxifen dosing relevant to CYP2D6 variants.[53] The evidence base will grow and the use of genomic information to make therapeutic decisions can be expected to continue to expand in the future.

CONCLUSIONS

Clinical cancer care has experienced an innovation boom in recent years through the utilization of genomic sequencing of malignancies to allow for individualized, targeted therapeutic treatment. Indeed, clinical oncology, perhaps more so than any other medical specialty, has realized the promise of advancing genomic technologies.

The future that we have projected here is contingent on the continued development of evidence across many areas of clinical cancer genetics. New challenges that we expect to emerge as we move further into the twenty-first century will include those that come with increased lifespan including increases in elderly cancer survivors who have special care needs, as well as increases in new cancers in those who are very old.[54] Unfortunately, longevity will be accompanied by increases in later age cancers, a problem for which the healthcare system currently has limited clinical management experience. It appears that the type of cancers that occur in centenarians are quite familiar, namely breast cancer, colorectal cancer, prostate cancer, lung cancer, and kidney and urinary tract cancers. However, we will need to learn more about the biology of these tumors, their responsiveness to therapeutic interventions, and the tolerability of therapies in those of very advanced ages.[55]

The biggest potential impact on the future of clinical cancer genomics lies in a public health approach that screens populations for risk, identifies those risks, and then addresses those risks through prevention or very early detection and eradication of malignancy. This sort of population-wide preventive management will require not only advancements of the scientific evidence, but it will also require the engagement of public health institutions (e.g., state departments of public health and the Center for Disease Control and Prevention). The expansion of the role of institutions of public health beyond cancer epidemiology and tracking to include cancer genetic screening and prevention, in a manner similar to newborn screening (NBS), will provide a platform that is available to the whole society, not just those with a particular insurance or provider.[56,57] Just as with NBS, cancer prevention through DNA-based screening for cancer risk can become one of the greatest public health achievements in this century.

References

1. Siegel RL, Miller KD, Jemal A. Cancer statistics, 2020. *CA Cancer J Clin.* 2020;70(1):7–30.

2. https://obamawhitehouse.archives.gov/precision-medicine. *The Precision Medicine Initiative.*

3. Denny JC, et al. The "all of us" research program. *N Engl J Med.* 2019;381(7):668–676.

4. Guttmacher AE, Collins FS. Welcome to the genomic era. *N Engl J Med.* 2003;349(10):996–998.

5. Owens DK, et al. Risk assessment, genetic counseling, and genetic testing for brca-related cancer: US preventive services task force recommendation statement. *JAMA.* 2019;322(7):652–665.

6. Sudlow C, et al. UK biobank: an open access resource for identifying the causes of a wide range of complex diseases of middle and old age. *PLoS Med.* 2015;12(3):e1001779.

7. Nicora G, et al. Integrated multi-omics analyses in oncology: a review of machine learning methods and tools. *Front Oncol.* 2020;10:1030.

8. Yu KH, Snyder M. Omics profiling in precision oncology. *Mol Cell Proteomics.* 2016;15(8):2525–2536.

9. Richards S, et al. Standards and guidelines for the interpretation of sequence variants: a joint consensus recommendation of the American College of Medical Genetics and Genomics and the Association for Molecular Pathology. *Genet Med.* 2015;17(5):405–424.

10. Harrison SM, Rehm HL. Is "likely pathogenic" really 90% likely? Reclassification data in ClinVar. *Genome Med.* 2019;11(1):72.

11. Landrum MJ, et al. ClinVar: public archive of interpretations of clinically relevant variants. *Nucleic Acids Res.* 2016;44(D1):D862–868.

12. Miki Y, et al. A strong candidate for the breast and ovarian cancer susceptibility gene BRCA1. *Science.* 1994;266(5182):66–71.

13. Friedman LS, et al. Confirmation of BRCA1 by analysis of germline mutations linked to breast and ovarian cancer in ten families. *Nat Genet.* 1994;8(4):399–404.

14. Wooster R, et al. Identification of the breast cancer susceptibility gene BRCA2. *Nature.* 1995;378(6559):789–792.

15. Narod SA, Foulkes WD. BRCA1 and BRCA2: 1994 and beyond. *Nat Rev Cancer.* 2004;4(9):665–676.

16. Kohlmann W, Gruber SB. Lynch syndrome. 2004 (February 5 [updated April 12, 2018]). In Adam MP, Ardinger HH, Pagon RA, et al. (Eds). GeneReviews® [Internet]. Seattle: University of Washington; 1993–2021; Petrucelli N, Daly MB, Pal T. BRCA1- and BRCA2-associated hereditary breast and ovarian cancer. 1998 (September 4 [updated December 15, 2016]). In Adam MP, Ardinger HH, Pagon RA, et al. (Eds.). GeneReviews® [Internet]. Seattle: University of Washington; 1993–2020.

17. Murray MF, Giovanni MA. Bringing monogenic disease screening to the clinic. *Nat Med.* 2020;26(8):1172–1174.

18. Feuk L, Carson AR, Scherer SW. Structural variation in the human genome. *Nat Rev Genet.* 2006;7(2):85–97.

19. Walsh T, et al. Spectrum of mutations in BRCA1, BRCA2, CHEK2, and TP53 in families at high risk of breast cancer. *JAMA.* 2006;295(12):1379–1388.

20. Shannon KM, et al. Which individuals undergoing BRACAnalysis need BART testing? *Cancer Genet.* 2011;204(8):416–422.

21. Imai K, Kricka LJ, Fortina P. Concordance study of 3 direct-to-consumer genetic-testing services. *Clin Chem.* 2011;57(3):518–521.

22. Stadler ZK, et al. Genome-wide association studies of cancer: principles and potential utility. *Oncology.* 2010;24(7):629–637.

23. Khera AV, et al. Genome-wide polygenic scores for common diseases identify individuals with risk equivalent to monogenic mutations. *Nat Genet.* 2018;50(9):1219–1224.

24. Fahed AC, et al. Polygenic background modifies penetrance of monogenic variants for tier 1 genomic conditions. *Nat Commun*. 2020;11(1):3635.

25. Harper AR, Nayee S, Topol EJ. Protective alleles and modifier variants in human health and disease. *Nat Rev Genet*. 2015;16(12):689–701.

26. Schwartz MLB, Williams MS, Murray MF. Adding protective genetic variants to clinical reporting of genomic screening results: restoring balance. *JAMA*. 2017;317(15):1527–1528.

27. U.S. Preventive Services Task Force. Genetic risk assessment and BRCA mutation testing for breast and ovarian cancer susceptibility: recommendation statement. *Ann Intern Med*. 2005;143(5):355–361.

28. Guttmacher AE, Collins FS, Carmona RH. The family history—more important than ever. *N Engl J Med*. 2004;351(22):2333–2336.

29. Murray MF, et al. Comparing electronic health record portals to obtain patient-entered family health history in primary care. *J Gen Intern Med*. 2013;28(12):1558–1564.

30. Manickam K, et al. Exome sequencing-based screening for BRCA1/2 expected pathogenic variants among adult biobank participants. *JAMA Network Open*. 2018;1(5):e182140.

31. Grzymski JJ, et al. Population genetic screening efficiently identifies carriers of autosomal dominant diseases. *Nat Med*. 2020;26(8):1235–1239.

32. Murray MF. The path to routine genomic screening in health care. *Ann Intern Med*. 2018;169(6):407–408.

33. Buchanan AH, et al. Early cancer diagnoses through BRCA1/2 screening of unselected adult biobank participants. *Genet Med*. 2018;20(5):554–558.

34. Evans JP, et al. We screen newborns, don't we?: realizing the promise of public health genomics. *Genet Med*. 2013;15(5):332–334.

35. Levy HL. Ethical and psychosocial implications of genomic newborn screening. *Int J Neonatal Screen*. 2021;7(1).

36. Moyer VA and U.S. Preventive Services Task Force. Medications to decrease the risk for breast cancer in women: recommendations from the U.S. Preventive Services Task Force recommendation statement. *Ann Intern Med*. 2013;159(10):698–708.

37. Owens DK, et al. Medication use to reduce risk of breast cancer: U.S. Preventive Services Task Force recommendation statement. *JAMA*. 2019;322(9):857–867.

38. Drew DA, Chan AT. Aspirin in the prevention of colorectal neoplasia. *Annu Rev Med*. 2020.

39. Nikas IP, Paschou SA, Ryu HS. The role of nicotinamide in cancer chemoprevention and therapy. *Biomolecules*. 2020;10(3).

40. Hartmann LC, Lindor NM. The role of risk-reducing surgery in hereditary breast and ovarian cancer. *N Engl J Med*. 2016;374(5):454–468.

41. Pijpe A, et al. Exposure to diagnostic radiation and risk of breast cancer among carriers of BRCA1/2 mutations: retrospective cohort study (GENE-RAD-RISK). *BMJ*. 2012;345:e5660.

42. Siravegna G, et al. How liquid biopsies can change clinical practice in oncology. *Ann Oncol*. 2019;30(10):1580–1590.

43. Hofman P, et al. Liquid biopsy in the era of immuno-oncology: is it ready for prime-time use for cancer patients? *Ann Oncol*. 2019;30(9):1448–1459.

44. de Wit S, van Dalum G, Terstappen LW. Detection of circulating tumor cells. *Scientifica*. 2014;2014:819362.

45. Bettegowda C, et al. Detection of circulating tumor DNA in early- and late-stage human malignancies. *Sci Transl Med*. 2014;6(224):224.

46. Leon SA, et al. Free DNA in the serum of cancer patients and the effect of therapy. *Cancer Res*. 1977;37(3):646–650.

47. Romero R, Mahoney MJ. Noninvasive prenatal testing and detection of maternal cancer. *JAMA*. 2015;314(2):131–133.

48. Pon JR, Marra MA. Driver and passenger mutations in cancer. *Annu Rev Pathol*. 2015;10:25–50.

49. Martínez-Jiménez F, et al. A compendium of mutational cancer driver genes. *Nat Rev Cancer*. 2020;20(10):555–572.

50. Tie J, et al. Circulating tumor DNA as an early marker of therapeutic response in patients with metastatic colorectal cancer. *Ann Oncol.* 2015;26(8):1715–1722.

51. Corcoran RB, Chabner BA. Application of cell-free DNA analysis to cancer treatment. *N Engl J Med.* 2018;379(18):1754–1765.

52. Evans WE, McLeod HL. Pharmacogenomics: drug disposition, drug targets, and side effects. *N Engl J Med.* 2003;348(6):538–549.

53. Goetz MP, et al. Clinical Pharmacogenetics Implementation Consortium (CPIC) guideline for CYP2D6 and tamoxifen therapy. *Clin Pharmacol Ther.* 2018;103(5):770–777.

54. Bluethmann SM, Mariotto AB, Rowland JH. Anticipating the "silver tsunami": prevalence trajectories and comorbidity burden among older cancer survivors in the United States. *Cancer Epidemiol Biomarkers Prev.* 2016;25(7):1029–1036.

55. Joseph SC, et al. Common cancers in centenarians. *Med Sci Monit.* 2014;20:18–23.

56. CDC. Ten great public health achievements—United States, 2001–2010. *MMWR Morb Mortal Wkly Rep.* 2011;60(19):619–623.

57. Murray MF, Evans JP, Khoury MJ. DNA-based population dcreening: potential suitability and important knowledge gaps. *JAMA.* 2020;323(4):307–308.

Index

Note: Page numbers followed by f or t represent figures or tables respectively.

A

ABO blood group, 218
Abortion, 77
ACMG. *See* American College of Medical Genetics and Genomics
Adenoma malignum, 188
Adenomatous polyposis
  constitutional mismatch repair deficiency syndrome, 128
  familial. *See* Familial adenomatous polyposis
  MUTYH-associated. *See MUTYH*-associated polyposis
  serrated polyposis syndrome, 127–128
ADH. *See* Atypical ductal hyperplasia
Adolescents, 422
Adrenocortical adenomas, 120
  cortisol-producing, 308
  description of, 306–307
  nonfunctioning, 308
  risk assessment of, 309
Adrenocortical carcinoma
  description of, 306–308
  in Li-Fraumeni syndrome, 309–310
  in Lynch syndrome, 309
  risk assessment of, 309
  syndromes associated with, 309
Adrenocortical tumors
  management of, 306–307
  risk assessment of, 306–307
Advanced Tele-Genetic Counseling, 38
Alcohol
  breast cancer and, 75
  pancreatic cancer and, 221–223
ALH. *See* Atypical lobular hyperplasia
Allele, 4t
Allele frequency, 65
Allelic heterogeneity, 4t, 5
Allelic loss
  definition of, 4t
  description of, 10
Alternative care delivery models, 54–56
American College of Genetics and Genomics, 37

American College of Medical Genetics and Genomics, 53, 66, 193, 382, 385
American Society of Clinical Oncology informed consent, 46–47
Americans with Disabilities Act, 393
American Urological Association, 256–257
AMP. *See* Association for Molecular Pathology
Amsterdam criteria, for Lynch syndrome, 31, 171, 194, 195t
Anaplastic lymphoma kinase protein inhibitor, 235
Anastrozole, 104–106
Aneuploidy, 1
Anxiety, 397–400
APC gene
  cloning of, 11
  discovery of, 10–11
  inheritance of, 2
  mosaicism, 21
  mutations of
    in familial adenomatous polyposis, 2, 117, 143, 221
    germline, 5, 12
    missense, 2
    somatic, 13
  structure of, 2
APC protein, 2, 5
Apert syndrome, 258, 258t
Aromatase inhibitors, for breast cancer, 105–106
Ashkenazi Jewish ancestry, 35, 42, 44, 68, 191–192
Association for Molecular Pathology, 66
Association for Molecular Pathology v. Myriad Genetics, 395
Ataxia-telangiectasia, 100, 221, 343, 345–346
ATM, 84t, 99–100, 345
Attenuated familial adenomatous polyposis, 5, 117–118, 121, 124, 127, 277
Atypical ductal hyperplasia, 76
Atypical lobular hyperplasia, 76
Autism spectrum disorders with macrocephaly, 170
Autonomy, 379–380, 381t
Autosomal dominant diseases, 2
Autosomal recessive diseases, 2

B

BAM files, 62
Bannayan-Riley-Ruvalcaba syndrome, 94, 130,
       133, 169. *See also* PTEN hamartoma
       tumor syndrome
BAP1 tumor predisposition syndrome, 249t,
       253, 328t, 337
BARD1, 84t
Basal cell carcinoma
    characteristics of, 321t, 322
    clinical features of, 324f
    early detection of, 322
    epidemiology of, 325
    management of, 339
    prevention of, 327
    risk factors for, 326
    in solid-organ transplant recipients, 327
Basal cell nevus syndrome, 328t, 330–331, 331t,
       351
Base excision repair, 8, 15
Bazex-Dupré-Christol syndrome, 331
BCRAT. *See* Breast cancer risk assessment tool
Beckwith-Wiedemann syndrome, 310–312, 364
Beneficence, 380, 381t
Benign prostatic hyperplasia, 259
Bethesda guidelines, for Lynch syndrome, 31,
       145, 194, 195t
BHD. *See* Birt-Hogg-Dube syndrome
Bilateral salpingo-oophorectomy
    in breast cancer prevention, 45, 104, 158
    risk-reducing
        description of, 177
        in Lynch syndrome, 177
        ovarian cancer risk reduction with, 91, 99,
            101, 201–202
        primary peritoneal cancer after, 202
Bile duct cancer in familial adenomatous
       polyposis, 121
Binary sequence alignment files. *See* BAM files
Bioinformatics, 62–63
Birt-Hogg-Dube syndrome, 249t, 252, 253t
Bishop, Michael, 8
Bladder cancer
    Apert syndrome and, 258, 258t
    clinical presentation of, 256
    Costello syndrome and, 258, 258t
    description of, 255
    epidemiology of, 255–256
    genetic counseling for, 258
    genetic risk of, 255–256
    genetic testing for, 258
    hematuria associated with, 256
    hereditary causes of, 249t, 257–258
    hereditary retinoblastoma and, 258, 258t
    in Lynch syndrome, 151, 257, 258t

management of, 259
physical examination of, 256–257
risk factors for, 256
squamous cell cancer, 256
urothelial cell carcinoma, 255–256
Bloom syndrome, 329t, 333–334, 346
BMPR1A, 130–131, 155, 280, 354
BOADICEA model, 82
Body mass index endometrial cancer
       and, 162
Bohring-Opitz syndrome, 350
Boveri, Theodor, 1, 8
BPH. *See* Benign prostatic hyperplasia
BRAF V600E mutations, 68, 148–150
Brain tumors, in familial adenomatous
       polyposis, 121
BRCA1
    in breast cancer, 5, 84t, 87–92, 88t–89t
    in colorectal cancer, 143
    discovery of, 17
    in hereditary breast and ovarian cancer
        syndrome, 219
    multigene panel testing, 52
    in ovarian cancer, 88t, 184, 201
    in pancreatic cancer, 88t, 92
    in prostate cancer, 88t, 261
    urgent testing for, 48
BRCA2
    in breast cancer, 84t, 87–92, 88t–89t
    discovery of, 17
    in hereditary breast and ovarian cancer
        syndrome, 219
    multigene panel testing, 52
    in ovarian cancer, 88t, 201
    in pancreatic cancer, 88t, 184
    in prostate cancer, 88t, 261
    urgent testing for, 48
BRCAPRO model, 82
Breast atypia, 76
Breast cancer
    ATM, 84t, 99–100
    BRCA1, 5, 84t, 87–92, 88t–89t
    BRCA2, 84t, 87–92, 88t–89t
    BRIP1, 84t
    cancer genetics referral for, 33–35
    CDH1, 84t, 95–96
    CHEK2, 84t, 101
    Cowden syndrome and, 170
    early-onset, 34
    epidemiology of, 71
    familial, 80–83
    family history of, 73, 102–106
    genetic mutations associated with, 73
    genetic predisposition for, 73
    genetic testing for, 35, 77–79

in hereditary breast and ovarian cancer
  syndrome, 184
in hereditary breast syndromes, 106–109
HER2 gene expression in, 24
heritability of, 18
lifetime risk of, 73
Li-Fraumeni syndrome and, 93–94
Lynch syndrome, 159–160
male, 35, 73, 92, 184
NBN, 85t
outcomes of, 107
ovarian cancer and, 90–92
PALB2, 85t, 98–99
in Peutz-Jeghers syndrome, 129, 129t
prevalence of, 34
prevention of
  anastrozole, 104–106
  aromatase inhibitors, 105–106
  bilateral salpingo-oophorectomy for, 45, 104
  chemoprevention, 104
  exemestane, 104–106
  lifestyle modifications for, 106
  raloxifene, 105
  selective estrogen receptor modulators,
    104–105
  tamoxifen, 105
prior history of, 76
PTEN mutations, 85t, 94–95
RAD51/C/D, 85t
risk assessment of, 71–83, 102
risk factors for
  abortion, 77
  age, 73
  age at first full-term pregnancy, 74
  age at menarche or first menstruation, 74
  age at menopause, 74
  alcohol, 75
  breast atypia, 76
  breast density, 76
  breastfeeding, 74
  description of, 72, 72t
  diet, 75
  diethylstilbestrol, 77
  ductal carcinoma in situ, 76
  ethnicity, 73
  family history, 73
  gender, 73
  genetic predisposition, 73
  hormonal, 74–75
  hormone replacement therapy, 75
  lifestyle, 75–76
  lobular carcinoma in situ, 76
  long-term night shift work, 77
  obesity, 75
  oral contraceptives, 74–75
  personal history, 76–77
  physical activity, 75
  radiation exposure, 76–77
  recognition of, 73
  reproductive, 74–75
  tobacco use, 76
  weight gain, 75
screening for
  magnetic resonance imaging, 88–89, 103
  mammograms, 103
  in pregnancy, 104
  recommendations, 83
  ultrasound, 104
self-examinations for, 96
STK11, 86t
susceptibility genes for, 87f
TP53, 86t
treatment of
  aromatase inhibitors, 91
  breast-conserving surgery, 107–108
  breast reconstruction after, 90
  chemotherapy, 109
  lumpectomy, 109
  mastectomy, 108
  medications, 90–91
  platinum-based chemotherapy, 109
  poly-ADP ribose polymerase inhibitors, 109
  raloxifene, 91
  risk-reducing mastectomy, 107–108
  risk-reducing surgery, 89–90
  systemic, 108–109
  tamoxifen, 90
  triple-negative, 34–35, 42
Breast cancer risk assessment tool, 82–83
Breast-conserving surgery, 107–108
Breast density, 76
Breastfeeding, 74, 104
BRF1, 154
BRIP1, 84t, 186, 201
Brooke-Spiegler syndrome, 328t
BWS. *See* Beckwith-Wiedemann syndrome

C
CA 125, 198–200
Calcitonin, 295
Calcium channel blockers, 311
Cancer
  driver mutations of, 7–8
  familial predisposition to, 9
  family history of, 37
  future of, 25
  genes involved in, 8–9
  as genetic disease, 1
  leading sites of, 33f
  mutations in, 9–10
  somatic genetic testing of, 24–25
  susceptibility genes for, 18

Cancer cells, 24
Cancer genetic counselors
    finding of, 38
    referral to, 37–38
Cancer genetics
    breast cancer referral, 33–35
    colorectal cancer referral, 33
    counseling process for, 42–47
    endometrial cancer referral, 33
    pancreatic cancer referral, 33
    referral to, 31–34, 37–38
Cancer genomes, 7
Cancer genomics, 7–21
    driver mutations, 7–8
    passenger mutations, 7–8
Cancer risk identification
    DNA-based screening for, 438
    family history for, 433
Capillary gel electrophoresis, 64f
Carboplatin, 109
Caretaker genes
    definition of, 4t
    description of, 9
    loss of, 9
Carney complex, 264, 293, 310
ß-Catenin, 2
C cells, 295
CCS. See Cronkhite-Canada syndrome
CDC73, 253–254
CDH1 gene
    in breast cancer, 95–96
    in diffuse gastric cancer, 95
    in gastric cancer, 272
    management of, 84t
    mutation of, 53
CDKN2A, 219
Celecoxib, 125
Cell-free DNA, 440
Centers for Medicare & Medicaid Services, 67
Cervical cancer, in Peutz-Jeghers syndrome,
        97–98
Cervical embryonal rhabdomyosarcoma, 189
CFLE. See Confocal laser endomicroscopy
CFTR, 221
Chédiak-Higashi syndrome, 329t
CHEK2
    breast cancer, 84t, 101
    definition of, 142
    in hereditary nonpolyposis colorectal cancers,
        142, 161
    management of, 84t
    mutation of, 51
Chemoprevention
    for breast cancer, 104
    for endometrial cancer, 177–178

for familial adenomatous polyposis, 125–126
    for Lynch syndrome, 162
    for ovarian cancer, 200–201
Chemotherapy
    for breast cancer, 109
    for pancreatic cancer, 234
Children
    cancers in. See Pediatric cancers and conditions
    genetic test result discussions with
        age-specific resources, 420t–421t
        developmental considerations in, 418–422,
            419t
        "five Ws" for, 422–425
        healthcare provider's role in, 426–428
        overview of, 416–417
        post-result disclosures, 425–426
        preparation for, 417–418
Chompret criteria, 354
Chromosomal abnormalities, 368–369
Chronic kidney disease, 251
Chronic pancreatitis, 222, 228
CHRPE. See Congenital hypertrophy of the
        retinal pigment epithelium
Circulating free DNA, 235–236
Circulating microRNA, 236
Circulating tumor cells, 440
Circulating tumor DNA, 440
Cisplatin, 109
Claus model, 82
Clear cell carcinoma, 188
CLIA. See Clinical Laboratory Improvement
        Amendments
ClinGen, 65
Clinical Laboratory Improvement Amendments,
        67, 80, 384
Clinical Pharmacogenetics Implementation
        Consortium, 441
ClinVar, 65, 432
CMMRD. See Congenital mismatch repair
        deficiency syndrome; Constitutional
        mismatch repair deficiency syndrome
CMMRDS. See Constitutional mismatch repair
        deficiency syndrome
CMS. See Centers for Medicare & Medicaid
        Services
Colon adenomas
    in familial adenomatous polyposis, 118–119,
        125
    treatment of, 125
Colon cancer
    lifetime risk of, 187
    in Lynch syndrome, 169
    PTEN mutation in, 95
Colonic polyps, in PTEN hamartoma tumor
        syndrome, 132

Colonoscopy
  familial adenomatous polyposis screening
    uses of, 122
  Lynch syndrome surveillance uses of, 157
Colorectal adenomas, in Lynch syndrome, 149
Colorectal cancer
  allelic loss in, 10
  BRCA1 in, 143
  cancer genetics referral for, 33
  diet and, 163
  early onset, 144–145
  familial adenomatous polyposis as cause of,
    12, 118–119, 122
  familial colorectal cancer type X, 142, 161
  genomes of, 7
  hereditary cause of, 35
  heritability of, 18
  Lynch syndrome as cause of, 24, 35, 141–142,
    276
  MUTYH-associated polyposis as cause of, 126
  obesity and, 162
  screening for, 122, 161
  surgery for, 123–124
Common variable immunodeficiency syndrome,
  370
Competency, 382
Complementary DNA, 395
Computed tomography
  kidney cancer evaluations, 254–255
  pancreatic cancer screening, 226
Confocal laser endomicroscopy, 236
Congenital hypertrophy of the retinal pigment
  epithelium, 120
Congenital mismatch repair deficiency
  syndrome, 346–347
Consortium for Pancreas Screening, 224
Constitutional mismatch repair deficiency
  syndrome, 21, 128
Contrast enhanced endoscopic ultrasound,
  236
Copy number variants, 432–433
Correa's cascade, 269
Costello syndrome, 258
Cowden syndrome. *See also* PTEN hamartoma
  tumor syndrome
  breast cancer associated with, 170
  definition of, 169
  description of, 43, 94, 130, 169–170,
    253, 281
  diagnostic criteria for, 174–175
  germline testing for, 174
  PTEN hamartoma tumor syndrome, 169
  renal cell carcinoma in, 253
  skin cancer associated with, 328t, 335–336
  skin lesions associated with, 170

  trichilemmomas associated with, 43, 132, 170,
    253
  uterine tumors associated with, 170
CpG islands, 22
CpG sites, 6
CPIC. *See* Clinical Pharmacogenetics
  Implementation Consortium
Cronkhite-Canada syndrome, 131–132
Cryptorchidism, 262
CTRC, 221
Curcumin, 125
Cushing's syndrome, 307–308, 310
Cutaneous lichen amyloidosis, 298
CVID. *See* Common variable immunodeficiency
  syndrome

D

DCIS. *See* Ductal carcinoma in situ
"Deep sequencing," 7–8
De novo assembly, 62
De novo germline mutations, 15, 50
Denys-Drash syndrome, 364–365
Depression, 397–400
Dermoscopy, 320
DES. *See* Diethylstilbestrol
Desmoid tumors
  in familial adenomatous polyposis, 119–120,
    123–125
  management of, 124–125
  screening for, 123
DFMO. *See* Difluoromethylornithine
Diabetes mellitus, 222
Diamond-Blackfan anemia, 365–366
DICER1, 294
DICER1 syndrome
  in children, 366
  description of, 188–189, 294, 436t
  diagnosis of, 366
  genetic testing for, 197–198
Diet
  breast cancer and, 75
  colorectal cancer and, 163
  gastric cancer and, 270
Diethylstilbestrol, 77
Diffuse gastric cancer
  CDH1 gene in, 95
  hereditary, 95, 271t, 271–275, 281t, 423t, 436t
Difluoromethylornithine, 125
DiGeorge syndrome, 370–371
Direct-to-consumer genetic testing, 67–68, 80,
  183, 384–385
Distress, 397–400, 406t
DNA, repetitive sequencing of, 7
DNA hypomethylation, 21
DNA methylation, 21–22

DNA repair, 8–9, 13, 15–21
DNA sequencing, 7, 61
Dominant, 4t
Dominant negative effect, 2, 4t
"Double duct" sign, 211
Double-strand break repair system, 8, 154
Down syndrome, 368–369
Driver mutations, 440–441
   classes of, 10
   definition of, 4t
   description of, 7–8
   signaling pathways of, 10
Ductal carcinoma in situ, 76
Duodenal adenocarcinoma, 119
Duodenal adenomas, 126
Duty to disclose to patient, 388–389
Duty to recontact, 387–388
Duty to warn at-risk relatives, 389–392
Dyskeratosis congenita, 329t, 366–367
Dysplastic gangliocytoma of the
      cerebellum, 133

E
Early onset colorectal cancer, 144–145
Early stage genomic cancer diagnosis, 439–440
Edwards syndrome, 368
EIF3H, 153
Electronic health records, 385
Endometrial cancer
   body mass index and, 162
   cancer genetics referral for, 33, 36
   chemoprevention of, 177–178
   clinical management of, 176–178
   hormonal contraceptives and, 178
   incidence of, 36
   lifetime risk of, 187
   Lynch syndrome and, 36, 142, 158, 167
   in Muir-Torre syndrome, 169
   oral contraceptives and, 178
   Peutz-Jeghers syndrome and, 98
   PTEN mutation in, 94–95
   screening for, 176
   uterine serous cancer, 177
Endoscopic retrograde
      cholangiopancreatography, for pancreatic
      cancer screening, 226
Endoscopic ultrasound, for pancreatic cancer
      screening, 226
Endovascular ultrasound elastography,
      236–237
EPCAM, in Lynch syndrome, 152–153, 186
Epidermis, 320f
Epidermodysplasia verruciformis, 329t, 334
Epidermolysis bullosa, 329t, 334, 335f
Epigenetic alteration, 22

Epigenetics
   definition of, 4t, 6
   description of, 21–23
Epimutation, 22
Equity, 386–388
ERCC6, 154
ERCP. *See* Endoscopic retrograde
      cholangiopancreatography
Ethical and legal issues
   direct-to-consumer genetic testing, 67–68, 80,
      183, 384–385
   duty to disclose to patient, 388–389
   duty to recontact, 387–388
   duty to warn at-risk relatives, 389–392
   equity, 386–388
   informed consent, 381–382
   minors, 383–384
   overview of, 379–381
Ethnicity, 73
Exemestane, 104–106
Exosomal biomarkers, 236

F
FAF1, 155
Familial adenomatous polyposis
   adrenal adenomas associated with, 120
   adrenal tumors associated with, 311
   advocacy resources for, 423t
   APC mutations in, 2, 10, 117, 121, 143, 221
   attenuated, 5, 117–118, 121, 124, 127, 277
   autosomal dominant inheritance of, 2
   bile duct cancer in, 121
   brain tumors associated with, 121
   characteristics of, 10, 117–118, 271t
   chemoprevention for, 125–126
   in children, 350–351
   clinical phenotype, 118–121
   colon adenomas, 118–119
   colorectal cancer caused by
      description of, 12, 118–119, 293
      screening for, 122
      surgery for, 123–124
   congenital hypertrophy of the retinal pigment
      epithelium associated with, 120
   definition of, 117, 277
   desmoid tumors associated with, 119–120,
      123–125
   duodenal adenocarcinoma associated with,
      119
   extracolonic tumors in, 118t, 119–120
   gallbladder cancer in, 121
   Gardner syndrome, 118
   gastric cancer in, 271t, 277–278, 281t
   gastric polyps, 119
   genetic testing for, 121

hepatoblastoma associated with, 120
incidence of, 117
management of, 123–126
osteomas associated with, 120
pancreatic cancer associated with, 121, 221
papillary thyroid cancer associated with, 120
risks of, 5
screening for, 121–123, 122t, 278
small bowel tumors associated with, 119
stomach tumors associated with, 119
surveillance for, 121–123
thyroid cancer in, 293
upper gastrointestinal screening in, 122–123
Familial atypical multiple mole melanoma, 219,
    220t, 328t, 336
Familial cancer, 41–42
Familial cancer syndromes, 2
Familial colorectal cancer type X, 142, 154–155,
    161
Familial hypocalciuric hypercalcemia, 305
Familial isolated hyperparathyroidism,
    305–306
Familial medullary thyroid cancer, 299
Familial non-medullary thyroid cancer,
    292–293
Familial pancreatic cancer, 218, 224, 225t
Family history
    of breast cancer, 73, 77
    for cancer risk identification, 433
Family tree, 43f, 43–44
FAMMM. See Familial atypical multiple mole
    melanoma
FAN1, 154
FANCD2/FANCI-associated nuclease 1, 154
Fanconi anemia, 92, 219, 329t, 347–348
FAP. See Familial adenomatous polyposis
FASTQ files, 62
Federal Employees Health Benefits Program, 47
Ferguson-Smith syndrome, 332
Fibrofolliculomas, 253f
Fine-needle aspiration, 290
Fitzpatrick skin type, 320, 321, 325–326
Follicular thyroid carcinoma, 291
Folliculin, 252
Fordyce spots, 169
Frameshift variants, 60
Functional DNA repair, 17

G

Gail model, 82–83
Gallbladder cancer, in familial adenomatous
    polyposis, 121
GALNT12, 154
Gametogenesis, de novo mutations in, 21
Gardner syndrome, 118

Gastric adenocarcinoma
    classification of, 269
    signet ring cell, 271, 273f
    subtypes of, 270
Gastric adenocarcinoma and proximal polyposis
    syndrome, 271t, 278–279
Gastric adenomas, 278
Gastric cancer
    diet and, 270
    diffuse, 269
    epidemiology of, 269–270
    in familial adenomatous polyposis, 271t,
        277–278, 281t
    familial intestinal, 271t, 275–283, 281t
    in gastric adenocarcinoma and proximal
        polyposis syndrome, 271t, 278–279, 281t
    genetic counseling of, 283
    genetic predisposition to, 270–271
    genetic testing for, 272f
    in hamartomatous polyposis syndromes,
        279–283, 281t
    Helicobacter pylori and, 270
    in hereditary breast and ovarian cancer
        syndrome, 271t, 281t, 282–283
    hereditary diffuse, 271t, 271–275, 281t, 423t,
        436t
    in juvenile polyposis syndrome, 271t, 279–
        280, 281t
    in Lynch syndrome, 271t, 276–277, 281t
    in MUTYH-associated polyposis, 271t, 279,
        281t
    overview of, 269–270
    in Peutz-Jeghers syndrome, 97, 271t, 280, 281t
    in PTEN hamartoma tumor syndrome, 271t,
        280–281, 281t
    risk factors for, 270
    risk reduction for, 283–284
    screening of, 281t
    subtypes of, 269–270
Gastric polyps, 119
Gastric type intrapapillary mucinous neoplasms,
    213–214, 214f
Gastroenteropancreatic neuroendocrine tumors,
    304
Gastrointestinal polyposis syndromes
    Cronkhite-Canada syndrome, 131–132
    definition of, 117
    familial adenomatous polyposis. See Familial
        adenomatous polyposis
    Peutz-Jeghers syndrome. See Peutz-Jeghers
        syndrome
Gastrointestinal polyps, in Peutz-Jeghers
    syndrome, 129–130
Gatekeeper gene, 4t
G396D mutation, 15

Gender, breast cancer risks, 73
Genetic aberrations, 1
Genetic alterations
    large-scale, 60
    order of, 11–12
    small-scale, 59–60
Genetic counseling
    advances in, 54–55
    barriers of, 54–56
    bladder cancer, 258
    hereditary breast and ovarian cancer
        syndrome referral for, 189, 190t, 191–194
    limitations of, 54–56
    pancreatic cancer, 223–224
    prostate cancer, 261
    psychosocial assessment in, 54
    telephone-based service for, 38
    testicular cancer, 264
Genetic counselors, 392
Genetic discrimination
    definition of, 393
    federal law regarding, 393–394
    state law regarding, 394–395
Genetic diseases
    cancer as, 1
    clinical heterogeneity in, 3–6, 4t
Genetic exceptionalism, 385
Genetic heterogeneity, 4t, 5
Genetic Information Nondiscrimination Act, 47,
    56, 80, 394–395, 395t
Genetic pleiotropy, 4t, 5
Genetic predisposition, 73
Genetic risk perception, 398
Genetic terminology, 2–6, 4t
Genetic testing
    at-risk family members, 50
    bladder cancer, 258
    circumstances for, 48–49
    DICER1 syndrome, 197–198
    direct-to-consumer, 67–68, 80, 183, 384–385
    familial adenomatous polyposis, 121
    familial atypical multiple mole melanoma, 220t
    hereditary breast and ovarian cancer
        syndrome, 42, 44–45, 47, 52, 220t
    hereditary breast syndromes, 77–79
    hereditary pancreatitis, 220t
    ideal candidate for, 47–48
    informed consent for, 382
    kidney cancer, 254
    laboratory for, 49–50
    for Lynch syndrome, 171–174
    for men, 405
    of minors, 383–384
    multigene panel testing, 52–54
    newborn screen, 382
    pancreatic cancer, 223–224

Peutz-Jeghers syndrome, 196–197
    positive result of, 50
    prostate cancer, 261
    PTEN hamartoma tumor syndrome, 132–133
    regulations for, 67
    result report for, 66–67
    results of, 50–51
    skin cancer, 339–340
    testicular cancer, 264
    "true negative" result of, 51
    uninformative negative result of, 51
    variant of uncertain significance result of, 51
Genitourinary tract cancers
    bladder cancer. See Bladder cancer
    hereditary types of, 248t
    kidney cancer. See Kidney cancer
    overview of, 247
    prostate cancer. See Prostate cancer
    testicular cancer. See Testicular cancer
Genome Medical, 38
Genome-wide association studies, 142, 386, 433
Genomic sequencing, 438
Germ cell tumors, 262
Germline alterations
    definition of, 1
    somatic mutations versus, 1
Germline mutations
    in APC gene, 12
    definition of, 4t
    de novo, 15
    for Lynch syndrome, 24
    in p53 gene, 12
Germline panels, 23–24
Germline risk
    identification of, 433–438
    preventive action for, 439
Germline testing, 23
Germline variants, 432–433
GINA. See Genetic Information
        Nondiscrimination Act
GNAS mutation, 217
Gorlin syndrome, 131, 351
GREM1 gene, 127
Griscelli syndrome, 329t
Gut epithelium, overgrowth of, 3
GWAS. See Genome-wide association studies
Gynandroblastoma, 189

H
Hamartomatous polyposis syndromes
    gastric cancer in, 279–283, 281t
    juvenile polyposis syndrome, 130–131
    Peutz-Jeghers syndrome. See Peutz-Jeghers
        syndrome
    PTEN hamartoma tumor syndrome. See
        PTEN hamartoma tumor syndrome

Haploinsufficiency, 3, 4t
HBOC. *See* Hereditary breast and ovarian cancer syndrome
HBOC syndrome. *See* Hereditary breast and ovarian cancer syndrome
HDGC. *See* Hereditary diffuse gastric cancer; Hereditary diffuse gastric cancer syndrome
Helicobacter pylori, 160, 222, 270
Hepatoblastoma, in familial adenomatous polyposis, 120
Hereditary breast and ovarian cancer syndrome. *See also* Ovarian cancer
   advocacy resources for, 423t
   BRCA1 mutations in, 219, 261
   BRCA2 mutations in, 219, 261
   BRCA testing in, 191–193
   breast cancer risks, 184
   characteristics of, 184, 219, 434t
   definition of, 184
   description of, 34, 37
   gastric cancer risks, 271t, 281t, 282–283
   genetic counseling for
      options for, 191–194
      referral for, 189, 190t
   genetic testing for, 42, 44–45, 47, 52, 220t, 415
   multi-gene panel testing for, 193
   non BRCA-associated, 186–189
   pancreatic cancer risks, 219
   prostate cancer risks, 261
   risk assessments, 189–194
Hereditary breast syndromes
   breast cancer management in, 106–109
   genetic testing for, 77–79
   management of, 83–102
   recognition of, 77–78
   "red flags" for, 78t
Hereditary cancers
   cellular processes involved in, 59
   characteristics of, 184
   classification of, 59
   Cowden syndrome, 169–170
   DICER1 syndrome, 188–189
   distress associated with, 401
   DNA repair and, 16t
   incidence of, 41
   Lynch syndrome. *See* Lynch syndrome
   Peutz-Jeghers syndrome. *See* Peutz-Jeghers syndrome
   polymerase proofreading associated polyposis, 170–171
   predisposition syndromes for, 49
Hereditary diffuse gastric cancer, 95, 271t, 271–275, 281t, 423t, 436t
Hereditary hyperparathyroidism jaw tumor syndrome, 253–254

Hereditary leiomyomatosis and renal cell carcinoma, 249t, 252, 252f
Hereditary leiomyomatosis and renal cell cancer, 351–352
Hereditary mixed polyposis syndrome, 127
Hereditary neuroblastoma, 362
Hereditary nonpolyposis colorectal cancers
   CHEK2 in, 142
   epidemiology of, 141–145
   etiology of, 141
   low-susceptibility alleles, 142, 145
   Lynch-like syndrome. *See* Lynch-like syndrome
   Lynch syndrome. *See* Lynch syndrome
   microsatellite stable, 142, 154–155, 161
   moderate-penetrance genes in, 142–145
   penetrance-modifying genetic defects, 153–156
Hereditary pancreatitis, 220t, 221, 225t
Hereditary papillary renal carcinoma, 249t, 251–252
Hereditary paraganglioma-pheochromocytoma syndrome, 352–353
Hereditary retinoblastoma, 258, 258t, 353
Heritability, 18
Hermansky-Pudlak syndrome, 329t
High-penetrance genes, 52–53
HIPAA
   history of, 393
   privacy rule of, 392
Hirschsprung's disease, 298–299
HLRCC. *See* Hereditary leiomyomatosis and renal cell carcinoma; Hereditary leiomyomatosis and renal cell cancer
HMPS. *See* Hereditary mixed polyposis syndrome
Homologous recombination, 8
Hormonal contraceptives, endometrial cancer and, 178
Hormone replacement therapy
   breast cancer risks, 75
   breast density and, 76
"Hot nodules," 290
HOXB13, 261
HPRC. *See* Hereditary papillary renal carcinoma
HR. *See* Homologous recombination
hTERT rs2075786, 153
Human Genomic Project, 21
Human genome, 6–7
Hyper-immunoglobulin M syndrome, 371
Hyperparathyroidism
   familial isolated, 305–306
   hereditary, 303, 304t
   in multiple endocrine neoplasia 2A, 305
   primary. *See* Primary hyperparathyroidism
Hyperparathyroidism jaw-tumor syndrome, 305–306

I

IBIS risk model, 80–82, 81t
Ileal pouch anal anastomosis, 123
Ileorectal anastomosis, 123
Illumina, 61
Immune checkpoint therapy
   description of, 25
   pancreatic cancer treated with, 235
Immunohistochemistry, for Lynch syndrome,
   147–149
Incidentalomas, 250, 307–308
Infants, juvenile polyposis syndrome in, 131
Informed consent, 46–47, 381–382
InformedDNA, 38
Intestinal-type intrapapillary mucinous
   neoplasms, 214
Intrapapillary mucinous neoplasms, 213, 213f,
   216–217, 227
Intrauterine device, 74
Ion Torrent, 61
IPAA. *See* Ileal pouch anal anastomosis
IPMNs. *See* Intrapapillary mucinous neoplasms
IRA. *See* Ileorectal anastomosis
IUD. *See* Intrauterine device

J

JAK-STAT pathway, 3
JPS. *See* Juvenile polyposis syndrome
Junctional epidermolysis bullosa, 329t, 334
Justice, 380, 381t
Juvenile polyposis syndrome
   animal model of, 3
   characteristics of, 354–355
   description of, 130–131
   gastric cancer in, 271t, 279–280, 281t
   Smad4 in, 9, 280
Juvenile polyps, 280

K

Keratitis-ichthyosis-deafness syndrome, 328t
Kidney cancer. *See also* Renal cell carcinoma
   BAP1 tumor predisposition syndrome, 249t,
     253
   Birt-Hogg-Dube syndrome, 249t, 252, 253t
   CDC73, 253–254
   clinical presentation of, 250
   epidemiology of, 247, 249–250
   genetic risk of, 247, 249–250
   genetic testing for, 254
   hereditary leiomyomatosis and renal cell
     carcinoma, 249t, 252, 252f
   hereditary papillary renal carcinoma, 249t,
     251–252, 254
   hereditary syndromes, 249t, 251–255
   imaging of, 250–251, 254–255

magnetic resonance imaging of, 255
   management of, 251
   physical examination of, 250–251
   radical nephrectomy for, 255
   risk factors for, 249–250
   succinate dehydrogenase-deficient renal cell
     carcinoma, 249t, 254
   surgical interventions for, 255
   TSC, 253
   von Hippel-Lindau disease, 249t, 251, 254
Knudson's two-hit hypothesis, 2, 21, 45,
   46f, 353
KRAS mutations
   description of, 11
   in pancreatic cancer, 221
KRAS oncogene, 216–217

L

Laboratory
   for genetic testing, 49–50
   next-generation sequencing, 61–63
   variant classification, 65–66
Laboratory-developed tests, 67
Landscaper effect, 3, 4t, 9
Large-scale genetic alterations, 60
LCIS. *See* Lobular carcinoma in situ
Leading sites of cancer, 33f
Lhermitte-Duclos disease, 131–133, 170
Lifestyle factors, for breast cancer, 75–76
Li-Fraumeni syndrome
   adrenocortical carcinoma in, 309–310
   advocacy resources for, 423t
   breast cancer and, 93–94
   characteristics of, 353–354, 435t
   in children, 353–354
   clinical features of, 282
   description of, 12, 309
   diagnosis of, 309
   gastric cancer and, 271t, 281t, 282
   genetics of, 282
   management of, 282, 310
Likely pathogenic variants, 66
Linitis plastica, 269, 273
Liquid biopsy, 439–441
Lobular carcinoma in situ, 76
Locus heterogeneity, 4t, 6
Long-term night shift work, 77
LS. *See* Lynch syndrome
Lung cancer, Peutz-Jeghers syndrome and, 98
Lynch-like syndrome
   age of diagnosis, 144
   cancer surveillance in, 161
   characteristics of, 144
   extracolonic cancers and, 156
   mismatch repair mutations in, 144

Lynch syndrome
  adrenocortical carcinomas associated with, 309, 311
  age at diagnosis of, 168
  Amsterdam criteria for, 31, 171, 194, 195t
  Bethesda guidelines for, 31, 145, 194
  bladder cancer in, 151, 257, 258t
  BRAF V600E mutations in, 148–150
  breast cancer and, 159–160
  cancer risks in, 150–153
  characteristics of, 167–168, 219–220
  chemoprevention of, 162
  clinical criteria for, 145–147
  clinical features of, 276–277
  colonoscopy for, 157
  colorectal adenomas associated with, 149
  colorectal cancer associated with, 24, 35, 141–142, 276
  definition of, 141, 167, 186
  description of, 3
  diagnosis of, 168
  endometrial cancer associated with, 36, 142, 158, 167–168, 176–178
  EPCAM in, 152–153, 186
  epidemiology of, 141–142
  extracolonic cancers associated with, 142
  family history-based screening for, 171, 194
  gastric cancer associated with, 271t, 276–277
  gene-specific approaches to, 160–162
  genetic testing for, 171–174
  germline mutations in, 24, 186
  germline testing for, 173–174
  hereditary endometrial and colon cancers caused by, 168, 187
  immunohistochemistry for, 147–149
  incidence of, 145
  microsatellite instability, 31, 147–149, 168, 172–173, 187, 194–195
  mismatch repair deficiency in, 148, 168, 186
  mismatch repair genes in, 17, 68
  MLH1 in, 141, 151–152, 159–160, 277
  MSH2 in, 141, 151–153, 159–160, 277
  MSH6 in, 141, 153, 160
  Muir-Torre syndrome variant of, 168–169, 169t
  National Comprehensive Cancer Network guidelines for, 146–147
  ovarian cancer associated with, 158, 187–188
  pancreatic cancer associated with, 159–160, 219–220
  PMS2 in, 141, 153
  prediction models for, 145–146
  prostate cancer risks, 261
  risk assessment of, 171t, 171–174, 194
  risk prediction models for, 173–174
  risk-reducing surgery in
    bilateral salpingo-oophorectomy, 177
    description of, 177
    hysterectomy, 177
  screening for, 171, 194
  sebaceous neoplasms in, 150
  surveillance for, 156–160
  testing algorithm for, 172–173, 173f
  tumor testing for, 147–150
  Turcot syndrome variant of, 121, 169
  universal tumor testing for, 173
  variants of, 168–169

M
MADH4/DPC4, 130
MAF. *See* Minor allele frequency
Magnetic resonance cholangiopancreatography, 226
Magnetic resonance imaging
  breast cancer screening, 88–89, 103
  kidney cancer evaluations, 254–255
  pancreatic cancer screening using, 226
Male breast cancer, 35
Mammograms, 103
MAP. *See* *MUTYH*-associated polyposis
MAP Kinase, 10
MCNs. *See* Mucinous cystic neoplasms
Medical geneticists, 392
Medullary thyroid cancer
  disease-specific approach to, 297
  epidemiology of, 296–297
  external beam radiation therapy for, 296
  familial, 299
  fine-needle aspiration for, 295
  management of, 294–296, 299–301
  microRNAs for, 297
  radioactive iodine ablation for, 296
  RET mutations associated with, 296–297
  risk assessment of, 294–296
  total thyroidectomy for, 295
Medulloblastomas, 121, 123
Melanoma, 92
  ABCDEs of, 323f
  characteristics of, 321t
  clinical features of, 323f
  conditions associated with, 337–338
  deaths caused by, 325
  epidemiology of, 325
  family history of, 327
  invasive, 325
  management of, 338–339
  prevention of, 322
  risk factors for, 326–327
Menarche, age of, 74
Menin, 303

Menopause, age of, 74
Menstruation, age of, 74
Messenger ribonucleic acid, 2
MGMT, 17
Microarray-based comparative genomic
    hybridization, 63–64
Microsatellite, 147, 172
Microsatellite instability
    definition of, 187, 194
    description of, 9, 13, 25, 68
    for Lynch syndrome, 147–149, 168, 172–173,
        187, 194–195
Microsatellite stable hereditary nonpolyposis
    colorectal cancer, 142, 154–155, 161
Minimally invasive parathyroidectomy, 301
Minor allele frequency, 18
Minors, genetic testing of, 383–384
Mismatch repair
    description of, 6, 15, 17
    in Lynch syndrome, 148
Missense mutations
    definition of, 4t
    description of, 2
    oncogene activation by, 8
Mitotic heritability, 22
MLH1
    germline mutations in, 3
    in Lynch syndrome, 141, 151–152, 159, 277
    methylation, 68, 148, 149
MLPA. *See* Multiple ligation probe amplification
MMRpredict, 145–146, 173
MMRpro, 145–146, 173
Moderate-penetrance genes, 52
Molecular probe-based imaging, 237
Molloy v. Meier, 389t, 390–391
MRCP. *See* Magnetic resonance
    cholangiopancreatography
MSH2
    germline mutations in, 3
    in Lynch syndrome, 141, 159, 277
MSH6, in Lynch syndrome, 141, 153
MSI. *See* Microsatellite instability
MTS. *See* Muir-Torre syndrome
Mucinous cystic neoplasms, 213, 215, 215f, 217
Mucinous pancreatic cysts, 218
Muir-Torre syndrome, 168–169, 169t, 328t, 333
Mulibrey nanism, 362–363
Multigene panel testing
    description of, 52–54, 61
    for hereditary breast and ovarian cancer
        syndrome, 193
Multiple endocrine neoplasia syndrome 1
    adrenocortical tumors associated with, 310
    advocacy resources for, 423t
    carcinoids in, 304

characteristics of, 355, 434t
clinical management of, 305–306
description of, 303–304
Multiple endocrine neoplasia syndrome 4, 304–306
Multiple endocrine neoplasia syndrome 2A
    characteristics of, 435t
    in children, 363
    cutaneous lichen amyloidosis associated with,
        298
    Hirschsprung's disease associated with,
        298–299
    hyperparathyroidism in, 305
    pheochromocytomas associated with, 298,
        313, 315
    RET mutations associated with, 297
Multiple endocrine neoplasia syndrome 2B
    characteristics of, 435t
    in children, 363
    classical, 298
    description of, 299
    RET mutations associated with, 297
Multiple ligation probe amplification, 63–64, 64f
Multistep carcinogenesis
    definition of, 4t
    description of, 10–11
    in pancreatic cancer, 13f
    schematic diagram of, 12f–13f
Mutagenic insult, 8
Mutational signature, 4t
Mutations
    accumulation of, 10–11
    number of, 9–10
MUTYH, 15, 16t, 126, 143, 155, 161–162
MUTYH-associated polyposis
    characteristics of, 271t
    clinical presentation of, 126–127
    colonic phenotype of, 126
    colorectal cancer risks, 126
    definition of, 126
    description of, 50, 143, 435t
    duodenal cancer in, 126
    duodenal polyps in, 127
    extracolonic phenotype of, 126–127
    gastric cancer in, 271t, 279, 281t
    management of, 127
    natural history of, 126–127
MYC, 8
Myriad Genetics, 395

N
Nanopore sequencing, 62
National Cancer Institute Cancer Genetics
    Services, 38
National Comprehensive Cancer Network, 77,
    128, 176, 323

National Familial Pancreatic Tumor Registry, 219

National Institutes of Health Roadmap Epigenetics Consortium, 21

National Society of Genetic Counselors, 37, 382, 391

NBN, 85t

NBS. *See* Nijmegen breakage syndrome

NCCN. *See* National Comprehensive Cancer Network

Neonatal severe hyperparathyroidism, 305–306

Neuroblastoma, hereditary, 362

Neurofibromatosis, 314–315, 356, 434t

Neurofibromatosis 1, 356

Neurofibromatosis 2, 356–357

Newborn screen, 382

Next-generation sequencing, 61–63, 68, 79

NFPTR. *See* National Familial Pancreatic Tumor Registry

NGS. *See* Next-generation sequencing

NHEJ repair. *See* Nonhomologous end joining repair

Nijmegen breakage syndrome, 348–349

Niraparib, 109

NMP22, 159

Nonhomologous end joining repair, 8

Nonmaleficence, 380, 381t

Non-medullary thyroid cancer
   epidemiology of, 291–292
   familial, 292–293
   management of, 289–291
   radioactive iodine ablation for, 291
   risk assessment of, 289–291
   sporadic, 292

Nonsense mutations, 4t

NSGC. *See* National Society of Genetic Counselors

NSHPT. *See* Neonatal severe hyperparathyroidism

NTHL1 gene, 127

Nucleotide excision repair, 6, 15

Nucleotide variants, 60f

NUDT1, 155

Nursing, breast cancer screening in, 104

O

Obesity
   breast cancer and, 75
   colorectal cancer and, 162

Oculocutaneous albinism, 329t, 335, 336f

OGG1, 155

Olaparib, 109

Oncocytic-type intrapapillary mucinous neoplasms, 214

Oncogenes
   definition of, 4t
   description of, 8
   list of, 19t–20t

Oral contraceptives
   breast cancer risks, 74–75
   breast density and, 76
   endometrial cancer and, 178
   ovarian cancer risk reduction with, 91

Ornithine decarboxylase, 125

Osteomas, in familial adenomatous polyposis, 120

Osteonectin, 211

Ovarian cancer. *See also* Hereditary breast and ovarian cancer syndrome
   age of onset, 186
   BRCA1 in, 88t, 184, 201
   BRCA2 in, 88t, 201
   breast cancer and, 90–92
   CA 125 screening for, 198–200
   chemoprevention for, 200–201
   epidemiology of, 183
   epithelial subtypes of, 183
   hormonal contraceptives for decreased risk of, 200
   incidence of, 36
   Lynch syndrome-related, 158, 187–188
   management of, 198
   mortality rate for, 183
   PALB2 and, 99
   pelvic ultrasonography of, 198–200
   risk factors for, 183–184, 184, 185t
   risk prediction models for, 198
   risk-reducing bilateral salpingo-oophorectomy, 91, 99, 101, 201–202
   risk stratification for, 198
   screening for, 91, 198–200
   single-nucleotide variants, 186

Ovarian sex cord stromal tumors, 188

Ovarian tumors, Peutz-Jeghers syndrome and, 98

P

PALB2, 85t, 98–99

PancPRO, 218

Pancreatic cancer
   age of diagnosis, 225
   ATM, 100
   biomarkers
      circulating free DNA, 235–236
      circulating microRNA, 236
      exosomal, 236
      novel types of, 235–236
      screening uses of, 226–227
   BRCA1 in, 88t, 92

Pancreatic cancer (*Cont.*)
  BRCA2 in, 184
  cancer genetics referral for, 33
  confocal laser endomicroscopy of, 236
  contrast enhanced endoscopic ultrasound of, 236
  ductal adenocarcinoma. *See* Pancreatic ductal adenocarcinoma
  endovascular ultrasound elastography of, 236–237
  epidemiology of, 209–210
  familial, 218, 224, 225t
  future directions for, 210, 235–237
  genetic counseling for, 223–224
  genetic testing for, 223–224
  gene-to-environment interactions in, 222
  germline mutations in, 225t
  histopathology of, 210–217
  imaging modalities
    novel types of, 236–237
    screening uses of, 226
  incidence of, 36, 210
  lifetime risk of, 217
  Lynch syndrome and, 159–160
  molecular probe-based imaging of, 237
  molecular progression of, 210–217
  mortality rate for, 210
  multistep carcinogenesis in, 13f
  PALB2 and, 99
  in Peutz-Jeghers syndrome, 97
  risk assessment of, 217–223
  risk factors for
    ABO blood group, 218
    alcohol intake, 221–223
    anthropometric factors, 222
    ataxia-telangiectasia, 221
    chronic pancreatitis, 222
    classification of, 217
    diabetes mellitus, 222
    diet, 222
    familial adenomatous polyposis, 221
    familial atypical multiple mole melanoma, 219
    family history, 218
    genetic syndromes, 218–221
    Helicobacter pylori infection, 222
    hereditary breast-ovarian cancer syndrome, 219
    hereditary pancreatitis, 220t, 221, 225t
    inherited, 218–221
    Lynch syndrome, 219–220
    modifiable, 221–223
    mucinous pancreatic cysts, 218
    non-modifiable, 218
    Peutz-Jeghers syndrome, 220
    smoking, 223
    tobacco exposure, 221, 223
  risk stratification for, 224
  screening for
    age of initiation, 225–226
    biomarkers, 226–227
    computed tomography, 226
    economic burden associated with, 228
    endoscopic retrograde cholangiopancreatography, 226
    endoscopic ultrasound, 226
    imaging modalities used in, 226
    indications for, 225t
    magnetic resonance cholangiopancreatography, 226
    magnetic resonance imaging, 226
    pancreatic juice, 226–227
    program appraisals, 228, 229t–233t
    psychological stress caused by, 234
    risk stratification for, 224
    survival benefits of, 228
    termination of, 225–226
    treatment based on, 227–228
  single-nucleotide polymorphisms associated with, 222
  somatic mutations associated with, 12
  sporadic nature of, 209
  survival statistics for, 209–210
  susceptibility genes for, 219
  treatment of
    anaplastic lymphoma kinase protein inhibitor, 235
    chemotherapy, 234
    immune checkpoint inhibitor, 235
    platinum-based therapies, 234
    poly adenosine diphosphate-ribose polymerase inhibitor, 234–235
    screening-based approach, 227–228
Pancreatic cyst biomarkers, 226–227
Pancreatic ductal adenocarcinoma
  characteristics of, 211
  "double duct" sign associated with, 211
  gastric type intrapapillary mucinous neoplasms, 213–214, 214f
  genetics of, 215–217
  intrapapillary mucinous neoplasms, 213, 213f, 216–217, 227
  mucinous cystic neoplasms, 213, 215, 215f, 217, 227
  pancreatic intraepithelial neoplasms, 212–213, 213f, 215–216, 228
  precursor lesions for, 211–212
  progression of, 211f, 215–217
Pancreatic intraepithelial neoplasms, 212–213, 213f, 215–216, 228

Pancreatic juice, 226–227
Pancreatitis
  chronic, 222
  hereditary, 220t, 221
Pancreatobiliary-type intrapapillary mucinous
    neoplasms, 214
PanINs. *See* Pancreatic intraepithelial neoplasms
Papillary thyroid cancers
  in familial adenomatous polyposis, 120
  thyroid lobectomy for, 290
Paragangliomas
  hereditary causes of, 313t, 313–314
  hereditary paraganglioma-
    pheochromocytoma syndrome, 352–353
  management of, 311–312
  risk assessment of, 311–312
Parathyroid adenomas, 302
Parathyroidectomy, 301
PARP inhibitors. *See* Poly-ADP-ribose
    polymerase inhibitors
Passenger mutations
  definition of, 4t
  description of, 7–8
Patenting, of genes, 395–396
Pate v. Threikel, 389t, 390
Pathogenic variants, 66
Patient Protection and Affordable Care Act, 394
p16/CDKN2A pathway, 216
Pediatric cancers and conditions
  ataxia telangiectasia, 343, 345–346
  Beckwith-Wiedemann syndrome, 310–312,
    364
  Bloom syndrome, 329t, 333–334, 346
  Bohring-Opitz syndrome, 350
  characteristics of, 344t–345t
  congenital mismatch repair deficiency
    syndrome, 346–347
  Diamond-Blackfan anemia, 365–366
  DICER1 syndrome, 366
  dyskeratosis congenita, 366–367
  familial adenomatous polyposis, 350–351
  Fanconi anemia, 92, 219, 329t, 347–348
  Gorlin syndrome, 351
  hereditary leiomyomatosis and renal cell
    cancer, 351–352
  hereditary neuroblastoma, 362
  hereditary paraganglioma-
    pheochromocytoma syndrome, 352–353
  hereditary retinoblastoma, 353
  juvenile polyposis syndrome, 354–355
  Li-Fraumeni syndrome, 353–354
  Mulibrey nanism, 362–363
  multiple endocrine neoplasia syndrome 1, 355
  multiple endocrine neoplasia type 2, 363
  neurofibromatosis, 356–357

  Nijmegen breakage syndrome, 348–349
  overview of, 343
  Perlman syndrome, 367
  Peutz-Jeghers syndrome, 357–358
  PTEN hamartoma tumor syndrome, 358
  RASopathies, 358–359
  rhabdoid tumor predisposition
    syndrome, 359
  Rothmund-Thomson syndrome, 329t, 333,
    349
  Schwachman-Diamond syndrome, 367–368
  Simpson-Golabi-Behmel syndrome, 359–360
  tuberous sclerosis, 350–361
  von Hippel-Lindau disease, 361
  WT1-related syndromes, 364–365
  xeroderma pigmentosum, 328t, 332, 339,
    349–350
Pedigrees, 43f, 43–44
Pelvic ultrasonography, for ovarian cancer
    screening, 198–200
Pembrolizumab, 172, 195
Penetrance
  definition of, 3, 4t
  variable, 6
Periampullary adenocarcinoma, 124
Perlman syndrome, 367
Peutz-Jeghers syndrome
  adenoma malignum associated with, 188
  animal models of, 3
  breast cancer associated with, 129, 129t
  cancer risks associated with, 97, 129t
  characteristics of, 128–130, 220, 263, 436t
  in children, 357–358
  definition of, 128, 188
  diagnosis of, 130, 188, 196, 280
  epidemiology of, 128–130
  gastric cancer associated with, 97, 271t, 280,
    281t
  gastrointestinal polyps associated with,
    129–130
  genetic pleiotropy in, 5
  genetic testing for, 196–197, 220t
  ovarian sex cord stromal tumors associated
    with, 188
  pancreatic cancer caused by
    risks for, 220
    screening indications, 225t
  polyps associated with, 129–130
  STK11 mutations in, 3, 96–97, 188, 196–197,
    263, 280
  surveillance for, 130
  testicular cancer risks, 263
  treatment of, 130
p53 gene, 12
Pharmacogenomics, 441

Pheochromocytoma-paragangliomas
    description of, 311–312
    hereditary, 314–315
Pheochromocytomas
    description of, 298
    epidemiology of, 312
    hereditary causes of, 313t, 313–314
    hereditary phenotypes, 312
    management of, 311–312
    in MEN2, 313, 315
    metastatic, 312
    risk assessment of, 311–312
    susceptibility genes for, 312
PHPT. *See* Primary hyperparathyroidism
Physical activity
    breast cancer and, 75
    colorectal cancer and, 163
Pigmented ocular fundus lesions, 120
PI3K, 10
P16INK4A, 219
Platinum-based chemotherapy
    for breast cancer, 109
    for pancreatic cancer, 234
PLCO. *See* Prostate, Lung, Colorectal, and
        Ovarian Cancer Screening Trial
Pleuropulmonary blastoma, 189
PMS2, in Lynch syndrome, 141, 153
POLD1, 127, 170
POLE, 127, 170
POLE2, 155
Poly ADP-ribose polymerase enzymes, 18
Poly-ADP ribose polymerase inhibitors
    breast cancer treated with, 109
    description of, 35, 69
    pancreatic cancer treated with, 234–235
Polygenic risk scoring, 433
Polymerase proofreading associated polyposis,
        170–171, 176–177
Population-based genomic screening,
        438–439
PPAP. *See* Polymerase proofreading associated
        polyposis
PPB. *See* Pleuropulmonary blastoma
PPNAD. *See* Primary pigmented nodular
        adrenocortical disease
Precision medicine, 431
Predictive testing, 383
Pregnancy
    age of, breast cancer risks and, 74
    breast cancer screening in, 104
PREMM5, 145–146, 174
Primary hyperparathyroidism
    epidemiology of, 302–303
    management of, 301–302
    parathyroidectomy for, 301
    risk assessment of, 301–302

    symptoms of, 301
Primary immunodeficiency disorders
    common variable immunodeficiency
        syndrome, 370
    definition of, 369
    description of, 369–370
    DiGeorge syndrome, 370–371
    hyper-immunoglobulin M syndrome, 371
    severe combined immunodeficiency,
        371–372
    severe congenital neutropenia, 372–373
    Wiskott-Aldrich syndrome, 373
    X-linked lymphoproliferative disease,
        373–374
Primary pigmented nodular adrenocortical
        disease, 293, 310
Principle-based ethics
    autonomy, 379–380, 381t
    beneficence, 380, 381t
    definition of, 379
    justice, 380, 381t
    nonmaleficence, 380, 381t
PRKAR1A, 293
Programmed death receptor-1, 235
Prostate, Lung, Colorectal, and Ovarian Cancer
        Screening Trial, 199–200
Prostate cancer
    description of, 259
    epidemiology of, 259–260
    genetic counseling for, 261
    genetic risk of, 259–260
    genetic testing for, 261
    hereditary causes of, 18, 249t, 260–261
    HOXB13 and, 261
    imaging of, 260
    incidence of, 36
    management of, 262
    physical examination of, 260
    prostate specific antigen screening for, 260
    risk factors for, 259
Prostate gland, 259
Prostate specific antigen screening, 260
Proteus syndrome, 280
Proto-oncogenes, 10
PRSS1, 221
PS. *See* Perlman syndrome
PSA screening. *See* Prostate specific antigen
        screening
Psychosocial assessment, 54
Psychosocial issues, 396–407
PTEN, 43, 85t, 94–95
PTEN hamartoma tumor syndrome. *See also*
        Bannayan-Riley-Ruvalcaba syndrome;
        Cowden syndrome; Proteus syndrome
    advocacy resources for, 423t
    characteristics of, 131–132, 249t, 435t

in children, 358
definition of, 131–132
description of, 94, 169
diagnostic criteria for, 175t
epidemiology of, 131–132
gastric cancer in, 271t, 280–281, 281t
genetic testing criteria for, 132–133
syndromes related to, 133

R

RAD51/C/D, 85t, 201
Radiation exposure, 76–77
Radical nephrectomy, 255
Radioactive iodine ablation, 291
RAD51 paralogs, 186
RAF, 8
Raloxifene, 105, 439
RAS, 8, 10
RASopathies, 358–359
RB, 2
Read-count methods, 62
Read-pair methods, 63
Recessive, 4t
Recessive dystrophic epidermolysis bullosa,
    329t, 334–335
Renal cell carcinoma. *See also* Kidney cancer
    in Cowden syndrome, 253
    PTEN mutation in, 95
Restriction fragment length polymorphism, 10
Retinoblastoma, hereditary, 258, 258t, 353, 434t
RET mutations, 296–297
Rhabdoid tumor predisposition syndrome, 359
Ribonucleic acid
    messenger, 2
    nonsense-mediated, 2
Risk communication literature, 416–417
Risk perception, 398–399
Risk-reducing hysterectomy, 177, 201
Risk-reducing mastectomy, 96, 108
Risk-reducing salpingo-oophorectomy
    bilateral
        description of, 177
        in Lynch syndrome, 177
        ovarian cancer risk reduction with, 201–203
        primary peritoneal cancer after, 202
    for ovarian cancer, 91, 99, 101
Risk stratification
    for ovarian cancer, 198
    for pancreatic cancer, 224
RNA. *See* Ribonucleic acid
RNA sequencing, 61
RNF43, 217
Rombo syndrome, 329t, 331
Rothmund-Thomson syndrome, 329t, 333, 349
RPS20, 154

S

Safer v. Pack, 389t, 390
Salpingo-oophorectomy, risk-reducing bilateral
    description of, 177
    in Lynch syndrome, 177
    ovarian cancer risk reduction with, 91, 99,
        101, 201–202
    primary peritoneal cancer after, 202
Schöpf-Schulz-Passarge syndrome, 328t
Schwachman-Diamond syndrome, 367–368
SCID. *See* Severe combined immunodeficiency
SCN. *See* Severe congenital neutropenia
SDH-RCC. *See* Succinate dehydrogenase-
    deficient renal cell carcinoma
SDS. *See* Schwachman-Diamond syndrome
Sebaceous carcinomas, 169
Secreted protein acidic and rich in cysteine, 211
Segmental overgrowth lipomatosis arteriovenous
    malformation epidermal nevus, 170
Selective estrogen receptor modulators, for
    breast cancer prevention, 104–105
SEMA4A, 155
Serrated polyposis syndrome, 127–128
Sertoli-cell testicular tumors, 129, 263–264
Sertoli-Leydig cell tumors, 189
Severe combined immunodeficiency, 371–372
Severe congenital neutropenia, 372–373
Sex cord stromal tumors, 262, 264
Sex-linked diseases, 2
Sigmoidoscopy, for familial adenomatous
    polyposis screening, 122
Signet ring cells, 271, 273f
Simpson-Golabi-Behmel syndrome, 359–360
Single-base nucleotide variants, 59
Single nucleotide polymorphisms
    definition of, 4t
    description of, 6, 433
Single nucleotide variants, 15
Single-strand breaks, 15, 18
Sipple syndrome, 298
Skin
    anatomy of, 319, 320f
    Fitzpatrick skin type classification, 320, 321,
        325–326
Skin cancer
    basal cell nevus syndrome, 328t, 330–331,
        331t
    clinical management of, 319–322
    early detection of, 322
    economic impact of, 325
    epidemiology of, 324–325
    family history of, 327
    Fitzpatrick skin type classification and, 320,
        321, 325–326
    genetic syndromes associated with, 328t–329t

Skin cancer (*Cont.*)
  genetic testing of, 339–340
  lifetime risk of, 325
  management of, 322–323, 338
  melanoma, 321t
  nonmelanoma, 324–325
  prevention of, 322
  risk assessment of, 319–322
  risk factors for, 320, 321t, 326–328
  Rombo syndrome, 329t, 331
  screening for, 323–324
  types of, 319
Smad4
  in juvenile polyposis syndrome, 9, 130, 280, 354
  in mice, 3
  in pancreatic cancer, 216
  in T cells, 3
Small bowel tumors, familial adenomatous
      polyposis and, 119
Small insertions or deletions, 59
Small-scale genetic alterations, 59–60
SMARCB1, 359
SMARCB2, 359
Social media, 422
SOLAMEN syndrome. *See* Segmental
      overgrowth lipomatosis arteriovenous
      malformation epidermal nevus
      syndrome
Somatic genetic testing, 24–25
Somatic mutations
  in *APC* gene, 13
  definition of, 1, 4t
  germline alterations versus, 1
  rate of, 15
  signatures of, in cancer, 13–15
  tumor locations and, 14f
Somatic tissue testing, 68–69
SPARC. *See* Secreted protein acidic and rich in
      cysteine
Spigelman classification, 119, 119t, 122, 124, 278
SPINK1, 221
Split-read methods, 63
Sporadic cancer, 41–42
Sporadic non-medullary thyroid cancer, 292
SPS. *See* Serrated polyposis syndrome
Squamous cell cancer, 256
Squamous cell carcinoma
  characteristics of, 321t, 322
  clinical features of, 324f
  early detection of, 322
  epidemiology of, 325
  management of, 339
  risk factors for, 326
SRC, 8
STAT, 10
Stauffer's syndrome, 250

STK11/LKB1
  mutations in, 3
  in Peutz-Jeghers syndrome, 3, 96–97, 128,
      188, 196–197
Stomach tumors, 119
Stromal cells, 3
Structural variants, 432–433
Subtotal colectomy, 127
Succinate dehydrogenase-deficient renal cell
      carcinoma, 249t, 254
Sulindac, 125
Superoxide dismutase 2, 223

T
Talazoparib, 109
Tamoxifen, 105, 439
Tarasoff v. Regents of the University of California,
      389t, 390
T cells, *Smad4* in, 3
Telephone-based genetic counseling service, 38
Telomere shortening, 216
Testes, 262
Testicular cancer
  Carney complex and, 264
  epidemiology of, 262
  genetic causes of, 263
  genetic counseling for, 264
  genetic risk of, 262–263
  genetic testing for, 264
  hereditary causes of, 249t
  imaging of, 263
  management of, 264
  in Peutz-Jeghers syndrome, 263
  physical examination of, 263
  risk factors for, 262
Testicular tumors
  classification of, 262
  Peutz-Jeghers syndrome and, 98
TGFBR1, 155
Thyroid cancer
  anaplastic, 291
  familial, 292
  familial adenomatous polyposis as cause of, 293
  follicular, 291
  medullary
    disease-specific approach to, 297
    epidemiology of, 296–297
    external beam radiation therapy for, 296
    familial, 299
    fine-needle aspiration for, 295
    management of, 294–296, 299–301
    microRNAs for, 297
    radioactive iodine ablation for, 296
    RET mutations associated with, 296–297
    risk assessment of, 294–296
    total thyroidectomy for, 295

non-medullary
  epidemiology of, 291–292
  familial, 292–293
  management of, 289–291
  radioactive iodine ablation for, 291
  risk assessment of, 289–291
  sporadic, 292
poorly differentiated, 291
prognosis for, 291
PTEN mutation in, 95
screening for, 123, 293
well-differentiated, 291, 296
Thyroidectomy, 293
Thyroid function testing, 289–290
Thyroid lobectomy, 290
Thyroid nodules
  description of, 289
  fine-needle aspiration of, 290
  medullary thyroid cancer and, 295
  prevalence of, 291
Tobacco use
  breast cancer and, 76
  pancreatic cancer and, 221, 223
Total proctocolectomy with ileostomy, 123
TP53, 86t, 216, 353–354
Transforming growth factor-ß, 10
Transgenerational heritability, 22
Trichilemmomas, 43, 132, 170, 253
Triple-negative breast cancer, 34–35, 42
Trisomy 18, 368
Trisomy 21, 368–369
TSC, 253
TSGs. *See* Tumor suppressor genes
Tuberous sclerosis, 350–361, 423t
Tumor growth, 9
Tumor suppressor genes
  definition of, 4t
  description of, 8–9
  list of, 19t–20t
  promoters of, 22
Turcot syndrome, 121, 169
23andMe, 68
Two-hit effect, 4t
Two-hit hypothesis, 2, 21, 45, 46f, 168, 184, 353
Two-hit Knudsonian dynamics, 2–3
Tyrer-Cuzick model, 80

U
UCC. *See* Urothelial cell carcinoma
UK-FOCSS. *See* United Kingdom Familial
    Ovarian Cancer Screening Study
Ultrasound
  breast cancer screening uses of, 104
  endoscopic, for pancreatic cancer screening, 226

Uninformative negative result, 191
United Kingdom Familial Ovarian Cancer
    Screening Study, 199
Upper gastrointestinal screening, in familial
    adenomatous polyposis, 122–123
Urothelial cell carcinoma, 255–256
USC. *See* Uterine serous cancer
Uterine cancer
  in Cowden syndrome, 170
  diagnosis of, 167
  epidemiology of, 167
  risk factors for, 167
Uterine serous cancer, 177

V
Variable expressivity, 4t, 5
Variable penetrance, 6
Variant call format files. *See* VCF files
Variant of uncertain significance, 51–52, 66, 79,
    404
Variants, 65–66
Varmus, Harold, 8
VCF files, 62
Veliparib, 109
Vogelstein, Bert, 10
von Hippel-Lindau disease, 249t, 251, 312–315,
    361, 423t, 435t
VUS. *See* Variant of uncertain significance

W
WAGR syndrome, 364–365
Weight gain, breast cancer and, 75
Well-differentiated thyroid cancer, 291, 296
Werner syndrome, 328t
WES. *See* Whole-exome sequencing
WGS. *See* Whole-genome sequencing
Whipple procedure, 124
Whole-exome sequencing, 53, 61, 193
Whole-genome sequencing, 53, 193
Wild-type protein, 2
Wiskott-Aldrich syndrome, 373
WRN, 154
WT1-related syndromes, 364–365

X
Xeroderma pigmentosum, 328t, 332, 339,
    349–350
X-linked lymphoproliferative disease, 373–374

Y
Y179C mutation, 15

Z
Zollinger-Ellison syndrome, 304